ILLNESS IN THE ACADEMY

ꙮ ILLNESS IN THE ACADEMY ꙮ

A COLLECTION OF PATHOGRAPHIES BY ACADEMICS

EDITED BY
KIMBERLY R. MYERS

Purdue University Press
West Lafayette, Indiana

Library of Congress Cataloging-in-Publication Data

Illness in the academy : a collection of pathographies by academics / edited by Kimberly R. Myers.

    p. cm.

  Includes bibliographical references and index.

  ISBN-13: 978-1-55753-442-2 (alk. paper) 1. Health--Miscellanea. 2. Healing--Literary collections. I. Myers, Kimberly Rena.

  RA776.5.I454 2007

  616--dc22

                          2006032653

For my mother,
Marilyn Higdon Myers,
whose radiance remains my guiding light

and

In loving memory of my father,
Richard Zane Myers,
who embodied grace in life and through death

Contents

Foreword

ANNE HUNSAKER HAWKINS

I first met Kimberly Myers, a petite, dynamic woman with a winning smile and a soft south-ern burr of an accent, four years ago when she attended an NEH Summer Seminar called "Medicine, Literature, and Culture" that I co-directed. The seminar sought to expose teachers of humanities to the actual practice of medicine in a tertiary care medical center by "shad-owing" doctors and nurses, observing ethics case conferences, and attending departmental grand rounds and other medical presentations. These were some of a range of activities from which we expected participants to choose what most appealed to them. Kimberly distinguished herself early on by wanting to do everything!

Kimberly arrived at the institute with a powerful interest in the patient's experience of illness; she left with an idea for an anthology of narratives by patients about such experi-ences. A few years earlier, I had published a second edition of my own book about patient illness narratives, a genre I have called "pathography." Kimberly had read *Reconstructing Illness* and asked if we could talk about its theoretical and practical uses in medical educa-tion. When we did, I confessed to her that it was difficult to use these narratives in teach-ing because of their sheer size: almost all were book-length autobiographies. In response, Kimberly conceived the idea of a collection of shorter, chapter-length narratives. With her characteristic energy, she transformed this notion into reality by soliciting personal accounts of illness from scholars and teachers all around the world. The culmination of this project is *Illness in the Academy: A Collection of Pathographies by Academics*.

Kimberly's interest in the patient perspective was driven in part by her own chronic ill-ness. A gifted writer, she could easily have written her own book-length pathography. I am impressed, though, that she chose instead to solicit the stories of fellow academics whose experience with illness has shaped their lives in meaningful ways. Because of the wealth and variety of issues addressed under a single cover and the relative brevity of individual chap-ters, *Illness in the Academy* is more useful than longer pathographies to those who most need this information—medical students and practicing physicians. I know that I will be assigning this book to the medical students in my courses!

Pathography is both a relatively new and a rapidly growing genre of life-writing, and there are several reasons why. For patients, these narratives provide a kind of map, offering some guidance in the bewildering and often frightening terrain of serious illness. Reading the experiences of others creates for the sick and their caregivers a kind of vicarious support group. But these first-hand accounts can also prove useful and compelling to general readers, most of whom will someday themselves undergo serious illness. The greatest importance of pathography, however, may be its potential impact on "medical culture," affecting how doctors are trained and the way they practice medicine thereafter. Pathography serves to remind healthcare personnel that it is the patient, not the disease or treatment, that is at the center—what Kimberly rightly calls the "heart"—of the whole medical enterprise. In an age of increasingly technological medicine, pathographies like those in this book eloquently testify to the crucial human dimensions of both illness and healing.

Acknowledgments

Having the opportunity to thank those who have helped bring this project to fruition is my genuine delight. I am grateful to the National Endowment for the Humanities for their wisdom in sponsoring the "Medicine, Literature, and Culture" Institute during the summer of 2002, and to co-directors Anne Hunsaker Hawkins and Susan Squire for their vision in designing such a comprehensive and creative experience. Thanks to the faculty, physicians, staff, and patients of the Milton S. Hershey Medical Center, Penn State College of Medicine, for integrating twenty-five fellows into the daily life of the hospital, and to the Fellows themselves for the many ways they enriched my thinking during our time together. I would especially like to thank Dr. Shirley Eoff and Dr. Ernelle Fife for weeks of invigorating conversation in our apartment and for friendship that has gone beyond that summer.

At Anne's house the first night of the NEH, my fortune cookie read, "A new friend helps you break out of an old routine." It was actually much more than that: Anne inspired the sea change that has altered my professional course; without her, this book would not exist. Several other colleagues in medical humanities have furthered my commitment to our work. Talking with Dr. Rita Charon for the first time was a pivotal moment in my understanding of the real-world value of narrative medicine. Thanks to Ms. Martha Rodriguez, Dr. Tess Jones, and the members of the physician writers group of the University of Texas Health Science Center at San Antonio for allowing me to join them during the summer of 2005, and especially to Dr. Abraham Verghese for inviting me to participate in the art of bedside medicine and to share in the broader medical and medical humanities activities of UTHSCSA.

My deepest appreciation goes to the generous people who contributed their stories to this collection—especially for their willingness to make public important dimensions of health and illness that were fundamentally private—and to Margaret Hunt, managing editor at Purdue University Press, whose expertise and great good humor have made this project a pure joy. I also appreciate the work along the way of the following colleagues: Dr. Lynn Z. Bloom, Dr. Wendy Cater, Dr. Christine S. Davis, Dr. Yolanda Gamboa, Dr. Laura Hinton, Dr. Catherine Kasper, Ms. Therese Semonin, Professor Brendan Stone, Dr. Jean A. Wagner, Dr. Norman Weinstein, and Dr. Chris White.

For their generous contributions to this project, special thanks to Seamus Heaney, whose words quicken both pulse and impulse, and to Abraham Verghese, whose stories continue to inspire medical and lay readers alike.

I am also grateful to the following physicians whose wisdom and compassion have enriched my life: Dr. Craigan Gray, Dr. Charles Hammond, Dr. George Mulcaire-Jones, Dr. William Peters, Dr. Robert Sandler, and Dr. Steven Shaneyfelt. Special thanks to Dr. Brentley Jeffries for fostering a partnership in care from day one and for being on the other end of the telephone when I really needed him; to Dr. Michael Herring, who embodies every good thing medical humanities hopes to cultivate; and to Dr. Leigh Anne Townes, who was willing to enter the wound in order to help me heal.

Colleagues from Montana State University have supported my work in valuable ways. Thanks to the Office of the Provost and Vice President for Academic Affairs, the Office of the Vice President for Research, Creativity & Technology Transfer, and the College of Letters and Science for generous grants that contributed to this and related projects; to Dean Sara Jayne Steen for her unfailing insight and encouragement; and to Michael Miles, whose mere presence betters everyone he touches, mind and soul. For working with me to establish a medical humanities component in the WWAMI medical program, much appreciation to Dr. Linda Hyman and Dr. George Saari. I am also very grateful to the many students in my Medicine, Literature, and Culture and Poetics of Healing courses over the years whose enthusiasm and intelligence have affirmed my belief in the vitality of this field. Warm thanks to Brian Johnsrud for helping prepare this manuscript and for his loyal friendship, to Jenn Volz for designing the perfect cover for this volume, and to Teresa Klusmann and Carolyn Steele for keeping everything afloat day in and day out.

William Butler Yeats once wrote, "Think where man's glory most begins and ends / And say my glory was I had such friends." Any glory I might possess is God-given and friend-inspired. Deepest gratitude to the following people who have illuminated my journey: to Ann Simpson, who lit the spark and sustains the fire, who is (still) my hero; Dr. Pat Verhulst, woman warrior and ever Goldmund to my Narcissus; Nancy Williams, irreverent wit who would not only help me move, but also move the body; Bob Washel, who opened a world of yellow snapdragons and orange coffee; Dr. Aaron Butler, who shares "Life, like a dome of many-coloured glass"; Dr. Deborah DeRosa, my fellow wench; Bill and Dianne Chapman and Dayle and John Payne, who loved me even when I was broken; Michelle Miles, whose soulfulness is deep blue water in summer; the force that was Bop; Cathy Adkins, for much lake-lapping Zen; Billy Doswell, gifted playwright and my soulmate in words; and Dr. Earl Leininger, muse for too many years to count, whose steadfast friendship has shown me that all things are, in the end, possible.

I am blessed with a wonderful blended family: Marie Fulford, whose kindness is an abiding gift; Philip Thomas, who came to care for us, bearing food and rich, layered conversation; Jason Thomas, who possesses more courage and sweetness of spirit than I'll ever know; Dr. Laura Thomas Blanchard, lyrical confidante, gifted physician, and the sister I never had; and Matt Blanchard, who brews a wicked cup of hazelnut java.

And to my immediate family: my brother and sister-in-law, Kevin and Dr. Veresa Myers, light-bearers in the realm of medicine and the wider world; Brayden Zane and Kyndal Gray Myers, whose simple trust and love of stories have reminded me of the magic of childhood; my father, Richard Myers, whom I miss every day of my life and whose selflessness and courage live on in the lives of those fortunate to have been loved by him; and my mother, Marilyn Myers, whose faith in God, belief in me, and joy in living are the bedrock of my existence.

And finally to my husband and partner, Jim Thomas: your love, encouragement, unqualified support, and selfless care keep me living and alive. Thank you for the adventure of a lifetime together.

Introduction

⤠ KIMBERLY R. MYERS ⤟

I have just returned from my Medicine, Literature and Culture seminar, where we enjoyed a lively debate about ideas presented in two of the narratives collected within these pages; so tonight seems an auspicious time to begin this introduction. This is the last part of the book to be written because it has been the most difficult to write—primarily, I think, because it seems nearly impossible to convey succinctly the myriad ideas underlying a collection like this, and to speak to such a wide variety of readers in ways each of them will find meaningful. These introductory remarks provide a basic overview of certain terms, concepts and sources important to any reader interested in stories of health and illness, the doctor-patient relationship, and issues of advocacy in contemporary medicine. Some readers will need less information than I provide, and some will want more. In considering how I might best address, on one end of the spectrum, scholars in medical humanities who possess much specialized knowledge of the issues raised in and by this text and, on the other end, students (in medical schools and otherwise) and general readers who might be completely new to this field, I hope that I have hit a happy medium.

In her seminal text *Reconstructing Illness: Studies in Pathography*, Anne Hunsaker Hawkins illustrates how many people envision illness as a journey into a foreign country, where none of the customs are familiar and they don't speak the language.[1] Often they have come without preparation or warning; and along the way, they have lost agency and voice, no longer able to act and speak for themselves. Far from the familiar comforts of everyday reality, they clamber to reclaim the resources they had once regularly possessed, to make sense of their new lives. Many people rely on family and friends in new ways for support, encouragement, and mere human presence. Many seek a sense of spiritual purpose in life or cultivate an existing faith in increasingly earnest ways. And many people use the tools of their intellectual training to cope with the disruption and dis-ease that comes with living in the alien and alienating land of illness. The selections in this volume are snapshots of different dimensions of this journey.

The idea for this collection was born in the summer of 2002 during the National Endowment for Humanities Institute "Medicine, Literature and Culture" at Penn State College of Medicine, a gathering of 25 scholars committed to furthering the mutually advantageous

1

connections among our disciplines and the field of medicine. I was interested to learn what brought us all there, compelling us to give up our summers to do this intellectually and psychologically demanding work. In addition to the discussion sessions and presentations we had every afternoon and the substantial reading we did every night to prepare for these meetings, we also participated in clinical activities with physicians and nurses throughout the morning—attending grand rounds, rounding with physicians in various intensive care units, observing medical procedures, talking with patients and families about end-of-life issues. Some fellows had come mostly for professional reasons; they published and taught in the field of medical ethics, for example. But most of us had come for personal reasons, too, and we told the stories about our own illnesses or those of close friends and family. The events recounted in these stories had reshaped our professional interests and commitments. Conversely, our professional interests informed our personal responses to illness. Hearing how a historian used her knowledge of history to grapple with breast cancer was eye-opening to me—even more so when I considered her story alongside that of a feminist who used her training in gender and cultural studies to contend with the same disease. It became obvious to me that one's academic training—indeed, even one's identity *as* an academic—has much to do with the nature of his response to illness: which aspects of illness he focuses on, how he reasons through treatment options, what he chooses to do during recuperation. I started to think: If I found these connections so enlightening, perhaps others would, too—especially since an ability to read other people's stories with accuracy and sensitivity is critical for those working in many fields, including medicine, anthropology, social work, psychology, history, and literature. Thus began my plan for a collection of illness narratives, or *pathographies.*

Hawkins coined the term "pathography" to indicate "a book-length narrative about the author's illness" (*Reconstructing,* xiv). But perhaps a new kind of pathography, one specifically devoted to the intersection of health and career, would be useful. And perhaps another innovation was in order. While fine pathographies are currently available, many are impractical for classroom use because of their length; there is little time for book-length works in courses that must cover a large volume of material, and excerpting passages compromises the integrity of the narrative as a whole. Shorter illness narratives, on the other hand, can easily be read in their entirety. A diverse collection also exposes students to a wider range of diseases—and the challenges and coping strategies peculiar to those diseases—than single long texts can. Convinced of this need for shorter narratives and mindful of the illuminating perspectives offered by academics because of their disciplinary training, I put out a call for submissions by scholars about their own illness experiences or those of family members or close friends.

I had no idea what to expect in terms of colleagues' willingness to share such intimate stories publicly, so I was pleased when I started receiving inquiries. At first, there were a dozen or so emails; then the correspondence increased dramatically. Several times, email conversations progressed into telephone conversations, some lasting for more than an hour. These exchanges confirmed what I'd long felt: that a surprising number of academics, typically held to (specious) standards of objectivity in their work, often want to break through what we believe are the artificial boundaries between the personal and the professional and allow who we are as human beings to more fully inform our scholarship. For some of us, this desire reflects a growing dissatisfaction with postmodern self-irony and poststructuralist views of an impossibly disintegrated self. Especially in the domain of acute and chronic illness, subjectivity and wholeness *must* be taken for granted on some level because the first priority is to heal the self, body and soul.

Perhaps I shouldn't have been surprised by the overwhelming response to this project. As numerous scholars from a wide cross-section of disciplines have shown through quantitative and qualitative research, the very act of telling one's story is therapeutic.[2] Psychologist James Pennebaker has shown that "the evidence of dozens of studies over a decade of research strongly suggests that there are significant, positive, consistent, and identifiable relationships between writing and speaking about difficult or emotional experiences and physical health" (7) in part because in order to speak or write, one must confront the traumatic experiences head-on. One of the possible explanations Pennebaker offers for the salutary effects of writing is that

> the act of converting emotions and images into words changes the way the person organizes and thinks about the trauma. . . . Once a complex event is put into a story format, it is simplified. The mind doesn't need to work as hard to bring structure and meaning to it. . . . Translating distress into language ultimately allows us to forget or, perhaps a better phrase, move beyond the experience. (8, 12, 13)

Similarly, Virginia Woolf writes in her essay "A Sketch of the Past," "It is only by putting it into words that I make it whole; this wholeness means that it has lost its power to hurt me" (72). The story of a thing distances us from the thing itself, thereby becoming a buffer against, in this case, the trauma of illness. Inasmuch as we have to stand outside an experience to construct a story about it, we are removed from it. And as Woolf also implies, something in the very act of constructing a story provides a sense of empowerment, of creating something worthwhile out of something senseless and destructive. Physician-scholar Rita Charon explains how this process works specifically in the genre of pathography:

> the patient records and interprets his or her own illness. This recording empowers the patient to control and define the process of pain, suffering, and even the pathophysiology leading to the illness. In this genre, the professionals are consigned to the status of minor characters. . . . The important point is that the patient is active as the source of the narrative and as the interpreter of the narrative. This is genuine sole authorship. In this case it is the patient and not the doctor who learns and is shaped through the process of writing. ("Doctor-Patient," 138)

While the essays in this volume reflect such hope in the therapeutic power of narrative, several of the authors here would argue that writing is not the near-panacea some seemingly envision it to be. For instance, while psychologist Leslie F. Clark asserts that "conveying a story to another person requires that the speech act be coherent" (quoted in Pennebaker, 12), a few of the authors represented here make little attempt at "coherence." Although most people who suffer from serious illness try to divine the etiology and manifestation of their disease by constructing various narratives, these permutate along the way, resisting definitive cause-and-effect logic and defying closure. This does not obviate the *desire* to provide structure to an illness through a narrative; it simply means that in the end, the chaos of illness still exists. Physician-author Abraham Verghese clarifies this seeming paradox: "Can a story have no resolution? Indeed, yes. Many modern short stories do not have a clear resolution, and yet not having a resolution *is* the resolution. . . . The epiphany might simply be a coming to terms with the illness by all concerned—patient, family, and doctors" ("Physician," 1014). Sociologist Arthur Frank describes how such "chaos narratives" function: "the repetition of 'and then' events . . . grinds down time and space" and leads to disorientation. "The chaos narrative offers no guideposts, no numbered stages that lead to acceptance. In chaos narratives, nothing leads anywhere; home [or health] is a nostalgic memory, not a destination" ("Dwelling," 46).

While resolution might not always be possible, however, merely to speak for oneself "rather than being spoken for and to represent oneself rather than being represented or, in the worst cases, rather than being effaced entirely" is empowering (Frank, *Wounded,* 13). Further, the connection formed between teller and listener, even in a chaos narrative, is therapeutic. The essays collected here aren't merely some sort of private, cathartic writing; rather, the writers rely fundamentally on the presence of a reader to bear witness to their stories. In this way, writing is a form of "talking cure," and the interchange between writer and reader is a process of "empathic witnessing" or "therapeutic listening."[3] Some healing happens in the speaker's merely being heard and the listener's willingness to "enter the wound" *with* the speaker. This impulse is the source of Dutch theologian Henri Nouwen's image of the "wounded healer," the *best* healer because s/he understands what *needs* to be healed and is willing to enter the dark places, to bear witness. Frank conveys this truth metaphorically: "Some events tear a hole in the fabric of existence, and we knit the rough edges, so far as we are able, by telling stories about what happens. These stories cannot do their work of suture until they are witnessed. Our witness does not bring closure to suffering. It's just the best we can do" ("Dwelling," 46). As Verghese concludes, "The willingness to be wounded may be all we have to offer" ("Close Encounters," 192).

In this enterprise, the reader, too, benefits from a sort of bibliotherapy, or healing through reading.[4] Many of the authors whose stories appear here have spoken about their need to help others who are undergoing similar crises. This focus on helping others through their writing is yet another dimension of their own healing—a process I call "meta-healing." In much the same way that meta-analysis is an analysis of the analyses that have gone before, so is meta-healing a means of healing that occurs in observing the healing of others. This has also been an abiding goal of mine throughout the editing process. Ultimately, to further the democratic impulse in medical partnerships between doctor and patient, I advocate a kind of "feminist medicine" analogous to feminist pedagogy in which learning/healing transpires in community, and strict divisions between teacher and student / healer and healed dissolve. It is my belief that all of us are wounded healers—patient and nurse and physician, writer and reader—and that great power exists in recognizing the reciprocity inherent in our mutual needs and mutual contributions.

Indeed, the medical community is also increasingly aware of the importance of story and of cultivating a sense of partnership with patients, especially given the problematic history of physicians' relationships with their patients. A prevalent complaint today is that medicine is impersonal, insensitive to the desire for human compassion when suffering people need it most. But as Lilian Furst's scholarship reveals, this was not always the case.[5] Before the advent of "scientific medicine" in the mid-nineteenth century, physicians had comparatively few technological tools to aid them in treating sick patients. They relied almost exclusively on direct contact with the patient—listening to her story and observing, hands-on, the physical changes in her body—and they often functioned largely as bedside priests whose primary contribution was to provide comfort, if not cure, to a suffering patient. In short, a physician's regard was for the whole person. In the latter half of the nineteenth century, though, there was a dramatic expansion in laboratory sciences like chemistry and pathological anatomy, which caused physicians to move from the bedside to the laboratory. The distance between doctor and patient widened as physicians worked to keep abreast of increasingly sophisticated scientific advancements. Patients received less and less human touch and attention from their physicians, and instead spent more time with needles and machines that measured isolated dimensions of their physical bodies. In this way, over time medicine became depersonalized. Technology had opened up amazing potential for diagnosis and cure but in the process had also seriously compromised the human connection between doctor and patient. Broadly speaking, medicine shifted from comfort to cure, from patient specificity to disease specificity. Within a century, people had essentially been reduced to their bodies, even more minutely to individual organs, and at worst to their diseases.

By the late 1960s, widespread dissatisfaction with the state of medicine existed among patients and physicians alike, and in 1967, Penn State College of Medicine launched the first program in medical humanities. A primary goal of this initiative was—and still is, in dozens of similar programs in the finest medical schools here and abroad—to re-humanize medicine, to restore the dynamic and mutually rewarding relationship between doctors and patients. In discussion-based seminars, medical students examine various aspects of medicine through the lenses of literature, history, philosophy, film, and the arts in order to maintain a balance between the scientific knowledge they will require to treat the ailing body, and the human compassion necessary to care for the whole patient—in short, to unite the noble aims of comfort and cure. Programs in medical humanities also sponsor discussion- and writing-based colloquia for practicing physicians, nurses, and other health professionals so they have a community in which to address and process the human struggles inherent in their work with patients. The overarching aim of these related activities of medical students and health professionals is to foster good mental, emotional, and physical health in medical practitioners and their patients.

In addition to cultivating empathy, medical humanities programs aim to help future physicians hone skills of observation and perception so that they can pick up on important details in patients' stories, both those they tell verbally and those their bodies tell. Whether in the form of a patient history, lab report, or hospital chart, clinical medicine is, at core, a story; so presumably, the better a doctor knows how to read her patient's multifaceted story, the better she will be able to treat him successfully, body and spirit. An underlying assumption is that the "average" patient is sometimes not forthcoming with details that might be critical to proper diagnosis and treatment, and that the physician must find a way to enable the patient to "open up." The physician must then be able to interpret accurately the subtleties embedded in the patient's stories so that she has a sufficient quantity and quality of information to work with as she attempts to heal him. Rita Charon, a practicing clinician who also holds a Ph.D. in English, explains, "Not unlike acts of reading literature, acts of diagnostic listening enlist the listener's interior resources—memories, associations, curiosities, creativity, interpretive powers, allusions to other stories told by this teller and others—to identify meaning. Only then can the physician hear—and then attempt to face, if not to answer fully—the patient's narrative questions: 'What is wrong with me?' 'Why did this happen to me?' and 'What will become of me?'" ("Narrative Medicine," 1899). Charon calls this crucial ability to read a patient "narrative competence," which she defines as the "set of skills [textual, creative, and affective] required to recognize, absorb, interpret, and be moved by the stories one hears or reads" ("Narrative and Medicine," 862). Echoing what many gifted physicians recognize, Charon observes that "not only is diagnosis encoded in the narrative patients tell of symptoms, but deep and therapeutically consequential understandings of the persons who bear symptoms are made possible in the course of hearing the narratives told of illness" ("Narrative and Medicine," 862).

In medical education, therefore, stories of illness are important learning tools because, unlike "logicoscientific knowledge [that] attempts to illuminate the universally true by transcending the particular [,] narrative knowledge attempts to illuminate the universally true by revealing the particular" (Charon, "Narrative Medicine," 1898). Pathographies reveal not only much about patients' personal experiences in the land of illness and medicine, but also much about cultural mores, assumptions, and practices that significantly influence things like informed consent, treatment protocols, and patient compliance. Reflecting on and discussing ideas raised in pathographies can dramatically enhance narrative competence. Ultimately, physicians working toward increased narrative competence and patients working toward increased understanding of health and disease are promising complements: both are impulses toward revitalizing the human dimension of medicine. In assembling the stories for this collection, I hope to facilitate greater awareness and sensitivity among physicians (present and future) and patients as they try to meet in the middle, partners working toward the common goal of humanistic healing.

A NOTE ON SELECTION AND ORGANIZATION

Of the more than 90 submissions I received, I selected pieces for inclusion in this volume on the basis of the ideological, ethical, and practical issues they raise surrounding health and illness, and the potential they hold, in my estimation, for helping those who read them—whether medical professional, academic, or general reader. Inasmuch as possible, I tried to represent the widest array of diseases and academic disciplines and to achieve balance in gender, cultures, and ethnicities. In some of these efforts, I was limited by the venues available for publicizing the call for submissions, by the propensities of scholars in different fields to write in certain ways about certain topics, and by a willingness to discuss some kinds of illness and not others. Because my own discipline is English, I was more successful in securing advertising in journals devoted to languages and literature; understandably, the majority of submissions therefore came from scholars in these fields. Moreover, the kind of writing this collection requires is likely more familiar to scholars in the humanities, social sciences, and medicine. My experience with this collection indicates that women are perhaps more forthcoming about health issues than men. I should mention, however, that based on several conversations with female academics who were deliberating whether to submit their illness narratives, women feel more potentially threatened by admitting illness in the academy, especially given a perception that the academic world is still governed primarily by men who might view illness as a justification for reinforcing a glass ceiling when issues of promotion are at stake.

I received proportionately more pieces on breast cancer and psychological disorders than other diseases. The reasons for this tendency are doubtless complex. But my experience working with dozens of manuscripts and talking with hundreds of people who struggle with illness has led me to two rather simple—and hopefully not overly simplistic—conclusions. First, I believe that willingness to talk candidly about breast cancer reflects the emphasis on female community and support at the center of women's cancer organizations and, indeed, in what studies have shown to be women's preference for the collective, shared experience as a form of solidarity and empowerment.[6] I was completely surprised by the number of essays devoted to psychological disorders, especially in a collection explicitly about the academy, where one's professional worth is determined by the quality of one's mind. Reading the essays, though, clarified for me that the people struggling with these disorders are perhaps keenest of all to prove that their illnesses do not ultimately undermine their intelligence or effectiveness as teachers and scholars. That these individuals can reveal the difficulties of their situation while at the same time displaying how well they perform (especially in the act of writing, arguably a scholar's primary currency) is an assertion of professional and personal competence and healing.

To provide the best resources for expanding one's understanding of various dimensions of medicine, I have included two kinds of texts: those that *overtly* reflect how a scholar's heightened awareness of particular concepts affects the way he "processes" illness, and those that more *implicitly* reveal an academic's body of knowledge and patterns of perception. While pieces in both categories transcend the merely personal to present ideas germane to an eclectic readership, there are some key differences. In the former group, many writers practice what contributor Christopher Smit defines as "autoethnography," in which the author "uses the same principles of ethnographic writing (i.e., observation, analysis, storytelling, deduction, and theoretical exegesis, etc.), but the lens is turned back on the author rather than on another group or culture. This style of writing shifts between personal anecdotes and reflection, storytelling and analysis." Here, much of the interpretive work is done for the reader. The latter group contains pieces that are less analytical and in some cases more "creative" in their depiction of illness and the culture of medicine. These texts enable readers to sharpen their own powers of analysis not only through reading reflectively, but also by identifying the important questions for themselves. While some stories offer potentially effective patterns for coping, others reveal perspectives that some readers will surely consider problematic, even troubling. In all cases, I believe, the essays will raise consciousness and spark interested and invested discussion on a wide range of issues—from patient advocacy and social activism to intuition; from prejudicial treatment on the basis of economic status, ethnicity, gender, sexual orientation and age, to tenure and mercy killing.

The organization of this volume proved to be quite challenging, since many of these stories encompass multiple diseases and disorders and sometimes reflect the illness experiences of both self and other. In order to guide readers most efficiently to the topics of their choice, I have opted to group pieces within four broad categories and then into subcategories according to predominant concerns. Admittedly, this organization seems artificial and even reductive at times. The lyrical works of Irish poet and Nobel laureate Seamus Heaney and internationally renowned physician-author Abraham Verghese work remarkably well as anchors to the volume, spanning as they do the landscape of hope, disillusionment, and healing in medicine today. Reading them as companion pieces will provide a poetic comment on Verghese's belief that even "in having no cure to offer, we actually [have] everything to offer[:] to really understand the story that is playing out . . . [by] crossing the traditional threshold of a medical-industrial complex and beginning to engage with the patient, with their story, on their turf" ("Physician," 1015). May the stories collected in this volume guide us to new insight, new meaning.

NOTES

1. Another landmark study of the myths and metaphors of illness is Susan Sontag's *Illness as Metaphor*. See also chapter 1 of Arthur Frank's *The Wounded Storyteller: Body, Illness, and Ethics*.

2. For instance, see works by the following authors: psychologist James Pennebaker, sociologist Arthur Frank, humanist Anne Hunsaker Hawkins, physician-medical anthropologist Arthur Kleinman, and physicians Abraham Verghese and Rita Charon.

3. "Empathic witnessing" is Anatole Broyard's term (169). "Therapeutic listening" is Rita Charon's description of the physician's part in any successful clinical encounter ("Narrative and Medicine," 862).

4. In fact, Anne Hunsaker Hawkins calls pathography a "vicarious support group" (*Reconstructing*, xi). Dr. Ernelle Fife offers an important admonition, however: "Certainly, 'the writing cure,' as well as the 'talking cure' or the 'reading cure' or indeed any cure that promises a relatively quick or easy end to disease should not be accepted without critical analysis" (43).

5. The discussion that follows is an exceedingly brief synopsis of Lilian Furst's *Between Doctors and Patients: The Changing Balance of Power*. See also Furst's *Medical Progress and Social Reality: A Reader in Nineteenth-Century Medicine and Literature* and Anne Hunsaker Hawkins and Marilyn Chandler McEntyre's *Teaching Literature and Medicine*.

6. See Carol Gilligan's *In a Different Voice: Psychological Theory and Women's Development*; the work of feminist theologians including Rosemary Radford Ruether and Carol P. Christ; Sandra Zagarell's 1988 essay "Narrative of Community: The Identification of a Genre"; Kristina K. Groover's *The Wilderness Within: American Women Writers and Spiritual Quest*; and works on women's "circle groups," including Beverly Engel's *Women Circling the Earth: A Guide to Fostering Community, Healing and Empowerment*. Fictional sources include Alice Walker's *In Love and Trouble*, Louise Erdrich's *Love Medicine*, Amy Tan's *The Joy Luck Club*, and Diane Glancy's *Pushing the Bear*.

REFERENCES

Broyard, Anatole. "Doctor, Talk to Me." *On Doctoring: Stories, Poems, Essays.* 3rd edition. Ed. Richard Reynolds, M.D. and John Stone, M.D. New York: Simon & Schuster, 2001.

Charon, Rita, M.D., Ph.D. "Doctor-Patient / Reader-Writer: Learning to Find the Text." *Soundings* 72 (1989): 137–52.

———. "Narrative and Medicine." *New England Journal of Medicine* 350: 9 (26 February 2004): 862–64.

———. "Narrative Medicine: A Model for Empathy, Reflection, Profession, and Trust." *Journal of the American Medical Association* 286: 15 (17 October 2001): 1897–1902.

Engel, Beverly. *Women Circling the Earth: A Guide to Fostering Community, Healing and Empowerment.* Deerfield Beach, FL: Health Communications, Inc., 2000.

Fife, Ernelle. "*Seeds of Mortality: The Public and Private Worlds of Cancer,* by Stewart Justman: A Review." *The Montana Professor* 15: 1 (Fall 2004): 41–43.

Frank, Arthur. "Dwelling in Grief." *The Hastings Center Report* 34.1 (Jan.-Feb. 2004): 46–47.

———. *The Wounded Storyteller: Body, Illness, and Ethics.* Chicago: U of Chicago P, 1995.

Furst, Lilian. *Between Doctors and Patients: The Changing Balance of Power.* Charlottesville: UP of Virginia, 1998.

———. *Medical Progress and Social Reality: A Reader in Nineteenth-Century Medicine and Literature.* Albany: SUNY P, 2000.

Gilligan, Carol. *In a Different Voice: Psychological Theory and Women's Development.* Reissue ed. Cambridge: Harvard UP, 1993.

Groover, Kristina K. *The Wilderness Within: American Women Writers and Spiritual Quest.* Little Rock: U of Arkansas P, 1999.

Hawkins, Anne Hunsaker. *Reconstructing Illness: Studies in Pathography.* 2nd edition. West Lafayette: Purdue UP, 1999.

———, and Marilyn Chandler McEntyre. *Teaching Literature and Medicine.* New York: Modern Language Association, 2000.

Kleinman, Arthur. *The Illness Narratives: Suffering, Healing, and the Human Condition.* New York: Basic Books, 1988.

Pennebaker, James W. "Telling Stories: The Health Benefits of Narrative." *Literature and Medicine* 19.1 (Spring 2000): 3–18.

Sontag, Susan. *Illness as Metaphor.* New York: Farrar, Straus and Giroux, 1977.

Verghese, Abraham. "Close Encounters of the Human Kind." *The New York Times Magazine* (18 September 2005): 192.

———. "The Physician as Storyteller." *Annals of Internal Medicine* 135.11 (4 December 2001): 1012–1017.

Woolf, Virginia. "A Sketch of the Past." *Moments of Being.* Ed. Jeanne Schulkind. New York: Harcourt, Brace, Jovanovich, 1976.

Zagarell, Sandra. "Narrative of Community: The Identification of a Genre." *Signs: Journal of Women in Culture and Society* 13 (1988):

Brancardier

You're off, a pilgrim, in the age of steam:
Derry, Dun Laoghaire, Dover, Rue de Bac
(Prayers for the Blessed Mary Alacoque,
That she be canonized). Then leisure time

That evening in Paris, whence to Lourdes,
Learning to trust your learning on the way:
"Non, pas de vin, merci. Mais oui, du thé,"
And the waiter's gone to take you at your word.

Now Cathleen Conroy's in the corridor
Where you've been standing. *Vierge. Vivace. "Ma fille,"*
As Mr Conroy calls her, who calls you "ye"
And "Son". "Son, what's the time?" "Son, would ye shut that door."

Hotel de quoi in *Rue de quoi?* All gone.
But not your designation, *brancardier,*
And your little bandolier, as you lift and lay
The sick on stretchers in precincts of the shrine

Or on bleak concrete to await their bath.
And always the word "cure" hangs in the air
Like crutches hung up near the grotto altar.
And always prayers out loud or under breath.

Belgian miners in blue dungarees
March in procession, carrying brass lamps.
Sodalities with sashes, poles and pennants
Move up the line. Mantillas, rosaries

And the *unam sanctam catholicam* acoustic
Of that underground basilica—maybe
Not gone but not what was meant to be,
The concrete reinforcement of the Mystic-

al Body, the Eleusis of its age.
I brought back one plastic canteen litre
On a shoulder strap (*très chic*) of the Lourdes water.
One small glass dome that englobed an image

Of the Virgin above barefoot Bernadette—
Shake it and the clear liquid would snow
Flakes like white angel feathers on the grotto.
And (for stretcher-bearing work) a certificate.

—*Seamus Heaney*

⇜ PART I ⇝

ILLNESS AND IDENTITY: DYNAMICS OF SELF AND IDENTITY

Illness within a family often has a dramatic impact on personal identity. Roles shift and become more complex, multilayered. Whether positively or negatively—or both simultaneously—illness functions as a clarifying pool, offering new perspectives not only for those who are ill, but also for the family members who provide care.

The first four essays in this section are from adult children whose experiences with a sick parent were formative. Sharon D. King and Patricia O'Hara address the sense of mystery surrounding their mothers' suffering, respectively, from rheumatoid arthritis and mood disorders. King and O'Hara reveal the stress and guilt that serious, chronic illness creates for the parent *and* child, and their essays evince the poignancy of trying to reconstruct and reinterpret seminal childhood events many years after the fact. Ellin Ronee Pollachek and Moya Lynn Alfonso describe their experiences with mothers who developed gynecological cancer—ovarian and breast, respectively. Especially given the genetic component of such cancers, both women come to a new understanding of their own gendered bodies through their mothers' diagnoses and treatments. Pollachek's unflinching look at the complexities of a love-hate relationship between mother and daughter is a corrective to society's tendency to romanticize death as an avenue to reconciliation.

The next three essays concern other family members' illnesses. Michael Rowe examines his critically ill son's liver transplant and the aggregate medical oversights that ultimately led to his death. Exploring his dual role as father and medical sociologist, Rowe scours his memory for cues that might have enabled him to save his son. Michael J. Meyer chronicles his joint position as caregiver to his wife, who is dying of ovarian cancer, and as patient who suffers from colon cancer. At the time of his illness, Meyer also battles an analogous ethical cancer at his university; both lead him to a new sense of liberation and faith. Michael Verde explicitly addresses issues of self- and family-identity as he describes his grandfather's advancing Alzheimer's disease, and offers an uncharacteristically hopeful, lyrical perspective on the ravages of dementia.

The final two essays reveal the tensions inherent in situations where family members are also healthcare professionals. Tami L. Higdon discusses her attempt to be fully present as daughter to a father diagnosed with pancreatic cancer while also using her skills as a hospital chaplain to enable her family to come to terms with his prognosis. Emanating from various faith traditions, the observations she offers provide both critique of and argument for spirituality's central role in illness and death. Susanna Black finds herself in the untenable position of grieving sister and knowledgeable physician whose family looks to her for advice and encouragement when her brother's advanced prostate cancer is discovered far later than it should have been because of medical negligence.

Manzanita

⌒ SHARON D. KING ⌒

> *. . . udia continuo il vento*
> *tra le frondi del bosco e tra i virguiti*
> *e trame un suon che flebile concento*
> *par d'umani sospiri e di singulti . . .*[1]
> —*Torquato Tasso, Gerusalemme Liberata,*
> *Canto XIII, 40*

It is cold outside, the fog blotting out cars and houses across the street. Inside: the warmth of sputtering candles, carols from the old records, a smell of buttered cider. I stand in the kitchen coaxing back the past.

The once-bright blue orbs are faded now, and spotted; I turn them this way and that on the tiny boughs to hide their flaws. The little manzanita tree, cut from the tall twisting bush with its ruddy bark by my grandfather, has long had its knotty branches sprayed silver; every year since I can remember we have performed this rite at Christmastime. My mother has never ceased to be delighted at the sight of it, trimmed and gracing the walnut table, though her broken hands have not come near the fragile twigs for years, for fear of snapping them off. I do my best, under her gentle guidance. But I do not have her eye.

Behold the tree.

⌒ ⌒

She is in bed, lying still, bosom rising and falling with breaths drawn softly, poured out heavily. Her wrists and ankles are bound with strange foam claws. Her twisted toes are taped into place. There is a long scar, hidden by folds, across the base of her neck. More scars ring her breasts; one smiles across her stomach; still others are etched into her feet, her ankles, her wrists, her back. One shoulder is set higher than the other, and there are deep gouges in both from where bra straps have worn down into the bone.

She sleeps deeply, dragged off to slumber inevitably through the good offices of pharmacopia. Tonight it is Xanax. It shuts out the noise, the panic, the endless shrieks of guilt and recrimination. Tomorrow we will pay for the peaceful sleep, tomorrow when the lions crowd back and roar their way out. But tonight she is at rest.

I listen to her breath, watch the light-blue nightgown moving slowly, regularly, see the shadowmauve creases under her eyes and the silver roots at her brow. I lean over and touch the skin of her cheek: still velvet.

My mother.

e vidi gente per lo vallon tondo
venir, tacendo e lagrimando . . .
mirabilmente apparve esser travolto . . .[2]
—*Dante Alighieri, Commedia (Inferno),*
Canto XX

I have grown up alongside my twin, her illness—knowing its wanderings, flare-ups, cool-downs; sensing its torments, rejoicing in its wanings. Long before I was born it had been her companion, bodymate, faithful and undeserting presence. It defined her. It maddened her. At the beginning it sent her from doctor to doctor, sure cure to sure cure, friend to enemy. It set her apart, driving away bosses, colleagues, prospective boyfriends ("They wouldn't know me by the time the first movie ended, I was so stiff," she would whisper to me as we cuddled in bed on winter evenings. "I could barely walk out to the car. And they would never, never call again. They knew I was sick; they didn't want to have to deal with me. I would go home and cry.") It left her with an assortment of copper bracelets, a few jagged scars, a fearlessness of bee stings, and an utter contempt for psychiatrists ("What do you mean *whom do I hate?* I hurt. I'm sick. Not in the head. *I'm sick.* Why won't you listen to me? Why won't you help me?")

Then someone had listened. A specialist. Dr. Poisnick. I never met him. He was as close to Jesus as we got.

Rheumatoid, he told her. It's not like the ordinary kind. We're just learning about it. She learned with them.

And so did I.

She is in me and around me, guides me from breast to spoon, from warmth and depth to chill stretches of light. I do not yet know the realms of day, but I reach to her voice. Her laugh at the first word I utter.

Her hands, his hands show me off to the clouds, plant blossoms around me. I awake to the rhythm of cups on tables, songs teased out on a Hawaiian guitar, snatches of frogverse. She draws me into magic, the land of make-believe. I put on my green elf-hat and seek out my fellows amongst the bushes in the yard. The crab claws she was cleaning come to life and chase me squealing down the hall. I am a princess. She ties on my velvet-trimmed cape and sparkling slippers.

Her pride is in me, lying on the hall floor sucking apple juice. *She's normal. Perfectly normal.* Her power: *They told me never to hope for you. It was enough to be married; I could never raise a child.* Her relief. *I didn't have to take any steroids when I was pregnant with you. I was in remission. You brought that to me.*

Then the spell breaks; the glass slipper shatters.

≈ ≈

I don't know why you're crying
But here is a Kleenex
See, here's the whole box
See this pretty flower?
I picked it for you
It's just for you, Mama
This vase is for you
This picture's for you
They're all for you, Mama
Please, Mama, don't cry
I love you, Mama
I love you, don't cry[3]

≈ ≈

> *Oh, Rose, thou art sick!* ...
> —*William Blake,*
> *Songs of Innocence and Experience*

My fear is a lump in my belly, so no food will go down.

In the cafeteria, my friends prod me to eat. I cannot. I am in second grade and my mother is in the hospital. For an operation.

"She won't die," my grandmother, tiny and unbending, tells me. "She'll be fine."

My father, at home at night, is silent. He has known her sickness too, has watched her figure and her cheeks balloon out from the prednisone, has seen the huge scaly patches of psoriasis flare across her back, her legs. She is always tired, and he is always working.

"Here." One of my schoolmates, a ponytailed girl named Camille, hands me an orange Popsicle bar. "This will taste good, it's cold and it's so hot outside." It is spring in Fresno, and already there is not enough shade on the playground. I lick the Popsicle, my stomach leaping inside me. It is hard for me to swallow. I follow my friends out the double metal doors on wobbly legs. The light hurts my eyes.

I trail around the playground behind my friends. The grass smells sweet. At the far edge of the yard, I can go no further. I lean against a tree and throw up, orange juice bar and all.

My friends are busy gathering clods of hard soil and tufts of bermuda grass. The pool of vomit is quickly camouflaged. They tug me back to the yard monitor.

"She's real sick."

I follow the monitor into the principal's office. They call my grandparents, who come and take me home.

≈ ≈

"Just jump."

I am seated astride my mother's back. She has been lying down. I have been trying to rub her back, but my small fists cannot pummel her hard enough. Then she has an idea.

"Climb on top of my back," she says. "Like I'm a horsie."

I clamber up readily and seat myself in the small of her back. "Hey, Mom, you're my newest bucking bronco!" I giggle and bounce a little, then twist from side to side, unsure. Daddy sometimes plays horsie with me, but he is always tossing me around or dashing across the floor, and I have to hang on for dear life. Mom does not move.

"Jump, honey. Jump up and down."

I oblige. She gasps and groans under my thumping eight-year-old weight. "Move back a little bit, honey," she says, breathless. I adjust my seating; she gasps again, but there is relief in the sound. We ride for several minutes. I slow and stop.

"I'm tired, Mommy."

"That's all right, honey. You go play in your room."

And my father is amazed when she is fast asleep an hour later, when he gets home from the office. She who walks the house at night with the fiends at her back.

⌒ ⌒

> *O wretched caitife, wheder shall I flee*
> *That I might scape this endles sorowe? . . .*[4]
> —*Everyman, anonymous 15th-century*
> *morality play*

There will be no miracle tonight.

The house is still. My mother has gone to bed; my father fingers his stamp collection in the living room.

The arc of light from my desk lamp falls hot on my hands. I try to write but no words come.

I turn half around and twist the coverlet of my bed in my hands. The pale-pink chenille spots catch on the rough patches of my fingers. I tug it, lean over and grab my red velvet pillow, in which I keep my most secret writings. I hug it to my chest, open its zipper carefully.

The letter I tuck in is not one of my own.

It does not come from far, but far enough. It answers my own letter, a miracle in itself, but its answer has pitched me deeper into misery than ever before. A misery of my own making.

The letter says simply: She will not come. The wonder-worker, healer of body and soul, will not come to my city to cure my mother. She will hold her healing services elsewhere, and she enjoins me to bring my mother there, if possible.

It is not possible. My father does not believe in faith healers. Neither does my mother. Except that she has no choice. There must be hope out there, somewhere. Her life cannot be this mere condemnation of pain. I know this, and I believe.

But there is more in the letter. If we cannot come, it tells me, I should pray with the lady that my mother be healed on a certain Sunday. This very day. We will carry the victory, we will make it "HER DAY." The capital letters across the page shriek out my own capital sin.

For I am not faithful. When the day finally comes, I have forgotten. After church, I play with my girlfriend across the street all afternoon. Too late, after dinner, I remember. My mother, who has seen the letter, asks quietly if I have prayed at all for her that day, if I have forgotten her and my promise.

My ten-year-old mind creates excuses. I mumble something about the need to play on the Sabbath too. But she is right. I did not pray; she is not healed. And the healer, fast in her citadel, has been wronged as well. She was counting on me to hold up my end. She has prayed to no avail. God was waiting for me, and I was not there.

I turn the pillow over and slide it gently back onto my bed. Cold waves wash over me. I shiver and hold icy fingers to the desk lamp. I had pinned so many butterfly-hopes on that letter, arriving with its bright stamp and out-of-city postmark. The miracle-lady would come, and my mother would walk down the aisle and be delivered of her pain. She would heal the aching body and twisting fingers. She would free my mother from the tortures of tar treatments and sun lamps, the humiliations of prune juice, the relentless circle of soporifics and stimulants. And I would be my mother's savior, the good daughter.

I am instead one more betrayer.

A gulf between us never bridged.

⌒ ⌒

> *Si ne me vient del ciel la grace,*
> *Nem puis estre gieté de paine,*
> *Tel est li mals que me demaine . . .*[5]
> —*Service for Representing Adam,*
> *anonymous 12th-century French drama*

No known causes, no known cures. This was the mantra I was raised on, prompting gazes back on every possible misstep, pauses on each future choice. There were no exemptions from second-guessing what might have been the trigger: the loss of a fiancé after the war, the ravages of malnutrition during the Depression, even being not enough of an outdoors girl, as her sister had been, while she was growing up. *Maybe that was what brought it on. If only I had played more, been more carefree, like Margaret Ann, maybe I would be well today.*

We did know something about it, though: it was often brought on by a blow to one's immune system that turned it, part of your own body, against you. Like your heart refusing to beat for you, a pair of lungs closing down on you, the child once within you standing rebellious and obdurate. But it had to be a big shock. And such a shock she had had, during a trip taken while she was still very young. Fierce and independent, she had been desperate to shake off the horrors of losing a mother to bone cancer, eager to recover from the stigma of having a lover straggle home from the war only to tell her goodbye.

So one spring she, her sister, and a friend had packed their bags, piled into her car, and set off along the Blue Ridge Highway, the route that would lead them south to freedom from the snow of Toledo winters and the drudgery of postwar employment. As I heard the story, retold many times ("Is that tobackky?" my feckless aunt had mimic-queried a quizzical-faced field worker in Kentucky, as they bumped along innumerable back roads), all had gone well until they reached the terminus of their journey south: the palm-swept beaches of Miami. There they had staked out a day-long stand on the sunny shore. My mother, the fairest of the three, had no hat and the most daring of 1940s swimsuits. She did not burn. She melted.

"They had to cut me out of my suit," she would murmur to me as we snuggled together in bed, always her place of refuge from the relentless pain. "The nurses would whisper around me, but I knew how scared they were. At first I hardly cared if I lived or died, but then I wanted to live. And I told them to get me well enough, send me home."

When she did get home, brother and father did not recognize her. She was many months watching the new skin blossom under the burnt, the swollen features shrink back to their normal size. Her friends rallied around her, but it was as if she had shucked off her past along with her skin. The next year she took another car trip, this time to the West Coast. And the year after that, she moved to San Francisco, to work in a new branch of her old company.

And the following year, she began sensing a strange aching in her joints, which no doctor could explain.

☞ ☜

Pale blue pebbles skip
and in the dim unquiet, rise and strike
Nightmare calls: the crushing weight of pillows, the hum of
music down the hall, the hourly need for the toilet. A snort,
and then a snarl, awake again, with no easy falling back. A
slow crawl
tanglefeet stumble, water falls
and the house hold its breath, remembering
the knife flashing in the dark

☞ ☜

. . . a veces me acuerdo suspirando
del antiguo sufrir!
¡Amargo es el dolor; pero siquiera
padecer es vivir![6]
—*Gustavo Adolfo Bécquer, Rimas (1871), LVI*

We nearly lost her countless times. Most of her sufferings were, if not directly caused by rheumatoid, magnified by the stress of the disease. There was the time, during our family car trip to the Grand Canyon, when she came down with dysentery so severe she lay hospitalized in Vegas for a week. The time she had a hysterectomy for endometriosis, for a brief period more acutely painful than the arthritis. The time she underwent an operation to correct an aberrant thyroid, where they had to slice her neck open from ear to ear. The time she had breast reduction surgery because the vertebrae in her back had weakened so she could barely stand upright. The myriad occasions she ended up in the hospital with a broken arm, a dislocated shoulder, a rampaging bladder infection, a heart attack. There was the memorable episode when she was sent to the hospital for surgery on her contorted toes, which no shoes could contain. She was overmedicated into a stupor so horrifying that my father, red-faced and bellowing like a prizefighter, nearly throttled her doctor. One of the few rheumatoid specialists in the city, he had seemingly made a simple mistake in writing her orders; years later, after I became a candystriper, I found him drying out in the private wing of the hospital, as he apparently had done many times before.

Yet her life did not cease. Steadily, shakily, stubbornly, my mother clung to the quotidian. Her life was counted out not just in throbbing pain but in the joyous stanzas of "How Great Thou Art," the verities of Dr. J. Vernon McGee, the thoughtful cadences of a good sermon at church. It was gauged in the spaces between laughter. It was measured in the rumbles and ticks of dishwashers, clothes driers, water timers, the mental energy to read a short news article or make out a grocery list, the will to iron a shirt or cook a pot roast. Most of all, she spun herself along through her own relentless monologues: what she had to get done, what never got done, what she should be doing, why she couldn't do things, what things she would like to see, what she never would see. Her last words to me, in the wee hours of the morning before she died, were of her wish to see the just-released film *Jurassic Park;* she had always been taken with dinosaurs.

Her life was equally measured out in doses. To me, that which most marked her apart was her devotion to the host of drugs that kept her functional, even if marginally. She learned to take pills anywhere, everywhere, gulping them down with a tiny paper cup of water or no water at all, merely saved-up saliva. I was in awe of her technique, even more so after I tried it once myself, with aspirin. Of course it made me gag, the grainy feel of the dissolving pills lingering in my throat for hours. At one time I counted in her cabinet, she was taking fifteen different kinds of prescription drugs: drugs to wake her up and drugs to put her to sleep, drugs to make her move and drugs to slow her down, drugs to buffer her stomach from the drugs that kept the agony of her joints at bay. Drugs for her depression, which made her angry. Drugs for her anger, which made her obsessed. Drugs to drain off excess water. Drugs that stripped her of potassium, and drugs to replenish her of it. And later, many more drugs for a heart that had been worn down by over forty years of struggle.

She detested her dependence. She fought against it, waiting to take her lifeline, the painkillers, until she could bear it no more. During one of my years in graduate school, she was able to boast that she was down to six types of medication, and only half the prednisone taken ten years before. But by then the patterns were set: the drugs had dragged us down their spiritual path even as they spelled out our schedules. We rushed to doctors' offices for promises, pharmacies for fulfillment, home for respite and gentle oblivion. The next day, the next pill, the next pang and its hoped-for panacea. We were all hooked.

The best was the worst. It was a silent pain, insidious, unceasing, a vampire at the vein of motion that scorned the mirrored glass. No one looking at my mother, fixed with her morning's dose, would ever know her joints were crumbling away inside her, carrying precious nerves and muscles and tissue with them. She was plump, gracious, smiling and talkative in the few endeavors she pursued. "You look like you're doing so well," those who knew would tell her. For the people who didn't know, there was no revelation from her. It was hard to speak serenely when she wanted to scream a hundred times a day.

Ah! longues nuits d'hiver, de ma vie bourrelles,
Donnez-moi patience et me lassez dormir!
Votre nom seulement et suer et frémir
Me fait par tout le corps, tant vous m'êtes cruelles...[7]
                                    —*Pierre de Ronsard, Derniers vers (1586)*

I stumble across the wide black-and-crimson mat marking the threshold of the foyer of St. Agnes Hospital. In two seconds, the automatic door swooshing behind me, I am out of the artificial chill and into the shimmering heat of a Fresno summer.

It takes my breath away. The pale brown dirt is too hot for bare skin; the white concrete overwhelms thin sandals. The blacktop of the parking lot sometimes becomes liquid in the 105-degree heat of a good June; we carry its goo away on thick-soled shoes. The light is just as unrelenting. Yet I would not trade it for where I have just left: the cold room with its thin blankets, the frail wrist encircled by its plastic bracelet, the soggy food trays and somber bouquets. I hate this place no less than my mother does, this place where I was brought into the world and which has kept us both prisoner so many, many times.

For a moment I gaze at the brown hills of the eastern county across from me. Out there, beyond that ridge, my future awaits. If I can only earn it.

Behind me, above me, my mother lies helpless on her bed, her feet enclosed in casts, her mind engulfed in fear. She has just had surgery to cut off bone spurs on her feet and fuse the faltering bones in her ankles. I am about to set off on a five-week trip to the south of France—I, who, though a first-year college student, have never been away from home.

It does not matter that it is a study trip with the local university, led by my favorite professor and enrolling some of my better friends from college. It does not matter that I speak excellent French, that my study skills are peerless, that through years of tutoring I have earned most of the money needed for the trip. None of this matters. I know this.

What does matter is that I will not be there to help my mother when she comes home from the hospital. She is terrified.

And I, determined.

And we are both guilty: of stubbornness and selfishness and anger. My father will not stay home from work; her friends can only do so much. She fears for her life.

I fear for mine.

For nearly a month I have carried the burden of housewifery for her, as her broken bones were reknitting. I have done laundry, vacuumed carpets, mopped floors, ironed my father's work shirts, cooked him acceptable stodgy evening meals of steaks and potatoes and salad. I have shopped for groceries with a keen eye towards bargains, made up the beds though there was no mother to critique them, even flimsily stitched on a button or two. And every day, sometimes twice, I have visited my mother, bringing flowers from the yard, a few homebaked cookies, letters and cards and snippets of books to relieve the tedium of recovery for a few moments. I pay my dues. But for all this, there is no proving myself. My dreams of Provence are folly in both my parents' eyes. I am needed at home. How can I abandon them?

In the end, I do earn my trip. I turn my back, I step away, breathing a prayer that all will somehow go right. The jetplane I leave on sails me away to a lavender-brushed land where I see my first cloister, tour Roman ruins, hear exultant operas, taste the robustness of French wine as it flows around good food, good conversation. Even my descent to the beaches of the Côte d'Azur, so fretted over by my mother and aunt, leaves me unscathed, with but a little freckling and peeling at the shoulders.

But the price is high. Within an hour of being home, with treasures to share and pictures to show, I am brought back to accounts. My father leaves to go back to work, my mother leans over to show me her new ankles. She chokes back tears.

"Oh, honey, I thought I would never make it until you got back," and then the whisper-cry, "you'll never know how *mean* he was to me while you weren't here . . ."

⌒ ⌒

My father, my hero. Her illness exacted its own measure on him.

As I grew up, he was always the strong one. The courageous one. Small, but indomitable, witty without owning the word, upright in every way. He gazed levelly at the bleak future my mother mapped out for them should he marry her and said: I am not afraid. I want to make you happy.

In his own way, he tried. She wanted for nothing, except perhaps more of his time. He showered her with every request she made: special treatments for the psoriasis, a swimming pool to ease aching bones, money for each and every operation her doctor suggested. Even more absurd: a chance at a normal family life. She was not ungrateful. But he could not do what he had promised. No power on earth could bring happiness to someone in such pain.

He worked harder as she grew older, frantically trying to keep her mobile, stable, coherent. The disease tore at the fabric of friendships, gnawed at the edges of rationality. He would steer her from conversations turning too acerbic, guide her gently towards rest even when she didn't think she was tired. She would snap at him, and if he snapped back, he would recover, mend the breach. He may have regretted his choice. He never said so.

Irony wore his face in my family. My father, the hardworking healthy one of the household, had prided himself on his clean living, never touching a drop, never smoking or taking drugs, eating a cornucopia of fruits and vegetables, getting seven good hours of sleep each night. All to no avail. While I was away at graduate school, he was diagnosed with Parkinson's disease, the worst case his doctor had seen. No one knew where it came from, and, as with the arthritis, there was no cure. Six years later, he was dead. He was gone before my mother, who spent her five final days pining after him.

Long before he died, his own disease had robbed him of the ability to speak. But I recall one of the last things he said, while lips and tongue still obeyed his silent bidding. Gazing up at me, blue eyes in the gaunt face imploring, he grasped my hand just before they wheeled him into surgery, one of the many we had tried to make him right again.

"*Take care of your mother.*"

I gave my word. And this time, I kept it.

In the end, her heart caves.

At the gathering after the funeral, relatives sit stunned: they have just seen my mother, visited with her, at my father's memorial five days before. Now she is the one they mourn.

My youngest cousin, John, takes my hand, points to it and strokes it gently. I gaze up at him, questioning.

"Hers didn't look too much like hands anymore," he says quietly. "Now they are perfect, the way they used to be, the way she wanted them to be."

I nod dumbly. She had long agonized over the way the disease had twisted the bones of her hands, turning graceful fingers into curling claws, making it impossible for her to play the piano she had so loved. For most of my life she had worn bright nail polish to hide the crackling, misshapen fingernails, assaulted by psoriasis. Her hands had been a source of continual embarrassment to her.

But not to me. I had loved those hands, had grown to the touch of them, marveled how they still could be summoned to do her bidding even when they had stiffened into crooked place like the errant branches of a manzanita tree. For that is what they reminded me of, though I never told her: the scrubby, hardy mountain tree that masqueraded its resilience in pliancy. My grandparents used to make walking-sticks of manzanita, so hard was its wood. A tree most would take for a shrub, whose slip-smooth russet branches thrust upward with the arcs-en-l'air of a ballet artist, outward with the exquisite torsion of a baroque pearl.

Manzanita hands, rising up to the sky.

NOTES

1. unendingly he heard the wind
    amongst the branches and the bushes of the woods,
    making a mournful harmony
    that echoed with human sobs and sighs . . .
(All translations in endnotes for "Manzanita" courtesy Sharon D. King © 2006)

2. And through the curving valley I saw people
    Both silent and weeping, emerge, . . .
    All seemed incredibly contorted . . .

3. "I don't know why you're crying," from *The Four Corners*, by Sharon D. King.
(Copyright © 2000, Sharon D. King. Used by permission of the author.)

4. Oh wretched coward, where shall I run
    To get away from this endless sorrow?

5. If heaven does not grant me grace,
    I shall never be free from pain,
    So great the sorrow that overpowers me . . .

6. Sometimes I remember with a sigh
    My past sufferings!
    Misery is bitter, but at least
    To suffer is to live!

7. Oh, long winter nights, tormenters of my life,
    Bring me patience and let me sleep!
    The mere mention of you makes me shake and sweat all over,
    So cruel have you been to me . . .

QUESTIONS

1. What are some of the ways the narrative shows the illness presenting itself as an entity, a being in itself? as a rival to the narrator?
2. How does the ailment affect the life choices of the ailing woman? of the narrator? of others in the story?
3. Comment on guilt in this narrative. Whose is it? Why and how does it manifest itself?
4. Discuss the title and central image of the essay. How does manzanita function symbolically?

Some Questions to Consider
☞ PATRICIA O'HARA ☜

*"But no story is the same to us after a lapse of time;
or rather we who read it are no longer the same
interpreters."*

—*George Eliot, Adam Bede*

PREFACE

Okay, fair enough: no story that we tell or read stays the same over time. It's the nature of narrative; it's the nature of memory. But no matter how many times I come back to this one, it's always a sad story and one I don't understand. Even someone like me—an academic who reads and teaches and writes about stories for a living—even I can't wrest a satisfactory pattern of meaning out of this one. It's the master narrative of my past, but its lineaments shift each time I try to read it.

It's my mother's story I'm talking about here, or, let me say, a particular chapter from a long time ago.

From 1968 to 1970, my mother was institutionalized on three occasions—for periods of time that ranged from six weeks to eight weeks—in a Catholic mental hospital in Westchester County, New York. She was admitted for multiple suicide attempts, alcoholism, and depression. These mental breakdowns were not without some precedent in her life. In 1960, she spent time in a facility in Westport, Connecticut, and in her thirties it was a drying-out place or two somewhere. I forget where now. But the crack-ups at the end of the sixties—those were something else entirely. Or so it seemed to me then. And so it seems to me even now when I think about the lonely time in which the central fact of my adolescent existence, as I experienced it, was that I had a shameful, untellable secret.

My mother had come undone.

And all the king's horses, and all the king's men

She did get put back together again, however, in an imperfect sort of way. I left home for college in 1970, and her patch-up followed thereafter. Post-1970, no one in my family of three ever talked about those events. Or maybe my parents talked to each other about them, but neither talked to me. An occasional remark might slip loose from its moorings and glance off the side of The Past, but nothing ever hit the mark. There was no moment in a dialogue when I asked, *How did things get so bad for you* or that she offered *I was really losing my mind back then.*

So you see, sometimes it's been like it never happened, or like it happened in someone else's family, or to some girl who went to a different high school or who was the cousin of a friend of a friend. The strange otherness of the experience has served me well at times when it was useful—maybe essential—to misplace my family history and reinvent myself: as twentysomething free spirit, as somebody's girlfriend, somebody's mother, somebody's college professor. It has served me less well at other times, like nights when I lay awake wondering about the warning signs of adult-onset depression.

My mother died in 1995. It's not in the nature of our relationship for my father and me to let our conversations edge too far or deep into the past, and it will, therefore, never come up between us for the rest of his life. I intend for it to stay that way. Yet since her death, those massive nervous breakdowns in the sixties have become a story I can't lose. Maybe the consequence of long-term silence is a compulsion to narrate. Think Victor Frankenstein or the Ancient Mariner or Jane Eyre. My problem is not the compulsion to narrate, but I do feel compelled to understand what happened in the past. That compulsion, however, is accompanied by the knowledge that one can never know what really happened in the past, but only versions of what might have happened, each version with its own claims to the truth. That knowledge also keeps me awake nights.

This, then, is a telling of where I've been looking for my mother's past and how I've been trying to construct narratives out of old letters and medical records and memories. It's partial telling, of course, and I approach it here in the way I know best: as a problem of narrative and interpretation.

It's important to remember, however, that after a lapse of time, we who return to a story are no longer the same interpreters.

So the story changes all the time.

NARRATIVE PRACTICES

As of this writing, I have 572 files in a folder named TEACHING on the hard drive of my computer: syllabuses, exams, study questions, pop quizzes, teaching notes, course descriptions, book orders, and comments on papers. Some of the files I'll never use again; some I'll revamp before distributing them to a new crop of students.

There's one file, however, that I use in every course I teach: a handout designed to prod my undergraduates to think in interesting and analytically sophisticated ways about the stories I assign to them. It consists of a series of imperatives and queries meant to lead the students beyond mere elements like who did what and when and where.

I call the handout "Some Questions to Consider."

I like to believe that, used thoughtfully, these questions can light a way into even the most opaque of stories.

Question: *Identify different kinds of narratives: impersonal (detached) vs. personal (recognizably human).*

1.   Handwritten letters: personal and recognizably human.

> *March 3, 1968*
> *Dear Pat—*
> *It seems kind of funny to be writing you a letter but here goes. I meant to write sooner but just received this paper. I can say one thing about this place, it sure is <u>cold</u>. . . . Pat please write to me as I get so lonely for you . . . please believe I will soon be well & home & things will be very different. . . . Please take good care of yourself as I love you very much and I'm so proud of you in everything you do. Please excuse this writing. This is the worst pen I have ever used. All My Love, Mom xxx P.S. <u>Please write to me soon</u>*

This is one of two letters from my mother to me that I have from her hospitalizations—in fact, the only letters that I have from her from any time. There may have been more. I kept these two letters in a plastic bag that holds the sum of my high school mementos: notes passed to me during class, cards from friends, tickets from school plays, a graduation program. I am surprised that I didn't lose the bag over the years, having moved around so much. I have no recollection of preserving those two letters, but their survival testifies to the agency of the unconscious in directing our actions.

From this vantage point, after a lapse of decades, I experience the letter above as shot through with pathos, punctuated with all those *pleases* and written by a person (my mother, I remind myself) suspended in a cold and vacant place where there were no pens or paper. I imagine myself in my high school uniform reading the letter in 1968, sitting alone in the living room of a little house in a small town in New England.

I wonder whose pain I felt more acutely: hers or mine.

Please. Let it have been some of both.

> *March 12, 1968*
> *My Dear Pat—*
> *Hi love. Just received your sweet card. It only took one day to get here. I was surprised to hear you felt well enough to work so soon. Please try & do not overdo it. Nothing new here. Same old thing. But Pat it really is a very good hospital & believe it or not I do like the Dr. I just find it hard at times to talk to him. I'm making a hot plate in O.T. ha ha! I'll give the baskets a rest . . . tell everyone to write to me. Pat give the meat in the freezer to Mary. Be good and take care because I love you very much. Love, Mom. P.S. Water plant & change sheets often. Have Dad sweep sidewalks often.*

One thing I know for sure: my mother hated OT, occupational therapy. I assume that a patient's cooperation in occupational therapy was one measure by which the mental health care professionals gauged patients' recovery. This letter shows either that my mother knew how to please or that the staff effectively enforced participation in OT. She completed the hot plate, which I had for a long time. It was made of small, black and white mosaic tiles, glued on to a fiberboard backing and then grouted. She was not unhappy to part with it once I got my own apartment.

I doubt that OT helped with the process of recovery. I do, however, read her remembering the meat in the freezer and the houseplant in the living room as a positive sign that ordinary domestic life still beckoned her.

It's a relief, too, to know that I sent her a card.

2.   Psychiatric records: some detached, some recognizably human

On a warmish day in October 2001, a couple of months into a sabbatical designated for writing a book about various discursive representations of late-Victorian farm workers, I decided, with no apparent premeditation, to call the hospital in Westchester to request my mother's records. I have tried to reconstruct what chain of events or set of associations led me to pick up the phone to call directory assistance that day, but I can't figure it out. If I were reading this last sentence for the first time, I would suspect the writer of self-evasion. I accept that as a possibility, but I still cannot say why I called that hospital. But first-person narratives are the most unreliable and unstable, so any internal logic I might offer for my action that day is probably suspect anyway.

Yes, said the medical records officer, her records could be forwarded to me, but it would take some time to make Xeroxes from the microfilm and I would need first to provide a copy of the death certificate.

Yes, said the woman in the town hall, I should mail the request with five dollars and they would send me proof of death. She didn't ask why I wanted it. She might have known my mother, talked to her when she came in to pay her taxes or stood in line with her at the bank. I might have gone to school with her kids. I might have gone to school with her. It's a small town, and I have to remind myself that some people choose to live in their hometowns even after they're old enough to leave.

What arrived just before Christmas was a thick envelope, the kind that has visible fibers, like wisps of white hair, enmeshed in the paper. You could never accidentally tear open an envelope like that. It's the sort to which you have to take a pair of scissors and cut a crosswise gash to get at the contents inside.

The records that I removed from the envelope were both more and less than I expected. They comprise 212 pages, fastened into three packets, one for each hospital stay: February 28, 1968 through April 17, 1968; January 16, 1969 through February 4, 1969; and the final stay from November 23, 1969 to January 20, 1970. Each packet contains basically three types of documents. Medication charts and test results are book-ended between psychiatrists' reports (admission and discharge summaries as well as progress notes) and observation logs filled in roughly six times a day by staff and attendants.

The attendants' entries in the daily logs are the most compelling to me. They promise a plot, an unfolding of a narrative over time. They contain entries written in many different hands and thus offer multiple narrative perspectives.

The comments in the log range from the brief ("patient slept well") to the rather more extended, like this one from 5 a.m. on December 26, 1969:

> Pt stumbling down hall. In an attempt to take her back to bed, pt found to have safety pin in rt hand and scratching her left fore-arm longitudinally (not bleeding). Pt resisted when pin was taken away from her & started biting and scratching

(with nails) herself. Pt said she felt she had wronged the staff and therefore punishing herself. Reasoning failed to calm her so she had to be held down forcibly. Even after medications pt was still trying to harm herself so body restraints used and pt placed on 1:1 & secluded.

The entry column to the left of this summary indicates that she was given 50 mgs (it appears to say "mgs") of thorazine. The 6–7 a.m. entry notes that the patient was sleeping and the restraints were removed. An entry on the previous page records that the patient had been allowed a home visit to celebrate Christmas with her family, an event I cannot bring to the foreground of my memory. Try as I might, I can't remember that singular Christmas. Who bought the presents? Did we eat dinner at a restaurant? Did I put up a Christmas tree?

I daresay, there's a good reason for that particular lapse of memory.

In all of the documents that I received in the white envelope I am mentioned just a handful of times and identified only as "the patient's daughter."

And yet my past is embedded in the 212 pages of hospital records and the staggering number of stories that rise up like so many specters in the logs and reports—even in the easily overlooked stray pages. My father's signature in a visitor's log, for instance, indicates that on December 7, 1969 he visited my mother in the hospital but I did not go with him. I don't remember that occasion, but it must have registered with me at the time.

December 7, 1969 was my seventeenth birthday.

Even the medications logs—written in hieroglyphics incomprehensible to readers without medical training—call out to be heard. The pharmacological data voice the experience of mental illness. But it was somebody else's experience, and the shadows stretch too far and darkly for me to find my way into those stories.

I can only list in wonderment the names of pills and serums:

Elavil
Noludar
Mellavil
Sparine
Pyridium
Dilantin
Triavil
Librium
Seconal
Chloral Hydrate
Estrafon Forte

With a little ingenuity, I could probably transform that list into a poem.

A Psychotropic Haiku.

Question: *What is the narrator's relationship(s) to the characters?*
Psychiatrists' Reports and Daily Logs: clinical, complicated, contradictory

Dozens of narrators speak in the psychiatric documents: psychiatrists (three), attendants who filled in the logs six times a day, and RNs who initialed the meds charts. Theirs was a professional relationship with my mother. But sometimes I think I can hear more in their observations and diagnoses of my mother: sympathy, frustration, irritation. All the responses I myself underwent.

Some entries were neutral enough: "Patient slept well," "Patient was coughing during breakfast," "Patient requested a day pass." Others sounded like criticism, even dislike. One morning an attendant observed with approval that my mother was tidy and dressed in a "young modern style." An afternoon attendant noted, however, that my mother was dressed "immaturely for her actual age."

She was thirty-eight years old.

It must have been hard sometimes for her to make the right wardrobe choices. It must have been hard to guess the right answers to the questions being asked.

Question: *How does the narrative affirm or resist the society's dominant values & morals (gender, class, race, religion)?*

This is the ideology question, and one has to know some social history to know when a narrative mirrors with approval the values of the times in which it was written and when it critiques those values. I don't have a specialist's knowledge of the treatment of women's mental illness in the second half of the twentieth century in America, but those psychiatrists' reports and commentaries on my mother's conditions from 1968–1970 sound strangely out-of-date to me. They are full of phrases like "early oral fixation" and "pseudoneurotic pseudopsychopathic superstructure imposed upon underlying schizophrenia and paranoia" and "nexus of massive distortion projections." They refer to Bender and Figure Drawing tests and Rorschach examinations. Were figure drawing tests and inkblots the state of the art in psychiatry in 1968?

As I interpret them, the narratives in the records accept without question the psychiatric practices and teachings of the time. That does not stop me from resisting those practices and diagnoses as accurate representations of my mother's inner life, like when I read this pages from her discharge report of 1970:

> Mental status shortly after admission showed a distraught, hostile woman who was fairly well groomed. . . . At times, the patient was initially agreeable and compliant but at times she became demanding. In several instances, she became intensely hostile towards the therapist. Repeatedly, she misinterpreted, distorted, or used out of context ideas verbalized by the therapist and it was felt that the primitive mechanisms of distortion projection and denial were much in evidence. . . . During this admission, it seemed quite obvious that this patient is suffering from a schizophrenic illness which is felt to best be described as schizo-affective in type. Although many paranoid elements were recognized.

I cannot help but think of Sir William Bradshaw, the psychiatrist in Virginia Woolf's novel *Mrs. Dalloway*—a man who is said to be "a great doctor" yet "obscurely evil . . . extremely polite to women, but capable of some indescribably outrage—forcing your soul . . . with his power." As I read the psychiatric assessments, my mind calls up "The Yellow Wallpaper."

And I wonder this: if I had never read *Mrs. Dalloway* or "The Yellow Wallpaper," would my reactions to this psychiatrist's assessments be different?

But there are judgments. There was the psychologist who spun the inkblot test results into a narrative that is both humane and insightful:

> The poor prognostic picture of this patient is further established by the results of her Rorschach examination. What is suggested is that she has a poor self-concept. She sees herself as completely trapped and unable to spell out any goals for herself. She has tried to extricate herself but with no success, and although preoccupied with her failures, she sees no resolution to her conflicts . . . further testing into the Rorschach representations revealed a person who views reality as totally fragmented and disorganized. . . . She is a woman who has felt rejected, unloved, and bears resentment toward all the circumstances that have continually deprived her of happiness; a bad childhood, a bad marriage, and bad acting out behavior. By stamping a value quality upon things she is able to punish herself further.

I hear empathy in the words of this psychological evaluation. I doubt the psychologist really needed inkblots to reveal my mother to him, but if he found Rorschach tests helpful in articulating his understanding of the suffering of others, then I cannot dismiss out of hand the tools of this man's trade.

Which leads to my final question:

Question: *Do we assent to the judgments of the narrator(s)?*

No. Yes. Maybe.

I assent to some. I dissent from others.

Ask me today. Ask me tomorrow.

It all depends.

The last two entries in the attendants' logs written on the day my mother was discharged from her final stay at the hospital read: "Pt appears in good spirits. Prepared for discharge most of day. Socialized with other pts and staff in day room. Appetite good" and "Pt discharge[d] to husband. Appeared cheerful on approach."

But in his discharge summary written a week later her doctor says:

> It has been recommended to the family and to the patient that she be in the hospital for a number of months. It was felt that this would present the best chance for her . . . however it turned out that insurance coverage would not allow for this form of treatment . . . she is felt to be a very immature individual with intense dependency needs which show themselves directly through her demands on people and indirectly through physical symptoms . . . it is recognized that the outlook is quite poor and the patient's husband, sister and daughter were informed of this.

There are so many narrators.

So many stories.

So many mothers.

My mother in the records is Mrs. Darling at the opening of *Peter Pan and Wendy:* a woman with a "mind like the tiny boxes, one within the other, that come from the puzzling East; however many you discover there is always one more." The central emotional experience articulated in J. M. Barrie's children's story is the experience of absence, although most of us don't remember that part. We remember the Lost Boys running rampant in fields of Neverland. We forget the lost mothers.

It's a trick of memory.

Some days, it seems like all the stories I've ever read and all the stories I'll ever tell are nothing more and nothing less than variations on the theme of Mrs. Darling.

QUESTIONS

1. The author candidly presents many details, quotes, facts. What does she withhold? Why? To what effect?
2. Characterize the essay's tone. Does it remain consistent or change throughout the essay? Why?
3. Consider the essay's structure. How is it different from a traditional essay format? How does the form suit the subject matter?
4. How might mental illness be different from physical illness—to the one suffering from it and to the child?

The Book of Ruth
A Pelvic Space

⌒ ELLIN RONEE POLLACHEK ⌒

The memory of certain events, like that of certain smells and sounds, brings with it the rec-
ollection of a larger moment in time. George W. Bush's election was one such event. When
I boarded the plane to Florida, it had been declared that Al Gore had won the electoral vote.
By the time I disembarked at 2 a.m., the election was up for grabs; and when I awoke at 7,
George W. had been declared our new president.

Florida Medical Center is a university hospital in Miami. My mother had never been
to a university hospital before. She had preferred small community hospitals run by local
doctors and health-care professionals. But ovarian cancer is not a small-community illness.
It is global. And so, six months after my mother was diagnosed with stage 4 ovarian cancer
and told that she needed surgery, she chose the best gynecological oncologist in Florida and
he was affiliated with UM Sylvester in Miami. I flew down to be with her, to accompany her
through this procedure: a hysterectomy.

One way to conserve costs in this downsized economy is to create a do-it-yourself patient
community. Instead of having patients admitted the day before their procedures, hospitals
have patients do it themselves. So after filling out the paperwork, my mother and I went back
to the cheap, run-down motel across the street from the hospital, armed with instructions
about what to eat, drink and bring with her the following morning at 5:30.

She was to drink some concoction in order to make her bowels move. Whatever it was,
it seemed not to do very much for her bowels but it did make her scream her head off. She
screamed from the pressure; she screamed from the movement. She screamed from the lack
of movement. The more she screamed, the more I wanted to die. But there was nothing I
could do. I was a prisoner of her pain. I was there to witness.

When her pain was more than I could bear, I went out for a walk. The air was balmy
and the sidewalks were empty. I crossed the street and took the shortcut to the hospital. It
was midnight and I regretted my choice as soon as I moved from the light of the streetlamps
to the dark, starless path which would lead me to the hospital complex. A homeless man

was sleeping off to the side so that the security guards couldn't see him. I continued until suddenly I was in the hospital driveway—a big open area with lots of people and cars and guards. I didn't hear a word of English. This was the new America. The hospital cafeteria is open all night, so I headed there for some coffee and whatever else looked palatable. While waiting in line, I began hearing some of the war stories regarding the presidential election theft which the press would later cover.

When I got back to the room, my mother was still screaming. How could they have given her something that caused this much pain? How come preps are no longer done in the hospital? What is going on? As I lay in the bed next to her, listening to her scream—SCREAM—I could feel her agony. I wanted her to stop, but there was nothing I could do. And so she screamed. And screamed. I had never heard her scream in pain before. There had been moans but no screams. She was screaming like a wounded animal. I wanted to help her but she told me there was nothing I could do—which is what she had always told me: there was nothing I could do. I saw that I was still afraid of her. I would always be afraid of her because, in reality, once she got well nothing would really change. Not really. She still wouldn't have a good word to say about me. My hair would still be too long. I would still be too fat for her tastes. I was too mean to my husband. And how come I didn't have a real job? All of that would come back. But right now she was wordless and thoughtless. She was a scream, a human cry.

My mother had just completed six months of intensive chemotherapy. Nine hours every three weeks. Not only did she never throw up from the chemo, she actually drove herself back and forth to the sessions. And here she was, reduced to a whimpering, pitiful animal-like creature. For the first time, I realized she would leave me. Maybe now. Maybe during tomorrow's surgery. In a year. When?

Here is a secret. Something I've never told anyone. All of my life, all I've ever wanted was to live inside her. I once did, you know. Decades ago, I lived inside her and refused to come out. I was three weeks late when she finally got rid of me. She's been pushing me away ever since. When I was in kindergarten my mother enrolled me in an after-school ballet class, but I wouldn't go. I screamed and cried. I refused to leave her. She wanted me to be part of other groups, but I only wanted to be part of her. She tried to make me into her and she almost succeeded. Even now, if I could, I would swallow her whole and let her breathe through me.

Motherhood is much more rhetorical than ontological. We make assumptions about women and mothering, but those assumptions are no more real than are our generalizations about race or gender or age. If we look at the Old Testament, very little is said about mothering. What we know is who begat whom, but nothing is said about Eve's involvement with Cain and Abel. Haggar abandoned Ishmael when she felt that he was about to die in the desert. And Rebecca frequently complained about the war which raged inside her belly. Motherhood is not some unilateral bliss, as Hallmark would have us believe.

And so it was with my mother. I loved my mother with a kind of reverential love that is reserved for deities. I followed her around like a duckling follows its mother. The only problem was that my mother didn't want to be followed. I don't even think she wanted to be a mother. But she was. Twice.

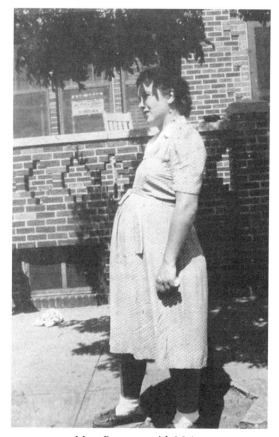

*Mom Pregnant with Me**

There has been much animosity between us over the years. I once told her that she would have done better if she had raised pot roasts instead of children. She answered that sometimes it's better to raise pigs than children; at least you can eat them when they're fully grown.

It was my father and his illness which brought us closer together. Now, six months into her diagnosis, the animosity was gone but not the edge. Her cancer, like some strident piece of steel wool, had scrubbed away the bad memories. But now with her screaming and crying it all came back. I didn't know how to let her be weak. All it would take would be a pillow. Quietly. Persistently. Just place it over the screams and it would all be over.

Sitting in a dark room, unable to sleep because of the screams of the woman who had been the strongest, most unyielding character I've ever known, I felt trapped. There was no escape. The only place to find retreat was in my work, my words, my release from the world. From the time I was eight years old, I had done this. From the time I realized that I had somehow come out wrong. During her eighth month of pregnancy, she fell down a flight of stairs and I shit. Literally. I've probably never forgiven her for making me live in shit, and she's probably never gotten over the fact that her daughter who inherited her beloved husband's curly hair was born with impetigo all over her body. My mother, obsessed with cleanliness and perfect skin, gave birth to a shitty daughter. On the other hand, it did wonders for my skin. Sort of like a homeopathic inoculation against dirt. After the sores healed, I never had a pimple. Not even throughout puberty.

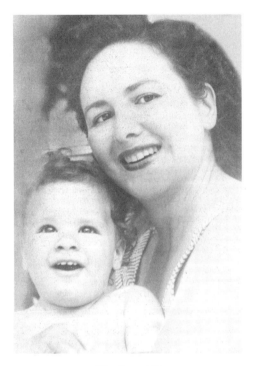

The Two of Us

CARETAKERS

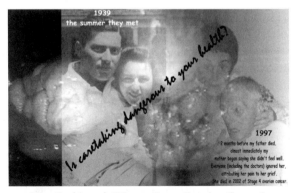

1939
the summer they met

1997
2 months before my father died,
almost immediately my
mother began saying she didn't feel well.
Everyone (including the doctors) ignored her,
attributing her pain to her grief.
She died in 2002 of Stage 4 ovarian cancer.

Is caretaking dangerous to your health?

Does Parkinson's Disease Cause Ovarian Cancer?

After my mother's death, I was tested for the BRCA1 or BRCA2 gene, which increases a woman's chance of getting ovarian and breast cancer from 13.2% to 36–85%. (Men carry the gene too and pass it on to their daughters.) But I did not have the gene. Did the stress caused by my mother's care for my father create the cells which killed her?

My father had died two-and-a-half years earlier. He had been ill for years—with Parkinson's for decades—but my mother kept him on an active schedule. Travel. Early-morning walks. Theater. This was the time for which they had worked and saved—she, by working one job for thirty years; he, by working two jobs for that same amount of time. But as the needlepoint pillow says in that fancy Madison Avenue shop, *Old age ain't for sissies*. My mother used to put it differently: *Screw the golden years*.

Taking control of his illness, my mother kept my father's Parkinson's disease at bay for as long as she could. Physical therapists were brought in; a woman came to live with them to help care for him. She did everything physically possible to take care of my father and then, when the end was near, she told me that she couldn't handle being with him when he died. She added that she didn't want him to die at home.

And so I began my monthly trips to Florida until he went into hospice, where I remained with him until he gently left this world at 1:35 in the morning on Dec. 21, 1997. I called my mother.

"Is she having someone drive her here?" the nurse asked.

"Nope. She's driving herself."

"How old is she?"

"Eighty."

It would have never occurred to my mother to call a taxi.

Shortly after he died my mother began complaining about having problems breathing. My brother's response was that she was a hypochondriac. He said she missed the attention she had gotten from being my father's caretaker. But I knew that was untrue. Ruth Pollachek never relied on her feminine wiles or helplessness. Strength was her drug of choice.

Once again, the same slow-paced sense of doom that had taken over my life during my father's final years began to resurface. It's a disquieting feeling, always waiting for the phone to ring. When it does, no matter how good the news, the assumption is that the next call will bring the bad news. When my father was sick, my mother protected me, shielding me from the direct rays of his impending death. But when she got sick, I had no one.

It was inconceivable to me that my mother could die. As irrational as that sounds, I didn't believe that it was possible that my mother, Ruth Pollachek, was capable of dying. She was always in control; she ruled the world around her through sheer, unrelenting nagging and insensitivity. Rarely, if ever, did she expose herself to a world in which she was not in charge. If she joined an organization, she became an officer. When she worked as a secretary, she was the best secretary possible and became indispensable to everyone around her. If she couldn't do the job perfectly—not good or great, but perfectly—she didn't do it at all. And so my brother and I, and even my father, were mere accoutrements. She was the centerpiece, and we, the rose petals and doily that announced her.

And then that changed. Suddenly her universe was not of her making. It became one of oncologists and surgeons and IVs and nurses. Even then, she was the perfect patient. Women half her age would have never been able to tolerate the dosage of chemotherapy that the doctors gave her. She was eighty-two and looked sixty. Even with cancer. If I needed any more convincing that she was omnipotent, this was it. And if that didn't do it, her ability to maintain an exercise program throughout the ordeal was the clincher. Every day—not every other day, but every morning—she walked two miles. Except for the third day after the chemotherapy. The third day was the worst day, so she only walked one mile.

A friend of mine who is thirty-seven and pregnant with her fourth child recently went to a new doctor. During the intake session, her doctor wrote the words "mature mother" on her chart. At eighty-two, my mother was also a mature mother. So what does the phrase actually mean? It points to the fact that the female body outlives its usefulness in its forties. Are udder-like breasts worthless? Should post-menopausal women take a gun to their heads and pull the trigger? What is a woman worth if she can no longer bear children or fuck without having to use KY Jelly? Women, once permitted wisdom, no longer are. Now we have to shoot ourselves full of hormones, silicone and botox. Hormones are good—for doctors. Cancer is a big business and hormones make it even bigger.

As a culture, we are enamored of death. I, too, have always had a fascination with the dead. Oftentimes I look for death in the woodlands of the Hudson River Valley region. What am I hoping to find? Nature's dominion over culture.

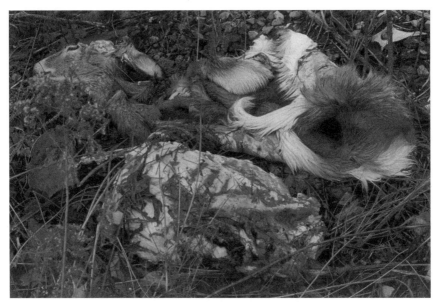

Nature's Dominion over Culture

The ultimate act of narcissism would be the ability to view our own deaths. We haven't figured out how to do it, so we watch each other die or look at the aftermath of death. Think CSI. Open coffins. Abu Ghraib.

While there is room in our culture for death, the same cannot be said for illness. Death gets buried or burned. An extreme makeover. Illness, however, is different. A reminder that we are mere flesh, in regular need of repair.

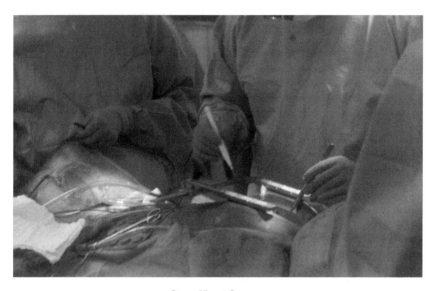

Open Heart Surgery

NOISE

Some of us even rot before we get to the grave. That is true especially if one is host to cancer.

Before my mother was diagnosed, I began getting phone calls from her friends. Morning, midnight, afternoon. They all had a similar ring to them. She couldn't breathe and became terrified; she panicked and called 911. I'd get a call every other week. Sometimes she'd be in the hospital for a few hours. Sometimes it was days. One day, about a year into the complaints, the doctors noticed some fluid around her lungs. A pulmonary specialist was brought in, but there was nothing wrong with her lungs.

And then something. It was in her lower abdomen. What did that mean?

They'll test the fluid and they'll probably find cancer cells, my sister-in-law told me in her oh-by-the-way tone of voice. She is a health professional and, typical of the health professionals I met during my mother's illness, she had a voice that was distant, compassionate but matter-of-fact. It's what Jean-François Lyotard calls noise. The noise (that pleasant "the doctor will see you in a few minutes" nonconfrontational voice) may keep away the feelings, but if you meet my sister-in-law you'll see that her expressed grief costumes her body. Every unshed tear is a pound, and each pound adds to a self-created impenetrability. But she was right. I have to give her that. The fluid showed cancer cells.

Something good. Once the diagnosis was made, an unexpected narrative began to emerge between my mother and me, one of love … as best either of us could actually love the other. But it was a start. We shed our skins and allowed something divine to emerge.

After they removed her ovaries and her uterus, the doctor told me that they tested the tissue around her ovaries and it tested negative. I was gleeful until the nurse told me that it always comes back. Cancer always comes back, she repeated.

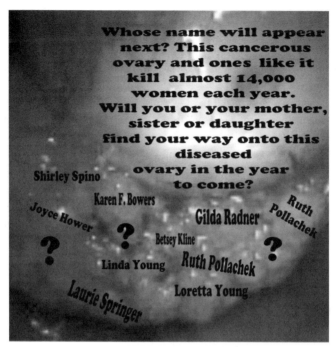

Who's Next

"What's the prognosis?" I asked her oncologist. This was not the surgeon but the doctor who gave her the chemo.

"When was she diagnosed?" he asked.

"In May of 2000."

"She has two years from then," he said in that matter-of-fact voice.

This is what dealing with death does: It turns you into a pod person. If you reveal a feeling, you are disqualified from receiving a license to practice.

"But the doctors said there was a 30 percent chance she could make it five years," I responded.

He was annoyed, this doctor with factory-like rooms and a demeanor more suited to a reptile than a human. How dare I slow him down with these questions! The problem is that the war on cancer has become a war on patients. Did I come up with that, or had I read it somewhere? I don't know, except that I do know it's true.

Two years was one year away. What do you do when you know your mother has maybe one year to live? Well I, for one, refused to believe it.

"I'm changing oncologists," she announced one day.

"How come?" I asked, making no attempt to disguise my pleasure.

"He never wants to do blood tests."

"What kind of blood tests?"

"To check my cancer levels."

The CA125 is one of the few blood tests which indicates the possibility of ovarian cancer. But the test is flawed; there are many false positives and false negatives.

"He's supposed to check it periodically, and now he tells me that he's not going to do it anymore. Who is he to tell me what tests he's going to do?"

"Good for you."

"I'm going to see the same doctor Sylvia saw. He's Indian and she said he's compassionate and concerned."

She was right. When I called him to see how she was doing, he was polite and kind and understood that the woman I was talking about may have been an old lady to him but to me, she was a mother.

I was flying down to Florida once a month and I was also trying to get my life together, but her illness was interfering. My brother only went down under pressure. He was too busy, he said. He ran his own business, he said. I had no business, so therefore it was assumed that I would be the one to become the caretaker. Being a photographer and writer and adjunct college instructor didn't count. It didn't earn me enough money to keep me home. Either that or let Mom fend for herself. I couldn't do it.

The second anniversary of her diagnosis came and went, and my mother was still around. We celebrated at Sweet Tomato, a great Florida salad bar.

"I've been reading about it," she said referring to the cancer. "Most people don't make it more than five years. But I'll take chemotherapy as long as they're willing to give it to me."

The word "death" was never spoken. Instead she filled her conversation with her disappointments. Surprisingly, I wasn't on the list. Topping the list were her daughter-in-law and granddaughter.

The breathing problems returned. This time it meant a pacemaker. "What else can go wrong?" she asked. A couple of months later the phone rang at 5 a.m. with the answer.

I shook as I picked up the receiver. A woman was speaking Spanglish. It took me a few minutes to figure out that it was my mother's next-door neighbor, Carmen. She had awakened me to tell me a story that I couldn't follow. What happened, Carmen? Your mother, she hospital. What happened, Carmen? She tell me to call you. What happened, Carmen? I sorry. My English not so good. What happened, Carmen? Hip broke.

Back down again. This time she was in a rehab center.

Jennifer, the woman who cared for my father, had come to take her home. Now there were two of us.

And then my mother said something that startled me.

"You've been wonderful throughout this. Just wonderful."

It was the second time that I recall hearing her praise. The other time was when, in 1999, I received my Ph.D. She had flown up for the graduation and she must have memorized every word of the ceremony, because she repeated it verbatim to my sister-in-law, who told me how annoying it was that my mother changed allegiances so easily. What happened to the daughter she hated and despised? my sister-in-law wanted to know.

"Your brother had always been the golden boy, and now it's you."

Her bitterness was palpable. I giggled and then later that day called my mother to ask her about it, but she totally denied ever saying a bad word against me. Of course I knew that what my sister-in-law had said was true, but I didn't care. As long as my mother loved me now.

Jennifer's presence gave me a reprieve. I could wait until late October to visit. Each trip was taking more and more out of me. Not just physically but emotionally as well. Jennifer was going to be a real help.

9 a.m., Friday, October 11, 2002. The phone rang. It was Jennifer.

"Your mother said to come down. She's said she's dying."

"She's not dying," I said. "I called the doctor yesterday and he said she's fine."

"What do doctors know?" my mother replied when she was given this information.

I called my brother. He said he was too busy to go down.

"I'll go down when she dies," he said.

"She won't need you when she's dead," I replied.

"Then I'll be here to collect the body," he answered in his smart-ass tone.

My mother had cared for her mother, my father's aunt and my father. And of course she cared for both my brother and myself throughout our lives. Now there was no one left to care for her. Not even herself.

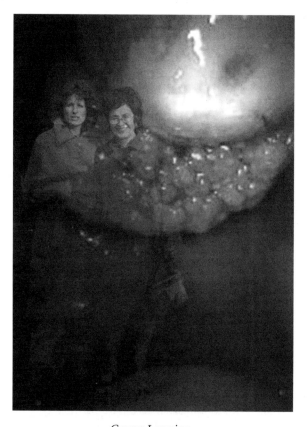

Cancer Looming

I called my mother throughout the day, but she wouldn't speak to me. I had a sick feeling all weekend. That and anger. I was beginning to feel like a yo-yo. What should I do? I'll fly down on Monday, that's what I'll do.

Sunday at 4:45 Jennifer called. I think you should come down. She's taken a turn for the worse. What do you mean? Her breathing has gotten very heavy and her eyes have begun to pop. Put the phone next to her ear, Jennifer. I was shocked at what I heard. She had that suffocating breathing. As if she were choking.

"Mom, I love you and I'm coming down. Please don't die. Please."

Later, after I arrived, after I visited my mother in the morgue, after I spoke to Jennifer, she told me that my mother opened her eyes when she heard my voice. It may have been the last voice she heard.

Jennifer got back on the phone. What should I do? Should I call 911? Your mother is shaking her head no. I knew my mother had a living will which indicated that she should not be resuscitated. But that was if her heart stopped. Her heart hadn't stopped. Call 911.

"She says no."

"Call me back when you get them."

When she called me back and the EMS workers were there I could hear them working in the background. They couldn't get a vein.

My husband and I were already en route to Kennedy Airport. It was a two-hour drive, but I decided I had to fly down. Jennifer told me they were taking her to West Side Regional Hospital. We were on the throughway traveling at breakneck speed. I called the emergency room.

My mother, Ruth Pollachek, was just admitted. Can you tell me how she's doing? The nurse tells me she will let me speak to the doctor who has been treating her. I don't remember his name.

"How is she?' I asked, barely able to speak.

He started telling me about the EMS workers, about the veins, about her heart. I knew she was dead. Doctors don't give you a history if the patient is alive.

"Did she die?" I asked. "Did she die?"

"Ruth had a hard day today," he said. "She died."

As I write this I have the same feeling of incredulity that I had then. She had a hard day? What kind of a lead-in is that? Maybe it was her best day. Now she doesn't have to be prodded and poked by the likes of you. Had he just said she's gone, it would have been fine; but telling me that she had a hard day . . . is dying hard? And then he added that she died peacefully.

"Keep her there for me," I said.

"When will you be down?"

"In four hours."

No problem.

There are drawers that hold people. Not the kind of silver, boxy drawers you see on TV but slender drawers. Drawers which seem barely deep enough to hold a person. My mother was in the third one down, the second from the bottom. The cabinet was beige. She would have liked that. Beige and blue were her favorite colors. But she was ice cold. How she hated to be cold. Whenever I visited her, we fought over the air conditioning. I liked it sub-zero; she wanted it about 78.

She doesn't look good, I said to my husband. And she didn't. This was not a peaceful

death. Her mouth was twisted. Her hair undone. Her arms were crossed, her lower jaw jut-
ted out. She reminded me of the figure in Andres Serrano's *Rat Poison Suicide.*

I thought back to Roland Barthes's *Camera Lucida,* in which he explored the nature of
photography as a result of his mother's death. He writes about trying to find his mother in
the photographs of her as a young woman. What he finds is his own "nonexistence in the
clothes my mother had worn before I can remember her."

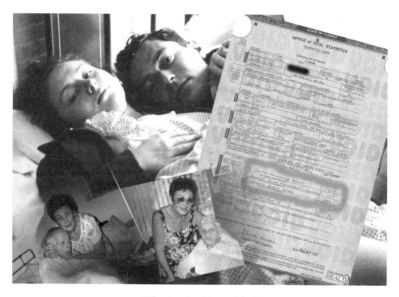

Who Am I without Her?

I had long ago come to know the woman who existed before I was born. There were
always photographs and stories. She was our star. The question for me was "who was I without her?" More specifically *was I* without her?

Her right eye was partly open and was already turning blue. It struck me as odd that it
was open. Many years ago I had written and published a short story about her eyes. In the
story "Daffodils" I am alone with her body in the funeral home. She is in a coffin, and I realize that I can't recall the color of her eyes. I need to know what color they are. I open her
lids and out pop two daffodils, one in each eye. I can hear my brother in the background.
When I try to close her eyelids, I am unable to do it; so I scoop out the daffodils and swallow them. Just like that. And then I leave.

In real life, I remember the color of her eyes. They are brown. Like mine. But now they
were blue. Her skin was turning yellow and her hair, which she normally combed over her
forehead, was standing straight up. She looked the same but worse. Not dead. Alive, but
sick. Her fingers had begun to swell. What I needed was a sense of goodbye. I knew I had to
kiss her. That would be my acknowledgment of my existence. A kiss. She was my mother.
Always would be.

QUESTIONS

1. Discuss the author's relationship with her mother. How does illness alter the response, if at all?
2. Comment on the author's use of photography and text. Why did she choose to include the photographs she uses, and why does she present them in this form?
3. Discuss the attitudes and behaviors of the various medical personnel as depicted in this story.

Breast Disease and Screening
My Mother's Story, My Story

⌒ MOYA LYNN ALFONSO ⌒

When I first enrolled in the master's degree program at the University of South Florida College of Public Health, I worked on a social marketing research project designed to increase breast cancer screening rates among low-income women. I served as an interviewer, going door-to-door to talk to women about their experiences with breast cancer and screening practices such as mammography. The survey was designed for quantitative data analysis, leaving no room for women to tell their stories. At that time, breast cancer was to me a distant threat—something other women in other families faced, not me, not mine. Mammography was a medical procedure and women who failed to comply with public health-recommended screening intervals were deliberately placing themselves at risk.

After the data collection phase, I was asked to help put together a publication based on the breast cancer project (Bryant, et al.). Through the process of putting the article together, I became increasingly familiar with breast cancer rates, treatments, and barriers to screening. I filled my head with anonymous information, detached from the women who underwent screening and thereby faced the potential for being diagnosed with a disease that hits at the heart of femininity.

While working on this publication, the abstract information I had gathered came alive through my mother's flesh. At fifty-six years of age, my mother was diagnosed with ductal carcinoma in situ, a noninvasive form of breast cancer—"the kind you want if you have to have one." My mother had for years followed her physician's recommendations for mammography and breast self-exams, particularly since she was diagnosed early on with benign fibrocystic breast disease. Her last mammogram was suspicious; a lump had changed and needed to be examined further. Based on the suspicious finding, my mother was sent to a surgeon, who recommended she have a biopsy. The surgeon reassured my mother that everything would be fine: "More than likely it's nothing." Results of the biopsy countered the surgeon's words of support. "Carcinoma," I heard. *I know that word. Cancer. Oh my God, my mother has cancer. No. Please God, no. Not my mother. My beautiful, sweet mother who has never done anything to deserve this.* The surgeon told her, "You need a second opinion.

You're entitled to that. Try not to worry. It's not breast cancer. Jackie, you don't have breast cancer. It's not invasive. It won't spread through your body." My mother's brain probably shut down. I knew she didn't understand what he was saying. *It's up to me. This is my background. Wait a minute. He said carcinoma but he said it's not breast cancer. That's not right. Say something. He's looking at me now. What does his look say? Perhaps he's saying, "If we tell her it's breast cancer, she will only worry needlessly. If we tell her it's not breast cancer, she won't worry as much."* In shock, I didn't argue with him. "Mom, it's okay," I told her.

When my mother went to have a follow-up mammogram, the technician asked her what her line of treatment would be for her breast cancer. My mother replied, "But I don't have breast cancer." The technician, not the daughter whom she trusted, told her, "Yes, you do." My mother asked me later, "Moya, why didn't you tell me? Did you know?" What could I say? I explained that I went along because I didn't want her to worry, and I apologized.

Wanting a second opinion, my mother scheduled an appointment with a well-known "cancer doctor" at Moffitt Cancer Center. She asked me to go with her even though I'm the baby of the family and typically ignored or dismissed. I was supposed to know about breast cancer. I'm public health. She trusted me and wanted me there. *I can do this.*

The day of the appointment, we arrived at Moffitt and passed through the giant revolving door. I couldn't breathe, and my eyes felt weird. We were led into a private room and the doctor and a student came in. As they talked to my mother, I heard their words, but my vision wasn't working right. I couldn't seem to focus. "We'll schedule surgery," the cancer doctor told her. She asked him, "Will I lose my breasts? If I have to, I will. Whatever it takes. My children and my grandchildren are the most important things in my life. I want to be here for them." The doctor touched her shoulder and said, "There is a chance, if it has spread within the breast. Radiation is a possibility. Odds are you won't need chemotherapy. Some women choose to remove the breast. Your insurance will cover the removal of the breast or both breasts . . . More than likely it has not . . ." I had a hard time following what the doctor was saying. The room was getting smaller. I couldn't breathe.

The day arrived for my mother's surgery. We were all there, except for my older sister, who lives in California. As they were getting ready to wheel my mother away, I hugged her. "I love you, Mamma." She told the nurse, "This is my baby. She's working on her master's degree in public health, and she's going to get her Ph.D." I clung to my mother and prayed. She looked pale. *Please God, let her be okay.* I couldn't breathe, but I couldn't cry in front of her. I was supposed to be strong. I stood up and told her, "It will be okay." They wheeled her into surgery; we were forced to wait. My dad talked to me about something; I wished he would just shut up. *You son of a bitch. This is partly your fault. You've never treated her right and you've put her through hell. It should be you, not her.*

After a while, the doctor emerged and led us to a private room. "The cancer spread outside of the duct. It was worse than we thought. We've talked to your mother and she said to remove both breasts." He kept talking but I couldn't hear what he was saying. *Oh my God, please. Please.* My dad broke down. My sister shook. My oldest sister, forever in control, asked questions. I couldn't hear. I couldn't think.

Surgery was over. Both of my mother's breasts had been removed. We asked, "When can we see her?" As we walked through the halls of Moffitt and entered the patient wards, I felt surrounded by cancer and death. I reminded myself that these people were alive; there was hope. As we entered my mother's room, we found my dad putting up our pictures for her. She wanted them in front of her, where she could see all of her babies and grandbabies. I sat beside her on the hospital bed and tried not to cry. I wanted to tell her it was okay, to comfort her, but she looked at me and said, "Mommy's okay darlin." I broke down and wrapped myself around her. I wasn't an adult; I was her little girl, who was scared to death. She let me cry and rubbed my back. "I love you mamma. I'm sorry. I was just so scared." "I know, baby," she told me. When I straightened up and looked at her, I could see how pale she was. I could also see the wraps around her skin where her breasts used to be. There were drains coming from each side where her breasts used to be. "The drains," the nurse told us, "will collect the blood until the healing process is complete. They'll need to be emptied."

I stayed with my mother that night. Although I tend to be emotional, she seemed to prefer me to be with her. In the days following her surgery, I tried to do anything to help her. I felt so helpless. We all did. I brought her special foods with natural estrogens. I tried to answer her questions. I emptied the blood from her drains. I helped her bathe. I listened to her. I changed her gown and tried not to look at the scars. But most importantly, I touched her face and her hands and breathed her in. I knew that she would be okay. She was getting better, but I felt like a wreck. I wasn't sleeping. I was crying a lot. I examined my breasts daily. Round and round, I felt the tissue, searching for lumps or anything unusual. I couldn't take a shower without checking my breasts. They told me it was normal. I've always been afraid of losing those close to me, but this was the first time in my life my mother's mortality was so vivid. Mine, too.

Shortly after my mother's diagnosis and surgery, I tried to retreat back into the protective coating of public health facts and figures: each year one out of eight women will be diagnosed with breast cancer. But I couldn't.

I have three sisters, two daughters, two nieces, and myself. That's eight.

MY STORY

In the months before my mother's experience with breast cancer, I noticed that every once in a while the front of my shirt or nightgown would feel wet. At first I thought I was just spilling stuff or splashing water on my shirt while cleaning the kitchen. Unfortunately, this explanation didn't hold during the times I hadn't been near water. It's amazing how the brain works to protect the self. One morning, after feeling the strange wetness, I lifted my shirt and saw clear fluid coming from my left breast. I looked it up in the women's health book I had for my public health work, and I searched the file cabinets in my brain for information. *Some women experience clear nipple discharge ... clear discharge is nothing to worry about ... normal. Nothing to worry about.*

During my next gynecological visit, the doctor asked me, "Has anyone in your family ever had breast cancer?" "Yes," I said. "My mother lost both breasts just recently. She had ductal carcinoma in situ." After hearing of my family history, she told me how important it was for me to check my breasts monthly and to have a baseline mammography when I was 35 years old. I reassured her, "I know." However, I didn't tell her I had checked my breasts daily since my mother's diagnosis, thinking it sounded kind of weird when said out loud.

I then told her about the clear fluid. She said, "It's normal, but it could be a symptom of a tumor." She sent me to have a blood test. The test results came back negative. "There's nothing to worry about," she said.

After about two years, the fluid wasn't clear anymore, and there was pain. One evening, after working for a while and trying to block thoughts of the pain from my mind, I told my husband, "Babe, my breast hurts. It's weird. Like a sharp pain through my nipple." He turned to me and asked tentatively, "Well, you're under a lot of stress. Are you sure it's not like the chest pain you've had before?" "No," I told him, "it's not anxiety. It's a weird pain." I held my breast, hoping the counter-pressure would make the shooting pain stop. I was right; in a few minutes it stopped.

A few days later, I took my bra off and noticed a weird brown spot on the inside of the left cup. I looked at it and felt sick. My breast was oozing bloody discharge. I went downstairs and searched the net for the phrase "bloody nipple discharge." Several hundred hits came up. I felt a little better knowing it was not just me. *Jesus. There's one with the word "cancer" in the same link.* I looked through several links that were attached to more legitimate sources of medical information and learned that bloody nipple discharge is indeed a sign of breast cancer 10 percent of the time. Although 90 percent of the time it's not cancer, my brain focused on the 10 percent. I kept searching for more information. One site said, "Most of the time it is not carcinoma. One possible explanation is a papilloma located within a duct in the breast." *That's what my sister had.* I looked up papilloma in my medical dictionary. I felt a little better after reading the academic definition, especially the word "benign."

Mom had benign tumors before the cancer. Instantly I tried to block this thought and called my new gynecologist. I told the nurse it was time for my annual checkup. "Plus, um, my breast is hurting and bleeding." I expected to have to wait a few weeks, but I was blessed with an appointment the following week.

The day of the appointment, I arrived at my new gynecologist's office and waited to be called. The time came, and I was led into a private room and asked to undress and put on a robe. I did as I was told, climbed onto the exam table, and waited. I listened to the baby crying in a room next door and thought about my girls. I laughed to myself when I thought how, although I worship my daughters, I never wanted to have to deal with a crying baby again. The doctor knocked and entered. He sat down.

"Well, you look thrilled to be here."

I laughed and scolded him for torturing the baby next door: "What did you do to that poor child?"

He laughed. "He's crying because he's now half the man he used to be," he explained.

The ice broke; the interview began. I told him about the discharge, the bloodstain on my bra, the hormone test two years ago, the pain, and my mother's bilateral mastectomy. He took notes while I talked. When he finished, he told me to lie back so he could examine my breasts. I lay back and thought about how funny it was to have another man touching my breasts. "No lumps," he said. *That's a good sign.* He then told me what I already knew: I needed a mammogram, but because of my young age, there was a chance that it wouldn't detect a problem. Mammograms only pick up about 85 percent of breast cancer cases in young women because their breast tissue is "lumpy, bumpy" to begin with, "but it's the best place to start." He wrote out a prescription for a mammogram and told me to have the results sent to him.

After I got dressed, I took a second to look at the prescription. It was for a baseline/diagnostic mammogram and had a hand-written note indicating my "family history" of breast cancer. I took a moment and thanked God that I had insurance that would cover a mammogram even though I was so young.

When I got home that afternoon, I called my sister. She told me to call Moffitt's Lifetime Cancer Screening, which is where she went for her mammogram. When I called the number, I was greeted by a very sweet woman who asked me a few questions and scheduled an appointment. I started to cry. I couldn't help it. "I'm sorry. My mother had breast cancer. She's okay now, but just hearing the name 'Moffitt' makes it all come back. I feel so stupid." "It's okay," she replied, "I understand." Despite her reassurance, I felt stupid and afraid.

After I hung up, I called my mother. I hadn't told her yet; I didn't want to worry her. When I told her I needed to talk to her, she sounded scared.

"Mom, my breast has been bleeding."

"Have you called the doctor? Don't let it go. You need to get in right away. Tell them about me."

"I know. I went to my gynecologist and he didn't feel anything. I have an appointment for a mammogram. I'm going where Terese went to have hers. She said they were really good."

"I'll go with you. Do you want me to go with you? Do you feel anything? Is there a lump?"

"No," I replied, "I don't feel anything. It's just bleeding. I'm sure it's just a benign tumor in the duct. There's a slim chance it's cancer, but 90 percent of the time it's nothing." I retreated into statistics.

She cautioned me, "Don't let them dismiss you because you're young. I'll go with you and tell them what I went through. You make sure they know you have a family history. Make them do a sonogram. Don't let it go like I did."

"You didn't let it go, Mamma."

"Yes I did. After the first biopsy, I let it go for a while because of the bleeding. Maybe if I had gone in sooner . . ."

"Mamma, that wouldn't have mattered. You always kept up with it." I tried to reassure her: "I'll make sure and push for every test they have. I won't let them dismiss me. I love you, Mamma."

"Mamma loves you too, baby. You'll be okay."

I hung up and cried.

I had to wait a couple of weeks before my mammogram. I had PMS the week before, and my breasts hurt. I felt the left breast leaking and looked down and saw the bloody discharge. I felt sick and angry and scared. I snapped at the girls and begged them to please stop fighting, knowing it was a futile plea, since they would probably fight if Jesus himself came down and asked them to stop. I tried to tell them, "Mommy's nerves are bad right now." They had heard me talk about my breasts, and I knew they were scared too. The house was filled with tension. At seven and eight years of age, they were old enough to know their mema had breast cancer; and at nine and ten years of age, they knew their mom was having problems with her breast.

Later that night, I went to bed and felt sick. I could feel the wetness on my nipple, and the room felt like it was spinning. I lay down next to my husband and touched his arm.

"Babe, I'm scared. I'm sorry I snapped at you."

He turned to me, "I know, baby. I love you. It will be okay."

I looked at him and thought about how much I had grown to love him and need him over the last decade. *Please God, life is too good. Let me be okay.*

The morning of my mammogram, I ran late. I had a hard time getting around. I felt sick on the way there. I had never had a mammogram, and through reading the research literature, I knew that a major barrier to repeat mammography is pain experienced during the first (Bryant, et al.). I grabbed my cell phone and started dialing numbers. No matter whom I called, no one was at home or at work. I was alone, just like I had wanted.

When I arrived at the building, I couldn't find a parking space right away. *I could just skip the whole ordeal and go straight to the library.* I drove around and unfortunately found a space. After parking the car, I walked up to the window and signed in. The woman at the desk told me to take a seat until I was called. I sat down and looked around. A mother and daughter were sitting across from me, both far older than I was. *That's good: further evidence that I'm too young to worry.* Next to them were another mother and daughter. The daughter was in her mid-teens and her mother was older and spoke rough English. The daughter was translating the forms into Spanish so her mother could answer the questions. *I hope I was a good daughter.*

They called my name, and I gave them my insurance information. "It will be just a minute." I sat and waited, staring at the door. *No one would care if I left. No one's here with me to stop me. I could leave and not deal with this shit.* I wanted to go, but I was too chicken to get up and walk out in front of everyone. Luckily, the nurse opened the door to the exam area. "Moya Alfonso?"

I was directed to a small dressing room and told to take off my shirt and bra and put on a pink cape. When I finished changing, I opened the door and followed the technician into the room where the mammogram would take place. She asked me about my symptoms and family history. I told her about the pain and the discharge and my mother's bilateral mastectomy. She started to explain to me what mammograms entail, but I cut her off by telling her that I'm a researcher at the College of Public Health and am prepared. I laughed, "I probably know too much." She laughed with me. The tension broke.

She placed my breast on the machine and told me how the upper part of the machine would lower and compress my breast for the X ray. My body prepared for the pain and discomfort I had read so much about. I realized I wasn't breathing only after she told me, "Okay, hold your breath and don't move." I thought about my mother and all of the tests she had endured. I thought of my little girls and prayed. The pressure came, but no pain. I tried to remember to breathe before the next X ray. The technician finished X-raying both breasts and said, "I'm going to take these to the other technician to read. You'll find out right away if they see anything suspicious." I felt sick. I didn't know I would find out so fast. My mind raced. *I don't want to know today. I want my funny doctor to tell me, not someone I don't know.* She told me, "Take a seat and relax." *Oh sure.* I sat down and read about celebrities and their assorted tribulations.

She came back a couple of minutes later. "I need to take a couple more pictures. This doesn't mean they saw something," she said. "It's of the left breast, but it doesn't mean they see anything wrong. They just want to get a couple more pictures. Because you're so young, your breast tissue is denser and it's harder for them to tell if what they're seeing is normal or something to be concerned about. Okay?" I replied, "Okay." *Shit.* The room spun a little while she took more pictures of my left breast. I noticed the pictures were of the exact area that hurt. When she was done, she told me to relax while she took the new pictures to be examined.

She came right back. *That was too quick.* "The films look good. The technicians didn't see anything. You'll get a letter and we'll send the results to your doctor. Do you have a surgeon? They'll probably send you to a surgeon now and recommend a ductogram. Do you know what that is? They'll inject die into your breast." I interrupted her: "Yes, I know. My sister had one and said it hurt like hell." We laughed.

I realized I wasn't breathing as I got in my car. I reminded myself to take a few deep breaths. I called my husband and left a voicemail. I called my mother and tried to sound convincing: "I'm fine, I'm sure. The mammogram showed nothing." She reassured me that the mammogram showing nothing was good news. I knew I should be grateful, but I felt negative: "It just means whatever's wrong is too small to be seen on an X ray." Sounding hurt, she tried to comfort me: "Your sister and I went shopping. We bought you a surprise. We left it hanging on your front door." Talking to her was too much of a reminder. Too real. I had to get off the phone with her, so I told her I had to work. I couldn't face the library, so I stopped by to talk to my friend Carol.

"I just had my first mammogram. Everything was okay."

"That's great, but why do you seem disappointed?" she asked.

I told her about the bleeding. "I almost wanted it to show something; that way I would know what was going on. Now I still know nothing. I'm ready to just have the damn things cut off."

"You know," she said, "that's not out of the question. Some women have them removed if they have a family history of breast cancer. Peter probably wouldn't like that, though."

I hadn't really thought of Peter. My wonderful husband who loves my breasts. The sweet man who loved to watch me nurse the girls and who loves to bury his face in my chest. I replied, "No, he probably wouldn't like that." I reminded myself that as a feminist I'm not supposed to concern myself with such things.

"Have they checked your hormones? What about medications?"

"Yes on both accounts. The next step is a ductogram, and I've heard it hurts. I'm going to be assertive and ask for drugs. Valium or Xanax. I know for a fact those work real well for me."

She laughed. "If breasts were meant to go through that crap, God wouldn't have given us Valium."

We laughed. I felt better.

It took several days to receive the results of the mammogram and several more weeks waiting for my gynecologist to follow up (which he never did). I eventually received the letter stating the mammogram was "normal." Over the years, one duct had filled with benign growths that were cutting off blood supply to the area. No cancer. Unfortunately, though, the pain and the bleeding continued. It took almost another year to meet with a surgeon, have a sonogram, and have the offending duct removed. I now have a small scar, but the pain and worry are gone.

The stress of not knowing, combined with feeling the periodic wetness in the context of the juggling act I do as a mom, wife, employee, and doctoral student, took its toll. Fortunately, I married a saint. I found that although my sister and mother had gone though a similar situation, my husband was the one I turned to. Only he could reassure me that it's me he loves (and not only my breasts) when I asked him how he would feel if I had to have my breasts removed. Only he could make me laugh when he grabbed his chest in sympathy pain when I told him my breast hurt.

Hearing the sound of fear in my family's and friends' voices when I talked about my breast bleeding helped me realize that my feelings of fear when coping with the threat of my mother's mortality were natural and understandable, not stupid. This sort of breathtaking emotion can be overwhelming; perhaps it turns some women away from pursuing tests that can expose life-threatening illness, while encouraging others, such as myself, my mother, and my sister, to pursue medical advice, procedures, and treatment (Hyman, et al.).

As a public health professional, I know that my health behaviors now will determine, in part, my daughters' future health behaviors. My oldest daughter's breasts have just begun to grow, and she is very proud. I look at her and wonder what her future holds. Will she be the one in eight? How have the experiences she has witnessed affected her health behaviors? I want my girls to take care of themselves, so I tell them how beautiful they are, talk to them about how to take care of themselves, and, most important, try to show them, as my mother showed me, the importance of screening, self-exams, and persistence—even in the face of breathtaking fear.

REFERENCES

Bryant, C., Forthofer, M., McCormack Brown, K., Alfonso, M., & Quinn, G. "A Social Marketing Approach to Increasing Breast Cancer Screening Rates." *Journal of Health Education* 31(6): 320–328.

Hyman, R. B., Baker, S., Ephraim, R., Moadel, A., & Philip, J. "Health Belief Model Variables as Predictors of Screening Mammography Utilization." *Journal of Behavioral Medicine* 17(4): 391–406.

QUESTIONS

1. How do cultural views of female sexuality affect breast cancer screening and treatment? What role does the culture of medicine, including ways of interacting with patients and specialized terminology, play in breast cancer screening and treatment?
2. How do the roles individuals play (e.g., wife, mother) impact understandings of illness and health behaviors? How did breast cancer, or the fear of it, impact the multiple roles the author and her mother played every day?
3. How can medical personnel deal with patients who are unable or unready to hear bad news about their health?

Unintended Research
A Sociologist's Experience with
Illness and Death

☞ MICHAEL ROWE ☜

I

Jesse, my nineteen-year-old son, lay critically ill in his bed on the pediatric intensive care unit of a New York City hospital. Two weeks before, on May 6, 1995, he had received a liver transplant. The operation seemed to have gone well. During the first couple of days after transplant, Jesse had gotten out of bed, sat in a chair, drunk some apple juice, and watched some TV—not spectacular progress but not so bad. By the morning of May 9, though, his heart rate, pulse, and blood pressure had crept up and his oxygen saturation rate and blood values had slipped down a bit. He had a slight fever. And he needed a lot of fentanyl, a narcotic, for pain. On May 10 he was taken back into surgery with a rising fever and severe belly pain. His surgeons discovered that they had inadvertently made a tiny perforation in his intestine during transplant surgery, while cutting through scar tissue that had built up after his surgery for ulcerative colitis two years earlier. Within days he was "in" sepsis and multi-organ failure. His body swelled up with fluid because his antibodies, which attacked the bacteria that caused and carried the infection, poked tiny holes in his blood vessels and capillaries. Water and protein and electrolytes leaked into his tissues and into his abdomen, lungs, hands, and feet. The fluid in his belly pushed up on his diaphragm, which pushed up and crowded his lungs, which pushed up on his heart. His lungs began to fill with blood and fluid. His doctors, worried that his left lung might collapse or that he might come down with pneumonia, cut a hole in his side and pushed a rubber tube through his ribs. Bloody fluid rushed out and down the tube along the side of the bed into a clear container with vertical cells that turned red one by one before our eyes. The doctor showed us the Before and After X rays. The Before was white from fluid, the After was pitch-black. Jesse had been breathing on a quarter of one lung, she said.[1]

A respirator *shooshed* and *haaahed* by the window, pushing oxygen into Jesse's lungs through a breathing tube in his mouth. He had IV lines—wherever they could find places to put them—for antibiotics, for pain meds, for the giving of blood and blood products, and for dialysis. Meds and blood hung from poles at the corners of his bed. Residents and lab technicians stuck him several times a day to measure his hemoglobin, hematocrit, and red blood cells and the antibiotics and immunosuppressants in his blood. A red light clipped to his index finger was attached to an oxygen monitor. Electrodes on his chest sent signals to another monitor, which measured his heart rate and blood pressure. Dr. Lanier,[2] the Chief of Gastroenterology, came in one afternoon and waved his hands around the bed. "Never add anything, never give anything, never treat anything," he said, "unless you have to. The more lines and poles and machines you see, the sicker the patient is."

Soon Jesse would stabilize and, in early June, receive a second liver transplant, sepsis having corrupted the first one. Two weeks later, though, another perforation, due not to a surgical accident this time but to his weakened condition, would be found. Another bout of sepsis would follow, with more downturns and rallies until his death in early August—after a total of thirteen operations, including two liver transplants and a splenectomy. But now, in the latter part of May, he lay waterlogged and unmoving on his bed, save for an occasional twitch of his left leg and faint hand squeeze.

If an ethnographer—a social scientist who immerses him- or herself in a new culture to try to understand it from the inside out—had walked off one of the elevators facing the lounge for the neonatal intensive care unit (NICU, pronounced nick-you), he might have seen me examining a long scroll of paper and recognized that I was at work on a primitive coding system. At the time we brought Jesse in to wait for his transplant, I was running a homeless outreach program for the Yale Department of Psychiatry and conducting ethnographic-sociological research on the encounters of homeless people and outreach workers. I had spent time out on the streets and in soup kitchens and shelters observing these encounters and talking to the participants. Shortly before bringing Jesse in, I had finished my fieldwork and had begun to code my transcribed interviews and field notes by noting key themes in the margins of their pages. I had then written my theme titles in two columns on lined paper, taping on extra pages as needed to create one long sheet of paper that I rolled up after finishing a coding session. Now, in the NICU lounge, I was grouping themes on a pad of paper for the next generation of coded notes. When I got to a computer again I would cut and paste thousands of pages of transcribed interviews and field notes according to my grouped themes. Eventually, all this material would become a book.

When the ethnographer (let's make him male, to match my gender) learned that I was the father of a patient on the pediatric intensive care unit (the PICU), he might have experienced an un-ethnographic moment of revulsion toward me. Here I was, working on my research while my son lay critically ill down the hall beyond the double fire doors of the PICU. And it's likely the image would have stuck with him. The ethnographer's learning curve is steepest during the early days of fieldwork. It is then that his eyes are open widest and he "sees" the most, shocked into awareness by an alien culture.

But the ethnographer, reporting for his first day of fieldwork on the PICU, would also know that while culture shock can force into consciousness the insights that may preoccupy him for years to come, it can also blind him to other patterns that do not announce themselves so boldly. Suppose he notes, while making his first rounds with the surgical team,

[handwritten: no faces, no persons. look out to a pitch black audience]

that the spatial arrangement of the fellows, residents, nurses, and medical students around the attending surgeon resembles an audience around the lead actor in a theatre. Reflecting on this observation later that evening while typing up his field notes, he comes up with the working hypothesis that a sense of performance among team members shields them from the suffering of their patients, who are performing the drama of their illnesses. Interesting enough for a start, and possibly on target. But what if this spatial arrangement is not repeated on subsequent rounds, which instead suggest a military image, that of the attending surgeon on point in the enemy territory of illness? Or suppose the theatrical image does repeat itself, but our ethnographer learns that before he joined the team that first day, the attending surgeon had said, "You know, I saw *Hamlet* last night with the mayor and I wondered, 'Is surgery a form of theatre?' With real-life consequences, of course. But if we're the actors in the OR, what does that make the patient? And back on the floor, does the patient *[handwritten: Lay d'an actor]* become the actor again? And what of it? Does this teach us anything about what we're doing? What do you think, Jones?" And so, unconsciously and only half getting the point (or getting the point quite well, knowing that the attending surgeon is always the lead actor), the team members had arranged themselves in an audience-like pattern that day and the next few days. The ethnographer, in turn, saw a performance motif, perhaps to the exclusion of others he could have observed.

But what if it were the ethnographer who had seen *Hamlet* the night before? Did Shakespeare lead him by the nose toward a nonexistent theatrical motif? Or did seeing *Hamlet* open the door onto a motif he could easily have missed? And even if the surgeon-patient interactions he observed bore it out, his insight would raise as many questions for him as it answered. Does this theatrico-medical motif or pattern say anything important about patient care, the overall structure of the unit, or the interaction among services? Could it be blinding the ethnographer to other, deeper patterns? In any case—whether he finds partial justification for his working hypothesis or discards it in favor of another—he will realize that his work has just begun.

In my case, the ethnographer would learn that he had caught me in a rare moment of quiet working on my notes, one he might not see again for days and would never see for more than twenty minutes at a time. He would learn from talking to me, or surmise from observing me and other PICU parents, that such an activity was a brief and fitful distraction that never truly caused the parent to forget the child's illness at all. He would also learn that the NICU lounge, enclosed by an elbow-high wood frame at either end and with its dark, soft, not-quite-clean blue couches and chairs and its dark blue rug and dim lighting only fifteen feet from the bank of elevators facing it, was more than a workstation or site of morning coffee breaks for exhausted parents. It was the place where parents like me met friends and family and had important conversations. Here, in the latter part of May, I told my mother the dismal good news that Jesse still had a fighting chance. The NICU lounge was also a campsite. Here we napped or slept many nights when we couldn't risk going back to the Transplant Respite Center, a large apartment in a high-rise nearby that the liver team kept for the families of their patients. And if the ethnographer gained my trust and spent some time talking to me, he might learn that the NICU lounge was, for me, a sanctuary, a place of meditation that, with its border of couches and elbow-high wood frames, formed a shroud to keep out intruding thoughts—my own and others'—and intruding people, outsiders who had not earned the right to stand with us, Jesse's parents, or with his doctors and nurses and thus were not part of the circle of sorrow in which Jesse was the irreducible center. Here, going into sleep or doze mode, I could follow my son on his quest, seeking beneath thought the wisdom of his body in my body and the secret that would lift him from his sickbed. The NICU lounge, in my sleep-deprived state, was a place for explorations beneath the surface of things to bring Jesse back.

The ethnographer, then, might conclude that the NICU lounge was what Erving Goffman called a "backstage" area[3] to the action taking place on the main stage, where life was being performed. For me that main stage was Jesse's room on the PICU. Here we would squeeze his hand and wonder whether we felt the hint of a squeeze in return. Here we taped up pictures of him next to the liver chart on his door, where the doctors gathered on their rounds, to show them who Jesse was and to remind ourselves. We knew what they would already know about him from reading his chart. That he was born in 1975. That he had three operations for hydrocephalus from the ages of three months to seventeen months and had been in remission ever since. That in 1991, at age fifteen, he had been diagnosed with ulcerative colitis. That in 1992 he had been diagnosed with a mild case of sclerosing cholangitis, a scarring and narrowing of the bile ducts going into the liver. That in 1993 an arteriogram, performed before an upcoming colitis operation, revealed early-stage cirrhosis of the liver. That his fatigue and other symptoms had been troublesome enough to lead to our wait-listing him for a liver transplant in January 1994.

Had they read the summary of his psychological testing, they would have known that Jesse was socially withdrawn and performed below his intellectual capacity in school. The chart would not have reported that he had a tendency to drift off into fantasies of superheroes and their heroic quests, or that he zealously guarded the privacy of his internal world and was a master at parrying adults' attempts to violate it. As one of his teachers said to me of this defensive gift, "It was mental sparring for him. I could look out the window and comment on how bright the sun was and he would smirk. He always knew when you were trying to get him to talk about himself." The chart would not have reported that he usually had one good friend at a time and that his loyalties to friends and those he admired, including athletes whose bodies did not betray them, were fierce.

Those who had seen him at the liver clinic during the year and a half of the wait-listing process would not have needed a chart entry to know that Jesse's vulnerability led many adults to be protective toward him. And they would have had a glimpse of his artistic talent in his self-portrait, which I insisted he bring in to show them. He had drawn it in early August 1993, the day before he was to have a subtotal colectomy at this same hospital. The surgeon would cut out his colon and the inner lining of his rectum but retain the sphincter muscle. He would then cut an incision in the side of his abdomen to create an opening, or ostomy, and pull the end of the small intestine through the hole to deliver feces to a plastic bag stuck to his skin with an adhesive flange that fit around the ostomy. In a second stage to be performed later on, the surgeon would remove the end of the small intestine from the ostomy, close off the ostomy, and pull down the intestine to the rectum. Using the last foot and a half of intestine, he would create a pouch to store waste, and sew it in just north of the anus. If successful, Jesse would have more frequent and, at best, toothpaste-consistency bowel movements, but would not have to wear a bag on his side.

He and his younger brother, Daniel, and I had been sitting at our kitchen table. Jesse picked up a piece of typing paper and a pencil and appeared to be doodling as Daniel and I talked and ate breakfast. Ten minutes later he put down his pencil. He had drawn a creature with many heads and eyes and mouths, certainly not human, though some of the heads and eyes and mouths were. It was a composite monster that the explorers of *Hakluyt's Travels* might have written about if they had known both the paintings of Hieronymus Bosch and the illustrations of artists toiling at the margins of late-twentieth-century comic-book culture.

Amid a menagerie of half-human, half-animal forms is a man's face in profile with rounded nose and puckered lips. His lidless, bulging eyes anticipate the unknown with a look not of horror, but of disorientation that might show on a face landing upright just after its beheading. Jesse's is a drawing of a body in uproar and astonishment over that uproar, as though the magician has just pulled a black egg from behind the ear of a healthy-looking volunteer from the audience.

Jesse put down his pencil. Daniel, sitting next to him, stopped talking and studied the drawing.

"What is it?"

"A self-portrait," said Jesse.

His doctors and nurses at the clinic did not know the full range of his comic vision, though, because they had not seen his carnivorous carrot with its mushroom-cloud green top swaying in a nuclear wind, bibbed for lobster but dining on humans. They had not read his stories about his alter ego, George 10 from the planet Eggnog III, who suffers from chronic tomatoed eggnog disease, an illness common to all Eggnogians, and must take specialized pills ten times a day to avoid turning into tomatoed eggnog substitute. And they did not see a bleaker side of his talent, because they had not seen the young man whose head he had drawn on tracing paper and superimposed on its skull, which he had drawn on heavy paper. The young man's hair is medium length and straight. A dark line for the hollow between jaw and cheekbone extends to the left side of his mouth like a gash from mouth to ear or a shadow grin. His eyes are feverish. The mouth opening on the skull is tight and wide and supports the young man's shadow grin. Jesse, alas, had been forced too soon to lift his own skull from the dirt, but had the courage to turn it in his hands and comment on it in the language that came most naturally to him.

II

There was much of sociological interest to observe on the PICU, if I'd had the time and focus for it. There was the fact that Jesse's suffering, and ours, were a privilege of sorts: he, and we, had the opportunity to contend with his bad luck because I had health insurance that paid for a liver transplant. Millions of Americans lack insurance to pay for primary-care visits and antibiotics.

There was the organization of intensive medical care teams and the interactions among them. The liver team made late-afternoon rounds with the attending surgeon leading the way and the attending gastroenterologist, or GI, at his side. A surgical fellow and GI resident followed, with the team coordinator, a social worker, and other residents and medical students bringing up in the rear. The GIs followed Jesse's medical condition, and the surgeons followed what they had done surgically, studying his liver and blood and kidney numbers written in pencil on the liver chart taped to his door.

Surgeons, to go by comments I heard and interpreted from the ICU residents, know how to cut and splice, take out old body parts, and put in new ones. They are highly skilled technicians, but they don't know how the body works when it's healthy and what disease is when health vanishes. Other medical specialists are drawn to their discipline because they want to care for the whole person, while surgeons are undersocialized individuals who lack the ability or inclination to deal with the person unless he's out cold on an aluminum table. I didn't buy this characterization, partly because it let the surgeons off the hook and partly because it didn't jibe with my observations of Jesse's surgeons from hydrocephalus days on. There was more than a kernel of truth to this lore, though. You could see it when the attending surgeon spent more time looking at the liver chart than he did at Jesse on his bed five feet away.

The PICU doctors followed Jesse's condition from minute to minute, making decisions about intubating and extubating, giving and stopping IV feeds, and giving or holding blood products. The GIs and PICU doctors spent time around each other and their patients, and knew that surgeons can cut, but only medicine can make whole. The liver surgeons looked down on the Gis, just as they did on the intensivists (M.D.s who specialized in intensive care), but from not so lofty a height, since they have to live with gut specialists. The GIs treated the surgeons with deference. When the attending surgeon came in, they watched as he cogitated, turned as he turned, and waited, like us, with bated breath for his assessment of the day.

There was the range of culture and class among patients and their family members and the question of whether differences in class and education were associated with differences in treatment—whether, for example, better-educated family caregivers get more or better treatment for their ill family members because they are more comfortable talking to, negotiating with, and confronting doctors. Minimally, if at all, I think. As the sociologist Charles Bosk observed in his ethnographic study of surgeons and ICUs, the democracy of suffering seems to call for a democracy of treatment on the ICU.[4] The big differences, I think, play out in the availability and use of health care outside the ICU. "Systems savvy" does make a difference on the PICU, but mostly in the realm of securing creature comforts for the patient. Comfortable beds, for example.

Jesse's bed had a standard-issue mattress with a green industrial-strength plastic cover and the usual push buttons for elevating and lowering the head and foot. During the latter part of May, his blood pressure was so unstable they decided not to transport him from the unit for a CAT scan, yet every night he had to be hoisted above his bed so they could see how much fluid he'd put on. The nurse would wheel in the Scale Tronix 2001, or the Tuna Scale as she called it, from its cubby next to the linen cart down the hall. An upright metal stand with a digital monitor rose from the back of its three-sided steel frame, open in front like a forklift on rollers to fit under the bed. The nurse would pull out a six-by-three-foot green plastic sling that was rolled up and lay the sling on the bed to Jesse's left. We, three parents and one nurse, would take positions, two on each side of the bed (the other parent would take a turn at getting in the way), and would roll Jesse onto his right side, push the sling snug against his back, and partially unroll it behind him. We would roll him over the hump of the sling onto his left side and hold him steady, then unroll the rest of the sling behind him, and finally roll him onto his back. When we had hooked the claws of the frame into metal rings at the four corners of the sling and checked Jesse for balance, the nurse would turn the crank on the metal stand, Jesse would clear the bed, and we would steady him and release. The nurse would push the monitor and call out a weight for one of us to remember. Then she would lower the sling onto the bed so we could roll Jesse in reverse to retrieve the sling and she could roll the Tuna Scale out of the room. All this to determine Jesse's weight.

You might think logic would dictate that a hospital which sponsored some of the most technically sophisticated and difficult operations known to humankind would have state-of-the-art beds for its sickest patients, but not so. These hospitals are in great demand because they attract the most skilled doctors to perform high-risk surgeries. Modest general hospitals, which vie for noncritical patients, are more likely to provide such creature comforts and hospitality—as a means of competition.

Jesse had survived the Tuna Scale, but by late June he was at risk of skin breakdown from lack of nutrition and bed sores from lying on his back for weeks. Too absorbed in his mere survival to focus on such things in May, we now began to think of a new bed for him. We'd heard about beds that could be adjusted for the body's pressure points and could even weigh the patient. Jesse's mother, Rachel, had worked in pharmaceutical sales and knew how to lobby doctors and medical systems. For two days she made his new bed her reason for living. We heard that the nursing supervisor was not pleased with her efforts. We gathered that she had something to do with the process of approving the bed and was miffed over not getting first shot at slowing things down. Rachel persevered and won for Jesse the very top-of-the-line bed she had picked out from a catalogue at the outset of her campaign. And it was a marvelous bed, to be sure—an airbed with a pillowed mattress. At its foot was a control panel with a touch screen to adjust for pressure points on the head, shoulder, buttocks, calves, and feet; to make the mattress firm or soft; to raise or lower the entire bed or parts of it; to weigh Jesse—no more rolling him from side to side and hoisting him on the Scale Tronix 2001—and to collapse the mattress like a popped balloon for a hard surface to work on if he coded.

Even when it comes to less essential items like a comfortable and more efficient bed, I wonder whether the democracy of suffering pushes the ICU system to compensate for parents less skilled in dealing with bureaucracy. Just as the nurses, for example, help to fill in the gap of caring and love when parents' work forces them to spend most of their time away from the unit, I suspect that nurses and other health professionals pick up some of the slack for parents less skilled at lobbying for their children.

I must have been observing these things at the time; they didn't just pop into my head years later. Yet I tried to avoid such observations and banish such thoughts. I had to be fully present for Jesse—personally, fully, father to son. Standing back to analyze things could dilute my presence for him. Years later, I see a certain illogic in such a notion. How could I be fully present for Jesse if I set aside a part of myself? But that part knew nothing about dealing with the critical illness of a child. Thought itself was a player in these proceedings, and

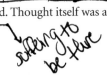

thought that separated itself from Jesse's body might tip the scales toward his dissolution. The horrible sanctity of his suffering demanded that its celebrants set aside all thoughts which would make of his suffering other than what it was—his body descending into itself to face what it had become—itself turned against itself, an organism seeking to effect its own dissolution. Our unspoken prayers were that, just as the miracle of health had transformed itself into the miracle of illness, it would, by the same process, transform itself again and leave Jesse whole and clear of infection. Or as Dr. Lanier put it, "If the infection in Jesse's liver turns around, his liver might turn around. If his liver turns around, his kidneys will kick in. And magically, everything will change. The swelling will go down, the bleeding will stop, and he will wake up and get better."

I did not lose my capacity for rational thought and action. I meticulously set down in my Jesse notebooks the facts of blood drawn and given, blood pressure, temperature, the level of oxygen in his blood, and the bare clinical statements his doctors made during their rounds. Yet this most rational activity was ruled in part by superstition. I limited myself to the facts during those days, eschewing description or interpretation. Having or writing down thoughts that removed me a degree or two from Jesse was tantamount to deserting my post and letting him slip out in the night through the cordon we had formed around him.

III

My experience with Jesse's illness and death has continued to unfold in my experience of grief and bereavement and in my writing about him. During that unfolding, my disciplinary training has asserted its influence.

A physician colleague asked me to write an editorial on medical mistakes for his online journal, hoping to start a dialogue with his fellow doctors on an unpopular but important subject. I wanted to do something more than simply list a series of individual errors or possible errors that his doctors had committed during Jesse's three-month hospitalization. In mulling over how to proceed, I thought about Kai Erikson's account of the Buffalo Creek Flood.[5] On February 26, 1972, a lake of sludge and water formed from the waste of coal-mining operations broke through its sludge-formed dam and careened down the valley into the town of Buffalo Creek, West Virginia, killing 125 of its citizens and destroying 80 percent of its homes. Two other disasters followed the flood: first, the owners of the coal-mining company hid behind their attorneys, avoiding contact with the survivors; and then the Army Corps of Engineers, in its well-meaning zeal to provide safe living conditions for the survivors, assigned them to trailer camps without attention to previous longstanding neighborhood ties, thus completing the destruction of the community. Erikson coined a new term and theory from these events—"collective trauma"—as a way of understanding how large-scale disasters affect both individuals and entire communities. The survivors of the Buffalo Creek Flood suffered, without a doubt, from what we call individual trauma, but these separate and personal traumas were shaped by the destruction of community.

I decided to look at medical mistakes as both discrete incidents of physician error and as a series of mistakes that, taken together, told a story of medical care gone awry. The singular mistakes were the surgical perforation of Jesse's intestine (a surgical "accident" rather than a mistake, but a necessary link in a chain); a cluster of missed signs—changes in heart rate, blood pressure, and oxygen saturation rates—during the first days after transplantation; a surgical resident's misdiagnosis of gas pain on the third night after transplantation, when Jesse was writhing on his bed in pain; and, three months later, the calls of condolence from Jesse's doctors that never came to us after his death. I noted that these singular mistakes became the cumulative mistake of Jesse's care and of my and my family's relationships with his doctors. I commented on the latter's resemblance to the collective trauma of the Buffalo Creek Flood survivors, and noted two further similarities. First, like the silence of the owners of the coal-mining company, which provided fuel for the lawsuit the citizens of Buffalo Creek brought against them, the silence of Jesse's doctors ultimately led me to conduct my own investigation into whether malpractice had occurred. (I did not sue, but that is another story.) Second, just as the survivors had considered the owners of the mining company to be integral members of their community and were thus more sharply wounded when the owners turned their backs on them, so the loss of trust that I and my family experienced with Jesse's doctors after his death was directly proportional to the sense of trust and collaboration we had with them while he was fighting for his life.[6]

This is only the beginning of a sociological inquiry. The next question, like that of the attending surgeon's after his monologue on surgery as a theatrical performance, is "What of it?" Is this similarity between personal and communal disasters forced or superficial, or are there elements of private disasters that mirror those of large-scale disasters, and vice versa? Put another way, what can we learn from cumulative "mistakes" in encounters between individual citizens and institutions that may help us understand the larger dislocations and disasters of modern society?

Let me give a second example of how my disciplinary training exerts its influence on me. Since Jesse's death, no part of his hospitalization has plagued me more than the evening of May 9, 1995, the third night after his first transplant. My wife, Gail, had left a few hours earlier for our home near Waterbury, Connecticut to spend some time with our younger children. A few hours later, Jesse's mother and stepfather, Will, had left for the transplant respite center to take their turn at getting a night's sleep. Jesse seemed to be doing well, although he needed a lot of fentanyl to take the edge off his pain. The ICU doctors were keeping an eye on what appeared, from his last belly X ray, to be an ileus, a condition in which the intestinal wall stops making contractions to digest food. An ileus can come from either a kink in the intestine or an infection. Doctors must watch closely to make sure that what looks like an ileus isn't an obstruction, where the part of the intestine above the obstruction keeps working and pressure from soupy waste builds until it bores a hole in the intestinal wall and escapes into the abdominal cavity. This can lead to peritonitis, an inflammation of the lining of the abdominal cavity, and that can lead to sepsis. As a precaution against possible infection, Jesse was given the first of a triple dose of three powerful antibiotics around 8 p.m. By eight-thirty he was writhing on his bed from belly pain. Dr. Bergman, the ICU resident, called the surgical team several times. She held off giving him more fentanyl because she was worried about peritonitis and didn't want to mask his symptoms before someone from the liver team could evaluate him.

At 11:30 p.m., three hours after Dr. Bergman's first call, Dr. Wolters, a surgical resident, walked into Jesse's room, examined his belly, and decided he had gas. He prescribed a bolus, a big dose, of fentanyl, discontinued the triple antibiotics after the first dose, and left. When the fentanyl finally kicked in hours later, Jesse was free from pain until early evening the next day, around the time that a belly X ray showed free air at one point along the loops of his intestine. He was taken back into surgery, where his surgeons found a hole in his intestine. He had begun a battle for his life that would end three months later.

My own investigation into these events, along with the informed speculation I've engaged in (since the principals were not going to talk to me) and a senior gastroenterologist's chart review after Jesse's death, persuade me that his severe pain on the evening of the ninth was a result of his intestinal perforation "opening up." While there is no way of knowing what would have happened had he been taken into surgery on the ninth rather than a full day later, it is obvious that the delay, during which intestinal contents were leaking into his abdominal cavity, did him no good, and it is plausible to say that it cost him his life.

The most obvious error was the surgical resident's misdiagnosis of Jesse's pain. Other errors, given the high likelihood that the surgical and ICU residents called their respective attendings, were the surgical attending's signoff on his resident's assessment and the ICU attending's signoff on that. As time has passed, however, I have concluded that the key to this disaster was Dr. Bergman's failure to transgress boundaries—horizontally, by bucking the surgical resident's assessment, and vertically, by bucking her own attending's instruction to follow the surgical team's lead. My assessment, of course, stands or falls on my conviction that Dr. Bergman strongly suspected an intestinal perforation that evening.

I think the "structure of the situation"—a basic sociological tenet which says social context, norms, and rules partly shape our actions—discouraged Dr. Bergman from taking action that might have saved Jesse's life. She committed no technical or legal error. If another resident had pushed harder, another still would have been more timid. Individual action is always important, but it takes place within social and institutional structures that shape and constrain action. I wish Dr. Bergman had pushed the envelope more than she did, but she should not have had to put her career at risk by opposing the surgical resident's actions, or demanding that the surgical attending come to the unit to assess Jesse, or refusing to discontinue his antibiotics. The structure of the situation, I think, could be modified to allow lower-echelon doctors to buck authority when they are convinced their patient's life is at stake.[7]

Learning and influence go both ways—from the professional to the personal, certainly, but also from the personal to the professional. If my disciplinary training lurked behind my personal experience during Jesse's hospitalization and asserted itself after his death, my continuing reflections on medicine and mortality have had an impact on my view of myself as a sociologist. I have a stronger sense of the tragic in life, using Walter Kauffman's idea of tragedy as a condition in which "even an exemplary devotion to love, truth, justice, and integrity cannot safeguard a man against guilt."[8] While efforts should be made to limit medical error, and while tragedy can be an excuse for inaction in the face of social or institutional problems that can indeed be solved or ameliorated, there is an unaccountability in the structure of things that can take our best intentions and make them the instruments of error. With the best of intentions we may learn, after the fact, that we were the last necessary link in a chain of events that ended in tragedy.

In the story I just told of the events of May 9, I did not talk about my own role. You see, I had come to think of myself as Jesse's protector. I was the point person with his doctors during the four years of his illness, which began in 1991 with the diagnosis of his ulcerative colitis, and took him to hundreds of blood draws and procedures and doctor's visits. So it was perfectly appropriate for me to stay with him on the evening of the ninth. What happened was "not my fault," but if advocacy is to be more than busywork to keep parents from going mad, then logic says it may be effective or ineffective, well or poorly timed, and may fall short of the mark because of fatigue or rationalization or belief that one is best equipped to chart a course between challenge and accommodation. This is the right course in many situations, but it may have been exactly the wrong one this evening, when the more emphatic style of a Rachel or a Will, pitching a fit, perhaps, demanding that the attending surgeon come to the unit to evaluate Jesse instead of taking their turn at the transplant shelter that night, could have made all the difference.

Sociology, as one of the social sciences, can take no position on the question of tragedy, although it can study its social meanings and provenance. Yet I cannot imagine doing sociological research in which tragedy is banned from the stage. Even here, though, my training offers some help. Years ago, Professor Erikson told a group of his students, of which I was one, that he was about to travel down to Buffalo Creek to give a talk on the anniversary of the flood, and wanted to say something "wise." The comment seemed out of character for this most unpretentious of scholars. As he talked about his trip, though, I understood what he meant. In his account of the flood and its aftermath, he had used his disciplinary expertise to give people a certain way of understanding large-scale human disasters. He knew, though, that in speaking to the survivors of the Buffalo Creek Flood he would be in the presence of an experience that neither sociology, nor perhaps any other discipline, can plumb the depths of, and he wanted his comments to reflect that knowledge. Paradoxically, his implicit acknowledgment of the limitations of sociological inquiry had already allowed him to give voice to suffering and embody it in his account of those tragic events.

Following this line of thought and to conclude, my title for this essay—*Unintended Research*—may be misleading, since I did not conduct research in any formal sense. In another sense, though, the title is apt, since it also refers to the unintended research of living and confronting the unaccountability of experience.

NOTES

1. Here and elsewhere, I have drawn and revised some material for this essay from my memoir, *The Book of Jesse: A Story of Youth, Illness, and Medicine* (Washington, DC: The Francis Press), 2002.
2. I have changed all names other than Jesse's and those on my side of his family.
3. E. Goffman, *The Presentation of Self in Everyday Life* (Garden City, NY: Doubleday, 1959).
4. C. L. Bosk, *Forgive and Remember: Managing Medical Failure* (Chicago: University of Chicago Press, 1979).
5. K. T. Erikson, *Everything in Its Path: Destruction of Community in the Buffalo Creek Flood* (New York: Simon and Schuster, 1976).

6. M. Rowe, "The 'Buffalo Creek Effect': Medical Mistakes from a Family Member's Perspective." *Dermanities* 1(1) (2003): 1–3.

7. M. Rowe, "The Structure of the Situation: A Narrative on High-Intensity Medical Care." *The Hastings Center Report* 33 (6) (2003): 37–44.

8. W. Kauffman, *Critique of Religion and Philosophy* (Princeton, NJ: Princeton University Press, 1978), p. 244.

QUESTIONS

1. The author makes a distinction between being the subjective participant and the objective onlooker. Where do these identities cross or merge in this essay? to what effect?

2. The author suggests that mistakes cost his son's life. Who made the mistakes? What different choices were possible, and how would they have potentially altered the outcome?

3. Discuss how the author conveys the sense of alienation and timelessness in this narrative.

Luck or Miracle
My Battle with Cancer

❦ Michael J. Meyer ❦

*People break down into two groups when they experience some-
thing lucky. Group number one sees it as more than luck, more
than coincidence. They see it as a sign—evidence that there is
someone up there watching out for them. Group number two sees
it as just pure luck, a happy turn of chance. I'm sure the people
in group number two are looking at those 14 lights in a very suspicious way. For them, the situation isn't 50-50. Could be bad,
could be good. But deep down, they feel that whatever happens,
they're on their own. And that fills them with fear. Yeah, there
are those people. But there's a whole lot of people in the group
number one. When they see those 14 lights, they're looking at a
miracle. And deep down, they feel that whatever's going to happen, there'll be someone there to help them. And that fills them
with hope. See, what you have to ask yourself is, what kind of
person are you? Are you the kind who sees signs, sees miracles? Or
do you believe that people just get lucky? Or look at the question
this way—is it possible that there are no coincidences?*
—*Mel Gibson in M. Night Shymalian's movie Signs*

As I reflect back on the late '80s and '90s and the serious illness I struggled with at that time,
two songs from different eras echo in my memory. They are "Stayin' Alive," recorded by the
Bee Gees in 1977; and "I Will Survive," by Gloria Gaynor two years later in 1979. Neither
song is related to physical health, but the specific phrases in the titles ran through my head
when I confronted one of the most difficult periods of my life.

The year was 1986, and I was fresh out of graduate school, a late-blooming Ph.D. who
had been lucky enough to land a tenure-track position in a religious college located just outside Milwaukee. Since my oldest son was about to graduate from high school, my wife and I

decided to postpone moving from Chicago, where we had lived for sixteen years, especially since the job materialized just a month before school was to start. The school arranged a schedule to suit my commute, and, caught up in the excitement of finally attaining a life-long goal, I settled into a one-and-a-half- to two-hour daily commute and an occasional layover in a college dorm room when I was either too tired to travel or when the weather made the drive home treacherous.

My wife was supportive as always, and we dreamed of a larger home in a more rural set-ting, where we would really enjoy our forties and the golden years that were to come. Those dreams failed to materialize. Instead, my wife, Loralee, began experiencing mild stomach and bowel discomfort, and by the end of my first semester as a college professor, her body had developed some suspicious swelling in the abdominal cavity. In addition, her appetite had begun to decrease, and she was experiencing strange cravings for food.

Since we had planned a post-Christmas trip to New York City, Loralee delayed her visit to the doctor, and we made the trip despite our apprehension, enjoying Broadway theater and an exciting four-day vacation without having to worry about our children. When we returned home, however, it was clear my wife was not in good health. After a hastily arranged doctor's appointment in January, Loralee's general practitioner immediately referred her to a specialist. By mid-January, a mass had been found on one of her ovaries, she had undergone an opera-tion, and had been diagnosed with third-stage ovarian cancer. Nine courses of chemotherapy were prescribed, one every four to six weeks depending on her tolerance. The battle for life and normalcy in our family had begun. Would we survive? Could we stay alive?

Suddenly the commute to Milwaukee became a heavier burden, and my own responsi-bilities increased. Our children—Kevin, 17; Craig, 15; and Christine, 11—were frightened. Their mom was only 41, and the prognosis for survival was not good. They had watched their grandmother die of uterine cancer seven years before, so it was difficult to maintain a positive outlook. However, we always told them cancer was not an automatic death sentence. Surprisingly, despite our fears about the worst possible scenario, Loralee began to recover. A second-look surgery, standard practice at the time, was done after the nine-month regimen was complete; thankfully, no metastasis was evident, and the original cancer seemed to be in remission. Mom and wife had been restored; our prayers had been answered.

We decided that I would commute to Milwaukee for another year, and we would see how the recovery progressed. Loralee's hair returned, she began teaching again, and our world began to return to normal. When the summer of 1988 arrived, we went house hunt-ing in Milwaukee and were delighted to find a four-bedroom home near a small lake. The subdivision was gorgeous, and our new home had a spacious backyard that offered a release from stress, a place to relax in nature.

Loralee decided to work in the children's section of the local library rather than return to the classroom. Essentially, we were trying to develop a slower-paced lifestyle, a sugges-tion we took from Bernie Siegel's book *Love, Medicine and Miracles*. We even developed an independent consulting service and set up programs in language arts for area grade schools, in-service activities that could be scheduled at our convenience. But by February of 1989 the bubble of prosperity, good health, and a dream home was rudely burst when Loralee sud-denly experienced intense headaches and double vision. She was rushed to a local hospital where a CAT scan revealed that there were three tumors on her brain. During a ten-hour operation, a neurosurgeon successfully removed the tumors, only to discover they were metastases from the original illness. Ovarian cancer cells had begun to spread to other parts of the body. We were doubly shocked because we had been told that if the cancer had spread at all, it would have been within the body cavity. Having carefully monitored blood antigens on a monthly basis, we had rejoiced when they proved normal; we had no suspicion that the cancer was spreading elsewhere.

In addition, my stress was double now because I had discovered that the college where I was employed was not only misrepresenting its curriculum but was recruiting students with false advertising. Having grown up with a solidly ethical background and deploring the willingness of my workplace to exploit others for profit, I wanted to expose such underhandedness. Nonetheless, I feared that to expose the university's duplicity would cost me my job, a job that might be essential if I were going to be the head of a single-parent family. I wanted to survive, to stay alive despite the odds that seemed mounting against me.

The intensity of my situation continued to grow. A struggle at work now accompanied the pain of illness at home. While my wife survived the operation, the fact that she had brain cancer made the situation even more grim. It was as though everywhere I turned there was sickness: a moral and ethical sickness in the workplace and physical sickness at home. I hardly knew where to turn. I went through the motions in the classroom, tried to appear cheerful and upbeat about my employer, even though I knew the corruption had infected not only the higher echelons of the administration but several of my closest colleagues as well. When I contacted supervisory organizations like the church body that operated the school and the accrediting agency that affirmed the college's viability, the people in charge seemed much more inclined to look the other way, to ignore the growing malignancy. I knew I could not tolerate such academic corruption much longer.

Meanwhile, cancer continued to spread in my wife's body. By summer it had spread to the spinal column, and the deterioration of her body began in earnest. Radiation treatments weakened both her physical abilities and her hope for recovery. By Christmas 1989, it was nearly impossible for Loralee to reach the second floor of our house by herself. Wheelchairs and walkers were necessary, and talents such as piano playing and intelligent conversation began slowly to disappear.

My sadness knew no bounds as I began to realize that my wife would not survive. Moreover, my new career, the one I had spent years studying to secure, was crumbling. My children were devastated, and it was more and more difficult to keep their mother's inevitable death from their consciousness. Little did they realize there was another cancer—the one in the workplace—that their father also was battling.

Soon after Christmas, Loralee required hospice care. A hospital bed arrived and was placed in the first-floor dining room. Loralee needed heavy painkillers, and her parents arrived to watch over her while I returned to a despised workplace. By now my function in the classroom and the home had become almost that of an automaton. I struggled not to feel anything—either about the impending loss of my wife or about the clearly immoral practices of the university. I was numb, trying to deny the events were occurring.

At about the same time my wife lapsed into a coma, I decided to expose the hypocrisy

I was facing in the workplace, no matter if it cost me my job. I contacted a local newspaper and felt the lump in my stomach harden. As I entered a new phase of battling two types of illness, survival and staying alive became even more important.

By Easter, my wife had died, and an exposé had been printed about the college's unfair treatment of students. Perhaps I initially thought that since the cancer at school had been exposed, it would be cured. But unfortunately, I found that my three-year contract at the university was not going to be renewed when it expired in 1992. Despite my admirable publishing record and my positive classroom evaluations, I would soon be jobless. I turned to drama to escape, tried out for community theater in the hopes that playing another role besides reality would help me come to terms with my slowing disintegrating personal and professional life. In the past this outlet had been helpful, and I sought it out anxiously as a way to cope with a situation that seemed hopeless.

As fall approached, I found myself feeling weaker and weaker. Emotionally, I was exhausted, and physically I found myself unable to do even the simplest household chores like mowing the lawn. I vividly remember trying to cut a small four-by-four square of grass in the backyard and being so tired that I was literally forced to my knees. A trip to the doctor revealed that I was anemic and losing red blood cells rapidly. I suddenly realized that illness was now not merely a family problem but an individual one as well; it had invaded my own body. Test after test was performed in search of internal bleeding: fecal occult test, proctoscopy, barium enema; the doctor thought a bleeding ulcer was the likely cause. Although all the results were negative, my G.P. persisted, ordering me to have a colonoscopy. He said that the stress of coping with my wife's illness may have caused my own present physical distress.

I can still remember the cold table and the probing scope winding its way up the convoluted passages of my colon, only to hit some sort of blockage that prevented it from going further. Although I was supposed to be sedated and unable to feel or hear anything, the sharp pain caused by the scope trying to continue its journey caused me to awaken enough to distinguish the doctor's voice: "Oh, here's the problem," the specialist declared. "It's a tumor." I don't believe his comment was intended to be flip or insensitive, but his bedside manner left a lot to be desired. My heart sank; the unthinkable had happened. I was also a cancer patient. It had hardly been six months since two cancers had caused devastation for me; now a third, this time personally life-threatening, was an integral part of me. Perhaps caused by stress, perhaps by emotional terror, the cancer had developed and was spreading. I gulped twice, stunned at the diagnosis, and left the office in a semi-daze.

Soon I was home, trying to take in the enormity of my condition. Realizing how vulnerable I was, I called my dad and step-mom and implored them to come and be with me during this traumatic time. I felt so helpless, unable to summon the strength that had sustained me during my wife's illness. My voice quavered, then broke as I stammered out the facts over the phone. My dad softly replied in reassuring tones, "Of course, Michael, we'll come! We'll help in any way we can." As I try to envision it now, he must have held his breath in disbelief that cancer had struck again; but then again, perhaps he intuitively knew how important his calming voice was to me. He had been a cancer survivor since 1980, and with his encouragement, I was determined to be one too. Relief engulfed me, and I was no longer able to restrain the pent-up emotions I felt. As I finished the conversation, my daughter arrived home. The tears flooding my eyes must have given away the diagnosis, and, as she rushed upstairs screaming "No! No!" I realized the nightmare of illness had only begun.

On a cold October day I had eighteen inches of my colon removed and began to face the fact that a full year of chemotherapy awaited me. Each week I was required to arrive at the cancer clinic and wait for my turn to have an injection of a drug called FU5. On alternate weeks I would supplement this with a solid pill called levamisol, a "curative drug" that inevitably caused me to be nauseous and to lose my appetite.

Although my mental condition was unstable, I was anxious to return to the classroom. Teaching was the one thing that kept me going, the one thing that motivated me when life seemed so dark that survival was even more scary than dying. One day, as I was lying in bed clutching a pillow against the lengthy incision that crisscrossed my stomach, it dawned on me that not once in this lengthy bout with my own illness had I given any credence to the fact that my cancer might be fatal. I always clung to the hope of life and survival. My faith flourished as I prayed fervently that God would not let the cancer spread or recur. As in the past, my spirituality became a place of refuge where I found solace and hope for survival.

In addition, having read *Love, Medicine and Miracles* while my wife was ill, I knew that holistic healing was becoming more and more important as an integral part of cancer therapy. Positive thinking and imaging were being advocated as a clear advantage to attaining full recovery, and I began to think about ways in which I might challenge and defeat the rebellious cancer cells that had invaded my body.

My intensely religious upbringing had been an important factor in my attitude about my wife's illness, and I found it even more important when my own body was under attack. Besides my religious beliefs, however, I found that the research I had done for my dissertation kept resurfacing as one of the most important elements in my recovery process. John Steinbeck's philosophy as expressed in *The Log from the Sea of Cortez* led me to see that my study of his fiction had implications beyond completing the requirements for a Ph.D. Steinbeck writes:

> Non-teleological thinking concerns itself primarily not with what should be, could be, or might be but rather with what actually is—attempting at most to answer the already sufficiently difficult questions of *what* or *how* instead of *why*. . . . In the non-teleological sense there can be no "answer." There can only be pictures which become larger and more significant as one's horizon increases. (139)

Here, Steinbeck seemed to be giving me advice about my real life as well as information to include in my dissertation. Instead of being frustrated by the seemingly unfair hand I had been dealt, I refused to ask *why*, a question which could not be answered satisfactorily anyway. It made me assess what was truly important, and I decided to make some changes that reflected my developing self-discovery. I realized that my illness was not a punishment, but neither was it a random occurrence Instead, it provided an opportunity to learn from a close encounter with mortality. Consequently, I concentrated on *what* and *how:* What will be my reaction to illness? Will I give in and let it depress and defeat me? Or will I assert my self-confidence in my ability to confront and defeat a diagnosis as grim as cancer? I began to see that there were choices out there. I realized that how I dealt with my illness emotionally was as important as the medicinal regimens I was following with such a passion. The diagnosis of cancer did not have to be a death sentence, nor did the impending loss of my job need to engender fear and despair. Instead, this rather black outlook for my future led me to acknowledge that even negative events in an individual's life can sometimes lead to a positive conclusion. As Steinbeck says in *The Log from the Sea of Cortez:* "Perhaps no other animal is so torn between alternatives—Man might be described adequately, if simply, as a two-legged paradox" (98). My illness was paradoxically life-threatening and life-enabling, giving me the opportunity to discard negative old habits and to reassess priorities.

Following Steinbeck's philosophical formula, I decided to accept my fate and face it head-on. My belief in Steinbeck's so-called "non-teleological thinking—accepting "what is" and not questioning its appropriateness—began to pay off. I began to follow the suggestions of Siegel and selected positive images to attack cancer cells mentally. These images were based on Steinbeck's keen interest in King Arthur, who successfully defended himself against the great evils of Mordred and Morgan LaFey. I purchased miniature plastic figures of knights in military garb and spent ten to fifteen minutes a day relaxing and focusing on wellness. While I was doing this, I concentrated on the knights as destroyers of cancer cells; their weapons—a battle ax, a spear, and a mace—were my defenses; and aided by their shields and armor, I felt protected from the physical attacks that the disease presented. Bolstered by faith, positive attitude, and concentration on imaging, my health slowly began to return. It no longer mattered that my employer was corrupt; all that mattered was that despite the fact that my job was at stake, I chose to be true to myself. I had chosen the ethical high road and had not succumbed to accepting a clear wrong in order to preserve my position.

I am alive. I have survived. It has been a challenge, no doubt, and the triumph is in large part due to a writer's perspective that I might otherwise never have carefully considered and to the assurance that God would not give me more than I could bear. As I looked around during my illness, I saw many people in dire straits, some far worse than mine. Therefore I could not whine or complain, could not place blame or feel hatred for what had happened. I truly believe God was essential and that he placed the writings of Steinbeck and Siegel in my life. Through their messages, He led me past dejection. He led me past sadness, past illness and death. It was in their words and stories that I found hope; and I realize now that words and stories are an important remedy, a potential cure that lifts readers and listeners above pessimism and toward the hope that leads to healing. Thanks to Steinbeck, Siegel, and my faith, I will continue to be a member of M. Night Shymalian's Group Number One: assured that there are no coincidences and that I am not alone in my struggle for life and happiness. Someone surely is watching and reaching out to help.

QUESTIONS

1. How does the author's identity as caregiver impact his role as patient?
2. Discuss the author's perspectives on how faith and illness intersect.
3. What complements to traditional medicine does the author offer as valuable?

Over and Under and Back
from Whence You Came
⌒ Michael Verde ⌒

Alzheimer's is sometimes described as an existential disease. It is said that people who have it slowly lose their connection to both the past and the future and live increasingly in the moment. I hope so. The idea comforts, illumining in the loss—which appears increasingly absolute—a gain. So conceived, dementia, meaning "mind away," blends romantically into the exquisite forgetfulness of undiluted Being. The face before us, though seemingly recognizing nothing, apprehends all. And so, unexpectedly loosed from time and space, we sit together, here and now, in a "place of no winds." Nirvana. It is a good story—and, like I say, I hope a true one—but when you look into the face of someone you love who is deep in what they call the late stage of dementia, the only insight into existence you are apt to have is that its retreat is terrifying. Or so it was for me as I watched my grandfather's face, once animated, slowly settle into a mask. By no longer reflecting my presence, his face mirrored my absence: I beheld in him myself utterly forgotten. And when I didn't turn away, the "no winds" I was privileged to know revealed that one day it will be as if I never was. If there is anything redemptive about Alzheimer's and like dementias, at least for me, it will have to include, not evade, this terror.

Fortunately there is nothing novel or religiously esoteric about redemptions of this kind. Often we are introduced to them as early as childhood, on the brink of sleep, a blink away from the extinction of light and life and the subsiding sounds of the day. "Once upon a time," says a voice we trust to know. And thus so spoken appears a bridge between ourselves and what preceded us, between the passing of time and the passage into time, the road we faintly remember arriving on. We never were in the first place, the bridge reminds us, and yet here we are. And though we may, tonight or tomorrow night or the night after, never be again, the bridge will be, will always be. Death is a fact, but life is a story—a bridge into and out of existence. As my grandfather's Alzheimer's grew worse and worse and his memory less and less, his stories, never missing a beat, reminded me to attend less to what he remembered and more to what, once upon a time, will remember all of us again.

⌒ ⌒

We had a lake down there that you couldn't catch anything out of hardly but catfish. My grandmother went fishing every day—I say everyday, I mean everyday that the weather permitted, she'd go fishing. And we go down there and pass the lake up because the only thing in the lake was moccasins, snakes, and catfish—catfish was the only fish I ever saw caught out of there, or turtles. Usually if you caught fish down there and you put 'em on a string and put 'em back in the water—well, you was feeding 'em back to the snakes. So she didn't fish down there much.

So when the doctor told my grandmother that the only meat my granddaddy could eat were fish, it was way late in the day by then and, well, she didn't have no fish for him. Back in those days you couldn't catch a whole bunch of fish and put 'em in the ice box—we didn't have no ice box—and there wasn't no refrigerators at'll then. We had a smokehouse where the beef and hogs and things was smoked to preserve 'em. But fish, there wasn't no such thing as keeping fish over night.

And so my grandma said, "Well, Dude," she said, "I'm going down to catch your granddaddy some fish, let's go." I was too little to have been left there to help my granddaddy—I wasn't older than five or six years old. So we went down to the lake, and I remember, ol' grandmother when she got down there, well, she talked to the Lord like someone else maybe is talking to a person, you know. She said, "Now, Lord, you know our need, and I depend on you"—that was the way she talked to the Lord when she prayed—"Now, Lord, you know our need." I don't remember the exact words, but I'm telling you about the way she prayed. She always either looked up to the Lord, or she sat down and bowed her head. And I remember her recognizing God as the Supreme Power, you know. She didn't say it the way we oftentimes hear it now. She said, "I know, dear God, I look to you as the Supreme Power, and I look to you to meet and care for our needs. And you know our needs, and my husband must have fish, so I'll ask you to supply that need, and I ask this in the name of Christ, my Lord, my Redeemer, my Savior. Amen."

Soon as she said that she baited her hook up and throwed it out there, and I'm telling you less time than it is taking for me to tell you this part about the fishing she drugged in her first fish. She put him on a string, baited the hook up again and throwed it out there, and I'm telling you what, in five minutes time she already had them two fish on a string. So now she baited two hooks—at first, see, she had one hook, but now she put another hook on there, up above the first one about that far. Here's a hook, there's a weight, then this far up the line, see, she put another hook. Are you with me? She baited them hooks up and she throwed 'em out there and she said, "Now Lord, you remember Tom will have to eat tomorrow and I'll ask you to supply his needs. Thank you." Stuck that pole down in the dirt, stuck it way down in the dirt real hard, and we went on back to the house. Now she didn't say nothing else to me about it. She just baited them hooks and prayed. So we took the fish back up there and cooked the fish for my granddaddy. He'd always eat more than one. Sometimes he'd eat one and a half, but she always had two for him. She was anticipating his need.

Next morning, after she took care of him that day, well, I was already up and I'm going to say that maybe it was eight or nine o'clock by then. But I was already up and my grandmother already had our breakfast and we went back down there and she got down there and pulled that pole up. Now normally, I'm telling you, there was no chance in the world for anybody to set a pole out there and catch a fish that the snakes didn't eat that fish off that hook—that's a fact—or a turtle. They eat 'em all. But she pulled it out and there they were, two big catfish about that long, each one of 'em. Looked like twins. "Thank you, Lord." Baited that up. "Thank you, Lord, for supplying our needs. I'll ask you to do it." Stuck that pole in the dirt real hard. Every morning she went down there and took two fish off the line. She wasn't fishing—her fishing days were over. She had to be with my granddaddy. He had to have somebody around hearing distance at all time to take care of him and I was too little. The only thing she done is just go down there and pick up what the Lord supplied her.

My granddaddy ate those fish until he got to where he couldn't eat anymore. That was the way things happened for a long time. We'd go down there and pick up two fish. We had to get back to the house, but they were there. And do you know what? I was beginning to know that there was going to be two fish down there. I'd hear my grandmother pray and then thank the Lord for having supplied her thus far, would he continue to bless her, bless my granddaddy as well as her, and then she'd thank the Lord for her faith in him, for her trust in him. Them snakes a lot of times would catch a fish right off the same line you were catching 'em on. But not now, not these fish. They were right there, every day, like twins—two fish and no skin breaks on 'em nowhere.

I'm telling you what, you see enough things like that when you are a little boy growing up and you begin to believe—believe there are things out there more powerful than snakes, that's for sure.

⌒ ⌒

I was twenty-two years old before I asked my grandfather a single thing about his life. At twenty-two, I was lucky to have a grandfather still alive and of healthy mind, but at that age who fathoms the value in a blessing like that? I was a student at the University of Texas at the time, preoccupied with finding myself, as my parents' generation called it, and not having a lot of success for my efforts. The intellectual breakthroughs that I imagined in high school would be my daily college fare—the cathartic all-night confessionals, the romantic whirlwind, the revolution in religious and political sensibility—none of these rites of undergraduate passage were materializing for me. Mainly it was memorizing photosynthesis, paying rent, and avoiding parking tickets. One day, while in the Student Union on an errand to drop one class and add another, the kind of sub-intellectual task that seemed to constitute nine-tenths of my higher education, I decided there had to be a better way to "know thyself." I started weaning myself from class and hanging out in Quackenbush, a pre-Starbucks coffee shop replete with rotating bad art and cerebrally heavy bathroom graffiti. I bought a used book by Heidegger, began penning "deep" poems on napkins. Though I couldn't make heads or tails of *Being and Time*, the more I read it, the less substantial everything that wasn't Being—which was everything—felt to me; and that had the curiously welcome effect of persuading me that the universe had to be bigger than a university. In my senior year of high school, I had won a national writing contest sponsored by *Guideposts* magazine and took the very generous money that came with the prize and invested it in stock, which did well. Three years later, in my hour of metaphysical discontent, I had a nice chunk of change with which to be spiritually creative. The call reached me in Quackenbush. Cloaked in second-hand cigarette smoke, looking but not looking at a collage vaguely resembling a tree with snippets of body parts for leaves, I decided to quit school and move to Paris.

My grandmother and grandfather had just married and they didn't have a home yet, so they were living with my Aunt Mary and Uncle Charlie Grubbs, who were also trying to build themselves a place. This was in Kansas, years and years ago. In those days they had what they called quilting parties and log rollings. And what they would do is all the neighbors would get together on a certain day and the women would quilt and the men would build a barn—or whatever some family in the community needed. So one day a new neighbor moved in there and they were going to have a quilting party and log rolling. My Aunt Mary wanted to do this thing, but she needed a clean dress to go to it. So on Thursday, a couple days before the party, Aunt Mary got her a big load of clothes and went down to the crick.

In those days people used to wash their clothes at the crick—we call it a creek now, but back then they called it a crick. All the women had a certain day that they did their washing, and my Aunt Mary's day was on Thursday. So that Thursday Mary goes down to the crick and a Polack woman is there washing her clothes. This was a great big woman. She was about 6' 1" and weighed 190 pounds. I told you my grandmother weighed 105 when she was plumb grown. And Aunt Mary wasn't any bigger than my grandmother—she was a little bitty woman too. Well Mary explains to the woman, very politely, that Thursday is her day and that she really needs to get her clothes clean because there is a barn-building and quilting party coming up that weekend. Sorry, that woman said, but I have to wash today because I'm going to the log rolling and quilting party tomorrow. My Aunt Mary said well I was going to go to that too. That woman said I'm sorry it just so happens I have to use this day.

All Aunt Mary could do was to go back up to the house, which she did. She went in the house and my grandmother was fixing the breakfast for my grandfather. When Mary came in she was crying because she wasn't going to get to go to the quilting party. She was heartbroken. My grandmother asked her, what are you crying about? And she told her. Well, my grandmother said, well, I'll be back in a minute. She got her apron and turned that apron wrong side out. She went in there and got my granddaddy's razor—back then everybody used straight razors—got that big straight razor and left. She went down there and that great big ol' woman was putting Blue In in the water to rinse her clothes out. My grandmother walked up behind her and put her hand on the back of her neck there, you know, shoved her down in that tub of water. Seven or eight times she ripped across there. Well the first time she went across, that woman couldn't get out. She cut the muscles. She didn't have no muscles to pull out with.

My grandmother turned around, cleaned her razor off, left that ol' girl laying over that tub with her head under water. Then she went to the house, and called Mary and my granddaddy in there; and they went down and got Uncle Charlie out of the cornfield, got him back up there and they hitched up the mules. Two to a wagon, then got two more to tie onto the wagon to follow behind them. See this happened at about 9 o'clock in the morning. They had no alternative. They got all their clothes and got 'em a lot of food, the food that they had there and loaded that wagon up and put as much furniture on the wagon as they could and headed out west. Oklahoma then was not a state, it was a territory. And if you could get into Oklahoma you was safe if you was tough enough to keep out a gunman that would come in there ever now and then to kidnap you. If they could ever get you out of Oklahoma they could try you. I don't guess those people ever found out where my grandmother and granddaddy and Aunt Mary and Uncle Charlie ever went.

In Paris, with neither job nor homework, I continued brooding over coffee and trying to work myself into a deep existential angst that would culminate (after who knew how many dark nights of the soul) in a life-changing insight into myself. And to accomplish as much, I went to fairly absurd lengths. For instance, among other makeshift exercises concocted off the cuff to effect enlightenment, I assigned myself a koan. A koan is a seemingly non-sensical saying that a Buddha master will give to a disciple who comes to him seeking enlightenment. "What is the sound of one hand clapping?" for example. Or, "how many lions are there in a single hair?" The idea is that wisdom runs deeper than logic and that by con-founding all rational explanation, a koan provokes one's conscious mind into yielding the floor so that one's deeper, wiser mind can get a word in edgewise. Paris, I suppose, wasn't foreign enough for me to find myself. I would have to make it all the way to the East, if only in the confines of my little studio, where I sat once a day on the thin carpet with the lights out and meditated on my koan, which read as follows: Show me the face you wore before your mother and father were born.

When I was five years old, my mother went over to Mexia, Texas and started her a boarding house. My daddy was a coal miner in Hartshorne, Oklahoma. They had decided that they would divorce. My mother was going to be in Texas and my dad was going to be in Oklahoma—in Hartshorne. It was my choice which one I was going to stay with. I know my mother thought I'd say, "I want to go with my mother." But my dad didn't want to deprive me of that privilege, you know—the privilege of making a choice. I remember they called me—I was playing out there with the little black buddy of mine, Haywood, we were playing out there with two or three others—my cousins were out there, and we were playing and they called me around the house. Boy, I hated to take out a little bit of playing to go talk to them, but you'd be surprised when your parents would call you in like that how you forget about that playing right now—that's a serious thing to a five-year-old kid, I guarantee you. I never shall forget, my granddaddy's car was parked on the right and my daddy's car was parked on the left. My granddaddy had an Asperson Jackrabbit and my daddy drove a Dodge Brothers touring convertible. They had run-ning boards on cars then; my mother and daddy were sitting down there, the cars were about five foot apart. One was sitting on one running board and the other was sitting on the other. They called me around there and I stood between them. My mother explained what was going to happen. "Oh," I said, "I don't want that at all. I want to live together." My daddy said, "Well, son, we can't do that." In other words, neither one of them was putting any pressure on me as to which way I went. But he said, "It is your choice. You can live with either one of us you want to." Well, we were at my grandmother's farm. I had to make a choice. No persuasion that I knew enough how to present would change it. So . . . I guess there was some gratitude in my heart to an extent because I remember I looked over toward the house and I made up my mind in a split second "Well," I said, "then I won't live with either one of you, I'll live with grandma."

Now I was fortunate that at least I had a pretty good out, you know. I praise God for it, because my grandmother was a queen of a woman, a fine Christian woman, a loving person. I tell you what, that was one of the greatest blessings I ever had, because you can't imagine when a kid has to make a decision like that, that's pretty doggone tough. That's why I told my wife when I asked her to marry me—I said, "Now, Babe, don't say yes too fast. There's one stipulation you need to consider. Up until the time we ever have children, if you want to leave me, or if I want to leave you, that's our prerogative. But," and I told her to listen carefully, "But," I said, "if we ever have children, we shall live together as man and wife as long as there is at least one child left in our home, or until one of us dies. Period." And I told her to take all the time she needed to think on it because once we were married, I wasn't changing my mind on that point if it hare-lipped Satan.

⌒ ⌐

Show me the face you wore before your mother and father were born. Six months of sitting quietly in a candle-lit studio for forty-five minutes a day trying to get my mind around how a person can even have a face before his mother or father are born yielded no epiphanies. For a while I reasoned that the answer to my koan hinged on reincarnation, an idea which my Southern Baptist upbringing strongly suggested was sinfully superstitious. I spent many meditative hours trying to get over my reflexive resistance to the idea that after you died you quite possible came back here for a second round, or a third, fourth, or ten thousandth. Funny enough, I found unsuspected visual support for this alternative narrative in a coffee stain.

I chose the discolored circle in my carpet as a meditative focal point because I thought it would help me to stop imagining life as moving up and down, as the cross suggests, and to start picturing it as moving in a circle. Silly though it was, my daily ritual harmed no one. After several months I discovered that if I narrowed my eyelids just so, I could get the candle light flickering in my peripheral vision to move closer and closer in the direction of the stain on my carpet, to the coffee mandala by which I was working out new geometries with eternity.

⌒ ⌐

My daddy was a prize-fighter—he made extra money that way—and in 1926 the World Champion Lightweight of America came to Hartshorne, Oklahoma to train in the mountains, and while he was down there his people set up an exhibition fight with my daddy, and it was such a big deal that the governor of the state came down to watch. Like everybody else that lived in Hartshorne, my daddy was a miner. He worked 363 days a year. The only days he didn't work was Christmas and Labor Day. And on this particular day, because the men that owned the mines had gotten together and declared it a holiday—they wanted to see the fight too, don't you know—they even had a newspaper man from out east come down, and he was there interviewing people. And he wanted to interview my daddy. This was a real educated man, the newspaper man, you could see that, and he kept asking my dad all kinds of questions about things that didn't have anything to do with boxing. He used a lot of big words. He asked my daddy what it was like growing up in the rural south. He asked him about racial strife. My daddy could barely read and he didn't know what words like "strife" meant. But after a while he figured out that the man was saying something about black people and what it was like living with them. Now just because a man isn't educated or can't read doesn't mean he isn't smart—there's all kinds of ways people know things, boy. My daddy told the man, "Mister, the man I came to knock out today is white. If a Negro jumps in the ring, I'll concern myself with the colored."

After eight months of growing increasingly frustrated with the whole interiorized proceedings, the answer finally surfaced: my grandparents. If my intent was to find myself, I had come a long way in the wrong direction. I wasn't in Paris. I was in east Texas, in the memories of the people in whose past my present was forged. Their history, of which I knew next to nothing, was the face I wore before my mother and father were born. Ten days later, I returned to Houston. On the way to my parents' house from the airport, I asked to stop at Wal-Mart, where I purchased a tape recorder and three packs of six, 90-minute cassettes. The next morning I called Grandpa Leonard in Barber's Hill, Texas. "How's the coffee, Old Timer?" "Good for your spondulicks," he said. "I'm coming to see you."

Over the next two weeks my grandfather and I drank a lot of coffee, I on the couch and he in his orange recliner. Between us, next to a paper towel-stuffed Folgers coffee can (his spittoon) a tape recorder whirred.

My daddy used to come over and sit and talk with me—this was after him and my mother had divorced and I was living with my grandmother and granddaddy. He smoked cigarettes, my dad did. He lit him up a cigarette, you know, with a match—there weren't no cigarette lighters in them days. Everybody used a match, tablebox matches. They were stick matches. He'd strike that match on his britches's leg and light that cigarette. He'd always just flip it over his shoulder like that, back over and out on the yard. He'd turn that stem, and before it'd hit the ground that match was out. I never shall forget, I was about six years old then.

My granddad was working 12-hour days. He was a blacksmith. He left home in the morning before daylight, but in the summer, in August, he'd be back home before dark. It was the latter part of May, June, July, and August and about half of September, I'd get to see my granddaddy. I wouldn't see him in the morning; he got up too early. But I'd see him in the evening when he came home from work. I never shall forget, me and Benny—she was my second-oldest sister— we were out shucking some corn for my granddaddy's hogs. He'd feed 'em when he'd come in. Of course, it was still daylight at that time of year when he got in around 6:30, or maybe it was 7:00 o'clock, but it was still broad daylight. We were shucking the corn. Throwing the corn over here and throwing the shucks in the backroom behind us. I decided to roll myself a cigarette out of corn silk. I rolled a cigarette, just like my daddy would roll it, except I used corn silk. I got me a match. I was sitting in the doorway of the barn with my back to where we were throwing the shucks. I fired a match up on my britches's leg—I knew how to do that. I lit my cigarette, and I was talking to Benny. She was sitting by me, shucking the corn. I just flipped the match over behind me. But, see, I didn't twist it like my daddy would—I didn't know how to do that part yet. Like I told you, this was some time in August. Well pretty soon that room got pretty hot to me. I looked back there and the corn husks were on fire. Well, boy, we got out of there in a hurry.

We went through the open door and we got out and ran and screamed to my grandmother and she came out there. And we lived close enough to my daddy's sharecropper, Uncle Jessie—it was a 60-40 deal—that my grandmother could call him. "We got a fire. Fire! Fire! Come on, Jess," and Jess run over there and when he got there that room on the barn was just about gone where all the corn husks were. Uncle Jess didn't even stop there. It was too hot for him to stop there. This barn had two big rooms here, and in the middle there was a shed for the wagons. We had some special hogs in the shed that we was fattening up to get ready to kill. There was six hogs in there. They weighed about 200 to 250 pounds apiece, the ones we were fattening up. They was young hogs. We were getting them ready for the wintertime. The wagon bed we put cotton in was sitting in front of the door to the shed where them pigs were. That way the bed made a gate. You put the hogs in there and then set that wagon bed across there. Boy, them hogs were screaming up a storm. But Uncle Jess couldn't get close enough to the hogs to move the wagon bed out of the way. So that old man had an idea. He ran up there and my granddaddy had a big ol' male hog up there that was his breeding hog. To give you an idea what size that hog was, that hog dressed out when we later on killed him—the next year we killed him—at one thousand and ten pounds.

George—that was the old big hog's name, George. We had an uncle and an aunt who lived up on the mountain and they were George and Idi, so my granddad had bought that hog when he was three months old, and he was about a foot high—I think he was three months old when my granddaddy bought him. He named him after Uncle George—Aunt Idi's Uncle George. He was a registered hog but my granddaddy had the prerogative of naming him, so that was on his papers—George. Anyway, Uncle Jess ran up there and threw that gate open and old George went through it. He went down there and he ran his nose under the bed, under one end of that bed, and I tell you what, he threw it around at least a 45 degree angle—left a hole there ten or more feet wide for them other hogs to come out of there. A pig is a strong animal, but, boy, a pig that figures he's got half a chance to burn to death is stronger than a mule—maybe two mules. And boy did them little pigs—they was little pigs to George—come out of there. They took off down to the lake—on fire. Looked like a string of burning bushes stretched out the length of the pasture. They was gone for three or four days, but finally they came on back. Some had their ears burned almost off, and all of 'em were missing hair. But they were still in pretty good shape. Didn't any of 'em die. They got down to the lake and that water saved them.

I don't know now how I got off on that story—oh, I wanted to tell you about the love.

About two bales of hay was all that Uncle Jess could save. All of my granddaddy's cotton for the year, and all of his seed crop for next year—it was all burned up. All my mother and father's furniture, all my grandaddy's firearms, all his farm equipment, and just about everything him and my grandmother owned that wasn't in their little house—burned to nothing. Me and Benny was out there sitting on a bale of hay, behind one of those two bales that didn't burn, and, boy, I was crying. I realized I had made a costly mistake. I was sad as deep as my bones that I ever picked up that cigarette. I was heartbroke. My grandmother had already heard from Benny how it had caught afire. When my granddaddy—he tried to save all he could, you know—but by the time he got there the barn was almost gone, but the room on the west end was the room they got a few things out of. He started helping Uncle Jessie and they was getting all they could out of there. But anyway, when it was all over—when they had given up and they couldn't get anything else out of there, I never shall forget, my old granddaddy come over there and as kind *as a person could ever say anything, he said, "Now that's alright, son. You made a mistake, but granddaddy's made a mistake or two." He patted my back, picked me up, and hugged me. Lordy lordy lordy. Now that's love, boy, you know it?*

〜 〜

And that's how it went, story after story, tape after tape. I listened, and when I thought I heard a thread that might lead my grandfather to a new set of memories, a new trail of tales, I asked a question. I kept them simple, and for the most part open-ended. "How did you meet grandma?" "What was my mama like when she was a little girl?" "What was your first paying job?" When I began the project I feared the tape recorder might distract my grandfather, freeze his tongue by putting him on the spot. It didn't. If he was saying something like, "We came up to the bridge" and the tape ran out, he would halt his story and while I flipped the tape he'd contribute to the spittoon. Then when I was ready, I would hit play, nod, and he would pick up right where he left off: ". . . and we crossed it." I now have, safely recorded, close to twenty hours of my grandpa telling stories. I took my grandfather's stories and wove them together into a novella that I entitled *Over and Under and Back from Whence You Came.* That was the ditty my grandfather's father used to teach him how to tie a tie: you take one end of the tie and go over and under then back from whence you came. You do that twice and knot it.

No one knew at the time that my grandfather had Alzheimer's. It is not a disease that hits you like a stroke or a heart attack. It happens to you after it has already happened to you—like growing up, but in the wrong direction. It started with names; it ended with faces. The last face to go was his own. It is a fact about Alzheimer's that seldom gets mentioned—maybe because when it happens so many other, more functionally relevant debilities have assumed center stage—but one of the signature symptoms of having advanced to the final stages of the disease is that one's face assumes a conspicuous absence. The term "plasticity" is often used to describe the change—or the "lion's face." The latter description is an exquisite example of the tenacity of myth, of why science, particularly medical science, is as informed by story as by number. The lion-bodied sphinx offers the pilgrim an inscrutable face, the riddle of an echoless gaze. The demented make us crazy because the answer to the "disease" is as simple as it is impermissible to say: *over and under and back from whence you came.*

〜 〜

The first thing my grandpa lost was his job. I'm inclined to think this loss hit him the hardest of the many that were to follow. From the time he was eleven years old, he worked every summer in the oil fields, and at seventeen, his schooling behind him, he worked year-round. He began as a "gopher," running after bull-plugs and water buckets, for 25 cents an hour. That was in 1926. He worked his way up the company totem pole until he reached the position that best suited his taste. For 34 years he was a "driller." When technological advances reduced the number of drillers needed on a lease, my grandfather was promoted to "gauger," and for another 30 years, he was the Sun Oil Company's Higgin's Lease gauger. Until 1991, when the Sun Company called him in and very compassionately let him go. He was 80 years old.

My mother, summoned by my grandmother, who had not in many years, if ever, seen her husband so defeated, arrived at my grandparents' house to find her father slouched in his recliner, lost. From the TV droned the familiar blare of a baseball game; neither the voice of the announcer nor the action on the field concerned him in the least.

My mother knelt beside his chair. She held his hand. She reminded him of how blessed he was, how he had provided for his family for many years. Encouragingly she asked him, "Daddy, how many men are able to work until they are 80?" He listened, without responding. "You have always been a workman worthy of your hire," she told him. That was a very special phrase to my grandfather—to be a workman worthy of your hire. He looked over to my mother, and though lost in pain, he found the strength to squeeze her hand. Then he rose from his chair, excused himself. He walked to the bathroom. My grandmother turned off the TV and the house fell silent. Moments later my mother and grandmother heard my grandfather praying. The prayer lasted at least ten minutes; it was a conversation—my grandfather was talking to the Lord, praying as his grandmother had taught him to pray. He addressed the Lord God Almighty by name, recognizing him as his savior, his redeemer, the source of his life, health, and joy. This was not perfunctory obeisance; this was establishing the god-defined architecture of the world. My grandfather had lost his job, not his understanding of what a job was, or should be, in God's larger plan. He was orienting himself to something beyond himself, and thus resituated, he spoke to his savior by name, Jesus, like a friend. Shortly after the prayer ended, the sound of running water could be heard in the living room. He was taking a shower. He returned several minutes later to the living room in a fresh pair of coveralls, the defeat in his face, in his body, gone.

Then he lost names—people my grandfather had known for years whose names he suddenly could not recall. "John Brown!" he would exclaim in exasperation. "What is that man's name? It'll come to me in just a second. The Lord has wiped my mind clean. Understandably, this loss bothered him the most when the name he forgot was that of the person he was speaking to. He would always apologize. "I know who you are, friend, but I can't recall your name. What is your name?" It made encounters with friends occasions of apology, embarrassment, shame. A trip to the post office, for instance—which in a small town means a trip to commune with neighbors—became a source of small dread, a gauntlet to be hazarded.

Next, it was the names of particular things that escaped his recall. The microwave became the machine. A key became that thing you start the car with. Hockey was that game they play on ice. With the slow but gradual loss of proper names, his vocabulary distilled down to basic words: *water, wife, day, night, Astros, coffee, little girl, may the Lord bless you, I love you, bye now.* He answered the telephone, "Hello hello hello." And if your choice of words when you answered exceeded his verbal limits, he would very kindly say, "Just a second, let me give you the wife."

Leaving the house made him uneasy, obviously uneasy. In fact it was his anxiety that next signaled to us that things were changing in his head. A visit to my mother's house might last 30 minutes before he'd say, "Well, Babe, we better get on back to the house." My grandmother's osteoporosis made traveling difficult. A car trip required loading and unloading her walker, sometimes even a wheelchair. My grandmother would have barely settled in when he would make the first announcement that it was time to leave. "We just got here,

Charlie," she would tell him. "Watch the ballgame." But this wasn't his house, his couch, his bathroom, his TV. The coffee wasn't his, nor the kitchen where he'd retreat to pace. Five minutes later: "Okay, Babe, we've got to go now."

"Shut up, Charlie," my annoyed grandmother was apt to tell him, buying herself five or so more minutes before he would come and take her by the arm, gently but insistently pulling her to her feet. When my grandfather was not at home, it was always time to go.

His walks were an exception to this rule. Leaving the house to walk did not make him anxious. To the contrary, as the dementia progressed, *not* leaving the house made him anxious. The family encouraged his walking, taking it as a measure of his enduring vitality. Two days after he retired, coaxed on by his son (my uncle), grandpa took his first walk. Interestingly, he took it at one o'clock in the afternoon. Texas at one o'clock in the afternoon is the suggested temperature for baking a pie. We did not, however, attribute this scheduling decision to any deficit in my grandfather's cognitive abilities. The truth is, my grandfather's take on things was never what you would call predictable. Very particular guideposts, rooted in the Bible as he understood it and the ethos of sportsmanship as he lived and coached it, authorized his judgments. He was oblivious to his neighbors' opinions. Decisions met with Scripture and the memory of the people who raised him: if a certain course of action passed muster in these sectors, it was beyond veto. I remember looking up during one of my cousin's soccer games and seeing my grandfather standing in a trash can. This was years before he retired, years before any hint of dementia. The day was bitter cold and the wind fierce. The few hardy fans brave enough to be at the game were huddled like sheep in the portable bleachers, more occupied by their discomfort than the play on the field. Except for my grandpa. A yard or so from the sideline, he stood waist-high in a metal drum, absorbed in the game. People around me began asking who was the old man in the trash can. Even the referee took a double take during one pass down the sideline. I'll never forget that moment, that day. Alone among us, one man, my grandfather, had more sense than the wind and more self-confidence than the flock. Hence, years later, when my uncle informed the family that grandpa had worked out a very definite reason why he did his "best" walking *exactly* 60 minutes after his noon meal, we were concerned about his health but not his thinking—the logic, however ill-advised, was singularly Charlie Leonard's.

But being a man of singular mind cannot forever disguise the progressive advance of cortical destruction. Grandpa, for instance, developed a thing about shoelaces: he liked them—his and yours—tied. Understandable. An errant lace can precipitate a fall. But he wanted *all* laces, *all* the time, properly tied. Guests were welcomed with a quick reconnoitering of their footwear. "Your shoes are coming untied," he might say. And if you thought you had time to make it to the couch, or wherever you were going, before you attended to the escaping lace, you were wrong. "Better tie them shoes," he'd insist, hounding you until you did just that. And there were other quirky things. Visitors, including family, needed to be out of the house by dark—this from a man who in a different state of mind wouldn't let anyone, family above all, leave. "Oh, what's your hurry?" he would say if you suggested it was time to go. He thrived on company, but now it vexed him. Similarly, one day he got it in his head that when he went to bed, Grandma needed to go to bed too. She could be wide awake, engrossed in a TV show, but if he was going to bed, she *needed* to go. He then began compulsively checking the locks on all the doors and searching all the closets—we presumed for intruders. His quirky behavior now, unlike his quirky behavior before, was not the fruit of an idiosyncratic, sometimes frustrating but ultimately always endearing parsing of the planet: the world according to Charlie Leonard. Now he did weird stuff, and he, least of all, could tell you why.

Unsettling, alienating, even annoying, obsessive behaviors are nevertheless seldom dangerous. You can learn to accommodate their oddness, sweep them under a rug of selective attendance—at least you can as long as they are the exception to behavior and not the rule. But cognitive impairment can have consequences that are not negotiable in this way. Grandpa could drive a car long after he could drive a car *safely*. And there came a day during this stage of increasingly conspicuous deterioration in his ability to coordinate his movements with the world outside him when decisions had to be made on his behalf. Invariably these decisions, like the one to terminate his driving, circumscribed the range of his freedom. This is the first obvious impact Alzheimer's disease has on the body: it gradually necessitates other minds' assuming its control. Where my grandfather could go, and when, and how, was increasingly being determined elsewhere—in his case, given my grandmother's own precarious health, by his children.

There were, however, even in the midst of the discomfiting changes, also moments to be cherished, instances when his impaired receptors of social sense yielded a pronouncement that, if not reflexively dismissed as a symptom, made him seem wise again in his own distinctively comic way. During a visit to his son's house, for example, Grandpa was introduced to his daughter-in-law's parents, people he had previously met on several occasions but did not now recall. "What's your name?" my grandfather asked his daughter-in-law's mother.

"Annette Messina," she replied.

"Annette Messina," Grandpa echoed her, "that's a pretty name. And what's your name?" he asked her husband.

"Charlie," Mr. Messina answered, "same as yours."

"Charlie same as yours?" Grandpa chuckled. "That's a funny name."

My grandfather's dementia altered his perception of himself in another remarkable way. The novella I wrote based on the stories he told me when I returned from Paris ceased to be for him what you and I would think of as a book *about* his life. For him, the commonplace boundaries between now and then, character and person—between reading and living—finally blurred beyond distinction. There was a period of time, an astonishing window of both obliviousness and total lucidity, when he could read the stories of his life and understand that he was the main character, know that the little boy "Dude" and pages later the grown man "Charlie" were him, and yet not remember how each story would end. And when he had difficulty reading himself, he would ask my grandmother to read to him his "book," as he called it; or he would retrieve it from its drawer when a visitor came to the house and present it to him, sometimes asking his guest to read it, sometimes apparently just to see it in his hands.

It was a bad day when my grandfather was no longer allowed to walk alone—bad for him and painful to us. He walked five times a day, at least. When he could do little else unassisted, he *could* do that. He was free to walk. The routine punctuated his day, and, more than that, it gave him a meaningful purpose. He lived in a new residential development throughout which houses were springing up almost monthly. The neighborhood construction gave him, in effect, a job. His daily path would bring him to the newly rising structure, and when the workers left for the day he would tidy up the place: stack the scrap wood into little piles, toss discarded cans into buckets, rotate a lone brick to face just so. The owners of the homes told us how much they appreciated his nearly constant presence at their property because the construction workers, believing he was part of the family monitoring their efforts, tended, among other things, to keep more accurate timesheets.

A portion of his path took him to a nearby park. As his cognitive abilities diminished, his commitment to an unwavering routine increased. My uncle heard from several of the high school kids who regularly played basketball in the park that Mr. Leonard—as all the neighbors knew my grandfather—would walk, at least once a day and sometimes twice if they played long enough, right through their ongoing game, seemingly following an invisible line that perfectly transected the court. My uncle investigated, joining his dad on his walk the next day. Sure enough, he did it. My grandpa would pass through the boys; they would politely halt their game. "Hello, Mr. Leonard," they would say. He would offer a friendly nod and continue on. On the other side of the court he would turn and pass behind a row of pine trees. On the other side of the trees he turned again, almost ninety degrees, and walked directly to a row of hobbyhorses. Each horse he would pat on the head three times, as if, said my uncle, "they were his buddies." At the end of the row, he would glance fondly back at the well-aligned herd, acknowledge their daily meeting, and take his leave. His path back to the house was equally certain. Once when my uncle was walking with his father, he tried to redirect his father's route across the court so that he went around, and not through, the boys playing basketball. Grandpa pulled his arm away from his son and stayed true to his committed path.

Because he attended the construction of every new house in the neighborhood from the pouring of its foundation to its completion, daily performing his supervisory and custodial tasks, my grandfather's attachment to each rising home grew deep. None was his home, but all were his responsibility. He would continue to visit a house even after the new residents moved in. The man across the street woke one morning to find Grandpa in his hallway, fiddling with the thermostat. "It's cold in here, boy," my grandfather informed his neighbor. Another family returned from church to find my grandfather seated at their kitchen table. He offered them coffee—he had a pot brewing. "I think you missed your house, Mr. Leonard," the man said recovering from his initial fright, and he helped my grandfather find his way home. Then one day a neighbor called because Grandpa was urinating in their front yard. Our family decided then that Grandpa could no longer be allowed to come and go freely. It was not a decision that he either understood or accepted. For weeks when he couldn't open his front or back door—they were now dead-bolted from the inside—he grew impatient, then angry. Often he had to be discouraged, or prevented, from trying to kick his way outside. To guests he would ask, "Where's that, uh, uh . . ." turning his hand as if trying to start the ignition of a car.

His desire to be elsewhere is precious to me now. The clear evidence of will tells me how alive he was at that moment, in those days. At the time it was his capacities—what he could still do—that measured for me the extent and depth of his *aliveness*. Checking up on Grandpa meant comparing current abilities with those from the last report and subtracting. I convinced myself that I could, in that way, arrive at a rough sense of how much time I still had to make contact with him before it was too late.

My reasoning was more metaphorical than logical: I equated capacity with presence, equated what my grandpa could still "do" with how much he was still "there." I recognize that my perspective constituted a cognitive posture toward life that was flawed. I cannot now hear the term "cognitive impairment" without thinking that its typical application to people with mental deficits is profoundly selective, indeed constitutive. We have reduced the realm of the *cognitive* to the domain of the *functional,* and the functional very nearly to the *efficient.* I do not know if this reflex is Western—a symptom of science, capitalism, or modern bureaucracy. I do know that when I listen now to my grandfather's stories, especially when I hear him tell them in his voice (on cassette, but also more intimately in the replaying of them through the speakers of my memory), I hear a spirit that does not recognize the boundaries of science or common sense—even space, and less so time. The spirit does not seem, as I hear it, either cognitively potent or impaired, for its reaches me in a current of awareness that contains but is not limited to cognition, at least in any scientific or commonsense understanding of that faculty. The spirit seems to be narrative through and through—to move in, on, and through stories, the sea of human sense out of which all our tales, the tall and textbook straight, have their origin. If you were to ask me through what medium, if not cognition, this story-born spirit reaches me, I would say that of the body. I hear my grandfather's stories in my bones, and out of my bones, in the body that embodies my family, and doesn't stop there. *kinesthetic response*

I believe now that my grandfather was trying to reach his houses and his horses, and that the key to the locked door between those bodies and his own is the story we are telling ourselves about where human presence ends and begins.

⸙

My grandfather's gray hair was once black; it flowed in thick rows of perfectly coifed waves from his forehead over his crown to the high end of his neck. He was on the brown side of olive, half Cherokee-Choctaw Indian. Neither tall nor short, he began thin, ended thinner; the girth, insofar as there ever was any, marked a middle age that was the most abbreviated period of his life. "Every old man is twice a child," it is said. My grandfather complicated this adage, like so many others: his childlikeness never sufficiently abated for it to be said it ever left, or returned. His eyes, for instance, were the same age all his life. That feature alone would have convinced Jesus, had they met on the shores of Galilee, that Charlie Leonard was a good man, a workman worthy of his hire. His small hands wore the history of that work elegantly. If people cared to see the hands of old men in print, his would have made excellent models, save for the trace stains of the oil field and his dipping tobacco. He had a bit of the build of the Scarecrow in the *Wizard of Oz,* and in the last three years of his life, when the waning of his mind was being dutifully mirrored in the waning of his body, the skeletal stake that held him upright surfaced through a very thin padding of straw. Like the

Scarecrow he was a dancer; and that too surfaced in the end. My grandfather withered away, but he never lost his balance; he grew weak agilely. He never smelled bad, never looked dirty (even when he was), and I never saw him exhausted. One had the feeling he was committed to a certain style of growing old, of dying with the dignity of a very modest gentleman asking you to dance. He was and he was not in a body, even when it seemed as if a body was practically all that he was.

Once he was confined to the house, my grandfather's mental deterioration seemed to accelerate. Previously he had been able to do small tasks for himself and my grandmother, serving mainly as their collective body while she served as their collective mind. But he could no longer be relied on to put a prepared lunch in the microwave, help her get to and from the bathroom, or check on her at night if she called out for help. It is this period of my grandfather's life that I associate so strongly with his body. I am reluctant to say—why, I don't know—that he became his body, but he became his body. And interestingly enough, the more he became his body, the more his body also became our body—to feed, to wash, to move: to care for. When I hear people say that Alzheimer's is a disease that robs you of your humanity—or as I heard one expert say on a recent television special, "Alzheimer's rips away your very sense of self"—I picture my grandfather at his frailest, when he could not walk unsupported, when his skin was bone and his bone skin, when the pink rims of his eyes were always bleary, when he wore diapers and was fed soft food with a spoon, when the only word he spoke, if he spoke at all, was "bye," and when he didn't seem to recognize anyone except (maybe) his wife and three children. I picture him at his physically and cognitively weakest and ask myself if I can still detect his humanity. My answer is that the question has no answer because it means nothing—except for what it reveals about the society for which such platitudes have conversational, and thus imaginative, currency. My grandfather's self, whatever it is, is not, like "humanity," an abstraction; and the disappearance of any self that wasn't as tangible as his body was in its final hour isn't worth mourning. What dementia actually rips away are our commonplace fictions about personal identity.

When I returned from Paris seeking myself in the history of my family, what I did not realize, among other things, was this: the teller of our story is himself returning, into the bodies his stories shaped into a family.

The recliner, his recliner, is orange. He could move it up and down electronically with its pneumatic controls. The invisible motor whirs softly, ascending and descending. There was a period when Grandpa would recline and incline himself incessantly, up/down/up/down, like a child at play. And his wooden chair around the kitchen serving bar, where he took breakfast, lunch, and dinner—he also sat there. And the commode. Occasionally, during a family holiday reunion, he was walked to and seated at the dining room table. But the family somehow seemed closer to dispersion when the head of its table (and in the rural south there is still such thing) was being fed by his daughter than when we scattered around the living room taking our meals on TV trays. It was, after all, Grandpa's prayers that blessed our food and made us, in its sharing, whole. Or at the edge of his bed, which in time was replaced with a hospital bed, to be dressed. Helen, or one of his other caregivers, or my mother, would put on his socks as he, bemused, watched his cold white toes disappear. Or in his shower seat, showering himself, or later, being showered. The only other place that I know he sat after we quit allowing him to leave the house alone was on the concrete floor of the washroom, where Helen said she found him once, sitting, not quite cross-legged, with his knees up. He had taken off all his clothes and moved his bowels.

He lay in his bed, but he didn't like to. Deep into the night Helen would struggle with him to keep him in his bed. He had no difficulty getting his shrinking frame over the bed's safety rails, or over the wheel-locked wheelchair that Helen once thought might keep him from wandering back into the living room if she parked it outside his door. As a boy, Grandpa ran track, and later he coached my mother, who set national records as a hurdler. Scaling a wheelchair, even at 86 with advanced dementia, isn't something a Leonard is afraid to do. Grandpa liked being awake, and he liked being in the living room, and he liked doing what he liked.

When on his feet, he walked the house—every carpeted inch of it that was not locked to keep him out—until he finally lost the strength even for that. Eighteen months before he died, he had kidney stones removed. When he returned from the hospital there was a noticeable difference in the degree of his lucidity. My uncle thinks that the experience of the surgery—perhaps his going under general anesthesia—disoriented my grandfather so that he never recovered. Thereafter when he walked, it was only to get from, say, his recliner to the kitchen bar, where he took his meals, and it was always with assistance.

Our grandfather, our father, our husband, our neighbor Charlie Leonard was dying. He was now with us like a portable ark, the temple of our familiar, a mute presence sinking away in his recliner on the circumference of our family get-togethers, watching us without expression, save when we greeted or parted from him with an "I love you," and a kiss to his forehead. Then he would, always would, give us his eyes and grin.

Three Christmases ago, my grandfather's last, my niece Ashley was sitting beside him in his recliner watching him watch us open presents. Since our arrival two days earlier, he had been sitting in that same silent, expressionless, almost motionless fashion. Who knew what he was thinking? At some point Ashley, patting his arm, remarked: "Grandpa, this is all your family. There are all your children, all your grandchildren, and all your great-grandchildren." A jaw dropped, lips pursed, and for the first time in five months Charlie Leonard spoke. "We done pretty good, didn't we?" he said. That was what he was thinking.

According to Helen, my grandfather knew when he was going to die. I am inclined to believe Helen. She has been caring for elderly people, in all kinds of ill health, for over thirty years. Besides that, she is Pentecostal, which doesn't necessarily mean anything, but in Helen's case it does. She believes in God and his son Jesus and the Holy Spirit in the same historically physically unmetaphorically literal way that my grandfather's grandmother did. In fact, in some ahistorical, intangible, entirely metaphorical way, I can see with utter clarity that Helen was my grandfather's grandmother—at least she was on the night she knew that he knew he was going to die.

That night he would not let go of her hand. She had put him to bed and was sitting in a kitchen chair at his side. He helped her, as he had never done before, put his oxygen tube in his nose. "He always watched me," Helen said, "but not like this. He was watching every move I made that night, and he wasn't letting go of my hand. 'Charlie,' I finally had to tell him, 'I've got to go to the bathroom because'—well, because I did. When I came back," Helen continued, "his eyes were turned up to me, waiting. I moistened his lips with a wash rag. I knew by then that he was going to die. I've been with lots of people when they died, and I can always tell when it's going to happen. When they know, I know. And Charlie knew. So I called Jabo (his son), and I said, 'Jabo, you better come on over to the house; your daddy's going to be with the Lord shortly.' And he came over. And when he got there, I told him to go wake up his mama and bring her in Charlie's room so that she could kiss him one last time. And he did that. He led her over in her nightgown and she sat in my chair and kissed his forehead; she kissed his forehead for about twenty minutes. And the whole time he just watched her. Then I told them they'd better get some rest, that I'd sit with Charlie until he fell asleep. That was about, oh about, one o'clock in the morning. He wasn't ready to fall asleep, not yet. He watched me and watched me, and I talked to him and finally he smiled at me, like he would, and after about four hours he let his eyes close. I sat with him another couple of hours watching him breathe until about 6:20 a.m. and then I got up to fix breakfast. I made oatmeal and toast and a little coffee. When I went to wake him he had passed. He fell asleep in his bed and never woke up."

The last time I saw my grandfather I had come home from Wisconsin, where I was working at a college-prep school. It had been over a year since he had given any clear indication of recognizing anyone in the family but my grandmother. He was sitting in his orange recliner. His eyes were wet, the features of his impassive face collapsed into their skeletal frame. He was wearing one of the jumpsuits that had served as his attire, in and out of the oil fields where he worked, for seventy-three years. Except now it was completely clean, lacking even the stains of chewing tobacco; and tied loosely around his neck was a terrycloth bib. When I arrived, Helen was trying to feed him a cracker. I sat beside him on the couch; there was neither a spittoon nor a tape recorder between us now. "Hey, Old Timer," I said, "how about I tell you a story?"

The night before my grandfather's funeral, our family, from parts near and far, gathered together in his and Grandmother's living room. The talk, mostly small and expressed in a cheerfulness that could not disguise the pall, was broken finally when my grandfather himself spoke up. My little brother had found one of the tapes I had made years ago and brought his boom box in from the car. "I never shall forget . . ." my grandfather began. And as we listened to the stories he told, you could see in the faces circling the room that he never would.

QUESTIONS

1. This narrative suggests in numerous ways that even in its most advanced expressions, Alzheimer's disease does not destroy one's self, although some aspects of personal identity are radically altered by it and related dementias. How would you characterize those aspects of identity that survive vast cognitive destruction? What constitutes selfhood?

2. How is this narrative organized? How does its organizational strategy inform your understanding of the disease?

3. Consider the degree of truth and embellishment in the grandfather's stories. To what degree are memories true? What makes a memory more or less true?

Reflections of a Chaplain and a Daughter
⌒ Tami L. Higdon ⌒

We rarely speak about death in our society. Even from the pulpits of religious institutions, where we might expect to hear issues of life and death articulated, speaking openly and honestly about death has remained taboo. We set death aside as if it's not a natural part of living. And when we do speak of death, it usually surfaces in jest. We laugh about people's experiences in the afterlife through the jokes we tell, enjoying the best of them and passing them on to others. This is not surprising; it's human nature to ease our anxieties by finding ways to laugh in the face of the realities we fear most.

One of the perplexing realities I see in my work as a hospital chaplain is how few people have given serious reflection to end-of-life decisions. Since 1990, when Congress passed the Patient Self-Determination Act, patients are asked upon admission to a hospital if they have an advance directive and are given the opportunity to learn more about them if they don't. Still, over a decade later, few have given earnest consideration to the end of their lives, much less made their wishes known in a written advance directive. How often I have watched families struggle with trying to make decisions for a loved one who is dying, having never had a conversation with him about what he wanted. I understand what's behind that silence, for who of us likes to go around thinking about our own death or the deaths of ones we love? Denial isn't always a bad thing. But neither is it a good thing to put aside thinking about death until you're in the midst of it yourself or with someone you love. Although not all people are religious, most of us search for meaning and understanding in our lives. And when an illness or threat of disease occurs—whether acute or chronic—it can shake the foundations of our world. Some of the ways we have previously made sense of our world may not hold up in this new reality. Consulting with a chaplain can be helpful at such a time.

I began my profession as a chaplain in 1989 at Shands Hospital at the University of Florida in Gainesville. As part of the health-care team, my role is broadly interfaith. To some patients and families, I serve as a representative of a Higher Power. To others, my presence speaks to the value they and the institution place on spirituality as an integral component to holistic care. The multicultural nature of a health-care complex like Shands makes it an exciting venue in which to work. I value the opportunity to accompany people in life-and-death situations who don't always share my worldview.

Shands HealthCare is one of the southeast's premier health systems. It includes nine not-for-profit hospitals, more than 80 affiliated University of Florida clinical practices, and a medical staff of 1,500 UF faculty and community doctors. A comprehensive center for basic and clinical research, Shands HealthCare is involved in more than 1,500 investigations into promising technologies and therapies aimed at improving outcomes for patients through prevention, diagnosis, and treatment of disease. Researchers, physicians, and staff deliver advanced diagnostic and medical treatments and provide highly specialized, complex health services that draw patients from Florida, throughout the United States, and beyond. As the flagship institution of the Shands system, Shands Hospital at the University of Florida is a 594-bed tertiary-care center that includes a children's hospital, a regional burn center, a transplant center, and 142 intensive-care beds.

The theological and psychosocial expertise of the chaplain is a blended perspective that is unique in the health-care setting. In a world where our ethical maturity has failed to keep pace with technological advances, patients and their families, as well as health-care providers, find themselves in dilemmas that are far more blurred than sharply defined. University medical centers benefit from the chaplain's professional contributions, especially as they relate to the fields of medical ethics and end-of-life care. One of the chaplain's most challenging roles is helping patients accept, if not embrace, the reality that death is a natural part of living. Short of coming to a place where we can embrace death, we will miss out on the richest of gifts it gives us for living.

One of Woody Allen's best-known lines is about death: "It's not that I'm afraid of dying. I just don't want to be there when it happens" (quoted in Gross, paragraph 1). Buddhists would say that being there is not the problem. Instead, it is the solution. The Buddha traced all our suffering to delusion, and our delusions about death are most common; many of us believe that we are impervious to death. Buddhist teacher Larry Rosenberg says that we all "know" we're going to die but that this information is only frontal-lobe deep. The Buddhist premise is that "the fear of death, snaked around the fear of aging and fear of illness, is burrowed into our unconscious, a chronic undercurrent of anxiety. The Buddhist method is to 'flush out these fears,' to invite them into consciousness, stare into their faces, and so release ourselves from their grip" (Gross, paragraph 3). This perspective is helpful in chaplaincy.

While having a body of knowledge she brings to bear on her work with a patient, as does any legitimate professional, the chaplain also values the ability to be a non-anxious presence. This is not passive inertia. To the contrary: it is an active, attentive presence, one that enables the patient to set the agenda. Everyone has a story s/he wants to tell. And it is the honed skill of the chaplain through this non-anxious presence that creates a hospitable space in which the patient's story can be told.

In addition to the image of a non-anxious presence, a second fitting metaphor for the profession of chaplain is that of the "wounded healer," a term coined by Catholic priest and writer Henri Nouwen. The chaplain knows she must first be willing to recognize and address her own wounds before she can help another address his. It is almost impossible to help others face their darkness if you've never faced your own (Nouwen, xvi). In this profession, one moves fluidly between being a teacher one moment and a learner the next. When the North Carolina church in which I grew up invited me to return and preach on Father's Day 2004, I accepted the invitation without hesitation. The people in that small-town congregation have nurtured me in mind and spirit, and I valued, with humility, the opportunity to give back to these people some of the fruits of their labor as reflected in who I had become. In his *Essays in Gratitude*, D. Elton Trueblood wrote a chapter of gratitude about each of the people who had helped to shape the person he had become. I saw this invitation to go back home again as an opportunity to express this gratitude. My parents still lived and worshipped in that small community, and it would be an added bonus to be with them on Father's Day.

So I began to weave a sermon, one that from the very beginning I knew would be an offering of some of the lessons I had learned from the sacred privilege of walking for sixteen years with patients and their families in the valley of the shadow of illness and death. I would take this taboo subject of death, and I would offer a different perspective—a perspective I would not possess so clearly were it not for the hundreds of critically ill patients and their loved ones who have been my teachers. By allowing me to be their companion as minister in their valleys, I have learned lessons that have dramatically changed how I live and, hopefully, how I will die.

As I began to write, I remembered an important lesson I learned during my first year as a hospital chaplain. A Jewish lady whom I came to know during her treatment for cancer shared with me a story from Chaim Potok's novel *My Name Is Asher Lev*. There is a wonderful scene in which young Asher and his father are returning one Sabbath day from synagogue and see a bird lying on its side against the curb near their house. The young boy is full of questions:

"Is it dead, Papa?" I asked. I was sick at heart and could not bring myself to look at it.

"Yes," I heard him say in a sad and distant way.

"Why did it die?"

"Everything that lives must die."

"Everything?"

"Yes."

"You, too, Papa? And Mama?"

"Yes."

"And me?"

"Yes," he said. Then he added in Yiddish: "But may it be only after you live a long and good life, my Asher."

I couldn't grasp it. I forced myself to look at the bird. Everything alive would one day be as still as that bird?

"Why?" I asked.

"That's the way the Ribbono Shel Olom made His world, Asher."

"Why?"

"So life would be precious, Asher. Something that is yours forever is never precious" (156).

There is something about running out of time—about recognizing that our lives on this earth are finite—that causes us to cherish the moment and the people we love. We're thus less likely to put off saying and doing the things that really matter. But most of us never benefit from cherishing the present, ordinary moment because we live our lives in a kind of denial, forgetting from day to day that we are here for such a short time. And it's when we forget, it's when we fool ourselves into thinking that we have all the time in the world, that we begin to use up our time complaining about things that one day we would surely long to have as our only problems.

I was having one of those days one Wednesday. I wanted to be anywhere but at work. Nothing was going according to plan. Before lunch, I was already wishing Thursday and Friday away and longing for the weekend, far from this place that was driving me crazy. This was my frame of mind when I went upstairs to meet a patient who had asked to see the chaplain. Her name was Cindy. She was 48 years old and in the midst of weeks of therapy for a nasty infection that would not go away. She was discouraged; she was lonely; and she was wondering if her life would ever be the same again.

We spoke at length. I hope I helped her that day. I don't know if I did or not. What I do know is how much she helped me, how she served as one of those teachers life sends our way if we stay open to learning. Cindy lamented with me how she longed to be able to work again. Her illness had necessitated a leave of absence from her job, and for seven weeks she had been unable to return. She wanted me to pray for her that if she were ever able to return to work, she would never take such a gift for granted again. She was longing for the day she could go to work. And I, healthy and well, was lamenting that I had to work.

This is an important lesson I wanted to include in my sermon. I had lost touch with remembering that my days are limited, and that because my days are limited, every day of my life, no matter how mundane or ordinary, is a sacred gift. Those who have personally faced the challenge of surviving a serious illness or have lived daily with a chronic condition that limits them in what they can do understand.

Unfortunately, most of us forget this until some kind of seminal event occurs that shatters our world. So when someone says to me, "Tami, how do you do what you do? I'd take it home with me every night," I want always to respond with what I've learned: I do take it home with me every night; I take home with me the incredible gift of knowing how fortunate I am to have my health while I still have it, to be able to go to work every day and contribute to my world, to be able to work in my yard without having to stop every other step to catch my breath, to be able to walk to the end of my driveway and pick up the newspaper without giving it a thought, to be able to come home for family gatherings and not see an empty chair because a loved one has died. *Acknowledge the gift*

I have a ritual I go through at the end of each work day. On my walk from the hospital to the car, which is mostly on cement and asphalt, there is one small haven that goes through a lush green hammock. The birds that live in that hammock sing day after day their beautiful melodies. Each day, I pause on the bridge that crosses the ravine, and I listen to the wondrous music of those birds, and I simply say, "Thank you." I know there will come a day when I will not be able to walk out of a hospital. But in this moment, I can. And so I want to—actually, I am compelled to—express my thanks. I wanted to impress upon the congregation this truth, which Cindy and Asher's father knew: Something that is ours forever will never be precious.

For most of us, if we've befriended death, if we've recognized the short time we're here, if we and those we love are safe and healthy, it can become second nature to live out of this spirit of gratitude. But what about when we and those we love are not safe and healthy? What then? How will we respond? Will we ever be able to see life as good again? Will it be possible then to live out of this deepest sense of gratitude?

That was as far as I had come in my sermon preparation on Wednesday, May 26, 2004. Until that moment, the lives of my immediate family had been untouched by critical illness or the threat of impending death. How quickly reality can shift. My family learned that day that my father had a mass on his pancreas.

Although my dad was not dead, I knew with certainty that there is no cure for pancreatic cancer and had heard physicians say that the average span of life between diagnosis and death is three months. So my reality was that Dad would be dead by summer's end. My grief, though anticipatory, began simultaneously with my mother's late-afternoon, tearful phone call. At that moment, I felt like theologian and writer C. S. Lewis in *A Grief Observed*, a memoir of his grief over the death of his wife. Lewis reflects, "No one ever told me that grief felt so like fear. I am not afraid, but the sensation is like being afraid. The same fluttering in the stomach, the same restlessness, the yawning. I keep swallowing" (1).

I was aware from the beginning that I carried a burden my family did not know. Because they did not work in health care, though they were devastated, they were able to hope in a way that is a gift of ignorance. When their questions to me began to surface, however, I chose to tell them what I knew: there is no cure for pancreatic cancer, as there are for many other malignancies. The irony did not escape me that for several weeks I had been writing a sermon for Father's Day about what I had learned from patients facing critical illness. Now here my family was, right in the throes of that journey. I called the church that last week of May to let them know I doubted I would be able to keep my commitment to preach in less than a month. Given the emotional devastation I felt and the unknown of the immediate future—not to mention my need to find energy somehow to finish writing the sermon—I wanted to be free of what now felt like an overwhelming burden.

From the earliest moments of this journey, I was also aware of both the personal and professional parts of me. I was a daughter. I was a chaplain. I did not want to confuse the two. It was more important to me in the midst of this new reality my family was living to be a daughter and a sister than it was to be a minister to them. Too often I have seen "therapist types" forget that you can not "heal" your own family. And yet, I had sixteen years of professional experience working with families in the depths of where we now found ourselves. I had gained such wisdom. What was I to do with all of that? Not find ways to incorporate that wisdom into my own family's saga? What a waste that would be! I began to realize that my profession and the perspectives it has provided have become very much a part of who I am as a person. Thus, separating my personal and professional identities was not as easy to do as I had once thought. I would learn in the weeks to come that my being a chaplain would bring its gifts as well as its burdens. I am still learning to accept that tension.

The mass on Dad's pancreas had been found "by accident" after he had a CAT scan to determine if he had passed a kidney stone. There had been no symptoms to alert us to worry; so with no warning, the news literally shook us into another reality. Dad had the CAT scan in a small community and without the use of contrast, so I hoped my parents would choose to come to Shands for a complete diagnostic workup. When I offered them this option, they readily agreed. In the ensuing weeks, my parents, two sisters, and brother-in-law joined me in Gainesville, and we embarked on that bittersweet journey of learning all we could about this particular cancer and what it means, and riding that dreaded emotional roller coaster you find yourselves on after this kind of news shatters the normalcy of your world. During the almost two weeks that we were gathered here, Dad had an initial workup with one of the best gastroenterologists at Shands, another CAT scan, multiple blood draws, and an endoscopic ultrasound and biopsy.

Wayne Oates, one of the early pioneers of pastoral care, wrote about the tendency of patients and families to begin a process of "protection maneuvers" with one another when a diagnosis of a terminal disease has been delivered. Each person knows and thinks about the worst, but neither patient nor family members want to hurt each other. The sad consequence is that both are cut off from the care and support they could receive from the other (Oates, 26). For whatever reasons, that kind of protective maneuvering didn't happen with us, at least not in those first days. During those initial days of testing, procedures, and waiting for results, my family had many painfully vulnerable yet incredibly healing conversations. Everyone was living these days understanding that if this was indeed pancreatic cancer, as we were being led to believe, our time together with Dad was most limited. Although my family has always been good about sharing our love for one another and finding ways of expressing that love, we used those rare ten days to the fullest. Our conversations were sometimes full of tears and sometimes full of laughter, but all that left nothing but sheer gratitude in each of us for having been a part of this family. And I'm convinced that the genuine times of laughter happened because we did not try to protect each other from the emotionally painful conversations. In fact, I found it was a cause-and-effect relationship. It was routinely after the most honest, heart-wrenching conversations that the silliest, most light-hearted times together occurred.

After having to wait for four long days for the results of the biopsy, we all met again with the physician to learn the lay of this new foreign land. I never realized that one could feel so elated to learn about a cancer diagnosis until that early June morning. We were told that Dad did have pancreatic cancer, but that it was a rare type called an islet cell tumor. Unlike the aggressive adenocarcinoma, the islet cell is slow-growing and can remain dormant and unchanging for years. Although Dad's tumor was already six centimeters in diameter and had spread to the liver, he had no symptoms that were impacting his quality of life, and we were told that it could remain that way for months or even years to come. We still did not know what the future held, but we had been given what looked like the potential gift of more time with Dad. It was a gift that was literally and figuratively life-giving. We celebrated that evening with a delicious home-cooked meal, the first that had not been prepared by friends. Purchasing the groceries and preparing the meal were sacred rituals of thanksgiving.

While lying in bed that night, I thought about how my friends, both physicians and nurses, had prepared me to receive the news that Dad had pancreatic cancer and how my own need to be prepared had made me leap to the conclusion that Dad would be dead by summer's end. It was a humbling lesson for me—and should be for all of us in the field of health care—never to be presumptive in the face of life and death. As it turns out, my sisters were no less ignorant to have had hope at the beginning than I was ignorant to have assumed that there was just one horrendous kind of pancreatic cancer.

Such presumption reminded me of an old archetype that appears in most every culture. I heard this particular Brazilian version told by John Claypool at a conference in Daytona Beach, Florida.

> Once upon a time, in the mountains of Brazil, there was a hard-working woodcutter. When his father died, he left him a beautiful white stallion, an animal that was the envy of all who saw it. One day, the king came through that village and was so taken with the stallion that he offered to pay the woodcutter any price in order to buy it. But the woodcutter said, "You need to understand this animal is not just a workhorse for me. He represents my inheritance. He has become my best friend. To sell the stallion would be like selling a member of my own family. I simply cannot do that."
>
> Well, when word got around the village what he had done, his neighbors came and said, "You are a fool, a pure fool! You could have been financially independent for life. You could have curried favor with the king. You've passed it all up just to keep a simple animal."
>
> And the old woodcutter said, "Whether or not I am a fool, it is simply too early to tell. I am content to know what I know. I do not presume to know what I cannot know."
>
> A few mornings later, he went out to the barn, and lo and behold, the stall where the stallion was kept was empty. He looked all around but couldn't find him anywhere. And so it was presumed that someone had come in the night and stolen the stallion. In fact, someone even suggested that perhaps the king had come and taken what he could not buy. Well, when the news of this got around the village, they came and said to the woodcutter, "This proves our point. You are stupid. Here, you could have been rich, and now you have nothing. You are a fool."
>
> And the old woodcutter said, "Whether or not I am a fool, it is simply too early to tell. All I know is, the stable is empty. The stallion is gone. I am very sad. I am content to know what I know. I do not presume to know what I cannot know."
>
> Well, a few days later, to his great delight, the stallion came back with twelve wild horses that he had met on the mountain. It turns out he hadn't been stolen but rather had simply run away. And so the woodcutter corralled all thirteen of the animals, and word spread to his neighbors and they came and said, "We were wrong. You're shrewd! You're brilliant! By not selling the stallion, now you're richer than you would have been at the hand of the king. You really are a wise person."
>
> And the old woodcutter said, "Whether or not I am wise, it is simply too early to tell. All I know is the stallion is back. I have twelve horses I never expected to have. I am very happy. I am content to know what I know. I do not presume to know what I cannot know."
>
> As time went on, the woodcutter decided to tame some of these wild horses. He put bridles and saddles on them. He was inexperienced at it. One of them bucked him off one day, and both of his legs were broken. And the neighbors came and said, "We were again mistaken. We thought these twelve wild horses were going to be a blessing, but now look. You've broken your legs. You're going to be crippled for life. You must be cursed by these animals."
>
> And the old man said, "Whether I am cursed or blessed, it is too early to tell."

All I know is that I've hurt myself. I'm going to try to get well. I'm content to know what I know. I do not presume to know what I cannot know."

Well, it turns out that a few weeks later, a war broke out in the mountains of Brazil. Every able-bodied man was conscripted. The woodcutter would have had to go except for his injury. And every man taken from the village wound up being killed. And lo and behold, the tragedy of having his legs broken turned out to be the saving of his life. And once again the truth. When anything happens, it's simply too early to tell. (Claypool, "Avenues to Hopefulness")

John Claypool, Episcopalian priest, writer, and father of a ten-year-old daughter who had died from leukemia, went on to conclude after recounting this story, "We never know enough at any point in our lives to despair, but we do know enough to hope."

After learning that Dad's death was not as imminent as we initially believed, I decided to follow through on my commitment to preach—no longer as one who had only been there for others, but as one who was now there myself. Through the years, I have seen a grace from beyond us be sufficient for others. The Psalmist of the Old Testament said, "God is our refuge and strength, a very present help in trouble" (Psalm 46:1). Would I experience that myself, though, when such a challenge entered my own family's life? Although this story has not ended, I can already give voice to a resounding yes. I found preaching from this confessional point of view to be incredibly therapeutic in my own grieving process, as well as being perhaps the most effective job of preaching I had ever done. Joseph Campbell once said that preachers would do well if they would stop trying to tell people what to believe and begin speaking instead to the radiance of their own journeys (Moyers, xvi.). How true!

Huston Smith is one of the foremost scholars in the field of world religions in this country, and one who has, as a Christian, found a way to weave many of the teachings of the different faith traditions into his own spiritual practice. He recently served as a featured speaker at a friend's church. As Dr. Smith was waiting to catch his plane after speaking to the people there, he entertained a question from a young reporter from the local news:

"Dr. Smith, can you sum up for our viewers what you have learned from your study of the world's different religions over the last fifty years?"

Huston Smith looked at the young man incredulously, and then asked him, "You want me to sum up the content of my life's work in a sound bite?"

"Yes, I do."

So Huston Smith said, "OK, here goes. My parents were Christian missionaries who spent their entire lives teaching people about the love of God. Everything that I have been about in my study of the religions of the world is not a negation of what I learned growing up, but rather an amplification of it—because when you get right down to it, the Christian faith is not about morals, nor is it about dogma. It is about this one thing: bearing one another's burdens" (quoted in Lucas, 4).

Physician friends of mine this past year experienced what has to be the greatest of griefs: the critical illness and subsequent death of their two-year-old daughter. Michael, a pulmonologist, and Eileen, a family physician, are still living daily in those dual realms: one of sheer gratitude that they ever had Keira, and one of agonizing grief at her palpable absence. Making sense of something seemingly so senseless, Keira's dad, Michael, spoke the following words at her funeral:

> When the avalanche of highly unlikely and inconceivable things became our reality
> in early spring, anger settled in deeply. Here we were, having been faithful through
> a harrowing experience with Keira's heart disease and now were faced with the sec-
> ond malignancy in as many months. What good was my faith? Why did I bother
> praying? Where was God?
>
> The question weighed heavily on my heart, and I asked it over and over when
> I was alone. I would drive home struggling with the question and would find my
> lawn mowed. I would ask the question as I lay in bed and I would get up, check
> the web page and find that one of you had left a message that touched our hearts
> deeply. The messages of support would shine just enough light into the darkness
> that surrounded us at times to see where we should place our next step. As the roller
> coaster ride with Keira continued in the summer, we were obviously being carried
> by hundreds of seemingly tiny acts of Grace. Whether it was people covering for
> me at work for months on end, bringing a red fire truck to the house for Ryan to
> play with, people cooking dinner, or your words of love and support, I began to
> realize that maybe I was looking for God the wrong way. No thundering voice from
> heaven, no burning bushes, just the subtle signs of Grace that let us know that we
> were not alone and that we would be carried through the unthinkable. God used
> you to carry us through the fire. (Lauzardo)

I and my family, too, can speak to having felt carried during those weeks, as can so many others who have walked through their own fires. It is not easy. But as with the He-brew people in the desert, to whom God gave just enough manna to make it through one day and no more, so we are given just enough grace to make it through each day, sometimes moment by moment, in our times of trouble.

My parents were flooded with love and support before coming to Gainesville. And once all of us were gathered at my house, for over a week, my support community took over. My lawn was mowed, food was delivered every night, friends who had the ability to get Dad in to see the specialists he needed to see did so with utmost speed. And I was kept busy receiv-ing phone calls and mail that let us know that we were not alone.

None of us likes the challenge that change requires of us, and certainly not the change that critical illness and thinking about our own deaths bring. Reuel Howe was an Episcopa-lian priest and one of the great minds in the field of pastoral care. The story is told that Dr. Howe was called back to the parish where he began his ministry some forty years earlier to visit a dying parishioner. Charley said to him, "Reuel, I've wondered all my life what it's go-ing to be like to die. And now that I'm up close to it, lo and behold, what I'm discovering is simply an old friend in new garb." Dr. Howe listened as his friend continued:

> All my life I've had to let go of things that have served their purpose in order to
> empty my hands that I might move on to something that had even greater poten-
> tial to bless. When I was six years old, my mom came in that first morning of Sep-
> tember and said that I wasn't to put on my play clothes because, "Today you start
> school." I didn't know what school was. I knew it was a big building down on the
> corner with ominous windows and doors. I had no idea what it entailed, and as I

dressed, I looked out in the back yard. There was the swing, the sand pile, that secure place where I had spent so many happy childhood hours, and I had this terrible sense of sadness at being taken out of that. But it turned out after I ventured into it, that school represented the place where I grew in ways I would have never grown had my parents left me in the back yard. I experienced books, music, people. It became an incredibly enriching context.

Six years later, after I'd gotten used to elementary school, suddenly I had to do the same thing all over again. I had to leave what I had already come to experience and go to an even more threatening thing called junior high. Three years later I had to die to junior high school that I might be born to a thing called high school, and after that to a thing called college and after that, the world.

Reuel, in all of this, I have learned that every time you walk out of something, you walk into something greater. As once I had to die to the womb to enter this world as a baby, so must I die now to enter the next. But I believe that the change I'm going to experience, the letting go of what I have, is going to be the prelude to something that is genuine gain. (Claypool, Hope in the Face of Grievance)

I tell this unfinished story, this journey still in process, because I need to for my own healing and in hopes that it will help someone else. Mom and Dad have gone back to their home, my sisters to theirs. Even though the tumor has spread throughout Dad's abdomen, he has no symptoms that would prevent him from going back to live his life as he was already doing. There is no cure for Dad's diagnosis at this stage, and as long as he stays symptom-free, the oncologist's protocol is to do nothing in terms of treatment. Since it is a slow-growing cell, chemotherapy would serve little purpose other than making him terribly sick.

Dad could live for months or he could live for years. No one can tell us. In some ways, nothing has changed in terms of the living of our days. In other ways, everything has changed. We all now have more than a "frontal lobe" knowledge of death. Carlyle Marney, a Baptist minister who outgrew the provincial limits of his tradition and became an ecumenical pastor-theologian, reflected in his most popular sermon, "In the Meantime," that we live most of life waiting for something. Conditions are never exactly right. We live in that expectation of something which lies ahead (Carey, 178). I resonate with Marney in these days. It seems I ask myself daily how we are to live in this meantime. What do we do now?

I guess we follow Dad's lead. We go back to working and loving and enjoying where each of us has planted our lives, except we do so now having befriended death, remembering that nothing that lasts permanently can ever be precious. So we take what is precious, today, in the moment, and treasure it.

REFERENCES

Carey, John J. "Carlyle Marney as Ethicist." *Theology Today* 37.2 (1980): 170–182.

Claypool, John. "Avenues to Hopefulness." Sermon delivered at the Meeting of the Twenty-Sixth Annual Halifax Pastoral Care Institute. Daytona Beach, Florida. February 2002.

———. "Hope in the Face of Grievance." Talk given at the Meeting of the Twenty-Sixth Annual Halifax Pastoral Care Institute. Daytona Beach, Florida. February 2002.

Gross, Amy. Nirvana in the Midst of Everyday Life, n.d., http://www.beliefnet.com/story/27/story_2752_1.html (accessed 21 July 2004).

Lauzardo, Michael. Eulogy delivered at Keira Lauzardo's funeral. Creekside Community Church. Gainesville, Florida. January 2004.

Lewis, C.S. *A Grief Observed.* New York: The Seabury Press, 1961.

Lucas, Steve. "2004 Convocation: Summing It Up in a Soundbite." *Connections* 7.4 (April 2004): 4.

Moyers, Bill. *The Power of Myth: Joseph Campbell with Bill Moyers.* New York: Anchor Books, 1991.

Nouwen, Henri J.M. *The Wounded Healer: Ministry in Contemporary Society.* Garden City, NY: Image Books, 1972.

Oates, Wayne E. *Your Particular Grief.* Philadelphia: The Westminster Press, 1981.

Potok, Chaim. *My Name Is Asher Lev.* New York: Anchor Books, 2000.

Trueblood, D. Elton. *Essays in Gratitude.* Nashville: Broadman Press, 1982.

QUESTIONS

1. Discuss the author's dual position as family member and chaplain. How has this dual identity been an advantage and a disadvantage for her and her family?
2. The author represents different faith traditions in her essay. What does each have to offer in terms of its perspective on illness, death and life?
3. How have your own experiences with serious illness affected communication among family members? within your circle of friends?

Stay of Execution

⮷ SUSANNA BLACK ⮶

Driving home from work one evening, I hear a story on NPR about a physician who misses a diagnosis of fatal colon cancer in a long-term patient. Although the physician routinely recommends a screening sigmoidoscopy—a test for colon cancer—to his patients over 50, he fails to bring it up with this man. Perhaps he forgets; perhaps the patient has other issues that always seem more pressing. Several months later, the physician is shocked when, instead of hearing about a pending lawsuit brought on by the patient's wife, also a patient of his, she shows up for an appointment. He realizes that not only does she like him and trust him, she forgives him.

Before everything happened with my brother, I could understand this. I can imagine the doctor's fear and guilt because I have shared it. In my internal medicine practice, I have had patients like this, patients with a plethora of other active issues with whom I never seem to be able to find the time to discuss preventive measures. All doctors make mistakes; most of them, thankfully, do not cause major harm. The medical literature tells us that when a mistake occurs in the context of a good doctor-patient relationship, an apology from the doctor can help lead to forgiveness. A simple apology not only demonstrates concern; it humanizes a physician. As an internist and educator, this is what I teach my residents and students, and what I practice myself. But now I understand that a physician's apology is far from a magic phrase that will grant absolution.

What if the patient's wife forgives the physician only because the notion of having no familiar primary care doctor is worse than having one who has made a mistake? That she can't tolerate the idea of being alone, without a navigator, in the overwhelming ocean of health care?

⮷ ⮶

"Hey, Susanna, it's me . . . can you call me back soon?" says the voice on the answering machine. It's David, my older brother. I'm scrubbing last night's casserole dish and I can't get to the phone in time. Something is different. Usually, when David calls from work, he rambles—live or on the machine—about office politics in the financial world or the latest accomplishments of Phil, his twelve-year-old son. He rarely is so specific about wanting a call back so quickly. I put the dish on the drying rack and dial his office number. He picks up immediately.

He wants to be straight with me, David says. He tells me that his father-in-law had withheld information about his health from him and Dana, his wife, until he was very sick, and he has always sworn to himself that he would never do this.

"I have prostate cancer," he says. — *brother*

Prostate cancer! But he's so young! I'm overcome with a panic—it's cancer—then relief—it's not lung cancer, pancreatic cancer, a brain tumor. Early prostate cancer is quite curable. His internist, Dr. Wolf, must have picked it up by a routine PSA screening. A few years ago, David had mentioned that he was considering having his PSA checked early because of our family history of prostate cancer; I'm grateful that Dr. Wolf agreed.

"I've known for a couple of weeks but didn't want to tell you right away . . . you understand," he continues. His PSA level was high—15, he explains. Dr. Wolf found a nodule on his prostate and sent him to Dr. Contento, a urologist, who performed a biopsy a few weeks earlier. He will have a bone scan and CT scan later in the week to look for evidence of metastatic disease. Jesus! I feel slightly nauseous but cannot imagine any other scenario than localized, curable disease. From my own practice, I know that it is extremely unlikely for patients who have regular PSA tests and who end up having prostate cancer to have metastatic disease. Since most patients have a biopsy as soon as there is a bump in the PSA, most cases of prostate cancer are discovered early enough that treatment is usually curative.

"Oh, and the PSA had actually been higher than normal—I think he said 7—even nine or ten months ago," he adds. "Dr. Wolf didn't realize it until last month."

What? I'm flabbergasted. And angry. Dr. Wolf is a medical school professor and has a national reputation for both his research and incredible clinical acumen. My husband and I were the ones who had recommended Dr. Wolf so highly when my brother was looking for an internist more than ten years ago. How could such a canny physician have let something slip for almost ten months? Apparently, the printout of the lab results never made it onto his desk.

My brother keeps apologizing, as though it is his fault. I try to buoy his spirits and my own. I explain to him that his PSA is really not that high, though I don't tell him that it is close to the borderline for an increased risk of advanced disease. David's chances are still good that it's localized. Metastatic disease, I explain, can send PSA's up into the hundreds, even thousands. His other blood tests are normal, so the chance of bony disease is certainly lessened. He appreciates this. Dr. Wolf hasn't been as reassuring.

I ask David if Dr. Wolf ever apologized to him. He did, but David says it barely registered. To me, it seems like a useless gesture in the face of possible serious disease. It would be worse, though, if Dr. Wolf had simply made excuses and never accepted responsibility.

I try to go about my usual activities without getting overwhelmed by the news, but it's a challenge. Old people suddenly seem like the luckiest folks in the world. At the video store, I see a white-haired couple poking fun at each other while looking at the new releases. Even if they both drop dead tomorrow, I think, they've had the gift of a full life. They've experienced what David might not: watching their children grow up, having grandchildren, retiring, looking back over the expected three score and ten, at the least. Trying to escape by reading the newspaper doesn't work either: I become obsessed with the obituaries, jealous that so many others have had the opportunity to live into their 80s, their 90s. It's so unfair. David, a vegetarian for over twenty years, has always been very health-conscious, and he's a regular at his gym. His downfall was placing his trust in Dr. Wolf. Though I've always kept tabs on my sister's and parents' health issues, I had no question about Dr. Wolf's competence, so I never bothered asking David about his.

David calls the following week with the initial test results, which he reads to me from his notes.

"The bone scan was negative, the CT scan: no bony disease, but," he says, and I hear the paper crinkling, "there were two pelvic nodes and some hazy streaking around the prostate."

My sister, visiting from Chicago, mouths "What? What? What?" from the couch across the room.

"Not in the bones!" I scribble with a shaking hand on a scrap of paper, trying to look optimistic, though I'm terrified. You really screwed up, Dr. Wolf, I think to myself. You missed the PSA and now it really is too late. The cancer has gone outside of the prostate, He can't be cured. I tell David and my sister that we shouldn't read too much into an initial report. After all, it isn't unusual for an attending radiologist to disagree with the first interpretation. I say this out loud as if to convince myself that the report may indeed be wrong. I dread telling my husband about this report, as I fear he will say that I'm not being realistic.

By the time David calls the next morning with a printout of the official report, the nodes have been downgraded to "insignificant" and the streaking is thought simply to be a conglomeration of veins.

"It's fine; it's negative!" I stage-whisper to my sister, brimming with relief.

". . . but," my brother continues, "they saw a nodule in my lung." This doesn't make sense. Prostate cancer doesn't go to the lung. My sister and brother are worried, but I feel confident, this time, that this is nothing more than a red herring.

My brother goes to another urologist for a second opinion. Dr. Patel agrees that the tumor seems to be contained in the capsule and should therefore be surgically curable. Just to be sure, he wants to schedule another test, an endorectal MRI, which will give more information than the CT about any spread to local areas. Unfortunately, this cannot be scheduled for six weeks. Dr. Patel seems unconcerned about the timing. He is, however, troubled by the lung nodule and wants my brother to undergo a CT scan of his lungs. Fine, I say, but I'm anxious—not about the CT but about waiting so long for the endorectal MRI. I wish he could have the surgery now and get it done with.

A few days after the CT, David calls.

"The news isn't good," he says. I gulp.

"There were nine nodules," he says. Nine? This is bizarre. I still am convinced that this is not cancer. There are certainly many other diseases, many relatively benign, that can mark the lungs with multiple nodules; in fact, one of these, sarcoid, has occurred in several of our relatives. Dr. Wolf has told David that he should have a lung biopsy before proceeding with the prostate surgery, just to make sure, and Dr. Patel agrees. I understand their reasoning and caution, but I remain confident that the lung nodules are unimportant. Again, I make the round of family phone calls, trying to convince everybody not to worry. Dana is not convinced; she says he has been losing weight. I haven't realized this, but don't give it very much thought.

Off David goes for the lung biopsy. The procedure seems as complicated and risky as the prostate surgery will be. He has general anesthesia, a chest tube, and an inpatient stay for several days, including one miserable night without proper pain medication. The lung lesions, as I have promised, are benign. The last glitch, I think with relief. We will wait for the MRI, and then he will finally have the surgery.

During the six weeks between the lung biopsy and the endorectal MRI, David calls me several times to report that he is worried about the conflicting opinions. Dr. Wolf and Dr. Contento are concerned about the "high" PSA and the possibility of metastatic spread; the radiologist and Dr. Patel, whom David now considers his main urologist, are not.

I do some research, read articles on the Internet, try to sift through the evidence. For an internist with little background in the subtleties of urology, it's overwhelming. I read myself into a daze about tumor markers and staging systems. It's quite technical and it's difficult to concentrate on the information, much less absorb and apply it to David's situation. I resent the internal pressure I feel to take an active role as an interpreter of divergent opinions.

David has decided, finally, that he does not want anything to do with Dr. Wolf anymore. But without a primary care physician to help him sort through the information, I find myself even more entrenched in the awkward position of sister/doctor. I have seen several physician friends become overly involved in a family member's care (including one who ended up examining his own mother's cancerous breast when he couldn't reach her doctor) and don't want to do the same.

It's an awful feeling to lose my trust in medicine. You can't trust individual doctors, who may make mistakes like Dr. Wolf. You can't trust medicine as a whole, because so much is unknown. How do you know when to believe one doctor's opinion over another's? I don't want to be my brother's doctor, but I can't leave everything in the hands of multiple unknown specialists. I don't even know if I want to be anybody's doctor. Trying to help patients amidst uncertainty and possibly devastating error suddenly seems unbearable.

Wouldn't it be easier, I wonder late one night in front of the computer, eyes aching from fatigue, if I weren't a doctor? If I didn't know that doctors and medicine were fallible? Then I could just go with a gut sense of what was right. I find myself longing for what modern medicine has trained me to avoid: a paternalistic physician, a Marcus Welby type who would put a gentle arm over our shoulders and tell us, with a firm, confident kindness, what exactly is the right thing to do.

What I decide to keep from David at that time would likely make him even angrier at Dr. Wolf. David had a copy of his medical records sent to me, and my husband and I are stunned when we look at his PSA results from the last several years. Dr. Wolf did not just miss the most recent PSA; he ignored a trend of rising PSA's over the past three years. My brother could have had the surgery and been cured three years ago. This story could have been long over.

Several weeks later, the day after the MRI, I sit in a dentist's chair having my teeth cleaned and clenching my beeper in one sweaty hand. David is supposed to page me when he gets the results. As the hygienist scrapes my teeth, I focus on how much time has elapsed since this all started, and in my mind I imagine hundreds of gray metastatic cells loosening from the prostate like dandelion fluff freed by the wind. My pager still hasn't gone off by the time I leave, and I am sure the news isn't good. I call my husband to express my worry, but he says that David has just called him; everything is fine. There is no spread. There is still hope for a surgical cure. Again, reprieve and relief.

My brother travels to a business conference for a week. The surgery is scheduled for two days after his return. He has just made the difficult decision to hand over several large accounts to a colleague and has prepared himself psychologically to undergo the surgery with all its potential complications and the hope of a cure. The cancer will be removed, and that will be the end of the story.

But that is not to be. He calls me upon his return to say that Dr. Patel's team has reviewed the films again. The initial MRI report had called a small mark on the bone an "artifact"—present, but insignificant—but now there is concern that perhaps the interpretation was wrong; perhaps the mark is significant, potentially a metastatic lesion. If it is metastatic, there will be no surgery, and no cure. Another MRI is scheduled to clarify the issue.

It doesn't make sense. Why should this MRI be more helpful than the last? Why aren't any of the urologists recommending a bone biopsy? Wouldn't this be the definitive way to see what the bone lesion is—or isn't? Hoping for some answers, I call Dr. Patel. I want him to say that a bone biopsy is the next step, and that it will finally give us the information we need. Instead, he says that the likelihood is that it is metastatic and that a bone biopsy is not worth the risks. I cringe and shake off the "m" word. This is not metastatic disease, and we will prove it. But there's no time to try to find someone to do a bone biopsy before the scheduled surgery, so David has the MRI. — wtf! why not get biopsy,

The ambiguous mark on the bone is still there on the repeat MRI. The surgery is postponed for another three months. David is to start hormonal treatment—a treatment usually reserved for metastatic disease—and will have another MRI at the end of the three-month period. If the mark changes, or doesn't change, David tells me with some confusion, he may still be a candidate for the surgery. Everyone is devastated, though my brother says he feels like at least he is doing something—taking a medication—instead of just waiting. The question remains: Is this metastatic disease or not? I am desperate to know but fearful of knowing. The uncertainty is torturous, but at least it's leaving room for hope.

We decide to seek another opinion. I have emailed several physicians about their recommendations for urologists and several have mentioned Dr. Omura, a well-known Boston urologist. David seems emotionally exhausted, so I volunteer to set up this appointment. There is more bad news. Dr. Omura's assistant says that he will not see him because he has started hormonal treatment. It turns out that many surgeons will not consider operating on a patient who has had even one dose of the hormonal therapy. The hormones shrink the nerves around the prostate, she explains, and this makes the surgery more challenging in terms of avoiding the not-uncommon side effects of incontinence and impotence. My brother is quite upset that he hasn't been told about this effect of the therapy. Perhaps, he says, he would have sought another opinion earlier; perhaps he has blown his chance to have one of the top surgeons operate. I try to explain that maybe the top were only the top because they exclude some higher-risk patients, but it is too late. He is distraught.

Over the next month or so, not content simply to take the medication and wait, my brother sets up appointments with a number of different specialists. I accompany him to a meeting with Dr. Casey, another New York urologist, so I can try to get a better picture of what's going on. David arrives a few minutes after me, his lucky Knicks tie flung behind his neck. In Dr. Casey's office, he hoists a hefty pile of medical records onto the table—this from a man whose medical history a year ago would have fit into a single manila envelope. Dr. Casey, like many of the other physicians, exudes competence and confidence. He believes that a bone biopsy will answer the question once and for all. Relieved that someone finally shares our opinion about this, my brother opts for the possibility of certainty and goes ahead with the test.

Incredibly, the results are still ambiguous. Dr. Casey recommends waiting to see how the bony lesion responds to the hormonal treatment. And so we wait.

In my own internal medicine practice, I become more fastidious, even paranoid, about checking results. My indignation toward Dr. Wolf can only be justified as long as my own record-keeping is flawless. Before, I had told patients to assume that their lab results were normal if they didn't hear from me. Now, I begin to urge my patients to call if they haven't heard from me, and not to assume that no news is good news. As my in-box quickly floods with messages that I can't keep up with, I return to rigorous record-keeping of every test ordered. But it isn't fail-safe. When I don't notice an abnormal kidney lab result until three weeks after it's been drawn, I panic. Am I just as reprehensible as Dr. Wolf? The phone almost slips out of my sweaty hands when I call the patient and apologize profusely for missing the result. I'm surprised when he tries to make me feel better about it, but only relax two days later when new labs show his numbers have returned to normal. Sometimes, when the pressure of responsibility for my patients' health feels too weighty, I think for a fleeting moment about leaving medicine.

I continue to feel uncomfortable about my involvement with David's case, though whether I'm overly involved or not involved enough is still not clear to me. I urge him to pick a new primary care doctor and hope this will allow me to step back. He meets and likes Dr. Fuller but cannot transfer his trust after a single meeting. I feel internal pressure to stay, at least temporarily, in an advisory role.

And so we wait, and wait, and wait, our fates creeping slowly up another rollercoaster track. The uncertainty and waiting seem so much more tumultuous than what my patients go through, but I know this is ridiculous: every patient and family dealing with a serious illness must go through some semblance of this hell. My seeming position of privilege as a physician has only served to make me cynical about apologies and leaves me more involved—playing primary care doctor for my brother—than I would like to be. I am too cognizant of the shortcomings of physicians, the deficiencies of diagnostic tests, and the lack of certitude in medicine. My brother's on death row without a lawyer. The stays of execution come and go.

NOTE

Names and other identifying features of the author and most characters have been changed for confidentiality.

QUESTIONS

Knowing the best ? to ask

1. What are some advantages of being a physician when a family member becomes ill? What are some disadvantages? *dependence*

2. When a doctor's family member falls ill, what level of involvement with diagnosis and treatment is appropriate? Should the author have been more involved or less involved with her brother's case? *↳ support Dr, more*

3. What might the author learn from the experience that she can bring to the care of her own patients? *imp of quick lab results + informing*

4. What should doctors do when they make mistakes? *give them priority for*

5. Discuss the interplay of certainty and uncertainty in the narrative. *surgeries (not 3 mo)*

⬿ Part II ⬾
Concealing Illness, Performing Health

The two groups of essays in this section address, first, processes of closeting illness, passing, and coming out; and second, issues of sexuality, body image, and gender in the context of illness. While it sometimes seems simpler and safer to hide disease and disability in order to pass as "normal," many who contend with illness ultimately reach a point of openly redefining themselves, of calling for a new aesthetic that accommodates their unique physical and mental conditions.

Barbara J. Jago describes the paralysis of depression specifically in the context of the academy, where the pressure to perform significantly compounds the problem. Her auto-ethnographic essay illuminates the challenges of coming out with both colleagues / administrators and students. Hilary Clark's "mild" version of bipolar disorder with dissociative episodes presents her with a decision similar to Jago's: pass as normal or reveal a condition that could seriously compromise her professional identity. She concludes that in forcing us to slow down and accept limits, illness affords a critical perspective on norms of academic culture, with its high-pressure teaching and competitive research. Rebecca Hogan's narrative about bipolar disorder and paranoia provides interesting perspectives on the surprising benefits of such illness. As is true for many others who write about mental or psychological illness, Hogan illustrates how illness affects one's identity but is not itself an essential part of identity.

Barbara J. Campbell, Fulvia Dunham, and Lisa Katz reveal the complexities of living with gynecological disease and disorder in societies that define people in large measure according to their sex. Campbell's essay on endometriosis takes a frank—and sometimes darkly humorous—look at chronic, excruciating pain that compromises a young adult's sexual identity as well as her ability to perform basic human tasks. Dunham's multi-layered narrative brings to light the rarely diagnosed, rarely discussed disorder vaginismus, and the stigma associated with an inability to "perform" according to sexual norms. Finally, Katz's poems provide insight into various dimensions of mastectomy, most notably how the aesthetics of the female body are culturally scripted.

Coming Out with My Academic Depression
ᗡ Barbara J. Jago ᗡ

September 2001. The school parking lot is Monday-morning packed, bumper to bumper with staff and faculty, diligently working inside at the task of higher education. A chill invigorates the air of this early-September day, high clouds sweeping overhead. I find an empty space, slide my car in, and turn the ignition key. My heart races at the prospect of going inside to confront the once-familiar faces. Gathering my strength, I sit staring at the red brick walls of the former mill building that houses the University of New Hampshire at Manchester.

I can do this.

Coming to school, an activity that was once mundane, now feels monumental; a place that was once a haven now feels dangerous. I take half the morning to get here, a pot of tea, a hot shower, the right costume, a stack of books to prop me up. One step at a time. That's the way through depression, one foot in front of the other—or at least that's what Sibylle, my therapist, says. After a year, I am not so sure.

Crossing the parking lot toward the back door, I walk past a former student, early twenty-something with long blond hair. A smart young woman if memory serves. She doesn't acknowledge me. Perhaps she is still angry I bailed out halfway through the semester last year when I was diagnosed, abandoning three classes, unable to do the teaching I loved, taking medical leave and then long-term disability. Perhaps my professor self has been rendered invisible, obliterated by a depression haze. Perhaps she just doesn't know what to say. My eyes seek the refuge of the ground.

The weight of the back door pulls against me and I yank myself inside just in time to almost crash into my colleague Jeff descending the stairs.

"Hi Barbara," he says, without missing a step.

"Hi," I respond, my words chasing him down the stairs. He probably has to get to a class, an appointment, something important.

Don't take it personally. Simple moments in the hallway are now ripe with meaning.

Jeff had to clean up my mess last fall. As director of our newly created major in communication arts, he scrambled to cover my three classes, taking on one himself, handling student complaints, and doing salvage public relations. A few weeks ago, sitting in his office discussing my eventual return to full-time work, he was hesitant, unable to express confidence in my ability to do my job.

"Students were angry when you left," he explained. He never actually says that he was angry too. But I feel it. He stays at a safe distance from me now. No more chatting about our lives, no more respected and trusted colleague. I understand. He has to hedge his bets in case history repeats itself.

Down the stairs, key in lock, door closes behind me. Tears form. I take a deep breath. *I can do this.*

My new plant sits on the windowsill, already wilted. A thin layer of dust has settled on my desk since my last visit. *Visit.* That's what it feels like now. Like I am a tourist who doesn't really live here anymore.

I conduct housework anyway. A few blasts of breath clear my desk of debris. The water from my mug races through the plant's soil onto the windowsill. The lamp switch rotates between my fingers. My computer screen awakens with a simple keystroke. A single wrong number message occupies my voice mail.

In an instant, I am out on the riverwalk behind the building, sitting on a bench. Breathing. Breathing. The water in the Merrimack River flows gently past on its way to the Atlantic, calming my panic. I love the arrival of fall, the deep blue sky and invasion of cooler winds, though they foreshadow coming frosts.

As winter approaches, I already feel a bit snowed-in.

◠ ◡

August 2000. He dumped me. August just arrived, school looming in the not-so-distant future, no writing toward tenure accomplished, no books ordered, no fall syllabi compiled. And he dumped me.

I can't breathe. A year together. Enough time to get attached, despite the circumstances, the clichéd affair. A relationship disappeared, yet still everywhere.

I let him define me in ways I can't even begin to understand. Me: better, smarter, funnier, more capable because of his touch (now, all at once, the *illusion* of his touch). "I never loved you," he writes in a late-night email, as if to erase time and intimacies. And me.

I drink the pain down. A brewery of beer drowning feelings, garbage bags bottle-clinking on walks to the trash cans, a reminder of my failures. Ten years of sobriety gone. I was here before, in my late twenties, when an unplanned pregnancy led to an unwanted abortion and inconsolable grief. I almost killed myself then—and now, again, the feeling resurfaces, obliterating me with its arrival, fed by something inside me and at the bottom of every bottle.

I sob through weekly therapy sessions, a mere month of establishing a relationship with my therapist when August crashes down. Sibylle sits upright in her chair, listening, watching, the signs of a balanced and composed life in her manner and dress, calm and comforting, well manicured. She in counterpoint to my tissue-shredding hysteria, an endless display of neuroses and narcissism, the diagnosed depressive.

"Recovery is a process," she repeats.

⌒ ⌒

September 2000. Miraculously, the syllabi mutate out of old course files. The books order themselves. Classes are taught by an imposter going through the motions of my life.

I am a fraud. I hide in the bathroom, awash in tears, shaking from fear, breathless, panic attacked.

Five minutes to class.

I find necessary refuge in John's office—dear, sweet John, an associate professor of history, a trusted friend. He wears the deer-in-the-headlights look.

"Can you cancel my 11:30 class for me?" I plead, the inability to perform my job manifest in my sobbing, shaking, hyperventilating body.

"Of course," he responds, reaching toward me. "Are you OK?"

"No." I look up at him, desperate to figure out how to get out of the building.

Three weeks later, in a depressed drunken haze, I slice a razor blade down my wrist.

⌒ ⌒

January 2004. Two years ago, I incorporated the first three scenes you just read in my autoethnography, entitled "Chronicling an Academic Depression." Using the methodology of emotional introspection (Ellis, "Sociological Introspection"), this personal narrative detailed my struggle with major depression within the context of my role shift from graduate student to assistant professor of communication at UNH-Manchester.

I wrote my depression story for a variety of reasons: as a therapeutic step toward recovery; to promote understanding of the lived experience of depression, especially for family, friends, and colleagues frustrated by futile attempts to help me; and to encourage the critical exploration of the highly stressful academic culture we create and inhabit. In short, my writing was—and continues to be—motivated by the desire to construct a space for transformative dialogue about depression.

Many kind people have thanked me for sharing my story; they tell me I am "brave" for being so honest. Perhaps I am.

In October 2002, I told my story to a "brown bag lunch" audience of faculty, staff, and students at UNH-Manchester. Two weeks later, I shared it again with colleagues at the National Communication Association's annual conference. In December 2002, "Chronicling an Academic Depression" was published in the *Journal of Contemporary Ethnography.* And now I am writing this companion autoethnography, revisiting stories (slightly edited) from "Chronicling an Academic Depression" and presenting new ones that explore what it means to come out. You see, I am moving forward, but the past still lingers.

Seems I can't stop coming out. Perhaps I need an audience to make my story real.

⌒ ⌒

October 2000. The dean sits at my kitchen table. She seems out of place, her tailored suit uncomfortable in my apartment. I make tea, feigning hospitality and normalcy, then sit across from her, stretching a long sleeve to cover my Band-Aided wrist, the evidence of my half-willed attempt at razor-blade suicide. I feel like a mental patient without the hospital. Clutching my knees to my chest to keep warm, I tug at my shirt sleeve.

Perhaps I shouldn't be hiding the evidence. After all, the razor blades brought the dean here. But I am ashamed.

"We will put you on medical leave effective October 22," she explains. "Don't worry about your classes. We will cover them. Just worry about getting well."

The scene feels surreal. *How did I get here?*

The dean is kind, concerned, careful. She asks a string of questions: "Have you spoken to your therapist?" "Do you think you should go to the hospital?" "Can I do anything to help?"

Yes. No. No.

As she leaves, I hug her, hungry for human affection, to know that I have not disappeared. She feels stiff beneath my arms, or maybe I am just imagining it. I worry that I have gone too far, been unprofessional. This is uncharted territory for both of us.

▷ ◁

November 2001. There are always gaps in the telling. Names withheld. Details left out. Conversations kept in confidence. Secrets protected. Intersecting with other lives as it does, this story isn't only mine to tell. So I can't tell you everything. But that doesn't really matter. The "truth" is still here, the essential elements of my story fitting together in what Spence describes as "an aesthetic finality" (Spence, *Narrative Truth*, 31). You have to trust that I am telling enough.

Committing these details to paper, putting my self on display, sharing my pain with family, friends, and colleagues, risking personal and professional humiliation, I wonder how you will read these stories. After all, some believe depression colors and distorts one's view of reality (Solomon, *The Noonday Demon*). In fact, depression could be described as an illness of perception, interpretation, analysis. Is my story being told through the lens of depression, and if so, what does that mean? Is it less true? Muddled and confused? Warped by my illness? Am I undermining my credibility (as an author, teacher, human being) by the very act of testimony?

Arthur Frank doesn't think so. In *The Wounded Storyteller* he suggests that, like my personal narrative, testimony itself is a construction. "The more that is told," he writes, "the more we are made conscious of remaining on the edge of a silence. . . . Any analysis is always left gazing at what remains in excess of the analyzable. What is testified to remains really real, and in the end what counts are duties toward it" (138).

So what are our "duties" toward my story?

My story is, in many respects, the story of the academy. We talk about the stressors facing junior faculty, the endless demands on our time, our intellects, our emotions. I look at other professors, at UNH and elsewhere, some reaching tenure's promised land, emotionally and intellectually burnt by the process, some maniacally speeding toward tenure, others stalling by the roadside with no rescue in sight. What marks the difference between success and failure? Between coping and crashing? How can we improve what we all know to be an excruciating process?

▷ ◁

November 2000. I spy the clock from beneath my covers. 9 am. 10 am. 11am. Beau and Walter's insistent cat screams drift in from the kitchen into half-waking stress dreams. I am back in boarding school at the age of forty. I can't find the final exam location for a college anthropology class. I can't locate the right NYC subway train to take me home. My mother tries to kill me. I toss and turn under the crushing weight of my down comforter.

"Meow! MEOW!" The cat screams intensify.

I have to feed them.

I slip into my nightshirt, fill cat bowls, move to the couch. Cocooned in the pink blanket. Flooded by tears. Speechless.

The machine answers the phone. "Barbara, it's Kris calling. We're just wondering how you are. Pick up. Barbara? Are you there? Please pick up. We are worried about you. Barbara?" Click.

Again. "Barbara? Hi. This is Sue. Are you there? OK. Call me when you get this message." Click.

Again. Click.

Again. Click.

Time is punctuated by the Lifetime television schedule. *The Golden Girls. Designing Women. Moment of Truth* movies. TNT shows reruns of *ER* three times a day. I push the buttons on the remote from tactile memory, smoke cigarettes, drift.

I consider all the ways I might end my pathetic life: razor blades, car crash, bullet to the brain. Every day I weigh my options. Who would care? But I am too tired to act. They say suicides tend to happen when you are coming out of depression, still caught up in the darkness but energized enough to take action (Solomon), the ultimate irony of recovery. Perhaps the worst is yet to come.

Guilt fogs my thoughts. Canceled classes. Angry students. Disappointed colleagues. The tenure clock stopped. Reputation ruined. My mother's worried voice on the phone, reaching across the miles from Tampa, wishing for any sign of affirmative response. "Are you okay?"

I am living a parenthetical life. An aside. Easily removed. Expendable.

⁀ ⁀

Paraphrased from the *Diagnostic and Statistical Manual of Mental Disorders:* The diagnostic criteria for a Major Depressive Episode require that FIVE (or more) of the following symptoms must be present nearly every day during a two-week period and represent a change from previous functioning. At least ONE of the five symptoms must include (1) or (2).

(1) depressed mood most of the day.

(2) markedly diminished interest or pleasure in all, or almost all, activities most of the day.

(3) significant weight loss when not dieting or weight gain, or decrease or increase in appetite.

(4) insomnia or hypersomnia.

(5) psychomotor agitation or retardation.

(6) fatigue or loss of energy.

(7) feelings of worthlessness or excessive or inappropriate guilt.

(8) diminished ability to think or concentrate, or indecisiveness.

(9) recurrent thoughts of death (not just fear of dying), recurrent suicidal ideation without a specific plan, or a suicide attempt or a specific plan for committing suicide.

November 2000. The cushions of the off-white couch in Sibylle's office sink beneath me. She
sits, slightly above, in her desk chair, asking questions on the insurance company request
form for more sessions, a list of "yes or no" symptoms. "Hopelessness?"

"Yes."

"Guilt?"

"Yes."

"Weight loss?"

"Yes."

"Suicidal ideation?"

"Yes."

YES YES YES YES YES!

"On a scale of one to ten, ten being the worst, how would you rate your depression?"

"Ten."

"At what point on a scale from one to ten would you feel like you will be recovered?

Never.

I pause to consider. "Three."

Depression is a kind of death. The chemistry of my brain unbalanced, betrayed by my
own body, my former self disappeared. Depression has taken her away and in her place is
a stranger I long to know. I grieve my loss, feeling frustrated, angry, sad, and confused, but
mostly scared.

Frank says, "serious illness is a loss of the 'destination and map' that had previously
guided the ill person's life" (1). I have lost perspective. Depression has double-crossed me,
transforming my body, my self, my relationships, destroying my ability to make sense of the
world in ways that used to seem so concrete and certain. I am not the same person I was a
year ago. I struggle to narrate a self that has been altered by disease, to reclaim my body, my
identity, to create a new place in the world.

Depression also brings about a heightened reflexive awareness, a sense of the steps I
take every day to create a habitable reality, a viable self, a livable story. My story feels con-
trived and contingent, a patchwork quilt of perception I stitch together with needle and
thread, trying to make the disparate pieces blend together into a solid whole, a safe and warm
home. I am more fully aware of the ways in which my quilt can unravel at a moment's notice. One of the worst aspects of depression is the ability to watch yourself disappear, unable to act in self-defense.

Time has become both friend and enemy, a paradox. Rebuilding takes time, time also
spent waiting for the other shoe to drop. A recurrence is likely (Kramer, *Listening to Prozac*).
Depression begets depression, my brain chemistry forever altered by past occurrences, an
open invitation to repeat episodes. Then the reclamation process will begin again. Perhaps
I will be better at it next time, more aware of the signs, the resources, the process, my abil-

ity to come out the other side. I see the future as perpetual efforts to keep disintegration at bay, a blend of success and failure. Fear and hope. How do I stop my story from becoming a self-fulfilling prophecy?

Perhaps that nagging sense of fear is what will ultimately protect me.

⌒ ⌒

March 2001. "On a scale of one to ten, ten being the worst . . . ?" Sibylle repeats.

"Seven."

⌒ ⌒

June 2001. Sitting in the dean's office, I wring my hands and twist the silver ring on my finger. My heart beats explosively. We are meeting to discuss my return to school.

"How are you feeling?" she asks.

"Better," I reply. "I'm feeling much better. I'm still trying to figure out what this depression thing is, this amorphous mass of symptoms. It's difficult. But I'm doing some traveling, getting out into the world more. I *am* better." Even as the words leave my mouth and hang in the air between us, I appreciate their insufficiency.

"Are you taking medication?"

"Yes. The antidepressants didn't work for me, but my psychopharmacologist, Dr. Potenza, put me on a low dose of an antipsychotic drug called Seroquel. It has been successful in treating long-term depression. The drug helps me sleep, and keeps my head clearer during the day so I can more rationally respond to stressful situations. It seems to help."

The dean looks at me intently, gathering evidence of my mental state. "Good," she smiles, "but I have to say you don't seem much different from last December. You still seem very anxious to me. As you can imagine, I am concerned about your returning to teach again. We don't want a repeat of last fall."

I swallow hard to absorb the tears. "Nor do I."

She continues. "There is another option. Instead of teaching, there's a possibility of your returning on a part-time basis to do research. We would pay you as an adjunct an amount equal to one-eighth of your salary to reflect the research responsibilities of your tenure-track line. This would give you the chance to ease back into work."

My throat constricts at the thought of research, the toughest, most stressful part of my job. I eke out an "OK."

She looks me right in the eye. "As we make this decision, I want you to consider whether a tenure-track job here, or anywhere else, is what you want. It's not for everybody."

I swallow harder and pause before answering, waiting for the Seroquel to work its magic. "I have thought about that a lot," I admit. Having come to no clear conclusions about my career, I can offer no concrete response. "I am ready to come back."

Did I just lie?

⌒ ⌒

August 2001. "On a scale of one to ten, ten being the worst . . . ?"

"Four."

⌒ ⌒

October 2001. I am supposed to be writing a paper based on my autoethnographic dissertation research about fatherless women like me as part of my agreement with the dean to return to work part-time, one-eighth time—pie time. But I can't. I can't face this work.

A lot of time has passed since I committed anything to paper, since I felt like—acted like—a scholar. Sibylle tells me to envision myself happily, successfully writing so I imagine myself seated at the keyboard, writing with passion, confidence, and the mysterious feeling of gratification that comes with knowing you are saying something of value, something solid and useful. I imagine the words filling the computer screen, poetic and insightful, illuminating. I imagine readers voraciously consuming every word, feeling, thought, idea, comforted and educated by the experience, hungry for more, yet satisfied.

This is the story I want, and need, to write, for other fatherless women and their families, for my sister Laurie, and for myself.

I am scared I can't do it.

⟲ ⟳

When I began my father-absence research five years ago, I *thought* I was examining others' experiences in an effort to understand my own, to heal deep wounds. And I thought I *had* healed. But today, I am not so sure. I can't shake the thought that I made one step forward and fell back three.

I know one thing for sure: I explored fatherlessness to get a Ph.D., and I was successful. I conducted the interviews, wrote the dissertation, and successfully defended my ideas. But on another level, the process was anything but academic. It was heartbreaking, gut-wrenching emotional work, and in the end proved to be less than I had hoped. I satisfied my adviser and my committee, but not myself.

Today, I remain unsatisfied. This nagging sense that I didn't get it right, that I still can't retell these six stories of fatherlessness in a way that comforts them or me or anyone else, paralyzes my efforts to write, to think, to feel. I hide the tales of the six other fatherless women brave enough to share their stories with me in a file cabinet in my office. I hide the "revise and resubmit" letter I received for an article I hastily wrote about one of them in a folder full of my UNHM annual reports. I bury their words, their ideas, their feelings, because I am—to use Ruth Behar's term—the most vulnerable of observers (*The Vulnerable Observer*), afraid of my own emotions. Perhaps I am trying to bury my father, an act that (at least today) feels cowardly and still, after a lifetime, premature. Writing will be like a funeral, the funeral for Walter Cooke Jago, Jr. that we never had. Like burying the living.

I can't do it.

⟲ ⟳

Another story begs to be told: my depression story.

Once I start writing, I can't stop.

⟲ ⟳

October 2001. When Erin pokes her head into my office, I am momentarily unable to make an identification, her short brown hair now long, her younger face more mature. But as an unmistakable smile breaks across her face, I jump out of my chair.

"Hi Erin!" I blurt out, reaching to hug her.

"I have *missed* you!" she says, taking a seat on my couch. "How *are* you?"

Talking to Erin, a familiar sense of self returns, an old friend. I have been here before, talking to a favorite student, listening to the details of her life, offering advice. But this time is different. I am not the same person who sat in this chair a year ago.

When I left school last fall, the dean and I decided to be forthright about the reasons, a strategy to quell potential rumors, but more important, a way to bring the unspoken illness of depression out into the open. For Erin, my revelation offered comfort. She too struggles with depression, though in her case depression is coupled with periods of mania.

I feel unsure about how to progress, how much of my personal life to share with this student. Again, I find myself negotiating that fine line between respected professor and vulnerable human being. Does her knowing the gory details about my struggle with depression enhance or hinder our relationship as student and teacher?

Quickly, we are into depression-speak, that intimate and comforting conversation between people who know life on the backstage of depression. I can't *not* talk to her.

Erin tells me about her life as a manic-depressive. "I tried nine different drugs before I found the right one," she explains. "Zoloft saved my life."

"I wish antidepressants worked for me," I say, and then I hear myself narrating my experiences of the past year—the guilt over abandoning my students, my months on the couch, the alcohol, an anxiety-laden return to school. The words gush out of me. "I'm so happy to be back. But at the same time, I worry people don't see me the same way. I am not the same person. For a year I have lived as 'Depression Barbara' and now I am fighting my way back to 'Professor Barbara,' unsure how the two might coexist. But perhaps there is no way back, the Professor Barbara I once knew gone forever. I don't know who will take her place, and where depression will fit in."

"I know," Erin jumps in. "When I first heard my diagnosis—manic-depression—I freaked! It sounded so big, so scary. To take on that label . . ." her words drift off.

I nod in recognition. Throughout the past year I have wished for a brain tumor, cancer, anything but a "mental illness." Despite the substantial efforts of the mental health community to educate the public about depression, many people still don't understand. Not surprising. Depression has a long history of shifting meanings, ongoing debates as to its causes: weakness of character, traumatic experiences, heredity, sexual repression, chemical imbalances, sin. A vague entity, depression still has no clear physical manifestations, no simple diagnostic test run on a blood sample, no concrete definition—and no clear-cut treatment. The doctors can cut out a brain tumor, rid the body of cancer cells with chemotherapy and radiation, but can they rid the mind, body, and soul of depression? And if they can, how can you be sure when it is gone?

People fear what they don't know and can't understand. "Depression is a disorder of mood," William Styron writes in *Darkness Visible: A Memoir of Madness,*

> so mysteriously painful and elusive in the way it becomes known to the self—
> to the mediating intellect—as to verge close to being beyond description. It
> thus remains nearly incomprehensible to those who have not experienced it in

its extreme mode, although the gloom, "the blues" which people go through occasionally and associate with the general hassle of everyday existence are of such
prevalence that they do not give many individuals a hint of the illness in its cata-
strophic form. (Styron, 7)

Over the past few years, not a week has gone by when I have not heard someone say, "I am depressed." Recent decades have turned "depression" into a catch-all phrase for everything from
sadness and melancholy to a full mental meltdown into madness. Pathologizing sadness not
only condones the (over-)prescription of antidepressant medications but also, and perhaps
more dangerously, reinforces the unattainable American dream of perpetual happiness.

So I am left wondering: What is normal? What marks the lines between everyday sadness and depression, and how far across that line have I gone? How did I get here? Am I the
victim of a troubled childhood? Heredity? Have I committed some unpardonable sin? Am
I lazy? *Crazy?* Crazy scares me, the view of me as unstable, incapable, incurable.

A few months after I was born, my mother was hospitalized for schizophrenia. The
year was 1960. They doused her with electro-shock and insulin coma therapies, and a year
later sent her home. She was fine, and the condition never recurred. Forty years later, we
believe she suffered from postpartum depression, a grossly misdiagnosed condition for
women of her generation. But even my mother's lifelong best friend, my godmother Jean,
with her Ph.D. in English and staunch feminist ideology, still describes my mother as a little
bit "crazy." Did I inherit Mom's madness?

Erin shifts her legs, and I am back in the moment. "Depression—the weight of the
word is overwhelming," I tell Erin, shaking my head. "How do you ever get out from underneath it?"

We both know the question is rhetorical. If we can't even articulate what depression
feels like, how can we expect others to understand?

June 2002. "Barb, whuddya get?" Ed's words evoke a familiar refrain. He sits in his cart, stubby
green eraserless pencil in hand, recording our golf scores.

I wince and try to cover with a joke. "I parred the hole, two maybe three times."

Later and again. "Barb, whuddya get?"

"Too much!"

Quick evasions on this glorious summer afternoon divulge my fear of the permanent
record—*my* permanent record. Test scores. Course grades. GPAs. Even golf scores. All marked
down somewhere, forever, available for the asking.

Tenure is all about evaluation. Assessment. Judgment. And it haunts the lives of assistant professors. Student evaluations. Annual evaluations. Manuscript reviews. Third-year
evaluations. You feel as if you must constantly be on guard, always playing to the evalua-
tors. I feel like I am back in junior high, desperately wanting everyone to like me but coming up ridiculously short.

So when I received *The Journal of Contemporary Ethnography* reviewer comments on
my story three weeks ago, I could barely read them. More evaluation. And this time on a
manuscript into which I poured my heart and mind. My stomach did flip turns, but a looming deadline gave me the courage.

One very concerned and compassionate reviewer cautioned me against going public with my story because of the possible damage posed to my career by the stigma of depression. (This reviewer also asked the editor to consider the responsibility of a journal to protect its authors.) Another reviewer voiced concern for those whose personal experiences were contained within my story, especially Erin. Was I outing Erin without her consent? In short, these reviewers were asking me to consider the ethics of autoethnography.

You can't do "good" autoethnographic work without constantly questioning the ethics of your pursuit. As soon as you put that "I" on the page, you can't avoid asking if your revelations might be harmful to you or anyone else. So I have thought a lot about ethics and about my motives for publishing this story.

And, of course, there are no clear answers.

Perhaps publishing my story is just another way of slitting my wrists, trying to sabotage my career by boldly wearing the label of mental illness. The stigma associated with depression is very real; I have seen it in the eyes of friends, students, and colleagues. If I am being self-destructive (a quality I have clearly exhibited in this story), then perhaps the reviewer is more than justified in his/her efforts to protect me (and others like me) from myself.

Perhaps. But I don't think so. There's a difference between taking a razor blade to your arm and risking the social stigma of depression.

I have spent a great deal of time examining my motives, and I keep coming back to the same thought. If publishing this story does damage to my career, if some react by questioning my credibility as an author, my capacity to teach, my mental stability, then I believe that's the best reason to publish my story. Being depressed means that I (and others like me) face a particular set of emotional challenges which make my life extremely painful and difficult at times. Being depressed *doesn't* mean I am untrustworthy, incapable, or crazy.

If I am writing for any reason, it is to demystify and demythologize depression; the best way to promote understanding and fight ignorance is to speak out, to make my version of the story part of the permanent record. Everyone represented in these pages (especially Erin) has read this story and agrees.

⌒ ⌒

January 2002. Coming out the other side of this major depressive episode, I am a different person in a new place. I don't see the world or myself in the same way. Solomon tells us that "depressives have seen the world *too clearly* [my italics], have lost the selective advantage of blindness" (Solomon, 434). When I began writing this story four months ago, I described depression as an illness of perception, a warping of one's *normal* capacity for interpretation and analysis. Now I am not so sure.

Depression offers me an opportunity to glimpse a reality beyond what Peter Berger and Thomas Luckmann describe as the paramount reality of everyday life, to become more acutely aware of the ways in which we craft lived experience into meaningful and livable stories, to take the blinders off. As I read what I have written here, I am reminded of the myriad ways available to us to construct our stories and our realities, and the profound implications those constructions have for our lives. What constitutes a livable narrative? Have I created one for myself here? To what degree have I bought into the dominant medical discourse, the canonical story of depression, which strands me in the midst of this ongoing battle with mental illness? In what other ways might I narrate this experience?

Of course, these are questions without answers. I embrace them, taking comfort in the words of the German poet Rainer Maria Rilke: "be patient toward all that is unsolved in your heart and try to love the *questions themselves* like locked rooms and like books that are written in a very foreign tongue. Do not seek the answers, which cannot be given to you because you would not be able to live them. And the point is, to live everything. *Live* the questions now. Perhaps you will then gradually, without noticing it, live along some distant day into the answer" (Rilke, *Letters,* 35).

September 2003. Thirty faces from my Introduction to Interpersonal Communication class stare at me from six neatly arranged rows of desks. My students have just finished introducing themselves: name, major, reason for taking the course. I stand in the front of the room, framed by the white board at my back, ready to deliver my "first day of class" autobiography.

"You are going to *love* this course," I tell my students with arrogant self-assurance. "Let me say that again: You are going to *LOVE* this course! *Trust me!*

I lean against the teacher's desk, and then slide into sitting position. My black heeled shoes kick back and forth through the air. I grasp the desk's edge with both hands, pushing up just slightly, cross my legs, and smile. "So, why *should you* trust me? Why should you listen to *anything* I have to say?"

And then I begin my story: "I was born outside NYC, in a town called North Tarrytown." I narrate my childhood, my years in boarding school and college, my graduate work in cinema studies, education, and communication. I talk about my family, my friends, my boyfriends, the ups and downs of my close relationships. "After I earned my Ph.D. in 1998, I came to UNH-Manchester," I say, moving into the present. "Then, two years later, in the fall of 2000, I left school on medical leave for major depression. I was a mess. I tried every antidepressant on the market and none of them worked. What *did* work was talking to a therapist, and talking, and talking, and talking. In the spring of 2002, I returned to the classroom, a much stronger person, and have been here ever since." I pause, looking from face to face, careful to make eye contact with every student. "I love my job! I get paid *the big bucks* to discuss relationships with the *best* students in the world."

I scan the room for reactions, always fearful of lost credibility. Some students smile and nod. Some wiggle in their seats, avoiding eye contact. Some stare back blankly.

Every semester I come out to a new group of students. And every semester, at the end of our first class, at least one student always lingers behind. "I just wanted to . . . ," the student begins, shifting weight from one foot to the other, pausing just a little *too* long. "I . . . ahhhh . . . I just wanted to thank you for talking about your depression."

"You are very welcome," I say, smiling with as much warmth as I can possibly convey.

Then I hear *another* depression story, reminding me that *every* story makes a difference.

REFERENCES

American Psychiatric Association. *Diagnostic and Statistical Manual of Mental Disorders, Fourth Edition.* Washington DC: American Psychiatric Association, 1994.

Behar, Ruth. *The Vulnerable Observer.* Boston: Beacon Press, 1996.

Berger, Peter. L., and Thomas Luckmann. *The Social Construction of Reality: A Treatise in the Sociology of Knowledge.* New York: Anchor, 1966.

Boice, Robert. "New Faculty as Teachers." *Journal of Higher Education* 62 (2) (1991): 150–173.

Ellis, Carolyn. "Sociological Introspection and Emotional Experience." *Symbolic Interaction* 14 (1991): 23–50.

Frank, Arthur. *The Wounded Storyteller: Body, Illness, and Ethics.* Chicago: University of Chicago Press, 1995.

Karp, David. A. *Speaking of Sadness: Depression, Disconnection, and the Meanings of Illness.* New York: Oxford University Press, 1996.

Kramer, Peter. *Listening to Prozac: A Psychiatrist Explores Antidepressant Drugs and the Remaking of the Self.* New York: Penguin, 1993.

Rilke, Rainer Maria. *Letters to a Young Poet.* New York: Norton, 1934.

Ronai, Carol R. "Multiple Reflections of Child Sex Abuse." *Journal of Contemporary Ethnography* 23 (1995): 395–425.

Solomon, Andrew. *The Noonday Demon: An Atlas of Depression.* New York: Scribner, 2001.

Spence, Donald. *Narrative Truth and Historical Truth: Meaning and Interpretation in Psychoanalysis.* New York: Norton, 1982.

Styron, William. *Darkness Visible: A Memoir of Madness.* New York: Vintage, 1990.

QUESTIONS

1. Characterize the structure of this narrative. Why did the author structure it in this way? How does the structure inform your understanding of her depression?

2. The author makes the point that her credibility might be compromised by her depression. How? Do you agree? Why or why not?

3. What does it mean to "come out" about an illness? What does the author risk by doing so? What do she and others gain?

4. What is the role of authoethnography in scholarly inquiry? How does it relate to quantitative research methods? to other forms of qualitative research?

5. How might academic culture be changed to make the tenure process more manageable for junior faculty? What can junior faculty do to successfully negotiate the tenure process? What can senior faculty and administration do to assist junior faculty?

Invisible Disorder
Passing as an Academic

⬿ HILARY CLARK ⬾

It was the summer of '67, summer of the Hollies and Van Morrison. She was the Brown-Eyed Girl, but no making love in the long grass; she was no one's girl, too young and too plain for the Summer of Love. Twelve years old, having returned to Vancouver after two years in London, England, she was a grammar-school girl in white knee socks and navy cardigan, and home no longer felt like home. She wore a child's vest over barely-there breasts, soft buds, no bleeding yet. Her former girlfriends were strangers—short cut-offs, dirty bra straps, mascara and eye-shadow—Monique and Barb in the tree house, smoking cigarettes and comparing their rings from Kenny and Kurt (Kurt on probation and Kenny picked up by the cops again). Her stomach was sinking, skin cold with sweat, as cold as when the Thoughts came, unstoppable, rolling round and round her head as she lay curled on her bed—"may kill myself, kill myself"—while her mother broke down and really did try to die, singing and moaning and running out of the house, and the girl locked her bedroom door, especially at night. On foghorn nights there was a stranger in her mirror who sometimes stepped through. Her father, a psychologist, called it "depersonalization" (apparently normal), but once at school it lasted all day: the stranger sat in the girl's desk conjugating French verbs, and at noon finished her lunch without her.

⬿ ⬾

How can I remember that summer of '67, the early teen years? What really happened? The obsessive, repetitive thoughts, the anxieties, the emptying of self—yes, and the foghorn moments—but the woman stepping through the mirror is pure gothic, a genre that has always appealed to me. I've written dark poems about that other girl or woman, who speaks in my mouth and writes my words, who would appear in my room as I lay between sleep and awakening. She is a fiction haunting my poetry and yet also a real aspect of the dis-ease that began at puberty, as I lost my mother (for some years) to mental illness and gained a body and face that were never good enough—not busty enough, not sparkly white-teeth pretty like Midge flirting with Kenny at the front of the row in math. I was a serious, studious girl who would cringe at her father crying (did he cry?) and her mother screaming, and would

escape to her friends' homes to drink tea and envy them their families. There are holes in
my memory, rips and tears.

$$\LARGE \sim \sim$$

*At fifteen, she was prettier. She took up the classical guitar and a boyfriend, discovering the
pleasures of arpeggios, tremolos and kissing. She would take her guitar on baby-sitting nights
and practice études after the children fell asleep. She would prowl the house for secrets, opening
drawers and kitchen cupboards, exploring bookshelves—eating, looking, reading—one night
discovering a book of art erotica (phallic Greek youths) tucked away. Her body was dangerous.
She had drawn boundaries, though her boyfriend's mouth and hands made her swoon. Her
employer, a balding psychiatrist, would drive her home in the family Volvo and in the darkness
advise her on the arts of pleasure: "You're a young girl, don't study so much, have fun with the
boys, make love . . ." It was the year of "Brown Sugar" and "After Midnight," parties of dark,
sweaty dancing and mattresses on the floor. But she had locked up her room and her body, so
she'd climb firmly out of the Volvo and shut the door.*

*At nineteen, in the autumn of 1974, she took a year off from university and did the Grand
Tour of Europe. In her North American outfit of blue ski jacket and orange backpack, often traveling alone, she was highly visible—and vulnerable to older men, who would follow her, call to
her in English and abuse her in their own language, follow her onto the subway train at night,
grope her breasts as they passed in a jostling crowd. Angry, aware of her sexual power, she spent
the autumn months seducing men. In castles, cafés, and art museums, through Amsterdam,
Paris, Venice, and Florence, her real itinerary was erotic—making a conquest at a hostel, boarding a train with him to arrive in a new city late at night, find a cheap room, and wake up in the
morning under a stranger. Many years later a psychiatrist told her this was a manic phase, but
at the time she only knew desire—life was vivid, risky; she wanted to be in over her head.*

$$\LARGE \sim \sim$$

Depression narratives frequently include a "first-time" story, like the story of losing one's
virginity. When did I first know something was not right? When did I first turn to doctors?
In his book *Speaking of Sadness*, David Karp suggests that most depression stories follow a
"career" in which "inchoate feelings" of a problem, one's difference from others, thicken to
the point where the sufferer thinks, "Something is *really* wrong with me" (57) and decides to
seek help. Of the beginnings of my own depressive "career," however, I can remember little. I
think I was eighteen—or twenty, or twenty-one—and the doctor (a psychiatrist? psychologist?) was with the student health service at my university. All I remember of him was that
he was killed later in a car crash in Portugal. Such are memory's quirks. I remember a sunny
day, picnicking with friends in a park overlooking Burrard Inlet, and being unable to sit down
and eat—walking and walking, feeling utter dread because I was not myself but someone
else; I was no longer able to pass as myself. Fears of "losing it," losing myself—through long
days of struggling to breathe and speak—continued on and off throughout my undergraduate years. Then one day, walking into the campus pub behind a dark-haired Englishman,
I knew my future husband and thought I might be free. But when we married three years
later, depression persisted; my fears dimmed our California honeymoon, our long walks on
Stinson Beach. My bedside reading was Lowen's *Depression and the Body*.

Almost every narrative of depression includes a first encounter with medication, usu-ally the first of many. In *Speaking of Sadness*, Karp shows, through the words of his respon-dents, that the process of accepting antidepressants into one's life is rarely a straightforward one (78–103). There is often resistance at first to the idea of relying on pills, especially for a "mental" condition. The old stigmas are still powerful, even while doctors draw analogies with diabetes and high blood pressure, and the drug companies push Paxil and Effexor in the media, promising new birth and life. When was I first told I would need medication for depression? What were my feelings? I cannot remember. During my two M.A. years in Toronto I began attending a therapy group, but when, with the therapist's encouragement, people collapsed on the floor and began screaming, I ran outside and never returned. I must have accepted medication (like accepting the Lord) after that. I do remember that the old antidepressants made my mouth dry. Even more than before, I felt I wasn't myself. Identity is definitely at stake in taking psychiatric medications, as the brain with its defective neu-rotransmitters is the house of the self, the memories that make up a life's story. Although doctors may argue that antidepressants can save, giving the sufferer a taste of her true self once more, not every patient is a believer at first. But the misery usually makes one cave in, especially if one has children who are frightened. Especially if one has children.

And so through my doctoral years I wrote comprehensive exams, papers and dissertation chapters, began teaching, and went on and off antidepressants laced with Valium and wine. I went off meds during my pregnancies; I didn't need them anyway. My pregnant body was invincible, a glowing shield of well-being. When, six months into my first pregnancy, I went into premature labour, I was confident my baby and I would pull through. But after thirty-six hours of misdiagnosed labour, after rejecting with a great heave the labour-suppressing drug they finally gave me, I gave birth to my oldest son in an emergency Caesarean. He was quickly lifted out and whisked away. He was born with purple bruises all down one side of his tiny body, the consequence of sharing his mother with a baby-sized tumor—this thing I had to carry for six more months until, finally, it was surgically removed and found to be benign. For three of those months my son lived in hospital nurseries, and I grew to know motherhood as loss: in the first days, weeping as the mother in the next bed nursed her full-term baby ("Oh, I have too much milk!"); then pumping what milk I could and taking it into hospital, only to have it deposited in the Milk Bank for other preemies until my son could take a little through a tube. Or having to watch as he howled silently in his Plexiglas box, the monitor above flashing *apnea, apnea*. Since that first child, I have had two more; my second and third babies were full-term and blessedly ready to nurse. The milk must have magically shielded me, for in each case depression didn't return for a time.

☙   ❧

In the Department of Women's and Gender Studies at my university, I occasionally teach a course entitled "Women, Depression, and Writing." What we teach is intimately connected with our history and our lives; that is why, although I would ardently wish to be free of this illness, I teach this material. Sometimes the course is hard on the students, who are almost always women and frequently depressed. Each time, one or two flame out, can't finish the course, and sometimes end up in hospital. (I always give them fair warning on the first day of class.) I am usually relieved when the course is over, and wonder why on earth I don't work in another area—medieval manuscripts, cyborg studies, anything. But it always comes around to gender and women's lives, which press upon everything I choose to read, write, and teach.

In the course, we read life writing and poems by women who have suffered from depression or manic-depression. We look at what may account for the fact that across many cultures twice as many women are sufferers, as men. One issue that often comes up is the link between motherhood and depression: in the form of postpartum depression, certainly, but more generally in the very real fear and melancholy that a new mother may feel over her loss of former identity, which feels like a loss of self. The discrepancy between her own conflicted experience and the cruel myth of the blissful madonna creates unnecessary shame and suffering, can make a woman ill—as we read Nancy Mairs's "On Living behind Bars," for example, in which the author recounts her own experience as a young mother who, unable to function at home, signs herself into a psychiatric hospital. In the course, we also look at the ways in which, through writing their own lives, women can come to terms with their suffering, with the meanings of diagnosis and/or medication. We explore the role of writing in negotiating the sentence (life-sentence, often) of depression, and in revisioning the self under its shadow.

At eighteen I began to scratch small self-conscious poems into small black notebooks, and continued intermittently through my undergraduate years as an English student. (The young men I adored sat smoking in cafés, frowning over shabby notebooks.) However, graduate school put an end to this nonsense. As I was switching to comparative literature, I had to extend and deepen my French, learn Spanish, read in several literatures and digest theory—at that time structuralism, semiotics, deconstruction, and psychoanalysis. The Russian formalists and Prague structuralists ruined my eyes for good; the French surrealists were more fun but made my occasional stabs at poetry seem pathetic. After defending my dissertation, however, and embarking on an ill-paying career as sessional lecturer in English, I soon knew what I had to do. With a hyperactive four-year-old (our former preemie) and a toddler daughter, money anxieties, piles of first-year essays to mark, and a bad case of teaching nerves, I began to feel hopeless; there was no end in sight. So it was back to the doctors and meds again. Then one October evening I opened the back door and heard geese honking overhead; looking up at them I knew that, to survive, I had to begin writing seriously again. That was a beginning I *do* remember.

In 1990 I snagged a tenure-stream job in English at the University of Saskatchewan, and felt as optimistic as when I first saw my husband; from now on, I thought, I'll be *fine*. From an itinerant sessional life, driving miles to teach first-year lit and comp at three different campuses, I moved into a job which included start-up funds for research, a pension, interesting courses at the senior and graduate levels and, most importantly, the privilege of teaching in one place. I stopped the meds I had relied on while finishing the dissertation and teaching in Vancouver, and put doctors behind me forever. I worked very hard, got my probation renewed, had a third child (taking one month off), published the articles I needed for tenure, got tenure and got promoted—in short, leaped through all the hoops, rushing home to take over from the babysitter, feed the baby, then head back out for night class. But in my late thirties, I began to buzz. Exhausted from being awakened through the night by a wandering toddler, I was writing poems full of night alarms, fires, babies shrouded and shut away in drawers. My credit card debts were rising as I sent off for more and more books and bought far too many new clothes. I began to get erotically restless, admiring male students and developing crushes at conferences. Finally, I fell in love, and the whole makeshift structure of my life crashed down.

I nursed my obsession for several years, and my marriage came close to breaking. The crash brought back darkness and paralysis, the old feelings of unreality. Finding a doctor, I finally received a diagnosis that made some sense—mild bipolar disorder—and medication that seemed to work: an antidepressant combined with a mood stabilizer. But what I could not swallow was the idea that my romantic feelings (like my European trysts twenty years earlier) had been merely a manic symptom. My poems were full of tears and ice, frozen rivers, earthquakes and collapsing houses. As poets have known for centuries, there is nothing like unrequited love to inspire poetry. Indeed, a dam burst. After four years, two books of my poetry were published in the same month, and I was well on my way into a third book. Since then, I have slowed down considerably in poetic production, and I wince at the florid, over-written grief. I have become comfortably numb, as Pink Floyd would say, on a long-term combination of meds, with only the occasional really bad day. I imagine I will be on the meds forever and ever. My psychiatrist finally sent me away several years ago, advising me to get my prescriptions from the family doctor. I had told and retold all the stories of my past; now it was time to "get on" with the present.

☞ ☜

I taught "Women, Depression, and Writing" again last fall term. This time we read Kay Redfield Jamison's *An Unquiet Mind*, a woman's memoir of coming to terms with manic depression and a life sentence of lithium. The book has a great deal of resonance for me because the author is an academic, a professor of psychiatry who wrote an important textbook on manic depression while suffering from the illness herself. She recounts the mood cycles—cosmic highs and infernal lows—characterizing her life as a sufferer, particularly dwelling on the excesses of mania, "unbridled and intense moods" (212) she recalls quite wistfully, now that she is safely medicated. My female students were very taken with her stories of swept-away love affairs and erotic adventures, though they hooted at the Harlequin-romance language in which she recounts them. Jamison speaks of the difficulty of "coming out" (not to mention speaking out) as an academic with "this quick-silver illness," manic depression (7)—especially in her particular profession, where besides teaching and supervisory duties, she must take responsibility for patients who are as ill as she herself has been: "My major concerns about discussing my illness . . . have tended to be professional in nature. . . . I worry . . . about my colleagues' reactions once I am open about my illness. . . . It is an awful prospect, giving up one's cloak of academic objectivity" (202–3). Despite these worries and the particularly pressing issue of whether she ought to apply for clinical privileges, she is determined to come out once and for all because, as she puts it, "I am tired of hiding, tired of misspent and knotted energies, tired of the hypocrisy, and tired of acting as though I have something to hide" (7).

Indeed, there is no illness, except perhaps AIDS, that bears the shame still attached to mental illness and that is hidden so well in the academy. Even the most highly educated academics shy away from those lonely souls who frequent campuses and can be seen drifting about clutching textbooks, gesturing and nodding. Sometimes I am asked what I am working on as research. Upon answering, "Narratives of mental illness," I have seen unabashed shudders and heard comments such as, "I wouldn't go there!"

With an invisible disability, a mental disorder controlled with medication, I too find it difficult to pass as an academic. I must struggle against a continuing low-grade (or sometimes excruciating) melancholy, a pain experienced somatically as a weight on the chest, frequent headaches, backaches and stomach cramps. These symptoms are mixed with a handful of low-grade manic symptoms such as irritability, distractibility, and racing thoughts, finished off with a pinch of OCD in behaviours repeated to the point of distress. Teaching has become easier over the years, but it is still quite often an ordeal. On bad days I dread looking at the class and have to force myself to speak in a breathless, heavy monotone. On good days I "cook" but can go too fast, rabbiting off into digressions and inappropriate disclosures. Research is still a pleasure although, locked in a pattern of obsessive procrastination and self-subversion, I end up throwing away opportunities for conference presentations and publications. When I do get down to work, I juggle at least ten things at once, starting projects and leaving them unfinished—an unproductive approach, and unfortunately one that the present "multitasking" academic environment only emphasizes further.

The present humanities research culture in Canadian universities is geared to and rewards a particular kind of academic: highly focused, organized, ambitious, skilled at writing grant applications and at coordinating large, collaborative programs of research employing a significant number of graduate students—in other words, programs based on the science model. Academics in the humanities who work more digressively, who follow where their interests take them, value serendipity, and do not want to plan five or more years ahead—who prefer to write individual articles, poetry or novels, or scholarly books based on solitary research and unconnected to grantsmanship—these members of the profession find the going harder now, I think. Academics like myself, who struggle with mood disorders, invisible disabilities of the mind, find themselves at even more of a disadvantage in this academic culture of relentless energy, forward-focus and able-mindedness.

It seems to me, in other words, that no one thinks much about the subtle and not-so-subtle exclusions of mental illness from the academy, even while disability advocates are becoming increasingly vocal and politicized, and disability studies are properly taking their place in the curricula of the humanities and social sciences. We are the silent sufferers, whose exclusion or marginalization is rarely recognized. When we identify ourselves, there is discomfort. If we were to request concessions (extra assistance with marking, for instance, or extra time to write papers) similar to those our disabled students apply for (Braille, note-takers, extra time to write exams), the reaction would undoubtedly be hostile, with the unspoken question, "What are you doing in this job, then, if you can't cut it like the rest of us?"

In her essay "On Being Ill" (1930), Virginia Woolf writes evocatively of the critical distance from everyday life that illness brings to the sufferer:

... in health the genial pretence must be kept up and the effort renewed—to communicate, to civilize, to share, to cultivate the desert, educate the native, to work together by day and by night to sport. In illness this make-believe ceases. Directly the bed is called for ... we cease to be soldiers in the army of the upright; we become deserters. They march to battle. We float with the sticks on the stream ... irresponsible and disinterested and able, perhaps for the first time for years, to look round ... (196)

Here Woolf is likely drawing on her own recurrent bouts of manic-depression, but she is also referring to illness in general, and to the ill as subversives. I like the active quality Woolf gives to illness here—how it forces one to cease the daily "genial pretence," to lie back and "look round" at the status quo with a "disinterested," even a critical, eye. Woolf's emphasis on illness as a temporary stay in the mindless "battle" of everyday life suggests that the margins are not a bad place to be, allowing one insights, perhaps, that those who are healthy and unthinkingly "functional" may never have.

Like other disabilities, mental illness occupies such a marginal position in the academy, the sufferer is able, often jolted, into looking around even as he or she must continue in the "make-believe," marching in the daily battle to produce, produce, produce. The little slights, the feelings of shame, are worth it if they mark a critical distance. Or so I assure my youngest son, now twelve, whose ongoing ADHD characteristics—constant physical restlessness, inability to concentrate, tendency to interrupt and say inappropriate things—leave him vulnerable to impatience of his teacher and his principal, and to his classmates' teasing and bullying. As I watch him endure the anxieties that darkened my twelfth year, I assure him that he will grow up to be a very special person. Inwardly, I wish him freedom from the battle. Inwardly, I wish him peace.

⁕   ⁕

She was a little girl who loved storms, relished the strange green light that preceded them and the winds that would spring up, swishing the cedars and whirling up scraps of paper around her. Electrified with excitement, she would watch the thunderheads massing. Jumping up and down, up and down, she wished she had an umbrella so she could fly away like Mary Poppins over the treetops. She didn't know that it is unwise to put up an umbrella in a lightning storm—and a good thing, too, as she was learning to fly, and the wind and the lightning would lift her and set her down, gently, on the other side.

REFERENCES

Jamison, Kay Redfield. *An Unquiet Mind: A Memoir of Moods and Madness.* New York: Vintage Books, 1995.

Karp, David. *Speaking of Sadness: Depression, Disconnection, and the Meanings of Illness.* New York: Oxford University Press, 1996.

Lowen, Alexander. *Depression and the Body: The Biological Basis of Faith and Reality.* New York: Coward, McCann & Geoghegan, 1972.

Mairs, Nancy. "On Living behind Bars." *Plaintext*, 125–54. Tucson: University of Arizona Press, 1986.

Woolf, Virginia. "On Being Ill." *Collected Essays,* 4:193–203. London: The Hogarth Press, 1966.

QUESTIONS

1. What is the relationship between the author's illness and her writing?

2. Why do sufferers write personal narratives about depression? Why should one read them?

3. Is mental illness as stigmatized as the author claims? Come up with some examples and/or counter-examples from your experience.

4. Where should universities "draw the line" regarding faculty with mental illness? Who should draw this line?

The Manic-Depressive Professor

⌒ Rebecca Hogan ⌒

I.

I can't resist telling the story of my breakdown first, because the way it happened and the shape it took are so closely linked to my profession as an academic. My husband and I had just returned from the Modern Language Association Convention in Washington D.C., a meeting where thousands of English and foreign language professors gather to give and hear papers, meet old friends from other universities, and make professional connections of various kinds. In the last few weeks of the semester, the department had been working on a set of new personnel rules delineating how much one had to publish, how many conference papers one had to give, and how many committees one had to serve on to get tenure and promotion. This had been a stressful time, and I had become more and more irritable—because I always hate these bureaucratic procedures for judging colleagues, I thought. I later realized my irritation was also a result of hypomania that presaged a later depressive attack. It was a relief to get away to Washington. But when we got back and began the preparations for the semester, I noticed that the symptoms of depression, which I had suffered from twice before, seemed to be coming back. Particularly horrible were the sleeplessness and the inability to concentrate on a book or piece of writing. If I couldn't read and write, how could I do my job? I remember a chilling incident when my husband and I were talking to a friend on the phone and I asked her, "Is this phone being tapped? Is this conversation being recorded?" She responded with calm self-control that it wasn't, that I probably was overhearing some sounds from her art studio, but what must she have thought? This conversation was a harbinger of things to come. I called my general practitioner and made an appointment to see about going back on Prozac, which had helped me greatly in an earlier depression. But the day before my appointment, the depression I had been trying to fight off struck with overpowering force.

As I paced up and down the hall of our house, too restless to sit, filled with a bottomless sense of misery, I began to imagine how to kill myself. I thought of the Roundup plant killer in the garage. It was a bitterly cold January day, and I imagined simply walking out in the snow and lying down under a bush to freeze to death. I took out of the drawer, but did not use, a large sharp butcher knife. All the while a complete paranoid fantasy took shape

131

in my head in which my colleagues in the English department—my dearest friends, most challenging conversationalists, warmest supporters of my work—became a bunch of investigators, watching my every move, seeking to show me up as a bad teacher, a bad writer, a fake scholar, in short as the phony professor. As my husband drove me first to the doctor and then into the hospital in Madison, I thought I saw the faces of fellow professors in trucks or cars that pulled in from side roads or passed us on the main road. These were really, I suppose, hallucinations. They seemed so real.

As we pulled into the emergency room entrance (it was now night), I was sure that a person I saw hurrying toward the door and lighting a cigarette was one of my colleagues. Once I had agreed to be hospitalized and began my ten-day stay, I did not want to see any colleagues because of my paranoia. I now became sure that the hospital staff was part of the conspiracy, monitoring my phone calls, watching me with cameras hidden in the shower head, the thermostat, and the exercise machine. Despite my fantasies of total surveillance, I managed to be out of the sight of the nurses long enough to swallow six thin, half-inch nails that came with a coaster frame kit I had been given in occupational therapy to give me something to do over the weekend. I can't even get back now the sense of whether I actually wanted to die, but I spent the next two days in a total suicide watch mode, sleeping with round convex mirrors (like the ones used to track shoplifters) trained on me and subjected to much checking. Fortunately, I did not include my husband or my two sisters in the conspiracy and therefore had someone to trust during this miserable time.

After a course of antipsychotic medication to control my "suspicious" thoughts, and the lithium and Prozac appropriate to my now accurately diagnosed bipolar disorder, I began to recover my balance and was able to leave the hospital. When in the throes of depression you cannot see yourself truly any more than you can be yourself fully, yet the illness is part of you. Some of the people I met in the hospital thought Jesus talked to them. I wonder whether the content of one's paranoia is always affected by the mental furniture she has available to her. In the film *A Beautiful Mind*, John Nash thought the CIA was sending him messages through the newspapers. In government-funded science, it would make a weird kind of sense to think you're being followed and monitored by the CIA. So he was crazy, but the content of his craziness made perfect sense. I think the same might be true of me. The manic-depression is caused by a chemical or genetic flaw in the brain (serotonin levels), but the form the madness takes is an expression of my identity, personality, and culture.

II.

Another aspect of "becoming" a manic-depressive has been the development of a whole new area of professional interest. For thirty years, I've studied autobiography and with my husband have coedited a scholarly journal, *a/b: Auto/Biography Studies,* which has been in existence since 1985. But now, because of our personal situation, we've expanded into something new which we, who have collaborated on several conference papers and one published essay on it, laughingly call "nut-case autobiographies." Because of my personal experience, I am less inclined to see mental illness as romantic rebellion, or as an example of the postmodern playful fragmentedness of identity. And I'm fascinated by the question of what role illness plays in identity. In our essay, we quote therapist Martha Manning, who captures the disturbing consequences of pathologized identity when she hears a patient referred to in a case conference as a "thirty-five year old manic-depressive":

> I think about the difference between *having* something and *being* something. They are only words, but I'm struck by how much they convey about the manner in which the shorthand of illness reduces the essence of people in ways that labels for other serious illnesses do not.
>
> People say "I have cancer." They don't say "I am cancer." People say "I have heart disease," not "I am heart disease." Somehow the presumption of a person's individuality is not compromised by those diagnostic labels. All the labels tell us is that the person has a specific challenge with which he or she struggles in highly diverse life. But call someone a "schizophrenic" or "a borderline" and the shorthand has a way of closing the chapter on the person. It reduces a multi-faceted human being to a diagnosis and lulls us into a false sense that those words tell us who the person is, rather than only telling us how the person suffers. (169–70)

As Manning suggests, when we say that someone *has* cancer the implication is that the cancer can be cured or removed. But when we say that someone *is* manic-depressive or schizophrenic, we imply that a chemical imbalance or brain flaw is who we *are*, our *essence*.

In producing a scholarly essay on two academic pathographies, Kay Redfield Jamison's *An Unquiet Mind* and Jane Phillips's *The Magic Daughter,* I satisfied both a personal and a professional interest in the autobiography of mental illness. Not yet including myself personally in an essay on madness, I nevertheless felt a close connection with both authors and explored my own identity by exploring theirs. In the essay we argued that writing a pathography is a way for the author to gain a certain amount of control over the illness and its relation to the identity. Regaining authority and thus agency over one's experience is more literal here than in many other forms of writing. For me, writing the scholarly essay was also a way of gaining a sense of perspective and agency in relation to my own disease, to my manic-depressive self. So the genre I professionally study represents me and tells other versions of my own story. To quote the essay:

> For sufferers of various forms of mental illness, writing a memoir represents a reclaiming of self, a gathering of a fragmented self back into a narrative unity, if not a psychologically unified whole. By literally authoring a life, one that retrospectively makes sense and holds together despite the fissures and aporias that are experienced in madness, the memoirist provisionally reconstitutes the self. The divisions and gaps created by madness become part of the history of illness and part of the improvised unity of the reconstituted self. Writing the story of the self becomes a way to reconceive and reclaim the self. And even though unity can never be complete, agency is in some measure restored through writing. (Hogan and Hogan 40)

This is the professional prose of academic criticism, but behind it lies the personal passion of the manic-depressive academic.

III.

It's been astonishing for me that as soon as I "come out" as a manic-depressive in class—which I usually do "opportunistically" in relation to a memoir we're reading, a character we're discussing, or the biographical or autobiographical writing of a student shared in a read-around—I become the recipient of all sorts of stories from students who are bipolar themselves or who have friends or relatives who are. Considering how much stigma is still attached to mental illness in our culture, I try to make the classroom a safe haven where it can be discussed, treated as part of the broad spectrum of human identity, and greeted with empathy. Because I am a tenured professor who took a whole semester of sick leave to get over my breakdown, the nature of my illness quickly became public knowledge, and of course I told my colleagues myself. In the academic environment, where there is considerable tolerance for eccentricity and where one is employed "for life," it is safer to reveal one's illness than in many other jobs or professions. I didn't have to worry that I would be fired or even put on permanent disability, because my illness is treatable with drugs. So the illness could become an opportunity for teaching and writing, for self-expression and for a way back to the self. The questions I ponder in both classes and in writing are: Is a pathography different from an autobiography because the story of the illness is added to the story of self? Is a pathography always the story of a *loss* of self through illness or trauma? Can the illness be separated from the identity of the manic-depressive or schizophrenic, or is it central to that identity? These are questions which have much more than an "academic" interest for me.

When I look back over my life, I see that I have always been a manic-depressive, even though the illness did not express itself in earlier life in the kind of florid madness I experienced at 48. Because I've always been a very high-energy, fast-reading, fast-talking, gregarious, outgoing person, I used to joke that I was a manic-depressive without the depression. Nevertheless, I can remember from high school periods of depression when I slept a great deal, isolated myself with books, and felt miserable. Some of this was just adolescence, but it was more intense than normal, I think. In my late twenties, I decided to go back to graduate school four years after graduation from college; and instead of applying to the University of Colorado, where my husband was going, I applied to my old alma mater, the University of New Mexico. He stayed in Boulder and I went down to Albuquerque to live at my mother's and go to school. When I look back on this now, there seems to be something insane about the whole thing. I can't even remember why it seemed so important to go away to school; it was a terrible idea to move to my mother's house after seven years of marriage. I was leaving Joe at a time when he was struggling with his comprehensive exams and really needed my support. And the nuttiness of the whole thing showed up almost immediately, because as soon as I got down there, I began to fall apart. I felt miserable with an almost physical pain most of the time. I literally could not concentrate on the texts I was reading for my classes. As a master's candidate, I was doing my first teaching; and although I related well to the students, I felt completely helpless to organize, focus, and direct a class. I can remember pacing from room to room in my mother's house, lighting a cigarette in one room, moving restlessly into another room, lighting another cigarette, unable to sit still, to rest, to relax, unable to read (usually one of my main solaces in life), unable to sleep. Perversely, I felt that my husband had abandoned me, when I was the one who had gone off on this independent educational track. Anyway, I fell completely apart. Unable to go on teaching or learning, I withdrew from school, and with great relief returned home to Boulder, to Joe.

But of course the disintegration of my sprightly, outgoing, smart, energetic personality scared the hell out of me. In Boulder, I stayed in the apartment for a month without going anywhere. I didn't want anyone to ask me what had happened. Finally, at Joe's urging, I called the local county mental health service and made an appointment to see a therapist, a clinical psychologist. Even though I now recognize that some of my symptoms were very much like what I suffered in 1997, the only therapy I used to come back from my breakdown was talking therapy. Probably also the reduction of stress, getting lots of rest, and having no responsibilities helped to restore the chemical balance in my brain. I can't say this for sure, of course. But I slowly came out of my depression, registered for graduate school at the University of Colorado, and picked up the threads of my personal and academic life. It's interesting and somewhat puzzling to me that graduate school—the preparation for and practice of the academic life—both drove me crazy and helped restore my sanity at different phases of my life. It was in graduate school that I first developed a scholarly interest in autobiography, and I wrote both M.A. and Ph.D. exams on this genre. Now I wonder how close the connection is between this new interest in stories of the self and my own pathological experiences.

At the end of *An Unquiet Mind*, Jamison ponders, if a genetic cure for manic-depression could be found, whether she would want it because of the intensity the illness can create: "Do we risk making the world a blander, more homogenized place if we get rid of the gene for manic-depressive illness?" (194). And she personalizes the speculation further, asking herself "whether given the choice, I would choose to have manic-depressive illness." She answers, "If lithium were not available to me, the answer would be a simple no" (217), because of course without the aid of lithium the depressions would be unbearable. Here Jamison plays with the notion of having a choice about something over which there really is no choice. While manic-depression has brought me too much suffering for me to look on it entirely as a gift, I know it has shaped me in a thousand subtle and direct ways. Where does my energetic, quick-talking, quick-thinking self leave off and my manic or hypomanic self begin? Many people who are not manic-depressive become professors, but for me this profession gave creative scope to my bursting energy and allowed tolerance for my eccentricities. And as I have developed as a scholar and teacher, I have moved closer and closer to my own identity, my own disease and how it has shaped me. Perhaps this essay is the first chapter of my own "nut case" autobiography as I continue the process of understanding and coping with my own manic depression through writing its narrative.

REFERENCES

Goodwin, Frederick K., and Kay Redfield Jamison. *Manic Depressive Illness*. New York: Oxford University Press, 1990.

Hogan, Joseph, and Rebecca Hogan. "When the Subject Is Not the Self: Multiple Personality and Manic Depression." *a/b: Auto/Biography Studies*. Special Issue: *Remembered Selves*. Ed. Carolyn McCracken and Jeanne Holland. 16.2 (2001): 39–52.

Jamison, Kay Redfield. *An Unquiet Mind: A Memoir of Moods and Madness*. New York: Knopf, 1995.

Manning, Martha. *Undercurrents: A Life Beneath the Surface*. New York: HarperCollins, 1994.

Phillips, Jane. *The Magic Daughter: A Memoir of Living with Multiple Personality Disorder*. 1995. New York: Penguin, 1996.

QUESTIONS

1. Why does the author begin the essay with the story of her breakdown before giving any definition or discussion of her illness?
2. Why does the author quote the diary she kept at the time of her breakdown?
3. Comment on the distinction between having a physical illness and being a mental illness. How and why is mental illness viewed as somehow more integral to "who we are" than physical illness—or is it?

The First Girl to Land on the Moon
⁊ BARBARA J. CAMPBELL ⁊

ZERO

I just steal small things, like alcohol pads, tongue depressors, and rubber gloves. I never take anything that is really important, that could potentially make the difference between life and death in the doctor's office or the emergency room. Admittedly, I often admire the blood pressure cuffs, stethoscopes, loops of clear plastic tubing and unusual-looking machines—all those buttons, lights, switches, gauges—the absurdly proportioned tools and gadgetry that although intended to examine particular orifices of the human body, make one shiver at the thought, since they simultaneously seem as if they would be an impossible fit. Most of the larger and more vital instruments, however, I do not take; I would feel bad if they were needed to perform an important exam to save a life, and besides, I can't fit objects like ultrasound machines into my bag anyway. The day I take the photos, though, is the day I have to face the truth—I am a thief.

I rationalize that I deserve these objects as souvenirs. When I was healthy, I never noticed the contents of the doctor's office or an ER, until finally learning, after years of painful gynecological exams, to politely request the pediatric speculum. After being misdiagnosed for months, they finally discover what is wrong with me; meanwhile, with each torturous exam, procedure, and surgery I feel that I should get something in return, particularly because I never get healthier. If I am not going to get well as they had all promised, shouldn't I at least walk away with something that is used to understand my body or do work on it? I mean, if that scalpel cut into me, isn't it now a part of me? Doesn't it belong to me? It seems only fair.

I need the plastic tubing, the model of the shoulder, or the poster of the urinary tract because of innate curiosity. I simply want to untangle the loops of tubes for closer inspection, take apart the model of the shoulder, and look up all the words on the urinary tract poster in my *Dictionary of Medical Terms*. Out of all the many objects that have magically made their way into my purse or brief case, however, it is, strangely, one of the most insignificant that I prize the most. No one noticed when it was gone. I took it because it insults me, offends me, this ten-point pain scale.

137

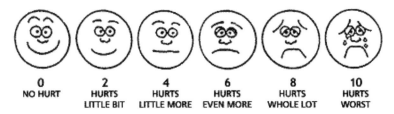

0	2	4	6	8	10
NO HURT	HURTS LITTLE BIT	HURTS LITTLE MORE	HURTS EVEN MORE	HURTS WHOLE LOT	HURTS WORST

Wong-Baker FACES Pain Rating Scale from M. J. Hockenberry, D. Wilson, and M. L. Winkelstein, Wong's Essentials of Pediatric Nursing, 7th ed. (St. Louis, 2005), p. 1259. Used with permission. Copyright, Mosby.

I hate the smiling face of the number zero. It looks so normal, so pleasant. The chart reduces my pain to something quantifiable and fixed—what is incapacitating for me on a daily basis is boiled down to one number on a predetermined scale composed by someone who has probably never even experienced a paper cut. I am 142 pounds, five foot six, blood pressure 112 over 72—just a body with an enigmatic but very common disease. Even on those days when I tell them pain is at a nine or ten, they refuse to give me painkillers. If one of them ever leaves a prescription pad in the exam room, I will surely take the necessary liberties to alleviate my pain.

My theft of medical objects is extremely ironic, considering I have never been good at science and am still trying to recover from the whopping 1.5 I received in my undergraduate biology class. What do I really want this stuff for anyway? I am in the humanities, not the sciences. I am a graduate student in English. Initially I concentrated in Renaissance drama, but now I focus on twentieth-century American literature. Throughout my graduate career I have been a teaching assistant, a research assistant, sometimes both at the same time. I am more an employee than a student. I am on the verge of taking my generalist exams but am specializing in academic novels written by women. All of my research about these texts and in the history of women's education illustrates that I cannot afford to be ill; otherwise, I might be proving all those men right who attempted to exclude women from receiving an education because of their supposedly inferior physical nature.

Of course, I realize that even if I were a waitress, an accountant, a veterinarian, I would still be sick. In fact, one of the few comforts I experience is the wholly arbitrary nature of my disease. People with chronic debilitating illnesses often create meaning for their disease through the belief that it is a test of their faith and relationship with a divine being, whereas I find great solace in the notion that I could have been anyone. Unlike many other people with my disease who I know pray to God for courage and guidance, I take a much more existential view. I had minored in philosophy as an undergraduate. My illness is not a test of strength of character chosen specifically for me—it just happened. It is as impersonal as a stranger entering my house demanding I feed him every day, let him read my books, and allow him to sleep in my bed. Moreover, he insists on following me around wherever I go.

At the same time, though, I also think that the pressures of graduate school—averaging over a thousand pages of reading per week, preparing for and teaching two classes, accumulating thousands and thousands of dollars worth of debt, and constantly being asked to prove whether or not one is worthy of this privilege for such little pay—certainly do not help my physical well-being. I find myself a little jealous of the waitress, accountant, and vet (not to mention the tenured professor) because there is a normalcy to their lives that mine lacks. To put it in academic terminology, graduate students occupy the quintessential liminal space—a sort of suspended animation. Of course, we are productive, engaged in our research and coursework, committed to our teaching, and making efforts toward publication and participating in conferences. Yet, we are also often caught on the threshold of becoming a full-fledged academic for years at a time as a prolonged rite of passage. If we do occupy such a liminal space, I have the perfect disease for a graduate student—it won't kill you, but you will never get well. Instead, you just suffer in limbo with chronic pain for the rest of your life, and various other systems of your body will simply fall apart without any cogent explanation. Are there any kinds of charts that can measure that? Can supposedly sophisticated medical machines assess the quality of that life? Pain changes you so you're not the same person anymore. My only wish is to leave my body. What does that stupid zero mean anyway? Does zero mean you are free of pain, or does it mean you don't feel anything at all?

They make me sign a form that says I will bring the photos back since they belong to them. I have no intention of bringing them back. They are pictures of my body. When I look at them in the car, they are hard for me to understand. I can only identify a couple of parts with certainty, but I do comprehend that even the average person off the street would be able to see that something has gone terribly wrong inside me. I am not normal. I am not zero.

NOBODY

This is not my body. I am not in my body. This is someone else's body, and I am simply looking on as an observer. There are no other bodies, just this body that I am not in. This hollow space—someone moves, drinks, nibbles, and naps. Someone hums, smokes. Watch this body; survey it carefully to make sure it moves correctly.

LOVE AND SEX

They are wrapped around each other in the dark. His body is a mystery to me, she thinks, while feeling his warm skin. She feels a familiar openness spreading from her navel, but something's wrong. She feels an odd pressure in her vagina. She shifts her weight and tries to ignore it, but with every motion from him it seems to increase. The pressure turns to stabbing pain which she can't ignore. She stifles the need to scream out. "I'm sorry . . . ," she whispers, rolling away from him. It hurts so badly, she is sure she is bleeding. She looks down there—nothing. Suddenly she sits up, he rubs her back. "I just want to be normal," she says and leans over, sobbing into his chest.

FADE TO BLACK

It is a couple of days before Christmas and she is sitting at her kitchen table eating Cheez-Its and smoking and talking to her friend Pearl, who had just flown in from Chicago for a visit. The girl is supposed to leave the next day to visit her family in Maine for the holidays, but it never happens. Pearl is supposed to stay in her apartment and watch the cats while she is away in Maine, but this doesn't happen. Instead, Pearl is talking and the girl is smoking, drinking orange juice and vigorously eating Cheez-Its and the girl's eyes slowly lose focus and she just sees Pearl's mouth moving and she can't make sense of the words—she feels hot—her temperature feels like it's shooting to 103. Pearl's face turns a dizzying blue, then green, and the girl suddenly blurts out, "I'm going to be sick."

"Are you okay?" Pearl asks. The girl runs to the bathroom and puts her head over the toilet. She can't throw up, despite the fact that her body tells her to. She stretches out on the bathroom floor. Strange tremors start; her body begins to shake violently against her will. She tries to make her brain control it, but the bathroom ceiling starts fading out, blue to green, then gray to black. She feels a sudden impulse to urinate—she crawls over to the toilet, and desperately tries to pull her pants down, but her fingers are like rubber and won't grasp the button on her pants because her hand is still shaking and she can't make it stop. Finally, she clumsily tugs at the button and yanks down her pants; she can only make out shadows, spinning outlines of shapes in her bathroom . . .

"Barb, Barb, are you okay?!" Pearl calls from outside the door.

The girl cannot respond, but hears urine streaming into the toilet.

"Should I call an ambulance?"

"Yeah." The girl feels all the muscles in her throat turn into concrete—her voice doesn't want to obey her commands either. Pulling her pants back up, she crawls back down on the floor hoping it will ground her. Her hands and her legs keep shaking but more than anything, more than anything, she doesn't want to black out.

It's funny when people say they blacked out, because it isn't really blacking out—it's fading into blackness.

OUTERSPACE

There is a young woman, about thirty years of age, sitting at a small round kitchen table cluttered with newspapers, books, and unopened mail. She looks up at the clock, which has a split on the face. She looks uncomfortable and tense. Occasionally she winces in pain. Exasperated, she lights a cigarette. She appears to be waiting for something impatiently. The telephone rings. She stubs out her cigarette, grimacing.

"Hello?" she says desperately.

"May I speak with Barbara Campbell?"

"This is she."

"This is Doctor—"

"I recognize your voice."

"You called earlier?"

"Yes, I'm having so much pain—"

"—where?"

"Lower left quadrant."

"Do you have a temperature?"

"I feel hot."

"But you haven't taken your temperature."

"No." The girl sounds impatient and confused. "No, I just don't understand why I'm still having so much pain. It's been three months since the surgery."

"I don't know—maybe you have some sort of IBS that is reacting in some sort of strange way. You shouldn't be in this much pain. I performed a LUNA procedure when I was in there, which should've helped—"

"—the moon?"

"No," she hears him laugh into the phone as if a small child had said something amusing. "Not the moon . . . Laparoscopic Uterosacral Nerve Ablation."

"Oh." She had no idea what that meant. "Isn't there anything you can do? I'm having so much trouble getting to school and to work. I'm in pain all the time." The girl's voice is rising. "I can't do anything . . . I still can't have sex, I have to urinate all the time." She feels herself starting to cry, but forces herself not to. "I thought the surgery was going to fix the pain, but I feel just as bad as I did before. I don't understand why I am still in pain. What could be causing this?"

"I don't know what to tell you, Barbara. I guess you're just a sensitive young lady."

She suddenly feels as if she's been kicked in the stomach—she can't breathe. She is transported down to the bathroom floor again. Apparently, it is her fault. She is "sensitive," she is delicate. There is more talk, but she doesn't hear what he is saying. He is miles and miles away speaking to her from a different time zone, across the ocean on the other side of the world. She tries to tune him in, but all she can hear are bits and pieces of a foreign voice coming through the crackling streams of a shortwave radio. The noise stops. She limply hangs up the phone and thinks that she cannot be the only one—there must be other people . . . other people living in bodies like hers.

> *Hi,*
> *I was recently diagnosed and my doctor said he performed a LUNA procedure during my surgery. I don't know what this is. Have any of you had this done during your surgery? What does it stand for?*
> *Thanks,*
> *BC*

> *Hi BC,*
> *Welcome to the message board. I hope it will be a good source of information and support for you. LUNA stands for Laparoscopic Uterosacral Nerve Ablation. Basically this means that the nerves from your uterosacral ligaments were ablated during the surgery which is theoretically supposed to help block pain if your disease returns. This is a very serious procedure, so I do hope that your doctor discussed it with you before he performed it. Personally, I'm not a big fan of cutting nerves. It is our nerves that tell us whether or not something is wrong inside our bodies.*

The following week she arrives at the doctor's office demanding her records and photos. They make her sign a form that states she will bring everything back because the materials are their property. She signs the form knowing that she will never bring them back—stealing other things never felt so deliberate. Plus, she thinks, they are allowed to take without asking, why can't she?

THE SICK ROOM

It is a bit like visiting your grandparents. You love your grandparents, but when you were a child and your family went to visit them you were always keenly aware that you had entered the sick-room, a mentholated world of Vicks, pill bottles, heating pads, coughing, and slow-motion. You want to run, to be young and screw around in the street with your friends playing kickball, but instead you have been dragged here against your will to listen to the many aches and pains that will someday become yours too. Now, at this age, it is as hard for you to conceive of being well as it is to imagine your grandparents when they were this old. Photographs never help either. You can see them, the youthful shadow and outline of the face, but to try and connect that image with the elderly version you knew in real-life just makes it seem superimposed. Looking at photographs of yourself from before you were sick produces the same response, so you never look at them anymore.

One day, though, you are in the grocery store. You buy some yogurt, bran, prune juice, Cream of Rice cereal, beets, and a six-pack of spring water. You try to put the six-pack into the basket you are carrying, but it won't fit. The basket is heavy, but the water is heavier. On days like these, you feel like you are drowning in a whirlpool of hot water and every time you come up for air someone keeps pushing your head down again. A brush with sharp metal tines is scraping at your insides and then the familiar dull throb in your pelvis becomes a wailing hammer plummeting against your left ovary. You hear a 10,000 Maniacs song in the organic foods section and nearly weep because it reminds you of a time when you were well, a long, long time ago in college when you and your friend Robert skipped school and drove out to a dairy place in the country to get ice cream and that song was playing on the radio. You miss ice cream, but you restrain yourself from looking into the freezer cabinet for chocolate chip because dairy makes more estrogen and will just make the disease grow. You stand in the express lane, the basket on the floor, kicking it periodically with your foot as the line progresses, sweating, sure you will pass out any second. You are so tired that the six-pack feels like a giant boulder. An old woman behind you with a cantaloupe and some strawberries in the front part of her carriage says to you, "You can put that in my carriage if that's too heavy for you, dear." The woman has a nice smile. "Oh, no, that's okay, thank you though." You feel yourself beginning to cry, in part because you forgot that complete strangers can be nice to each other, in part because she is an old woman, so you feel a maternal protectiveness from her, but also because you know she sees you for who you really are. Somehow, old people know when they look at you that you are just as much in decline as they are, diseased, in pain, with every organ on the fritz. How do they know? How can they tell? You look your age—to them your body appears young, but you don't fool them.

You wipe your eyes and try to chat small-talk with the old woman in line. She jokes with an old man with an oxygen tank who feigns several attempts to cut ahead of her in line. We laugh as they start a pretend feud, but when you hear yourself laugh it sounds funny. It doesn't sound like it's coming from you.

GOSSIP

"Pricking, pounding, beating, stabbing, thrusting, pinching, burning— Circle the one that best describes your pain."

While she is pleased that the list is at least made up of active verbs, she is disgruntled because to choose just one of these descriptors will not accurately describe her pain. She is tempted to circle all of them, but she suspects that this will just confuse them.

It is jarring to see a plastic model of endometriosis from the makers of Lupron Depot next to an issue of *Talk* magazine with Lara Flynn Boyle on the cover in a slinky, sequined outfit. The exam room is a dusty pink and the obligatory Monet painting hangs slightly crooked on the wall below a strategically placed dried flower-and-twig arrangement that she imagines was built by the birds that followed Snow White around during "Whistle While You Work." She is disturbed by the tendency of every OBGYN to transform the medical space into a domestic one. Her first gynecologist's office was decorated in a similar fashion, but had a painting of two women, back to back, both dressed in white, hair pinned up, pale, glowing skin, each with a baby. One woman is breast-feeding her infant and another is bottle-feeding, but both are happy and serene. Doctors always assumed that having a baby was her main objective.

She is just contemplating whether or not the plastic model of the uterus from the Lupron company will fit in her bag when it suddenly occurs to her that filling out forms with so many different doctors is like the game you play when you're a kid. You and all of your friends sit in a circle and you whisper something into one kid's ear, and he whispers it to the next kid, and so on, and so on, but by the time you get to the end of the circle the information is all garbled and there are pieces missing. Completing forms and intake interviews with nurses always made her feel as if she were playing that game. It is hard to tell her story in the same way every time with different medical professionals. She might forget, embellish, lose information—they always went so fast it was easy to do. Part of the problem is that they never ask for a story because the narrative methodology is already set. There are certain forms to be filled out, family history to be recorded, x's to be checked, items to be crossed out or through, words to circle from a list of verbs that have been chosen for you, like pricking, pounding, beating etc. She doesn't describe her illness and pain the same way every time, and the way they force you to tell it makes everyone's stories uniform.

She had hoped that the dysfunction in her pelvic organs would make the other parts of her better. She wanted the problem in one part of her body to make something else creative and wonderful happen somewhere else, as she had often heard occurred with the senses. When someone goes blind, supposedly the ears compensate for the loss and hearing becomes sharper and more acute; or when people lose the ability to move their legs, they work at developing their upper-arm strength. She tried to listen to the body, to hear where the hidden reward might lie. Considering the location of her disease and pain, she liked to imagine that maybe something incredible might happen—like she would get taller, or amazingly flexible, or her IQ would jump one hundred points—but nothing like that happened.

When she looks at all the completed forms together, she doesn't recognize them as a representation of herself and her pain. The parts are too disconnected to make a whole. It is like looking at herself in old photos from before she was sick—she looks like a stranger. She doesn't look like me.

INSIDE-OUT

Grammy knew there was something wrong with me but she didn't know what it was because in my family we are not supposed to talk about it. During a family visit to her retirement home, she pulls me aside when everyone else is getting their coats and says, "I sure hope you feel better soon. Don't you hate it when they tell you you look good? I tell you, nothing irritates me more!" I am surprised. It is as if she read my mind. Like her, I know that people are well-intentioned when they respond with "Well, you look good," when I am forced to tell them that I am ill. But I am also keenly aware of the fact that such a phrase unintentionally undercuts one's efforts to try not to limp down the hallway at school, or run to the bathroom every fifteen minutes to urinate, throw up, or change one's pad. After all, if you look good, you must not be in that much pain, right? Every day I try to remain vertical rather than doubling over with my hands folded across my belly, wailing like a new-born when attempting to hold polite and intelligent conversation with faculty and fellow graduate assistants. Some days, during these interactions, all I can do is smile and nod, smile and nod. I begin to worry that my colleagues will think I am stupid because I do not speak. All of my mental and physical energy is not invested in concealing my illness, but rather in forcing my body and mind to perform its daily requirements—to discipline it enough to do its job. If people could see the photos of the inside of my body, would they say I looked good then? If they turned my body inside out to take a real good look, how would they respond? It occurs to me that people in my field should know better than to make such remarks, but perhaps they just don't know what else to say. It is odd that they can capture the various subtleties of a narrative, commit to memory every known fact about a novel, possess an in-depth knowledge of the historical context in which a text was produced, but often misread people. I remember when I was an undergraduate and my advisor and favorite teacher came into literary theory class one evening, threw an open book on the seminar table, and asked, "Does this text exist if no one reads it?" It was an elementary question to begin our discussion of phenomenology. I think that a disease is like a text—a story—and not one produced in a vacuum but one influenced by the social and cultural circumstances in which it was produced. I am bewildered by the fact that many of my colleagues fail to grasp that like texts, the personal and political meaning of disease is at least partially socially constructed. I am thirty-four years old and trapped in Grammy's eighty-year-old body and nobody, including my colleagues or members of the medical profession, seems to understand this but Grammy and I—and Grammy never went to college.

THE FIRST GIRL TO LAND ON THE MOON

Endometriosis is a puzzling disease affecting women in their reproductive years. The name comes from the word endometrium, which is the tissue that lines the inside of the uterus and builds up and sheds each month in the menstrual cycle. In endometriosis tissue like the endometrium is found outside the uterus, in other areas of the body. In these locations outside the uterus, the

endometrial tissue develops into what are called nodules, tumors, lesions, implants, or growths
[which] can cause pain, infertility, and other problems.

I don't know how it happened, really. All I knew is that instead of looking in *American Literature* and the MLA database, I found myself searching for articles in MEDline and in the stacks at the library, picking up issues of *Gynecologic and Obstetric Investigation,* and *Fertility and Sterility.* Initially, I felt guilty about this behavior—certainly more than I ever did about stealing instruments from doctors' offices and hospitals. None of the research I was doing concerned literature. Nothing I did in the library had anything to do with my upcoming exams or my dissertation. My greatest fear was that one of my advisors, or, god forbid, the director of my graduate program, would catch me in the middle of a riveting new article of *Clinical Obstetrics and Gynecology* or *Immunology.* With all the afternoons I spent skulking around the library, you'd swear I was looking at porn.

> *Women with endometriosis may also have associated disorders related to autoimmune dysregulation or pain. . . . Compared with published rates in the general USA female population, women with endometriosis had higher rates of hypothyroidism . . . , fibromyalgia . . . , chronic fatigue syndrome . . . , rheumatoid arthritis . . . , systemic lupus erythematosus . . . , Sjogren's syndrome . . . , and multiple sclerosis. . . . Allergies and asthma were more common among women with endometriosis. . . . CONCLUSIONS: Hypothyroidism, fibromyaligia, chronic fatigue syndrome, autoimmune diseases, allergies and asthma are all significantly more common in women with endometriosis than in women in the general USA population.*

Ever since I bought my *Dictionary of Medical Terms,* I discovered that medical discourse is not so impenetrable.

Laparoscopic Uterine Nerve Ablation
(LUNA)
Uterosacral transaction is a relatively easy procedure to perform laparoscopically. A standard three-puncture technique is used (10- to 12-mm umbilical trocar, two 5-mm lateral suprapubic accessory trocars).
It is relatively easy.

> While genital tract involvement is the rule, endometriosis is also seen in the gastrointestinal tract, the urinary tract, lungs, scars, and nerves. Extrapelvic endometriosis is not as well understood as pelvic endometriosis. . . . Extrapelvic endometriosis is defined as endometriotic lesions found outside the pelvis and includes cervix, vagina, vulva, intestinal tract, urinary tract, abdominal wall, thoracic cage and lungs, extremities, and the central nervous system.

When I begin reading articles on my disease, I find that they stand in stark contrast to my own experience and those of others. I try to reconcile the language of the medical journals, and the charts and graphs detailing the various limited successes of Lupron, Danazol, and laparoscopic surgeries, with the women I have corresponded with and for whom none of these treatments worked. I compare myself to a woman who has had six laparoscopies, when I have had only two—would four more rid me of this disease? Would a couple of rounds of Lupron, complete with side effects, make me healthy again? Would yet another session with the behavioral pain therapist—who suggested that I put Post-its around my apartment describing what a good person I am in hopes that it would reinforce a positive self-image—really help? It did not take me very long to understand that I would never again be the person I was before I was ill. I would not be able to stay up late writing, take on an extra class solely for the love of teaching it, hop into my car and drive two hours to New York to do archival research because of some curious, deep-seated intellectual tugging in my brain, have parties on a whim, make love, drink, smoke, and eat whatever I want whenever I want or go for a run. I miss this person. Instead my career will suffer because my body will be unable to manage the workload, and my personal and professional relationships will become strained, at best. In essence, I will never be able to be spontaneous again. My life will be routine, planned out, plodded through, and predictable because I will always have pain. My disease is not confined to one portion of my body, even if that is where, empirically speaking, it resides—it is a part of my consciousness forever. I am outside your charts and graphs. You have your studies of us, but you do not have our stories. At the same time, I read your articles because I suspect you think that stories are not enough.

It is late at night and I am walking from the library to my office. The campus is empty—I am completely alone. The frozen air hits my stiff body. When I start to pull my scarf around me it begins to snow. I don't know why, but I feel like I am breathing for the first time. I look up at the moon and imagine that I can put in my pocket and keep it as my own.

REFERENCES

Ballweg, Mary Lou, and the Endometriosis Association. *The Endometriosis Sourcebook.* Chicago: Contemporary Books, 1995.

Murphy, Ann. "Clinical Aspects of Endometriosis." *Endometriosis: Emerging Research and Intervention Strategies.* Ed. Koji Yoshinaga and Estella C. Parrott. Annals of the New York Academy of Sciences, vol. 955 (March 2002): 1–10.

Sinaii, N., et al. "High Rates of Autoimmune and Endocrine Disorders, Fibromyalgia, Chronic Fatigue Syndrome and Atopic Disease among Women with Endometriosis: A Survey Analysis." *Human Reproduction* 17(10) (2002): 2715–2724.

QUESTIONS

1. Discuss the significance of the title and the reasons behind the author's stealing items from the doctor's office.
2. Where does the point of view shift in the essay, and how is that significant?
3. Why does the author choose not to name her disease until the end of the essay? How does that affect the way one reads the essay?
4. Examine the ethical questions raised by the LUNA procedure—in general and also particularly with regard to informing the patient beforehand.
5. Discuss the psychosocial effects of endometriosis.

A certain remoteness
telling vaginismus

⌒ Fulvia Dunham ⌒

"Down there? . . . I can't tell you this. I can't do this, talk about down there."[1]

I told you, it's closed down there; it's a damp cellar, off limits, a place you don't go.

I'm listening to Eve Ensler's *The Vagina Monologues*, marveling at the maturity of the students' performances. I'm glad that most of them don't know, and may never, what it is to have trouble with the vagina—vagina trouble. Arranged in crimson and hot pink costumes before the microphones, they handle the stories with wit, self-possession and apparent understanding. Fortunately, they will probably never have to understand the experience of realizing that the road is closed "down there," closed to all traffic, such that one can only go around. *When one goes around, obviates, circumvents, are the routes that one then travels merely compensatory detours, or are they part of a new frontier?* The Vagina Monologues urge us to become comfortable with our vaginas, rise to anger about how they've been ignored and maligned, talk about them, look at them, celebrate them, touch them. This is a noble, necessary activist project. *But is it valid, because of the pain, not to?*—to explore other erotogenic zones, distribute libidinal investments differently and elsewhere, redirect, reject the usual teleologies that tell us that, even if we choose not to choose heterosexual sex, we still should be in touch with, able to touch, our vaginas?

> *If we prefer not to—cannot—"parler femme" with our "two lips," are we still women?—can we enter the sexual economy?—are we still there at all?*[2]

⌒ ⌒

Before that performance of the *The Vagina Monologues*, I'd sent a couple of email messages to the organizers of the show. I was responding to a tip a student had given that they would be setting up an evening of panels to accompany the monologues—to address issues such as violence against women, health care for women, and sexual harassment. I knew some of the organizers; some had taken courses on women's literature with me, and they knew I approached texts from a gender studies angle. I asked if there would be any space for raising awareness about a women's health issue that many people didn't know about: vaginismus.

I didn't say I'd been contending with it for fifteen years; I didn't feel comfortable making it seem like a personal crusade. I wanted it simply to be an issue to which I was drawing attention in a university community in order to advance knowledge.

"**Vaginismus** occurs," I quoted from a pamphlet, "when there is an involuntary spasm of the muscles surrounding the outer third of the vagina resulting in painful, difficult, or the impossibility of any form of vaginal entry or penetration."[3] The rest of the pamphlet offers more information that I didn't pass along:

> The etiology of **vaginismus** is also unknown. It has been linked to factors such as chronic muscle tension of vaginal muscles resulting from painful experiences with (attempted) intercourse. The muscle tension worsens the already present painful conditions, the anxiety and fear concerning penetration and possible pain with penetration, or both.
>
> **Vaginismus** is related to a group of other forms of **vulvovaginal pain**—including **vulvodynia**, which is chronic pain (rather than pain that occurs when there is any contact with the vaginal area) and **vulvar vestibulitis**, which is characterized by sharp, burning pain at attempted vaginal entry including sexual intercourse, tampon insertion, and gynecological exams. It also involves significant pain upon Q-tip palpitation of the vestibule and in some women, increased redness or irritation of the vulva.

From what I can tell, I have suffered from both vaginismus and vulvar vestibulitis. Treatment for these conditions

> involves cognitive-behavioral therapy / pain management in a group or individual format alone or in combination with muscle training / physiotherapy and biofeedback, and surgical interventions.

The note I received in return from the V-Day organizers was courteous and professional. They provided background information about the V-Day projects:

> V-day is the name for the college initiative that gives the rights for the VMs to college students for free, provided the students donate all proceeds to a local women's charity. On —— campus, the Vagina Monologues group is [the same as] the V-Day group. So far we've had a Vagina Forum (women only) and are now planning on a Vagina Forum II to which we will specifically invite men. We've also started up a performance evening of original student works.

They invited me to participate: They wanted to set up "a debate among [university] faculty on any subject regarding Feminism in Performance, violence towards women, or any other VM relevant issues"—and asked me what I thought.

What they didn't acknowledge was that I'd mentioned "vaginismus" in my one of my emails. Quite possibly, they'd been busy and had overlooked it. But as the query I'd sent had focused principally on drawing attention to vaginismus, the lacuna was conspicuous—and I wondered if it might result from nervousness about what could be construed, in effect, as the lack of a hole ("girl without a hole" comes to mind; the phrase appears in a testimonial in Katz and Tabisel's *Private Pain*).[4] I wondered about the forms of anxiety that, even in an emancipated environment in which we were all working together to talk about vaginas, might prompt that kind of evasion.

Of course it's understandable: many women have never heard of vaginismus, and so when they do hear about it, they probably wish to proceed carefully, to ascertain how many people actually confront this, to refrain from comment for fear of saying something inadvertently insensitive. But that women don't know about it to begin with—that they, like many medical practitioners, have never heard of it—is the shame of the matter. *It's a shame*. And this is the difficulty: despite everything, it's still a shame—in most contexts, a cause for embarrassment and shame. Although some studies report that nearly 20 percent of women between the ages of 18 and 24 have experienced some form of vulvovaginal pain, there is nonetheless still little hospitality in our climate for this form of disclosure.

Why, in this era of sexual awareness, improved sex education, debate about sexual identity and queer power, might it still be stigmatized? Perhaps because, in the effort to validate sexual orientations and identities that have endured prejudice and violence in the past, and to celebrate new, hitherto unrecognized forms of sexual identity, what has emerged is a value system that valorizes sexual openness and frowns on sexual closedness. Vaginismus is likely to be regarded as a form of sexual closedness. Its etiology is unknown, but it is thought often to afflict women who have emerged from families that are repressed, unable adequately to talk about sex; perhaps, in this respect, it indicates dysfunction. *Dysfunction.* It may stem from experiences of sexual abuse. It does often happen to people who are anxious, though it remains unclear how much of the anxiety preexists and fosters—and how much results from—the vaginismus. *there was just terror, and weird involuntary cries* I remember listening to a lecture on vaginismus, delivered by a kind and sympathetic therapist, feeling like a prim prude, shrivelled spinster, uptight, old maid bluestocking, all the rest of that concatenation. It's difficult to feel otherwise.

and if your body is closed, if you can't let anyone in, if you can't talk about it easily because no one knows what you're talking about, if you're obliged to remain closeted because people often forget what you've told them, then you're simply repressed—closed—out of the loop—out of circulation—unable to come out because you can't let anyone in, because there's no language with which to come out, and because nobody cares

☞ ☜

Later, I did find people who were more willing to listen. In fact, miraculously, I found that in Montréal, where I had happened to move, there was a team conducting some of the most advanced research out there today on vaginismus and related vulvovaginal conditions. Fortunately, given the pioneering work being done in the city, there were a couple of physiotherapists who specialized in working with vaginismus sufferers; and at last, I signed up with one of them.

Recently, I've even been lucky enough to be able to get in touch with some of the researchers doing work on the subject. I was invited by one doctoral student, part of the research group, to give a brief talk on my experiences with vaginismus to some master's students in education— and I wrote the following. I was trying to make all this accessible **make this inaccessibility accessible** *to an audience who would, at best, be only mildly interested.*

I discovered it when I was 17, when I tried—and failed—to have my first GYN exam. I'd gone to the family doctor warned by my mother that I might be in for an unpleasant, but not intensely uncomfortable, experience. What I found instead was that, when the doctor first tried to approach my vaginal area with a Q-Tip, doing no more than touch gingerly, I felt a primal terror unlike anything I'd ever known. I remember writhing, almost thrashing, and crying, nearly losing consciousness, trying to stop this from happening—and beginning to make weird cries that didn't sound human, and that really didn't even feel as though they were mine. It was all involuntary, and it felt as though someone else were uttering the cries, as if I had lost control of my reactions and something else, some other force, had taken command.

Not surprisingly, the doctor was unsettled. He was old-school, well-meaning, mild-mannered, no doubt quite embarrassed by my response. Abashed, he told my mother, quietly, that I was somewhat "tight" down there and might consider getting a hymenectomy. It was only years later, after several other people had also suggested this to me, that I learned that a hymenectomy doesn't actually address the problem of vaginismus. Despite the widespread and erroneous belief that it helps women, "opens them up," at best, it would have been ineffectual, unrelated to the problem; at worst, it might have left significant scars that could have caused pain and discomfort in years to come.

And in fact, the funny revelation was that, when I finally reached the point in physiotherapy where my therapist was able to determine whether my hymen was intact or not, she found, inexplicably, that it was not. I had never been able to have penile-vaginal intercourse, but it wasn't there. So had a hymenectomy been attempted, there wouldn't have been any hymen to address.

It actually wasn't until some years later, when I was in college, that a clinician— with whom I had tried to have another unsuccessful GYN exam—gave me a name for what I was suffering from: vaginismus. I wasn't given the kind of detailed definition or informed scholarship that I've been able to find here in Montréal, but at least I had a term for what was happening—and that was a great help.

Women with vaginismus experience pain on attempted vaginal entry with intercourse, tampon insertion, gynecological exams.

It was true: I couldn't insert a tampon there, couldn't withstand a GYN, and couldn't allow a sexual partner there. Unable to find anyone I could talk to about this or who could help, I resigned myself to using sanitary pads, avoiding GYNs, and accepting that there were forms of sexual expression I simply wouldn't be able to manage.

Given my later training in gender studies, it became tempting to try to believe that this wasn't a "problem" or "dysfunction"; it was simply a "difference." But given the imperative we receive in our culture to express ourselves as sexual beings, the messages we're sent that suggest that we're incomplete, uptight, wound-

up, or repressed if we can't or don't, it doesn't feel like merely a difference; it feels like a deficit. It also doesn't feel like just a difference when the desire is there, but the means of expression are not. It feels like an insurmountable obstacle.

The most difficult part was not being able to talk to either family or partners about this. Exchanges with family members were uncomfortable; people were usually tentative and shy, occasionally asking if I'd fixed "my little problem," implying that it was a bad habit of aversion I had to correct rather than a problem or illness with which I needed help. They may not have wanted to intrude. I think the unspoken assumption in many of their minds was that if you can't perform normally in sexual terms, you're unfortunate—but not in need of a hand, as you would be if you had a recognizable illness. The worst part about it is that often people simply won't talk about it; they tend not to remember what you've told them about it; they betray nervousness when the topic is addressed; and they usually assume that some other family member has helped you out. Interchanges with partners, meanwhile, were uneasy and awkward—episodes I got through, often finding that derision lay on the other side of a period of polite acceptance—or sometimes, simply the stark truth that a male significant other couldn't stay because sexual needs weren't being met.

Under those circumstances, it's easy to feel like a freak. It is easy to feel that this obstacle will stand in the way of ever achieving closeness with romantic partners—and that the vaginismus is just one of many ways in which you're closed off from the vitality, the natural life cycles, of the world. Given the premium placed on sexual success by our society, it's easy to feel less than whole, less than adequate. It's easy to feel doomed, denied a chance at life and connection with others, and I readily admit that I more than once succumbed to bitterness.

When I was first talking with the research team doing work on vulvovaginal pain, looking into the possibility of setting up a support group for women who contended with various forms of it, an editor approached me, asking me for a personal testimonial. She wanted it for a newsletter, focused on sexual issues, that she was putting together for teenagers in the city. I wrote her a piece of about 500 words, using some of the language from the above account. She wrote back:

> *It's very good, with a nice arc and certainly the ring of truth, and I'd like to use it in the newsletter, but with some changes. The tone and phrasings, and sometimes the vocabulary, are often very adult, resulting in a certain remoteness. Also, in some places it's missing important elaboration; for example, how did you feel during that first GYN exam after your extreme and unexpected reaction? Labeling those feelings will make the piece more compelling and will help girls with similar experiences to identify.[5]*

It has a "nice arc"—and certainly "the ring of truth" (but not the actual truth?). It has "a certain remoteness"—is this because of the "nice arc"? Should this story be told without a "nice arc"? And how would I tell it?—how bring this into narrative? I'd like to help young

people to "identify" so that they can better understand, find support, and promote awareness. But it's too "remote" to be "compelling."

It is characterized by sharp, burning pain at the entry of the vagina

(burning burning o lord thou pluckest me out o lord thou burning

better to marry than to burn burning hurting)

or the impossibility of any form of vaginal entry[6]

⟜ ⟜

It is 1997. I am in northwestern Italy, in the mountains near Bolzano, travelling with a gay
male friend. We have met a boyfriend of his, a young Italian—I'll call him "Enzo"—who has
just cooked us a pasta dinner in his family's condo. Serving us espresso, Enzo talks medi-
tatively about when he plans to come out to his parents—soon, as his master's research involves work on gay male identity, and when he receives his degree, he will let them know.
He is somewhat worried—his parents have never suspected a thing, and they expect him
to get married soon—but he has confidence that everything will be all right. It's the truth,
after all. He loves them, and he must let them know.

We turn on the television. Gianni Versace has just been murdered—perhaps by the serial killer Andrew Cunanan: was this an act of homophobic rage? After a silence, Enzo just
says, quietly, simply, "So they've got Versace."

My friend and Enzo retire for the night. Enzo comes back into my room before I turn
in, asking if I have everything I need. Would I like a glass of water? Am I warm enough? Out
of the corner of my eye, I see my blue and white flowered summer nightdress. A stray word
from this afternoon's conversation at the *osteria,* among a group of other gay Italian men,
used about me, as they saw my expression in reaction to some of their stories, floats back
through my mind: *innocente.* I tell him I'm fine, and thank you for everything, *grazie,* and
buona notte. A few minutes later, in the dark, I hear them moving in the other room.

*I wonder if having what I have, being denied what is usually considered a rite of pas-
sage into adulthood, consigns one to an infinitely protracted childhood. What is the price
of innocence? What are its signs? I think about sexual repertoires—expanded repertoires. I
wonder what it would take for me to qualify as queer.*

⟜ ⟜

I am sitting at the bar, between two friends, also colleagues, near the school at which I teach.
Because of a family history of alcoholism, I don't drink; so at times, an environment like
this makes me uncomfortable. But this evening, I'm fine; I'm with friends, and glad to be
out for the night. My coffee is warm. One colleague begins talking about the relationship
she's having—unsatisfying, because sheerly about sex. She and this neighbor guy have nothing in common; it's too casual for her. The other chimes in. Sex, she says, is definitely over-
rated; and guys are in general. Then they ask me about the man with whom I have parted
ways two months before, after having been with him for two years. I say that things are fine;
everything's amicable enough, and he usually calls me every couple of weeks from Los Angeles. *when he told me, it was new year's eve, and then waking up in the middle of the night
just after, him near me, trying to tell him that it was all over for me, that i'd never have*

intimacy with anyone now, because no one would have the patience, that this was the last dance, impossible, that he was relegating me to life among those who remain alone—trying to explain—the words were broken—that although i wasn't sure i wanted children, i wanted the possibility I say that we're exchanging emails and phone calls fairly often. *and it would never be possible again and doomed no access cut off a certain remoteness—his looking at his watch to see if it was midnight yet* They have to catch me as I begin to fall backward off the chair. I remember both of them suddenly holding me at once—each one grasping an arm, keeping me from falling back. I must have begun to faint, but I still can't remember what happened.

☞ ☜

I remember being in their house. They had asked me to sit for their house and their cats while they were in Utah, then once again when they were in Israel—the lesbian couple with the three cats, the Victorian sofa, and the lovely ponds they'd just had installed in their backyard (with which, they said, they were "infatuated"). I remember the traces of ecofeminism, the ankhs in the study. The cats, too, I think, were used to signs of fecundity and sensuality, gestures of abundance. *and is this something I can do?* It has not been. This scene of contentment and fertility exemplifies what I'd like someday to have, and yet I do not think I would be able to go that route with another woman. It would have made everything much simpler had my desire traveled in that direction. *and the feeling that one evening, up in their bedroom on the quilted coverlet; no one around; I didn't know myself what was happening, until the silver cat had appeared on the bed and draped itself around my back, which was moving as though I were sobbing*

☞ ☜

The next year, at *The Vagina Monologues,* I take the opportunity to distribute some information about a support group for women with vulvovaginal pain that, in collaboration with someone else, I'm putting together. I set up pamphlets and posters. A young woman walks by, apparently a reporter for the school newspaper. "What is this?" she asks pointedly. I tell her. "And what does that have to do with the Vagina Monologues?" she asks.

I talk to a few people at other tables. There's a trans/gender alliance whose sign reads "No passing zone." There's an intersex group passing out info, trying to disrupt the equation between "woman" and "vagina." They object especially to the Ensler monologue in which a girl is born without a vagina, discovers it when she's fourteen, and feels she must have one: her father tells her not to worry, that he's going to get her "the best homemade pussy in America," and says, "when you meet your husband, he's gonna know we had it made specially for him."[7] The cultural ideology, as spoken through this monologue, is such that one must be either anatomically male or female; people are forced to choose; and often infants who are neither clearly male or female are subjected to surgery that decides for them, before they have a say.

I agree with the injustice of this. People who are marked as women in many respects can certainly live without vaginas—and should be able to if they wish to. *I wonder if it's the same as having one that doesn't work.* People should be able to live as they choose without being interpellated by the surrounding culture as either male or female. *Or is it that it just chooses not to comply?* I think then of Teena Brandon, of "Boys Don't Cry," who had been a girl all her life and then decided she wanted to be a boy—did not want to use her vagina, did not want to assign that part of her body significance as the culture told her she had to, did not want cultural codes to require her to construct her vagina.

am I succumbing to compulsory heterosexuality, the heterosexual imperative, the pressure to become more valid through an ability to participate legibly in the sexual economy? Their sign says, "No passing zone." Rather than seeking to overcome this, perhaps I should use this with which I have been fated to disrupt the usual equation between "intimacy" and "penetration." Should I question the usual assumptions about what constitutes sexual success and fulfillment?— challenge the commonplace equation between sexual fulfillment and fulfillment?

Is it wrong to want my vagina to open?

⌒ ⌒

It's 2003, and something has happened that I thought would never come to pass: I am largely free of vaginismus. Thanks to the expertise I've found in Montreal, I've been able to work with a physiotherapist who's among the most knowledgeable in Canada, and after a year of committed PT, I am at last able to have conventional heterosexual intercourse. I will probably be able to have children, should I want them, without recourse to artificial insemination. When working with one of the members of the research team, who understands the challenges of vaginismus, I can actually go through with a GYN. The "cold duck lips"[8] that one of Ensler's monologues talks of I still can't take, but I can get it done, and I am assured, at last, through my first pap smear, that I am cancer free. I feel as if I've finally addressed this, found language for it; I'm grateful for all the persistent work of those who have helped; and in unguarded moments, just as I thought I was through with all those glass slipper narratives, I even sometimes feel I've finally been able to go to the ball ("Vaginismus," I read in an account by Linda Valins, "has been described as the Cinderella of women's sexual problems"—because it's always been in the corner, ignored).[9] There's a wealth of information out there, I've discovered, for vaginismus sufferers. There's *Private Pain,* a book about vaginismus and dyspareunia by Ditza Katz and Ross Lynn Tabisel of the Women's Therapy Center in Plainview, New York. There's *When a Woman's Body Says No to Sex,* by Linda Valins. There's *The Vulvodynia Survival Guide.*[10] There's lots of new work being done to correct the erroneous impression given by researchers Masters and Johnson in 1970 that it's actually fairly easy to surmount vaginismus with a few simple exercises.

I am treating all that has happened to me in a fairly academic fashion: tracking down scholarship, accumulating a bibliography, researching the subject. And of course, my condition has been academic in other ways as well—because the lenses through which I have seen all this have necessarily been academic, the lexicon with which I express it academic. *But has my attitude toward it been academic enough?*—sufficiently aware and critical of the culture's normative narratives?

Perhaps I am at the point where I can—and even should—put all of this to rest. I remember a comment from a women's therapy center that offered treatments for vaginismus. The doctors there were talking about people who had "graduated" from their therapy process—"graduates" like me—who were talking to women still struggling with the condition:

> We found that "talking" beyond the necessary information/validation exchange leads to enhancing negative emotional turmoil, and more confusions/fears that will need to be "undone" as part of the actual treatment process.
>
> The "graduates" who spoke drew much satisfaction and validation [from] . . . having been cured, but only for a very short time before they were ready to move on with their own lives, putting the past behind them—our ultimate goal![11]

putting the past behind them I think it's crucial not to simply leave the past behind, simply to move on. As I now have the luxury of retrospecting about this, of choosing to engage in conventional heterosexual sex or not, I think it's crucial not to repress the questions that were raised, necessarily, by the condition. It's important to remember the distance ("remoteness") from so-called normal sexual practice that this whole experience has brought with it—perhaps has given me to use—and what I can see from that distance that others wouldn't. *she found me screaming it was the middle of the night my roommate didn't know what was happening—brought a damp cloth I was deeply embarrassed—couldn't explain why they were roiling out of me in the dark, these screams no hope couldn't stop she was kind, the daughter of a nurse I tried to say it was a nightmare only a nightmare*

The prospect of ceasing the practice of cultural critique at the threshold of the home space, at least keeping it in abeyance until one ventures forth again from the haven where one repairs at night, unquestionably has a certain allure (leave critique with the boots at the door). But it's important not to forget to bring to bear in one's private life the hard questions one asks elsewhere: important, even off the academic clock, to continue to problematize conventional assumptions about sexual success, completion, fulfillment. Fortunately, however much I may be tempted to do so, I cannot accept uncritically the assumption that women are most fulfilled when they are using their vaginas. Given all that's happened, it's simply not possible to take for granted the pleasure of what most people consider "normal" sexual interaction. It's also not possible to regard coitus, usually considered the telos of the male-female sexual narrative, as anything other than one option among many. The academic context has helped here—helped to cultivate this resistance, helped to reveal the potentially generative space that has opened up between me and the way things normally are and go, to find the reasons for dissent. I need to make something of all this, do something with it.

Eve Sedgwick notes that "queer" means thwarting the norm, moving at cross-purposes with the usual ideological currents that promote certain kinds of normalization, normative behavior.[12] It means interrupting those currents. *i am repeating what millions of others have enacted, but there is difference in this repetition, this citation, born out of the irony I was obliged for so long to maintain* Adrienne Rich ends her essay "Split at the Root" with phrases I've never forgotten: "If you really look at the one reality, the other will waver and disperse"—disparate aspects of one's identity that don't easily reconcile into a whole. *No passing zone* She encourages a "moving into accountability."[13] She asks such accountability of herself: "I know that in the rest of my life, the next half century or so, every aspect of my identity will have to be engaged."

I remember someone asking me a long, long time ago, "Are you gay?" I don't remember what I answered (actually don't remember—there's repression for you—and what else has been erased in this process?), but I remember thinking that whatever I answered would seem wrong. With that same kind of quizzical look—the one the person who asked me gave me—I might ask myself, "Am I a straight woman?"

I think the answer is no.

NOTES

1. Eve Ensler, "The Flood," *The Vagina Monologues: The V-Day Edition* (New York: Villard, 2001), 25–26.
2. I take these phrases from Luce Irigaray.
3. Monica Oala, "The Montreal Women's Vulvovaginal Pain Support Group" (pamphlet from support group, 2002).
4. Eve F., "The Girl without a Hole," in *Private Pain, It's about Life, Not Just Sex: Understanding Vaginismus and Dyspareunia,* by Ditza Katz and Ross Lynn Tabisel (Plainview, NY: Katz-Tabi Publications, 2002), 7.
5. Jane Pavanel, "Re: personal testimonial on vaginismus," email to the author, 4 November 2003.
6. The phrases here are adapted from those in from Oala's pamphlet on vulvovaginal pain cited earlier (see note 3); from T. S. Eliot's *The Waste Land*, part 3, "The Fire Sermon," which in turn references Buddha's *Fire Sermon* and St. Augustine's *Confessions*; and from St. Paul, *1 Corinthians* 7: 9.
7. Ensler, Preface to "Reclaiming Cunt," *The Vagina Monologues* 99.
8. Ensler, "My Angry Vagina," *The Vagina Monologues* 71.
9. Linda Valins, *When a Woman's Body Says No to Sex* (New York: Penguin Books, 1988) xxi. Valins credits Patricia Gillan, consultant psychologist, who used the phrase in an interview with Valins, 16 September 1987.
10. Howard I. Glazer and Gae Rodke, *The Vulvodynia Survival Guide* (Oakland, CA: Harbinger Publications, 2002). For the other publications, see notes 5 and 8.
11. Ditza Katz and Ross Lynn Tabisel, "Re: Query from McGill University in Montréal," e-mail to the author, 16 October 2003.
12. Eve Sedgwick, Foreword, *Tendencies* (Durham: Duke University Press, 1993).
13. Adrienne Rich, "Split at the Root: an Essay on Jewish Identity," *The Writer's Presence: A Pool of Essays.* Ed. Donald McQuade and Robert Atwan (Boston: St. Martin's Press, 1994) 111–12.

QUESTIONS

1. Consider the form of the narrative—how it embeds narratives within narratives. Explore the effects achieved by breaks in the narrative flow, interruptions, and shifts from one voice to another. What is the author trying to achieve with the different typefaces?
2. Reminiscing about her trip to Italy with her friend and Enzo, the author thinks, "I won-

der what it would take for me to qualify as queer." What does it "take" for someone to qualify as "queer"? Here, you might consider the etymology of the word "queer."

3. What is the author trying to achieve with the phrase that she culls from the pamphlet from the intersex group, "no passing zone"? For her, what would moving into "account-ability" entail?

4. Given what she has said throughout the narrative, why does the author say at the end that she "think[s]" she would say "no" to the question, "Are you a straight woman?" Note that she doesn't say what she is—only what she "thinks" she is not. Why might she have chosen to phrase it this way?

5. Note that the author has chosen not to write under her actual name. Why might she have made this choice?

Breast Art

⟡ Lisa Katz ⟡

BREAST ART

1.

Raphael's *La Fornarina* lives in a Roman palace now,
touching her left breast, holding it between thumb and forefinger
like a fruit she wants to prod in the market.
Perhaps the artist asked her to demonstrate
beckoning a lover
plumping up the smaller breast
showing off in front of the mirror.
You think she's coy.
Perhaps she wanted to touch
the lump she noticed yesterday.
Her eyes look surprised.

2.

In the church of the Frari in Venice
you look up at the ceiling.
You think you see the Virgin Mary
but it's just the artist's wife.
Her eyes roll upward.
She's transported with holiness
or her passion for Titian
and his for her,
but a gauze sash covers what's missing.
She'd rather look up than down.
The gaze is heavenward,
away from her flat earth.

RECONSTRUCTION

You say I should rebuild
with a sack of plastic, or
one part of the body
replaces another.

A woman might love
a man without a leg.
They can have children.
And men whose legs
don't work
make children
with women who climb on.
Sometimes a child disappears
like a lost limb.

Couldn't we have
a different aesthetic,
asymmetrical,
Japanese,
because of the war,
because islands get invaded.

Couldn't we
admire the ruined, the torn, the perfect
error, because the weaver
skips a row
for the sake of humility,
because your love
needs a few stitches?

See the scar,
the flat plain on my chest.
Connect the dots.
You won't get many chances
to look at an absence straight on.

SUPPORT GROUP

Five women are counting women
one by one, they want to count to five,
five cups, five eggs,
five oranges, five pearls,
five days a week to work.

Five women are counting women
one by one, they want to count to five.
And their children count the fingers on each hand:
father, mother, father, mother, father,
father, mother, father, mother, father.

There are so many new things to count.
The doctor who frowns *for your own good*
and the one who cuts
and the one who builds with plastic.
Time spent waiting.
For the first infusion
the second the third the fourth the fifth the last.
For hair to fall,
to grow back again;
cells and nodes and empty hands,
counts from bone and counts from blood.

How time dies in the waiting room:
months weeks
days minutes
seconds.

You'd counted on
longer, hadn't you?

Four women are counting women
One by one, they want to count to four.

THE FORM

Near Kastoria,
we were four kilometers from Metamorphosis
when I began to throw masks
out of the car window,
litter the road with my clothes,
infant, girlish, and grown-up,
foreign bra with one cup filled,
the new costume
of my lopsided middle age.
You ask me
not to throw my human shape away.

Three kilometers from Metamorphosis,
When we get there I will accept
the transformation, for worse or better:
the wife into bird, the mother into stone.
Not least of all I want the story meaningful.

Two kilometers from Metamorphosis,
and though my nakedness suits me now,
it won't be easy
to wear the body I've chosen,
the flat breastplate, no silicon or salt water.

One more kilometer. I tell you
everything here will be or was
human once,
the form I pick
is absence.

QUESTIONS

1. Find images of the paintings that the poet uses as the basis for "Breast Art: 1 and 2": Raphael's *La Fornarina* and Titian's *Assumption of the Virgin*. How do her interpretations of the women in each painting differ from more traditional interpretations? What does the poet suggest about the relationship among sexuality, spirituality, and breast disease?

2. Discuss reasons why losing a breast might be so disturbing—to a woman, to her partner, to society—even when the loss doesn't compromise her ability to function. Why are women encouraged to have plastic surgery following mastectomies? How are women who refuse such reconstruction viewed?

3. Discuss the poet's reference to Japanese art and war in "Reconstruction."
4. Discuss the poet's images in her invitation/challenge in the final three lines of "Reconstruction."
5. What is the significance of the objects in "Support Group"?
6. What is the tone of "The Form" and why does the poet choose it as her final "statement"?

☙ PART III ☙

AGENCY AND ADVOCACY

People who are ill find themselves struggling not only with difficult symptoms, but also frequently with the sense that they have lost control of their lives. Other people, even physicians, sometimes fail to validate the sick person's pain by listening carefully and acting promptly to mitigate suffering. Inasmuch as the academy is based on personal agency, scholars proactively seek effective means of communication and self-healing. The seventeen essays in this group are loosely divided into three sections: illness that is dismissed or trivialized; advocacy for self and others; and language as a special agent of healing.

Althea E. Rhodes argues that while they are not life-threatening, migraines have a profoundly negative effect on the daily life of oneself and one's family and should be taken more seriously by medical professionals; only then can the patient regain some of the control illness has taken away. Similarly, Susannah B. Mintz reveals how profoundly disorienting neck pain can be and how diagnostic language alone seems to legitimize it. She argues for narrative competence on the part of physician *and* patient as she wrestles with the locus of personal identity in a culture that insists on separating mind and body. Henry Abramovitch's story of his father's heart disease uncovers the alarming potential of ageism and implicitly argues that advocates are essential for the elderly in matters of health care. Rae Luckie's spirited essay on hysterectomy brings to light the all-too-common practice of infantilizing those who are ill and "of a certain age." Evelyn Scott's and Richard A. Ingram's essays highlight the disenfranchisement of those with severe psychosis; both reveal instances of profound loss of control but also unveil a certain logic that underlies erratic behavior.

Michael Edmond Donnelly, Jane E. Schultz, and Rebecca A. Pope narrate their highly focused, persistent attempts to become active partners with oncologists. Donnelly and his wife utilize their expertise as attorneys to secure the best medical care in the face of his diagnosis of testicular cancer. Similarly, Schultz navigates the "cancer industry" via assertive self-examination and self-advocacy throughout her treatment for the rare gynecological cancer pseudomyxoma peritonei. It is especially interesting to read original transcripts of her visits with physicians alongside her own interpretation of the information. When her mother develops colon cancer, Pope researches myriad alternative therapies—including nutritional plans and visualization—in an attempt to resist the Western "politics of medicine," which insists on aggressive chemotherapy. Chris Bell and Christopher R. Smit reflect different perspectives on political activism for those with disease and disability. Bell's diagnosis of HIV propels him on a life-altering crusade to inform others about the disease, while Smit resists being identified primarily as person with muscular dystrophy and only secondarily as a scholar of film and disability studies.

For many, language is central to the experience of illness, both in terms of accurately conveying information and imaginatively processing a new reality, privately and with health-care professionals. Andrea T. Wagner's essay about epilepsy exemplifies her inability to define or verbalize her seizures as she seeks words and narrative structure to give order to the physical chaos she experiences. Elena Levy-Navarro approaches the issue of verbalizing physical pain from a different perspective; she has language, but finds it too constraining and seeks alternate ways of speaking her illness. Kimberly R. Myers and Kristin Lindgren explore the role of language and literature as they narrate their quest for healing from inflammatory bowel disease and chronic fatigue syndrome, respectively. Both depict the leveling forces of disease that is not diagnosed with speed or certainty, and they use their professional training with words and images to anchor themselves to a semblance of their pre-illness reality. Roxana Robinson's story about a young woman's attempt to recover from an unidentified disease examines the ritualistic dimensions of medical treatment and the consequences of health-care workers who are insensitive to the power of language and how they use it. This story resonates beautifully with Raymond Carver's "A Small, Good Thing" in that it shows how those who are ill try to divine meaning from the slightest subtleties of the words and phrases health professionals use. So strong is her belief in the efficacy of writing that Ellen Samuels discontinues medication in favor of writing her way out of panic. She believes that illness is more than merely physical and contends that it should be viewed in broader, more creative contexts.

When Pain Is the Other Dancer
Living with Migraine

⌒ ALTHEA E. RHODES ⌒

Migraine. Even the name rhymes with pain. Let me describe a migraine morning. I wake after a night tortured by vivid Technicolor nightmares in which I am usually trapped or threatened in some way. The dreams duplicate themselves, so I get to relive the threat repeatedly throughout the night. While it is happening, I am, on one level, conscious enough to know it is a dream, although that doesn't buffer the emotional impact of the dream itself. The part of me that is awake knows what is coming as I struggle through the layers to full consciousness. The pain is there, lurking, greedy, waiting to pounce when I open my eyes. The light, no matter how dim, how diffuse, stabs my retina and pierces my brain; I know the second I make the slightest movement, the pain will engulf me. Of course, I move. I can't prevent it. I flinch and close my eyelids and then the pain comes. In waves. Thick, greasy waves that begin in the right back quadrant of my head and roll forward through the center of my brain to explode just behind my eyes. I can feel my scalp tighten and tingle, and even my hair hurts—until I am aware of the moment and placement of each individual hair shaft.

Slowly, gingerly, I force myself to roll out of bed, mouth clenched against the nausea. Because it's safer than walking, I make my way to the bathroom on my hands and knees. It seems to hurt less the closer I am to the ground. The journey to the medicine cabinet is a long one, one I endure only out of necessity. Once I make it, I sometimes curl up on the bathroom rug rather than make the tortuous return trip to the bed, a towel over my eyes to protect me from the light until the medicines kick in enough to make the return journey possible.

When in the grip of a migraine, all my senses are unnaturally sharp. I can feel my daughter walking across the kitchen floor downstairs. I can hear everything that happens in my condo and the condos on either side, as well as outside. I swear I can feel birds flying through the air, the vibrations of cars driving down the road. Television and radio are both torture devices. The explosion of sound buffets my eardrums and assaults my brain. The worst, however, are the smells. Unlike many migraine sufferers, I don't seem to have food triggers. But let me smell the wrong thing—cigarette smoke, particular perfumes, household cleaners—instant migraine! And when I actually have a migraine, my sense of smell is particularly acute. I can tell my husband is home before he opens the door because I can smell the cologne he put on that morning. We chose that cologne because most of the time it doesn't bother me. But on migraine days it's deadly.

Obviously, migraine doesn't affect just the person with the headache. Family members have to modify their behavior. That means muted TV and radio. No running, shouting, and please, no loud friends over. Mom has a headache, again. My daughters have had to make concessions. They both like potpourri and candles but are restricted to the scents that I can handle. They can never casually buy and wear perfume; they can wear only fragrances that I can tolerate. My husband and daughter have to do much of the household cleaning because I cannot tolerate the smell of household cleaners and chemicals. I can cook, make beds, do the laundry (as long as nothing requires bleach), but when it comes to anything that requires chemicals, forget it—they send me straight to the medicine cabinet.

The worst thing about the pain is what it does to my brain. I can't think. The pain is so severe that it disrupts my thought processes and all I can consider is stopping the pain. People talk to me and, sometimes, I don't answer them. They think I am ignoring them, but I am not. It's just that the words get mixed up in my brain, and it takes time to sort them out again and then make sense of them. The sound comes in, but it's just noise. I have to force the language center in my brain to sort the noise into words, and I don't always have the energy to do that. It's easier just to let the sound wash over me and let it go. The nausea brought on by the pain is so bad that I constantly have to guard against throwing up. All I can do is take my medication and try to sleep. All I want when one of these headaches hits is oblivion.

One of my friends also suffers from these debilitating migraines, and we have a nickname for this particular kind of headache: a brainfucker. A strong word, one not normally used in a forum such as this, but appropriate nonetheless because once a headache like this is over, which may take up to several days, that is exactly the way your brain feels: totally and truly fucked. It usually takes several days to recover, not only from the headache, but also from the medication, and from the inability to eat or exercise.

The medications deserve a separate note. When I first started getting severe migraines, all that doctors knew to do with them was give me heavy painkillers. At least now there are drugs specifically for migraines. Along with Topamax (a drug originally developed for epilepsy and found to be effective in migraine), I take an antidepressant daily for prevention. For pain relief, I have an arsenal of medications. There are several medications called "triptans," sold under various names, which work rather well. The drugs I normally use include Amerge, Maxalt, and Zomig. These drugs work by activating serotonin receptors in the brain, chemical pathways dealing with mood regulation. I also use Midrin to try to abort a headache if I catch it early enough. The really bad headaches sometimes require Demerol and oblivion. That, of course, is a last resort, after everything else has failed. If I depend on one medication too much, it loses effectiveness, and the migraine will rebound stronger than ever.

As the medications for fighting migraines have improved, the days I spend in bed have declined, and I have more headache days when I can take meds and continue with my life.

However, these days are somehow worse because, although I can go on with my day, I am in a befuddled state of mind and body. My synapses misfire and I am left wondering, what was I saying? What was I about to do? It is a surreal existence.

As a language teacher, I find this beyond frustrating. I teach English; my specialty is rhetoric and composition. Normally, I will have some combination of four composition courses, from beginning to advanced writers. I also teach technical writing and a course for students who are planning to teach high school English. I need all my brain cells to be operating all the time. Migraine and the accompanying pain interfere with that task by making it impossible for me to think. The pain shoulders everything aside and scatters my thoughts, and whatever seemed like a brilliant insight is lost. The pain acts as a thief by stealing language itself, by taking the words away from me and leaving me only with shadows that tease and holes where my ideas once existed. I have to work twice as hard to make them come back once the pain is gone.

Pain also steals time. Hours when I could be thinking and writing are relinquished to fight a migraine. Whole days simply disappear while I wallow shamefully in its grasp. I have tried working through the headaches, ignoring the pain and its attendant symptoms, but sometimes the results are not pretty. I have ended up in the hospital for several days on more than one occasion. That's the essence of living with migraines—with all the meds and all the modifications to your life, you can't stop them. If you are lucky, you can make them better and you can learn to live with them, but you can't stop them. No matter what, every once in awhile, they stop you in your tracks.

It is that loss of time that is so difficult for me. I am a natural procrastinator. In fact, I *need* to procrastinate. I need time in my writing process to let my thoughts develop between beginning a project and writing it. I realized how vital a role procrastination plays for me while taking an advanced composition course in graduate school. We were required to evaluate our writing process, and as I looked closely at mine, I realized that I wasn't wasting time, but writing in my head, subconsciously waiting until I was ready to commit to paper (or screen). As a result, I now write fewer—but better—drafts. I begin early, gather research, sit back, procrastinate, and then, finally, write furiously. How does pain affect this process? It robs me of that leisure time to reflect. Everything gets scrambled up, and I have to start over, reorder my thoughts. Or I lose so much time fighting the migraine that I get too far behind. Deadlines that were manageable are upon me and then gone before my brain can function again.

But there is—as there always is—another side to this pain. Sometimes the pain actually helps, gives me an edge, puts me in a place where everything is clearer, cleaner, sharper. Occasionally, instead of making me sleep, the migraine medications have the opposite effect and I cannot sleep; the combination of the medication and the pain makes my brain dance in overdrive. I am still unable to stand the light, so I have learned how to write in semi-darkness. With the help of a 25-watt nightlight, I scribble ideas on the legal pad I keep by my bed, ideas for class, ideas for a short story, ideas for an article. At these times the pain is almost sweet. I know at some point I am going to crash—extra sleep is necessary after a migraine—but I don't mind because I feel like I have actually accomplished something. Frankly, that doesn't happen often enough. It's usually just the opposite.

Productivity comes in another guise. The time leading up to one of these painful events is sometimes marked by an almost manic energy. I find myself in such a good mood that frankly I can't stand myself, and I am often abnormally productive. Writing at these times goes very smoothly, very quickly. The demands of a teacher's schedule do not always allow me to take advantage of this time to write for myself—I am often grading papers during these times—but even that form of academic writing comes more easily. I have only two complaints about these episodes of hyperactivity: I never recognize them for what they are, a precursor to a headache; and they are far too brief. While a migraine can last for days, these episodes never last more than four to twelve hours.

I don't know why I don't recognize that I am developing a headache. When I am feeling fine, I pretend migraines don't exist. I have to take my migraine medications every day, but I take them with my vitamins and don't give them a second thought. It's not at all unusual for my family members to look at me and say, "You're getting a migraine, take your pills." They say they can see it in my eyes, and certainly in my behavior. They tell me my whole face changes. One semester, my dean took one look at me and said, "You have a migraine today." I remember being very upset at his comment. First, I was mad at myself for not realizing I was getting a headache—again. Second, I was angry that someone with whom I have only a professional relationship could recognize the signs of a migraine, that this disease had intruded so far into my life.

I can't remember a time when I didn't have headaches, but like many women, I suffered an increase in severity and frequency after menstruation. I wasn't diagnosed as having migraines at that time, however; I just had headaches. When I complained of them while in the Air Force, the military doctors called them tension headaches or cluster headaches. They told me I had headaches because my mother did, or accused me of malingering, or simply gave me drugs. Very little was done in the way of diagnosis or treatment.

My headaches changed when I became pregnant with my second child, another hormonal stimulus.[1] I began having episodes of double vision which lasted for periods of twenty to ninety minutes and were sometimes followed by an intense migraine. Unlike the doctors I had seen so far, a neurologist I visited took my complaints seriously and performed a series of tests to rule out diseases such as multiple sclerosis and epilepsy. Since my test results were negative, he diagnosed migraine. He was the first to treat it as such, and I finally had a name for what I had always referred to as the monster in my head. But I still knew very little about it.

By this time, I was back in college. As a graduate student, I was constantly doing research on some literary figure or some aspect of rhetoric and composition. I added migraine to my list. At first, I found very little information. Much of what I did find, I couldn't understand because of all the medical jargon. Today, I still do periodic research on migraines. Much more information is available, and articles are being written for laypeople as well as medical practitioners. I was particularly interested in an article I recently came across on the American Medical Association website that discusses a theory about a "migraine 'pacemaker' or 'generator' located in the brain stem" that is responsible for stimulating migraines (Larkin). According to this theory, activity in the brain stem causes the attack, rather than acting as a response to the attack. The theory also explains why the medications now on the market cannot always prevent a rebound headache. Triptans decrease blood flow to the cerebral cortex and eliminate symptoms of migraine attacks, but the medicine does nothing to the brain stem. Therefore, the individual is vulnerable to another attack. Current medications cannot affect activity deep within the brain (Larkin). I hope Dr. Hans C. Diener of the University of Essen in Germany and his colleagues, who proposed the brain stem theory, find what they are looking for—and find a way to fix it. If they need a research subject, I'm here.

In the meantime, I am left to deal with migraines. Paradoxically, the pain has both hindered and helped my teaching, sometimes in unexpected ways. On the first day of class, while I am lecturing new students on being present for class, I have to tell them I suffer from migraines and that it is possible, at some point in the semester, I will have a headache and miss class. I have specific procedures for them to follow, and I tell them what I expect of them. Although I hate having to mention migraines, it shows students how to plan for contingencies.

Additionally, having to grope for language, having to struggle for proper sentence structure, makes me more aware of students' needs and difficulty with writing. Most writing teachers write at a level that is so far above their students that they have forgotten what it is like to be in their students' place. It doesn't hurt to be in that place occasionally. Finally, because I have this monster in my head, I am more compassionate towards students who have to deal with similar traumas in their lives. Pain defines and delineates my existence. Sometimes brutally, sometimes incrementally, it strips away the layers of civilization until all that's left is the animal core fighting just to cope with another day. Pain forces me into dependency—dependency on chemicals that can cause as many problems as they solve; dependency on the compassion and care of others who may or may not understand, who may view this uncontrollable pain simply as a "weakness." Pain deceives me, shrouding me in mist, sometimes giving me wondrous visions, but taking away my ability to capture them in language. My life is an intricate dance with pain as a demanding partner. I'd rather be a wallflower.

NOTE

1. When I had an emergency hysterectomy in my late twenties, my doctors predicted my migraines would get better. However, that was not ultimately the case. If anything, they worsened. Ten years later, when I went through menopause, they predicted that my migraines would improve or disappear. That hasn't been the case either. So hormones are involved somehow, but my doctors haven't been able to figure out just how.

REFERENCES

"Drug Profiles: Topiramate & Topiramate Capsules (AKA Topamax)" MAGNUM. n.d. 12 February 2003 <http://www.migraines.org/treatment/protpmax.htm>.

Larkin, Marilynn. "What Causes Head Pain in Migraine?" Migraine Information Center. 10 September 1997. *The Journal of American Medical Association.* January 18, 2003<http//www.ama-assn.org/special/migraine/newsline/briefing/pain/htm>.

Warner, Jennifer. "Epilepsy Drug Fights Migraine." *WebMDHealth.* 23 September 2002 <http://my.webmd.com/content/article/50/40479.htm>.

QUESTIONS

1. Discuss the ramifications of society's tendency to treat certain illnesses and conditions as "legitimate" while dismissing others as not worthy of serious attention. To what degree is this practice problematic?
2. To what extent should the author's family, colleagues and students cater to her needs as a person who suffers migraines?
3. Discuss the issues of control—who or what has it and to what extent—in this narrative.

Pain in the Neck

⌒ Susannah B. Mintz ⌒

The technician fastens a white strap across my face. He tells me it's to ensure that my head doesn't budge during the procedure, but the grip of that cold plastic cupping my chin makes me feel like a prisoner of madness. The aperture of the MRI machine gapes behind my head, silent and mean. The socks I wear with the thin hospital gown offer scant comfort against the chill air. In the locker-room prior to my appointment, I carefully removed anything metal from my body and now, on my back with head securely pinioned, I feel stripped of the little reassurances that hold me to myself—favorite rings and earrings, the barrettes that tuck my hair into a familiar style. The table is hard, the technician bored, and lying flat on the hard surface sends ripples of pain through my neck and shoulders. Just as he moves to slide me backward into the dark, narrow hold of the machine—so close, I can't imagine how it will not suffocate me—I tell him I cannot go through with this, and in shame I put my clothes back on and leave the building.

This pain brings me to a place I cannot see or touch. A slippery disk eludes my grasp, its maddening rub against the nerves impossible to halt through any instinctive manipulation. I press my fingers into the back of my neck, massage the muscles, stretch my head forward against the pain—all useless, even exacerbating. Before this happened, I had no conscious sense whatever of the structure of my neck, its lattice of vertebrae, disks, arteries, muscles, nerves. Now my neck has a serious hold on me, disrupting the smallest details of my routine.

The next day, I call my neurologist to explain what happened. He assumes I was claustrophobic, and to some extent he is right; I can't deny I feared the machine might trap me in its cylindrical grip. Yet I also need to convince him of the intolerable pain. I tell him I could not have endured thirty minutes flat on my back, but he isn't hearing me; he insists I try again, says he will prescribe something to calm me. We are engaged in a contest over meaning. Which of us knows me better in this moment? I wonder whose truth about my experience is more accurate, and if I had, in fact, been more psychologically than physically uncomfortable. Who is the "me" the pills will relax, and where does it reside—in my muscles or my mind? Could my fear be accessed through my body? Is it possible to unravel the two?

Despite our different accounts of what happened, the doctor and I collude in separating body from self. By focusing on my *physical* experience, I want to dissociate who I "am"—my character, my integrity, my worth—from the embarrassment of a phobic response to the MRI; by disregarding the physical component of my reluctance, the doctor exaggerates my *mental* ability to transcend the state of my body. He renders inconsequential the body's signals (my neck was meant to stay inert; it was there to be observed, not felt or "heard"), and simultaneously minimizes my reaction to the MRI as purely (and irrationally) emotional. Entangled in a question over knowledge, we both overlook the fact that my fear was a function of the pain I knew I would have to withstand inside the tight compass of the MRI machine.

I fret over the terrible responsibility of having to describe or defend my pain, as if I'll fail something, or someone. Whose needs are at stake in the telling? What makes me worry that I'll get it wrong, commit some kind of mistake? I am not fully in control of this discourse, and I do not trust that my version of events will be validated or heard.

This is a quest narrative to locate my neck.

With the help of a tranquilizer, headphones, and a sleeping mask over my eyes, I get through my second attempt at the MRI. Afterwards, the technician brings me into the darkened control room to show me the images of my neck. Stark patterns of black and white, like an infinite regress of Rorschach tests, hover in square screens, a geometric puzzle disconnected from the whole of my body or the totality of my "self." Yet they do reveal something fundamental and tangible about me, a structural cause, making me strangely and unfamiliarly visible. Cross-sections of my neck, a whole set of them, showing a tiny white bulge at the back, pressing into the spinal column. The guilty party.

Then, six years after the first incident, I have a second bout with my herniated disk, another summer spent in bed. But despite having been through it all before, I still can't figure out exactly what is happening inside my neck. I have trouble envisioning the structural problem, fail to grasp the implications of this or that course of treatment, can't explain to others my long-term prognosis. Why must we struggle so to ascertain the details? Do doctors assume we don't want to know, that too much information will overwhelm and perturb us? Is such withholding a sinister by product of the machinations of power? I see an internist, an orthopedist, a neurologist, a chiropractor, a bevy of physical therapists. They speak a garbled mix of medicalese and baby-talk, as if they can't decide how to patronize me most efficiently. But I'm in pain, and all I want is a crisp equation of cause, effect, solution. Of course, I recognize it isn't quite so linear. We expect doctors to have the answers; we get mad when they don't. The anger is a screen for fear, a fear produced by the expectation that we should be fully and unmistakenly aware of our physical selves. The doctors are saying to me: look, it's elusive, the body—despite your exercise, your green tea, your healthy diet and good work habits. These things happen and we don't know why; they happen and then they go away, simple as that.

But I need to know—for myself and for others. My zeal for technical information results from a need to prove I'm not making it up. I am a hypochondriac, but I haven't been fabricating my symptoms. I pore over the charts my neurologist forwards to me during the second flare-up, searching for language that will transform nebulous pain into tangible damage. The more technical it gets, the more legitimate I feel: "sagittal and axial cervical MRI performed using fast spin echo and axial gradient echo imaging." Findings: spondylosis. (Spondylitis is inflammation of the vertebrae, but this word is not in my dictionary.) Loss of cervical disk height. Mysteriously described "changes" that encroach on the opening for both nerve roots. Spinal cord "snuggly accommodated without deformity." "Focal cervical spondylosis at C5-6 with bilateral foraminal stenosis." Also: "a 2 mm, central, and right paracentral disk herniation which is just indenting the anterior aspect of the cervical cord." Further tests were recommended but never done: a kimatic examination of the spine and conventional oblique radiographs.

This is me in medical lingo, but I have trouble recognizing the self I meet in these records, where I am "the patient," "a 30-year-old right-handed white female." I am "ambulatory," a "graduate student," a set of mostly functioning muscles and nerves, "upset." Apparently I don't drink but do jog regularly, though the frequency of each of these activities does not accord at all with my memory of graduate school, and I wonder where the mix-up occurred. I feel guilty reading through all this, as if I'm spying, snooping in someone's diary, afraid I'll come upon something embarrassing about myself, some emotion or statement that I'll feel ashamed of.

I read: "abnormal needle examination of one of the muscles sampled." The neurologist never told me this, so I have no idea what it means. But I crave the authenticity it accords my pain.

⌒ ⌐

We're taught to be suspicious of depth metaphors of identity, "core" selves believed to reside at the center of something, the body as container of the self. But there really *is* a thickness to the body; it is not all surface. When my neck hurts I cannot touch ground zero; like an endless metonymic chain, I can attend only to the repercussions, the after-effects, the shadow.

It starts on a Saturday in June—the sixth, a perfect sunny day, Greg and I going to IKEA to look for a desk. I wake to the unmistakable sensation of disk against nerve, and I know I'm in for another long summer. I'd been in bed for weeks with an end-of-semester sinus infection, then spent several days hunched at my computer with encyclopedias and press materials in my lap, working on a magazine article due at the end of May. I figure it must have been the combined force of all that bad posture—the choreography of readers and writers, curved-over navel-gazers, human question marks, signifying what we do with our bodily ailments—that threw my neck out of whack. And I wind my way through the labyrinth of IKEA, afraid to speak of the agony I'm in, because pain, when it first strikes, comes as a surprise, and feels like a secret.

Can I describe for you how it feels? A toothache throb that weighs down my arm, a sour pain stabbing at the back of my neck, an awful friction deep within my shoulder joint. A hot prickle that encases my forearm and hand, pins and needles in my thumb and forefinger, a scarf of nettles, blood pressure cuff squeezing my bicep all day long. A lemony ache at the back of my throat. The sensation of something *right there* in the center of my neck, a feeling on the brink of choking me. A deep, unlocatable pain. It's all of this, yet none of it is accurate. Pain proliferates with endless variety. It reorganizes time; it brings my imagination to a complete halt.

For weeks, I can't sleep without muscle relaxants and pain killers, and only in one position, on my back with my head at a very specific angle. Even the slightest turn to either side causes pain. But sleeping is never as bad as waking up—that moment of truth. Some mornings the pain returns gradually, like a bad memory of some guilty excess indulged the night before. But more often it's immediate, an internal friction like tiny shards of glass rubbing the inside of my left shoulder, fire ants nibbling their way down my arm to the tip of my thumb. I promise myself, one day I will wake up and not have my first thought be about pain; I will wake up and not lie there in suspense, gingerly testing my neck, too afraid to move.

One night I dream pure pain. Pain in raw form, without narrative or visual imagery. I see nothing, remember nothing when I awaken but the impression of having dreamt a feeling of pain, of pain having entered my sleeping consciousness. I wake to a doubled effect: pain in the dream and pain in my neck. No story to relate, just the residue of a pain I'm still having, as if pain has obliterated any attempt to represent and stabilize it in language.

As soon as pain is gone, you cannot remember it. Just days after the most acute period of pain had subsided, even when I could still sense the disk against the nerve, I could not exactly recreate that feeling. This is the body's way of saving itself. If we remembered every sensation, we'd implode, fold inward under the weight of it all. Perhaps this is what it means to say that the body in pain is unrepresentable.

But is this true—that pain is unspeakable? If I tell you about my pain, will you feel it? Will I feel less pain? Will my pain become real and therefore tolerable? Why do I want to tell you how badly it hurts when I know that there's nothing you can do?

I want to make sense of it, how an experience so intense can evaporate so quickly. (I begin to understand how orgasm slides into pain, pain into pleasure.) I want to understand its significance to me, to figure out who this person is, this person in pain. I discover something new about myself: I am capable of great pain. I need to understand what this means.

Pain diminishes me, whirls me out of control, so I can't advocate for myself, don't ask the questions that might produce the answers I'm looking for. Because I depend on others to help me function with the least amount of discomfort, I can't afford to have anyone angry with me. You make nice when you're in pain; you can barely complain about your pain, let alone anything someone else is doing. You're beholden to people just to let you have your pain.

Bodies are intensely private things, but they're also communal. Some bodily subjects we cannot discuss in public (scatology, gynecology), yet when we're sick we invade each other's physical selves with the most ardent faith in our right of access, with our helpful remedies and hopeful explanations. We want to believe we know, that we can hold on to to something definable and firm. We share our ailments gladly; they are a point of contact, they lessen the irreducible distance between our physical selves. We take others' bodies to belong to us. Yet a chronically pained body that just keeps on and on, refusing to heal, threatens us terribly, provoking deep-seated, inarticulable anxieties. I know my friends want me to say I've improved. If I capitulate to that need, simply lie and say I'm feeling better, any discussion of my neck comes to a definitive halt.

Our bodies reside at a conflictual intersection. As Westerners, we're inculcated in the separation of body and mind. We construe our "selves" as pure consciousness, nothing but mind, yet we contemplate our bodies constantly: exercise obsessively, monitor what we eat, surgically alter what we don't like or can't subdue. We're encouraged to be medically savvy, and technology has introduced us to an unprecedented level of specificity about the interiors of our physical selves. We wax rhapsodic about the wonders of the human genome, about a future free of the depredations of aging and disease.

But pain shocks us with our own mortality. To confront our capacity for being hurt, our inability to fully control our physical state, is to catch a glimpse of death in the distance, there at the vanishing point of the hale and hearty selves we so long to remain. We congratulate ourselves for dominating the flesh, yet everywhere around us is manifest evidence of our inevitable decline, of the horrifying deterioration of vigor and viability. The disabled are punished for displaying the raw fact of physical breakdown we labor so strenuously to transcend; any form of incapacity, any change in motion or range, however temporary, seems the tip of a titanic iceberg, effecting a shift in social status, a diminishment of identity.

So we rage against the elusive causes of pain and our limitations as healers. We don't truly know what to say to the person in pain. It's not so much a failure of empathy, I think; it's our fear that makes us clumsy. We look upon the weak and recoil from that evidence of our own frailty; we shunt the runt to the margins. We equate worth with active doing and assume that physical limitations render a person inconsequential, a drain on resources, a detriment to the thriving social body. Perhaps we no longer euthanize disabled newborns in contemporary society, yet those primitive prejudices are entrenched in how we think about bodies, and they motivate the anxiety behind my frantic wish to *do* something about my neck and my pain.

We refuse to prepare ourselves for death and decay. Rather than fashioning a culture that guides us along that inevitable path, our medical technology and our obsession with form alienate us from any authentic relationship with our bodies, widening the gap. "I" is the task master, body the wayward pet.

☞ ☜

Two physical therapists evaluate my pain based on a scale they call "activities of daily living." Is getting dressed a six or a seven? They chatter back and forth as I struggle to assign a number to the shades of pain. Looking gravely earnest, they tell me that my insurance company will pay for another dozen sessions as long as my ADL pain ratings are above a certain number—but I can't remember which one, because they make it up for me to guarantee my return. I want to say, I have no activity, time is at a standstill, I'm not living: I'm underwater. I can't use the toilet, feed the cat, take a shower, do the dishes, or cook without some form of discomfort. When I lean over to brush my teeth or wash my face, my left thumb and forefinger erupt in prickly heat. I can't jot down a note on a piece of paper, write checks, or put on nail polish without the muscles at the back of my neck doing their angry twisted dance of pain. I laugh when they try to convince me of the seriousness of the scale. I say, it hurts when I turn my head, it hurts when I walk, it hurts when I reach for the butter with my left hand. It even hurts, I tell them, when I cry.

I'm suffocated with pain. I wander around the apartment as if I could stride my way out of my own body, but I end up back in bed, the only place that provides relief. Lying in bed is supposed to be bad, so I go to the couch, try to read, feel aggravated, lie on the floor, get discouraged, go back to the bedroom, lie on the floor again. I feel imprisoned in this body's ever-diminishing scope of movement—trapped in a body that refuses to cooperate, trying to make deals (with whom, exactly?), thinking about luck and breaks and wagers. I lie on the floor and stare at the ceiling, cracks in the foundation. The compass of my physical motion gets smaller and smaller. I spiral in place. I "make one room an everywhere." I cup my palms over my hip bones and frame my body's new house in my mind.

They show me how to do exercises called Mackenzie retractions—"chin tucks," colloquially. These serve an oddly parental function, separating the vertebrae in my neck like naughty siblings, so the disk can slide back into position. I do shoulder rolls and head circles and back stretches. I walk around like a swimmer before a race, or a nervous boxer, trying to relax. I'm supposed to put one hand on the side of my face and press my head against my palm to strengthen the muscles in my neck. I'm in a perpetual state of shock or awe, struck with a brilliant idea, or the fear that I've left the stove on.

I try powdered roots from South America, yoga on videotape, magnets. I don't believe any of it will work, but it provides some sense of control over my situation that all the mystifying conversations with neurologists, orthopedists, and physical therapists have denied me. There's defiant rebellion in such choices. Every time I apply the magnets, I feel empowered: just going to the drugstore, buying something, makes me feel better. I need hope, and I can satisfy the collective need to *do* something. Lying all day long on the floor, contemplating the precise angle at which the wall meets the ceiling, feels like drowning.

I want so badly to slouch, hunch my shoulders forward, let my gut go slack. I mourn the loss of sleeping on my stomach. I think, I will never again feel my body release itself so completely. I take excessively long, steaming showers, just on the verge of scalding. My neck vanishes in the heat. I imagine a trip to the beach, mounds of warmth cradling my neck. I would lie down in all that hot sand, and sleep and sleep.

My disk wields absolute control.

Pain is my constant companion, my own private habit. I'll admit, even though I think it's shameful, that I get a little apprehensive about the pain going away, about being back to my "normal," mundane existence, with no excuses for not getting work done or begging off social engagements, no justification for being needy. It's my summer of love with my neck, a tortured affair. I'm preoccupied with pain, the twist of desire that locked us in combat. I never worry about my neck abandoning me. It's always there, steady in its regard.

A dictatorial puppet-master. If my head strays too far out of place, my neck yanks a string and back swivels my head, front-center-and-tucked. I keep expecting my arms and legs to fly akimbo, jutting out in opposite directions, while I do a lurching dance for spectators transfixed by my pain. Please understand: this was not a normal kind of hurt . . . headache, scraped knee, menstrual cramps, paper cut, stomachache, burned tongue, splinter. These do not make you say to yourself: *I've never felt pain like this before.* They may discombobulate or inconvenience, but they do not take you by surprise with their irrepressible unfamiliarity.

I keep repeating the word "pain," so much that it seems almost meaningless, an empty signifier. I assume you'll know what I mean, but how can you? Our experience of pain is as individual as the bodies it affects.

Friends ask me, how's your back? And I have to correct them, again and again, *neck, not back.* My strange affliction, the inglorious neck—the stuff of zoos and soup stock, not case history or tales of debilitating pain told over drinks and a game of cards. Goose necks, giraffe necks, poultry gullets chucked in the garbage, turkey waddles indecently red. Certainly nothing sensuous or sexy about the *neck*—even the sound of it is graphic and harsh.

But the neck is a real workhorse. It supports the head! All ten pounds of it (imagine: your head perched like two bricks atop that solitary column). You can hold your head high, swallow food, breathe, look at a clock, get out of bed, turn to kiss your lover, drink a cup of tea, stay alive.

Just maybe, I suppose, there's something tender and vulnerable . . . the nape of a child's neck, the way it's always soft and cool. The neck as a place to nuzzle, hickies blooming like roses on Victorian wallpaper. *Necking,* they used to call it, as if a good kiss requires flex and twist, two bodies coiled around that singular axis, narrowing down to the deep interconnections of pleasure.

But something literally sickening is going on inside my neck, something that leaves me nauseous and weak. I want to sever myself from my neck. I want to reattach my head to the top of my torso. I have vivid daydreams about ridding myself of the pain, dark inchoate fantasies of surgery, someone cutting away the disk, or squishing it back into place—anything to relieve pressure on the nerve.

My neck is the cross I bear.

Pain does not usher me to the brink of conversion. But did I, after all, do something bad to deserve this? Disability is construed in our culture as a metonymy of wrong. When my sister and I were young, and my father would praise my ramrod-straight back as an object lesson to her teenaged slump, I'd feel terribly proud. But I've lost it now, some way that I was, some pure way embodied by good posture. I've gone slack, failed to stay upright; I haven't made good on something that might have been, lived up to some potential. Was it quitting the piano, neglecting my studies, hating my father and then forgetting to tell him I loved him again?

I feel ashamed, self-indulgent. Well, aren't I, lying in bed for two months? I know what you're thinking: that I'm exaggerating my symptoms, calling unnecessary attention to myself. That I should "get over it" or "work through the pain," that I should "forge on." I worry that I'm talking about it too much (and no one really knows what to say). I should fold the pain into my regular workday, stop obsessing. This is why I crave all that technical language:

because we're made to believe that we cause our own pain, because even our most intimate relations don't always take our pain seriously.

⌒ ⌒

"I felt," wrote F. Scott Fitzgerald, "therefore I was."

I roam, I re-experience myself. My thoughts tunnel inward toward that disk. Pain interrupted by periods of no-pain. What an awesome tapestry of word-eluding pains the body produces! I begin to doubt that I can tolerate any more of it. And if I can't—I wonder if I will dissolve, who I am anymore apart from pain.

My body is telling me a story only I can understand. We compose it together, in isolation. One day, we'll show it off as evidence.

QUESTIONS

1. Discuss the extent to which one must be able to describe pain or disease in order for it to become legitimate in the eyes of the patient and health-care professionals.
2. Who is the more valid judge of illness, the patient or the physician? In what ways?
3. Discuss how pain or disease dislocates us into an unfamiliar territory.

My Father's Illness
A Case Study in Ageism

⌒ Henry Abramovitch ⌒

This is the story of my father's illness and disease during the summer of 2001. It is based upon my direct participation with him, when I was his "case manager"; my diaries recorded at the time; access, sometimes surreptitious, to his medical charts; discussions with his many doctors, my sister, brother, uncle and especially my cousin, Dr. Martin Shapiro, Professor of Medicine, UCLA Medical School and past President of the Association of General Internal Medicine. It is also informed by my expertise as an anthropologist, clinical psychologist, and Jungian analyst and by the fact that I teach medical students the "human side" of medicine. In the course of my father's illness, I often felt like I was conducting a participant-observer project and relearning firsthand everything I teach my students.

DISEASE VS. ILLNESS

Medical anthropologists make a distinction between the illness, the patient's perceptions of what is wrong; and the disease, the doctor's understanding of what is going on. These two narratives may coincide as when a person is seized by a heart attack, or, to use the language of disease, when myocardial infarction (MI) occurs. Often, however, these narratives tell different tales, and a pathography is an account of the relationship between the story of the illness and course of the disease. The present narrative is also a story about "ageism," discrimination on the basis of age. From both the patient's and the doctor's point of view, the disease of a young person is not the same as illness in the elderly.

THE BEGINNING

My father was an extraordinarily healthy 92-year-old who had hardly known what illness was. He was still working as an accountant and running off as often as he could to his favorite activity: listening to lectures. His secret, as he told one of his doctors, was to choose the right parents. His mother had lived well into her nineties. He had two mottoes that also served him well. The first was "Stay away from doctors; they tell you that you are sick." And the second was "So far, so good!" This phrase was taken from a joke about an optimist who

179

falls from the Empire State Building and utters these words as he reaches the twentieth floor. My father lived alone in his own house in Montreal, Canada. His three children lived out of town: my brother and sister in New York City, and I in Jerusalem, Israel.

In the beginning, there was no illness, only a silent disease. My sister had come up for the weekend from New York City, where she worked in the Museum of Jewish Heritage. She had wanted to visit our uncle, my father's younger brother, at his lovely country house near the Vermont border. She also wanted my father, Harry, to come along. He didn't really want to go and, uncharacteristically, he told his brother on the phone that he was tired. His brother urged my sister to have him checked out by his doctor.

Dr. Dana Baran, or "Dana" as we knew her, had become Harry's doctor a few years earlier, at the suggestion of Harry's nephew, Martin, who had attended medical school at McGill University and now lived and taught in Los Angeles. Although a kidney transplant specialist, Dana agreed to be Harry's doctor because she and Martin were friends.

On that Sunday, Dana examined Harry and didn't observe anything unusual. "Just to be sure," she decided to do an EKG, which examines the electrical activity of the heart muscle. To her surprise, she discovered that Harry was suffering from a third-degree heart block. In this condition, the electrical impulses from the heart's own natural pacemaker do not reach the rest of the myocardium in proper sequence. The heartbeats continue slowly, independent of the pacemaker, causing a serious lack of oxygen in the blood—hence his tiredness. Without treatment, dementia and death normally occur within a year. Formerly, this condition carried an automatic death sentence; but today, it has an elegant solution: an implanted pacemaker, which sets the rhythm of the heartbeats and makes a life-killing arrhythmia less likely.

At the time, we joked that Harry had the wisdom to select a disease which still does not require him to take pills. With Dana as his protector, he was scheduled for emergency surgery at the Royal Victoria Hospital, where I myself had lain decades earlier in a coma, suffering from the life-threatening brain infection encephalitis. Harry had an initial temporary transplant before the permanent pacemaker was inserted near the clavicle under the skin. Because the latter was improperly implanted, it had to be ripped out and reinserted, which caused considerable bleeding; later, one could see giant blotches of red hematomas on Harry's neck and chest. In any case, the pacemaker took over and his heartbeat became strong and regular once again. I was not there, but followed his progress from afar by phone and email. After a couple of days, he went home, at first with some nursing care and then on his own. The doctors said he should be back to his old self very soon and scheduled a follow-up appointment for a couple of months later. Dana, unworried, went off for a long European holiday with her family.

THE HIDDEN DECLINE

I called often. We developed a telephone ritual greeting. He would say, "So how is Henry?" and I would reply, "So how is Harry?" He sounded weak but otherwise fine. I was not worried. He had never been sick. Why should he start now? He had a problem; it was fixed. End of problem. Little did we know that this was not the end, but only the beginning of his saga of illness.

Because he was living by himself, there was no one to actually monitor his progress. He would get dressed and eat some oatmeal, but then he felt so tired he would return to bed for the rest of the day. Instead of recovering, he was actually deteriorating. This fact came to light only when his brother came back to town and took him out for dinner. Harry looked terrible and barely ate. The latter was all the more shocking, since Harry was famous for his appetite. When asked what he would like to eat, he used to quote a Yiddish proverb: "A sick man you ask, a healthy man you give. So don't ask, give!" On this occasion, however, he fell asleep at the table and vomited. Sam was horrified.

My father had been widowed thirty years before, but for many years had had a companion. Harry used to say that she had the "gift"—the gift of being able to fall asleep anywhere. One Sunday, he went to buy bagels and found her asleep when he returned. But this time, he could not wake her. He drove her to the ER, but she died the next day. The dinner with Sam was around the first anniversary of her death, and our psychologically minded family wondered if this might explain his lack of usual zest. Sam tried to convince him to go to the emergency room, but he refused. He appeared confused and frail. When I spoke to Sam, I decided that I should just get on a plane and see what was going on. I knew from previous experience that my father would not be immediately pleased, and indeed, when I told him I was coming he said, "Don't!" Luckily, I also knew that despite his initial resistance, he would later be very happy that I had come. So I said, "I don't listen to fathers who say 'No!'"

I canceled all my commitments and flew through the night.

MY ARRIVAL

I arrived the next day and found my father both better and worse than I expected. He was able to get out of bed and come to greet me—that was the good news. The bad news was that when we embraced, he seemed fleshless bones pushing out flabby skin. He slept most of the time. He had no appetite, saying rather feebly that the food didn't taste good. The house had a sick person's smell and was even more disorganized than usual, which is saying an awful lot.

There was another factor: the heat. Montreal was undergoing the worst heat wave in a century. The rainless, torpid conditions had brought about parched fields, grasshoppers in plague proportions, and water usage restrictions. There were smog alerts, forest fires, and high electricity consumption. In such extreme conditions, the young and the old are most vulnerable. Sam had called Dana's replacement, a newly retired physician, who said the pallor of Harry's skin suggested that he was dehydrated. Because Harry also looked anemic and malnourished, the physician sent Sam out to buy Ensure, a dietary supplement, as well as bottles of water and multivitamins. The doctor took lots of blood for tests. He felt Harry might recover once the weather cleared.

My father and I had a frank, intimate talk about his living situation. Living alone, as he had done so well for so many years, was no longer an option. He had almost perished, and we could not allow any further deterioration. It was too risky. At the very least, he needed a live-in helper, if not relocation to a senior residence. I knew he was afraid that we would put him in a "home" against his will, and therefore he reluctantly agreed to consider a housekeeper. Through a cousin-social worker, we got the name of an experienced, sensitive, and reliable homemaker, Sheila, who was originally from Barbados. We believed we had solved the problem. Harry, however, continued to sleep all day and through the night. I saw that he could sound OK when he answered the bedside phone, and it was this momentary cheerfulness which had fooled all of us. I finally concluded that Harry was "going down the tubes." Without proper medical attention, he was going to die.

THE FIRST VISIT TO THE ER

I took him to the emergency room of Dana's hospital. Had Dana been there, I am sure things would have unfolded differently. There was only a single nurse and a single doctor doing double duty at the ER. Harry was not acutely in peril and we waited many, many hours until we were seen and many more hours as the various tests—EKG, chest X ray, urinalysis, blood work, and mental status—were slowly performed.

To our surprise, they discovered that Harry has a curvature of the spine, or scoliosis. Worse, they documented a definite cognitive decline. He struggled to remember the day of the week and missed the day of the month altogether. In the simple recall task, "Here are three words that I want you to remember. I will ask you about them later: apple ... car ... telephone," he remembered only "apple." After the test, with a mnemonic, he did manage to get "car" but never "telephone." The ER doctors asked whether he was depressed and, despite the death anniversary, his mood seemed fine. His prostate was once again enlarged, which might make it more difficult to urinate, and there were slightly raised white blood count (WBC) and neutrophils, suggesting a urinary tract infection. His lower limbs were swollen, indicating fluid retention. Interns, residents, and nurses of every shift all asked him about chest pains or difficulty breathing. I felt that they were almost hoping that he was having a heart attack, because that was something they knew how to treat.

All told, we spent over fifteen hours in the emergency room and, in the end, were sent home with a simple prescription for antibiotics. They did not even prepare a discharge note. It was a terrible disappointment. At various times during the long wait, Harry would start to dress and say, "We're leaving." It was only with difficulty that I managed to prevent him leaving prematurely, AMA: against medical advice. Now I wondered why I had bothered. The staff, harassed and overworked, didn't really know what was wrong with him and didn't have the motivation to find out. It was the first hint of "ageism" to come. We went home, and Harry went back to sleep.

MY FATHER IS DYING

After speaking with another cousin the next day, I realized that Harry was dying. The cousin recounted the final days of her father: sleeping all the time, no appetite, taking an hour to make a sandwich, which he then decided not to eat. The only result of his horrible visits to the ER just days before his death was that the staff sent him home wrapped only in a blanket against the cold winter night, not even making sure that there was someone at home to receive him. "Things slip through the system," my cousin said. "I imagine Harry will sleep more and more until that Great Sleep from which there is no waking."

The discovery of a urinary infection encourages my physician-cousin Martin, by contrast, because it might explain Harry's symptoms: sleepiness, fatigue, loss of appetite, and even the cognitive decline. I wish I could believe him. My more immediate problem is getting him to take the antibiotics (Cipro). He is unable to swallow pills whole. Only after much experimentation do I discover that I can grind them up in specially sweetened applesauce. I still feel that he needs more serious medical attention and in desperation send an urgent email to Dana in Europe. As soon as she receives it, she swings into action, and, with Martin's help, we are set to see her colleague and Martin's old teacher, Tom Hutchison. He makes the mistake of trying to help Harry get up to the examining table and has his hand swatted away. "I will do it myself," Harry snaps. Tom thinks there are several tests worth doing but explains that these tests can be done just as well on an outpatient basis. I know that Martin has always suspected a GI tumor, and I think of how often I have taught the ethical and psychosocial issues involved in treating inoperable cancer in an elderly patient. Is Harry really competent to give informed consent? Would he really want treatment? What is the balance between beneficence and malfeasance? Many years ago, my father told me that if he knew he was going to die, he would be afraid to go to sleep.

HOSPITALIZATION

Listening a second time to his heart, Tom discovers a very subtle "rub," a sign of "pericarditis," an inflammation of the sack around the heart. It is potentially a very dangerous condition, since fluid may suddenly accumulate, compress the heart, and cause cardiac arrest. Pericarditis, I learn, is usually caused either by heart problems or the invasion of an esophageal tumor. We go up to the cardiac care unit for an echocardiogram, which reveals water round the heart, as well as a transient arrhythmia and/or right-side heart failure. The doctors decide to hospitalize Harry, finally. I feel that with every new finding I get more of a medical education. Harry's difficulty lying on his back points toward heart failure, but his chronic hoarseness is suggestive of a tumor. Later they discover that he has an enormous amount of water in his lungs and will need a needle biopsy. I am relieved that he is finally in hospital and with 24-hour cardiac monitoring.

I am supposed to leave in a few days for a congress in Cambridge, England, where I am supposed to chair sessions, run groups, and even have a birthday party. I feel that my place is here with my father in hospital and send a flurry of emails trying to make alternative arrangements.

The cardiac intensive care unit is focused on heart problems, with little concern for the rest of the person. It is only with urging by Martin and myself that we "force" them to continue investigating. There is a concern that he may not be swallowing well and a danger that he may aspirate his food into his lungs. They do a "barium swallow," taking vivid pictures of how the meal goes down the esophagus. To our great relief, we are told everything is fine in that area, at least. Unfortunately, and with lack of foresight, the barium of this test has interfered with the more important upper GI series, which also uses barium for illumination. We will have to wait a few days before the barium clears, and Harry will have to go again without breakfast.

Another complication is that Harry's scoliosis makes it tricky to drain the water in the area around his lungs. The resident takes out 1300 cc of blood-colored fluid. He leaves another liter because taking it all out at once might affect the hemodynamic properties and lead to even worse problems. Martin says that the color can be deceptive, since only a few red blood cells can color the fluid. We must anxiously await the lab results. The pH level will give a clue. Reluctantly, the doctors finally agree to another chest X ray.

Martin notes the difference between the American and Canadian health-care systems. In the States, where the insurance companies call the tune, one is forced to do all the tests all at once in order to get the person out of hospital as quickly as possible. "If you are not on an IV line, the insurance company will not pay." In Canada, with universal health care, they practice "slowpoke" medicine, going about things much more slowly. Days go by when nothing happens. I realize we sound like Goldilocks tasting the porridge, saying first that it is too hot, then that it is too cold. Health care in the States it is too fast; in Canada it is too slow. I wonder where the health-care delivery is "just right," like Baby Bear's porridge.

THE DANGERS OF NEVER HAVING BEEN SICK

I spoon-feed Harry chocolate pudding. It is horrible to see him force himself to eat and hear him say, "I better eat, otherwise I won't be here." Harry is miserable in his understated way. Individuals like him who have never been sick often do very poorly in hospital, since they have no previous recovery against which to view the current episode. If you have been sick, there is a narrative of recovery; if you have never been sick, there is none and you are always skirting the abyss. Normally, a person ages gradually. I have my medical students do an exercise in which they list all the things they like to do; then they must cross off, one by one, those things they are unable to do as the aging process sets in. At 92, Harry is having his first crisis of aging. He complains, "You have a difficult patient. I am not what I used to be. I am a crab"; and when he lies back in bed, he sighs, "Look at me!"

WHAT A DIFFERENCE A DOCTOR MAKES

The head of service and Harry's cardiologist, Dr. Malcolm, has always been puzzled why Harry did not make a better recovery after receiving the pacemaker. Rereading the charts, he notices the botched job and the bad bleeding—"the worst I have ever seen for a pacemaker operation." He suggests that maybe the seeping blood caused the fluid in the lungs, the strain on the heart, and the general decline. Once the blood is reabsorbed and the fluid reduced, things may improve. Unfortunately, his week on service is ending and his job taken over by another, younger, and more arrogant physician. I will only mention one incident, which will stand for the rest.

During morning rounds, this physician, followed by his entourage, discusses each case and decides what is to be done. I wait patiently near Harry, hoping to finally catch the younger doctor and make an appointment to discuss Harry's progress. Politely, I ask if I can make an appointment. He asks why. I say to discuss my father's case. He replies tartly, "If I have something to tell you, I will let you know," and strides out of the room leaving me dumbfounded and shamed for even asking. I am vengeful and, in my mind's eye, draft a letter of complaint.

If there is something I have learned in this week-plus in hospital, it is just how necessary it is for patients and their families to have regular access to information. I feel like I am always trying to sneak or squeeze it out of the doctors. Once I am caught reading Harry's chart and am chastised. To avoid being treated like a naughty child, I offer to take him back from X ray or CT. Then I calmly read all there is to read. I see that they have scheduled another chest X ray and become convinced that they have found something terrible. When I share my fright with my friends, I am told that one of them had a biopsy rescheduled twice because the lab screwed up. "Nobody bothered to tell us."

FEEDING TUBES AND RESCHEDULED TESTS

Except for breakfast, Harry is hardly eating. He says the food has no taste. His Chinese dietician comes and tries to persuade him to accept a nasal-gastric feeding tube. Even with the supplements, he is getting only about two-thirds of his dietary needs. In fact, he has lost weight since coming into hospital. This is shocking. Her suggestion is also shocking, since the medical team has made no effort to investigate why he is not eating. An upper GI series, endoscopy, or CT would help, but these tests remain undone. Martin is outraged at the suggestion of a feeding tube: "It's psychotic!" he says. Frustrated, he tries again to get a lung and GI consult involved, but this ward has a macho sense of "We don't need help. We can do it ourselves." Or "We do heart. We don't do lungs and GI." He continues to suspect a massive tumor. My secret source, a tall Saudi Arabian physician, handsome as a prince, in confidence tells me that the young doctor thinks that Harry's loss of appetite is due to psychological factors; this is the real reason there is no work-up. He advises that we get him transferred to a medical ward. Dana, by email, agrees, and new tests are ordered. Some good news: The cytology of the lung fluid indicates there is no sign of cancer.

I spend the day looking at nursing homes and senior residences.

SERIAL SEVENS

When I return to the hospital the next day, I am pleased to see a geriatric consult. He is also from Arabia—from Oman. As part of the mental status exam, he asks "serial sevens": "Start with 100 and subtract 7; now subtract another 7; another 7. . . ." It is a standard test for concentration, the ability to hold numbers in your mind in order to do the simple arithmetic. Harry does not get even a single answer correct. The Omani switches to the simple version: "Subtract 3 from 20." Here, too, Harry stumbles. My father is, or perhaps now was, an accountant. Numbers are his business. He used to be able to add a list of numbers faster than anyone could tap them into a calculator. He does not appear to realize how poorly he has done. I try not to show how my heart is weeping.

HOSPITAL AS A PLACE OF ILLNESS

Another week has gone by. The arrogant young doctor has been replaced by a female physician, who is more compassionate and forthcoming. Soon, I must return to Israel, and the day before I am to leave, Harry says he is going to leave hospital. It is the weekend and no tests will be done. Maybe it would be better for him to be in a familiar setting. I see how "unhealing" the hospital is with its sterility, its noise, its noxious food, the enforced helplessness and the boredom. Sheila, the homemaker, starts visiting him in the hospital, bringing homemade chicken soup (the "Jewish penicillin"—even if she is from Barbados). I leave, not knowing whether I will ever see my father again.

While I am away, Harry goes home, but is soon back in hospital. My sister, up for the weekend, notices a change in breathing and this time, with Dana on hand, has Harry seen by a respirologist (as lung specialists are known in Canada), who starts him on diuretics and has him readmitted, this time to the medical ward.

Another liter of fluid is taken from his lungs. This time it is clear, a good sign. The new doctor thinks Harry might have gone into heart failure because of the pacemaker, causing fluid build-up everywhere—lungs, pleura, interstitial spaces, maybe even pericardium. Gradually, though, Harry is drying out. If the heart failure hypothesis holds, then his condition could be maintained via beta blockers and other heart meds.

Just as I am beginning to feel that he is in capable hands, I get a call from Sheila. She tells me that some doctor came by and said he was being discharged today. I rush to the hospital, where I am told that yes, he is going home, and the rest of the appointments will be made on an outpatient basis. I feel it is vastly inappropriate. No has sat down and talked to us, prepared us, proposed explanations, given a clear diagnosis, prognosis, treatment plan for the future . . . nothing. Over the weekend, my father had been able to walk around the floor, but today he hasn't wanted to get up at all. The lovely occupational therapist does get him up, but his oxygen saturation level sinks to a dangerous 82. His blood pressure is also low, at 90/45. Tests will later show that Harry's heart is pumping fine, but his carbon dioxide retention levels are dangerously high. Nevertheless, the head of this medical ward has determined now that Harry has dried out and he can go home, thus "turfing" Harry's care back to the cardiologist with an inconclusive diagnosis of "heart failure."

I call Dana and she is once again Harry's guardian angel. She stops the discharge and challenges the ageism implied in the rhetorical question, "What can you expect in a 92-year-old?" She organizes the lung and heart consults, which has not been done during the drying out. She proposes yet another hypothesis, namely that the phrenic nerve was injured during the pacemaker implantation, impairing the function of the diaphragm. Sadly, because her specialty is kidney transplantation, Dana does not feel herself competent to follow the heart-lung problems herself. She says with some humor, "Now if he needed a kidney transplant. . . ."

Martin calls for the fourth time today. He is very concerned about Harry's drowsiness, the lack of oxygen saturation, and low blood pressure. He describes another possible strategy: inserting a line directly into the chamber of the heart to monitor how the heart responds to different medications. He adds, "Why wasn't there a pulmonary consult from day 1?" I can only agree.

At night, Harry becomes anxious. A wrong number wakes him up. He becomes somewhat agitated: "Where is the phone? Where is the call button? What is this? Make sure they don't put up the handrail!" The night before, he tried to get out of bed to pee and was found climbing over the railing. He might easily have fallen. Hospitals are dangerous places.

QUARANTINE

The story moves now from the theatre of the absurd to farce. A patient who had been in Harry's ward for a few hours had been diagnosed with MRSA (methicillin-resistant *staphylococcus aureus*), a germ that is found on the skin or inside the nose of up to 20 percent of the general public; it usually causes no problems. In hospitals, however, the bug can infect surgical wounds, or cause pneumonia or blood infections. To avoid transmission, Harry's ward is put under quarantine. Anyone entering the room must wear gowns, gloves, masks. Whenever Harry leaves, he must wear the same. All the tests for lung function are suspended until the quarantine is lifted.

YOM KIPPUR

The next day is Yom Kippur, the Hebrew Day of Atonement, and it is the strangest I have ever had. Robed in my yellow isolation gown and latex gloves, I stand above Harry, who is listening to tapes of the all-important "kol nidre" chant on a borrowed Walkman. It is the first time he will not be in synagogue to join in the fasting and prayers. Harry is not a religious person and does not really believe in an Almighty God, but the tradition is important to him. We read the book of Jonah about that reluctant prophet. Harry's middle name is Jonah. Waiting for yet more test results, I feel like Jonah waiting to see what will happen to the Great City of Nineveh. My family arrives from Israel, and we spend days sitting all around Harry in robes and latex. It seems cruel that he cannot hold the hands of his grandchildren. We take photos. I think that these will be the last ones, but my kids are all staunchly convinced that "Grandpa" will recover. They say it is unfair for them to spend all day in the hospital, and I take them skating and bowling. It is for me a kind of play therapy, and I discover I can still laugh.

We again begin examining post-hospital alternatives: senior residences, supervised group homes, nursing homes. Research suggests that elderly people do worse and worse after every move, so we decide on a more expensive, but life-preserving option: to go to his home, with 24-hour supervision and a mobile oxygen unit.

He finally goes for his lung function tests, for which we have waited so long. And what happens? He is not able to breathe properly, so the results are useless. The specialist says they will try to do the investigation in some other way. I try to explain Harry's medical situation to him. He takes notes but the next day forgets. When the duty doctor tells him he has "a total heart block," he becomes agitated and asks, "So how am I alive?" I write out in big letters his six current conditions: heart block, for which he has the pacemaker; atrial fibrillation, when the heart fights the pacemaker; fluid around the lungs; his need for oxygen; his high CO_2 retention, still unexplained; and now also a suspected pneumonia, for which he is getting more antibiotics. I don't tell him that there is a serious decline in cognitive function, but I feel it again the next day, when he has me review his condition again from scratch.

A HAPPY ENDING

Despite all this anguish, there is a happy ending to the story. My children were right: Grandpa did not die. When a GI series was finally done, doctors discovered he had an ulcer. Once this was treated, his famous appetite reappeared along with his trademark "Don't ask, just give." He gained weight. Additionally, a test for oxygen at night revealed that he was suffering from "sleep apnea," a condition which prevents a person from breathing properly during sleep. In addition to his daytime oxygen, Harry makes use of a special mask which forces oxygen into his lungs all night. As soon as he started using it, his mental status recovered dramatically. He started handling his finances again. During income tax time, he was even able to work! He did so well that we reduced his care so that Sheila came only in the morning and her friend Carol helped him put on the mask at night and slept over, just in case.

Harry still resists the sick role. Looking back, he says that there was nothing ever wrong with his health. Often, he ventures out without his oxygen backpack, because he feels ashamed of being seen as sick. In the beginning, he would go out with sunglasses, even in winter. He continues to go for regular check-ups with his heart and lung specialists.

A year later, I came to visit Harry again with my family—to celebrate my son's bar mitzva. Harry still says, "I am not what I was." But he was there.

He even danced.

QUESTIONS

1. Define "ageism" and cite examples from the narrative.
2. What role, if any, does the family's ethnicity play in the story?
3. Discuss the attitudes and decisions of the various medical professionals in the story.

The Prolapse

⌒ RAE LUCKIE ⌒

The imaginary body is the body we anticipate, the body we behave as if we had, and it is constantly variable. It is also a socially constructed body because it is created out of the images and experiences which each particular culture provides.

—*Catherine Garrett*

24 JULY 1994

I really like Stephen King's writing. Not that I did much reading in hospital. I couldn't concentrate. Trish, my eldest, had armed me with horror books, but I only browsed through the *Women's Weekly*, *New Idea* and a couple of *Telegraph Mirrors*.[1] The sister brought the "tellies" around every morning. Trouble was, if you napped, the pink-uniformed cleaning duo whipped them away before eleven. Didn't like the room looking messy.

I was scared sick the couple of weeks before the operation. Half the time I couldn't sleep and the night before I went into hospital I played Tetris Max on the computer. All night. Tetris is supposed to be all the rage for women. It's not a "shoot the baddies" game. You try and stack different-shaped coloured bricks into neat rows, and work your way up the levels.

> *The higher the faster*
> *Click the brick right*
> *Click the brick left*
> *Down*
> *and*
> *down*
> *Each brick link makes a click*
> *Coloured links make a clack*
> *A full row makes a crash*
> *New level cow moos*
> *click clack crash moo swish swish click click*
> *husky flutes beating drums trilling chimes*
> *click crash moo beat beat beat dum de dum*

189

I was still wondering if I had done the right thing. Made the decision, that is. The gynaecologist always left it up to me. "You'll know when," he said, and I suppose I did, even though it took fourteen years.

It's amazing what you'll put up with, but it just creeps up over time. The back pain. Excessive bleeding. I remember October '91. I was organising my middle child Tracy's wedding and began bleeding. I was coping with a new job and travelling to the University of Technology to do my DipEd. Three hours each day in the car Mondays and Tuesdays, four hours a day on the train for the other three. At least I could study on the train.

Still bleeding at the wedding the week before Christmas, and on through the holidays at the beach at Hawks Nest. Visits to the GP—perhaps it was the hormone replacement therapy? Back to the specialist. Checks my history.

"How's the urine problem?" he asks. Of course we never talk about things like that, do we? Apart from "National Continence Week," and then it's really incontinence we're talking about.

It just sort of began when I was forty, with the odd drop when I sneezed or coughed. I needed to put a neatly folded Kleenex tissue in my breezeweight sensible full-brief flesh-coloured Bonds (Made in Australia) Cottontails. Just in case. Then at least two or three. What a relief when panty pads came on the scene! If I was on a health kick and tried to jog, I made sure I stuck in a full-size pad. By the early 1990s I began wearing pads all the time. Oh yes, I did the pelvic floor exercises, but I'll admit it: I hate dieting and exercise and I like food and wine (but not Chateau Cardboard, because you never remember how much you drink). Eventually I enjoyed a bottle to myself most nights—chardonnay because I often felt stressed and it helped the aches and pains. And I put on the weight. Although I didn't smoke—a good thing—I was fat, and the contraceptive pill wasn't considered a good idea. So I went into Jameston Private Hospital for a tubal ligation. The heavy bleeding began and I was back in again a few times for a D & C. I could never understand why hormone replacement therapy was a good idea if the pill was a bad idea, but I've been on HRT ever since the hot flushes began. I read in Germane Greer's book *The Change* that it's a bad idea, but I think maybe if I go off it now I'll crumble away to dust like an Egyptian mummy that has just been unwrapped. You've seen the movie haven't you?

Which brings me to "The Prolapse." Whenever I think of it I remember Frankie Howerd doing "The Prologue" in the 1970s English television comedy *Up Pompeii*. Now let's be frank—how would you like your insides beginning to fall through to the outside? The specialist tried to put it delicately.

"Do you feel anything poking outside your vagina at times?"

"Well," I said, "I don't go around feeling myself, but I think sometimes maybe I notice something not quite right when I have a shower or wipe after going to the toilet."

"Does it feel something like a nose?"

"I suppose so—I don't really know."

"Is it a hard little nose or a soft little nose?"

I burst into tears.

"I don't know—how hard is a nose?"

"Well, don't worry about it too much, but if it's more like a hard nose it's your cervix."

A nose is a rose.

But I kept ignoring things. More bleeding. More leaking. More dragging back pains. New GP. She looked and said, "That's a really significant prolapse you've got there—have you thought about getting something done about it?"

So she referred me back to the same specialist who first suggested the hysterectomy in the mid-1980s. It had to be my decision. I suppose it's because if anything goes wrong with the operation you can't say you were pressured into it. Specialists are worried about litigation.

To remove or not to remove? That is the question. The removal of my uterus. I haven't got any psychological hang-ups about it. At least, I don't think I have. I've had three kids, but I don't consider having a womb essential to my female identity. Being fat is. When I was little I had cute blue eyes and blonde hair. Then I got fat. I was the only fat kid I knew. I look around now and think I'd hardly be noticed in the McDonald's and KFC generation.

I remember the old advertisements on the wireless.

Are you too fat too fat too fat? Take Ford Pills.[2]

Inside my head I feel okay most of the time, but other times my body becomes all-encompassing. Especially when I'm still waking up with the same odd pains in the night and the morning.

Take a Bex or a Vincents APC for the pain you can't explain.[3]

Tracy, her husband, Tony, and our two grandkids were here in July, a few days before I went into hospital for the hysterectomy. Tracy was going through an old shoe-box full of photos waiting patiently in the bottom of the wardrobe. She pulled out our sepia hand-tinted wedding photo. I had on a short white dress and veil and white shoes with high heels and pointy toes. We both looked so young and happy and I was slim and pretty. Prescribed Dexedrine had done the trick. Take just one maroon and black capsule first thing in the morning. Wait for the little rush of energy and get through the housework like a dervish. But then I used to get this kind of anxious feeling in the afternoon and I often couldn't sleep at night.

Incontinence finally gets to you when you can feel the pad filling even when you're not jogging, sneezing or coughing and you begin to wonder if people around you can smell the odour. The ammonia smell of a baby's nappy. So you change pads every couple of hours. Then it gets worse. You get obsessive to ensure that you've always got a pad handy. Pads with wings. Supersize without wings at night. In bags, purses, make-up bags, in the car, in the drawers at work. I always have a spare in my bra. Just in case.

The final straw—being unable to control the dribble down my left leg between cleaning teeth at the basin and stepping towards shower. The majority of women in nursing homes are supposed to be there because of incontinence, so it couldn't just be happening to me. But nobody talks about it. My mother-in-law lost control of her mind but not her bladder. She died from a broken memory. What's worse?

So then it's back to the gynaecologist. Questions and recorded answers. Remove your lower garments. Lie down on the waterproof blue square. Cough. Don't feel embarrassed, cough harder. You know his hands are getting wet. "There's more than one problem," he said, staring over his half specs.

"The prolapse, bleeding and incontinence aren't necessarily related," he said, "so we'll get some tests done for the incontinence."

I love the way doctors say "we," don't you?

"They're not pleasant," he said. He explained the prolapse was caused by the weakening and collapse of the pelvic floor muscles from a number of causes probably related to childbirth (× 3), overweight, standing, and loss of oestrogen after menopause. "Just think of your pelvic floor like a hammock which is holding everything up—uterus, bladder, and bowel. After the uterus is removed, I'll do a suspension—stitch back the bladder and bowel and reconstruct the vagina. Your vagina will be as good as it was thirty years ago." He drew a diagram. "We'll cut here."

A song begins running around in my head. I imagine I'm in a crazy scene penned by Dennis Potter.[4] A group of blowzy middle-aged women are high-kicking in a chorus line.

> *A one two three four*
> > *link your arms and tap-hop-shuffle*
> > > *and tap and kick and step and kick*
> > > > *and step and kick and step and kick*
> *a one two three four*
> > *and turn your heads to the left*
> > > *and turn your heads to the right*
> > > > *and smile and sing and tap hop shuffle*
> > > > > *and a one two three four all*
> > > > *together now*

Enter stage right: Surgeon in top hat, white tie and tails—swinging a cane, dancing a soft-shoe shuffle singing to the tune of "Carolina in the Morning":

> *Nothing could be finer*
> *than to have a new vagina*
> *in the mor-hor-hor-ning*
> *Nothing could be neater*
> *than the stitching when I greet yer*
> *in the mor-hor-hor-ning…*

Well, it was nearing the end of semester and I had students facing the run up to final exams. I couldn't get an appointment out of class time with the urologist at the radiography centre, so I delayed for another month.

THE THINGS THEY DO TO DEAR (PART I)

"Drink at least a litre of water two hours before the appointment and don't go to the toilet, Dear." Dear wonders if she'll disgrace herself in front of the dozens of patients waiting. One of the staff is tidying years-old dog-eared magazines. "Would you like a cup of tea, Dear?" She smiles. Dear says, "No thanks," holds her knees together and tries to hold in the bulging hammock. Dear buries her head, wondering what is going to happen when it's her turn.

Nurse smiles and directs Dear to a small room with an ordinary toilet and a contraption like an upturned megaphone. She hands her a small, disposable blue gown. "Put this on, take everything off below the waist then wee in there, Dear," she says, pointing to the megaphone. Dear notices the megaphone has what looks like a microphone in it with a couple of leads disappearing under the door. Later Dear notices they're attached to a laptop.

The specialist is young, male and brash. He bombards Dear with questions, beginning with childhood illnesses. "Do you leak when you have intercourse?" Dear blushes: "Well I don't know I—er well I—er haven't—you know—er for a number of years. The questions go on and on. Finally he asks Dear if she is widowed or divorced.

"Um—er I've been happily married for thirty-three years," Dear says. She hides her embarrassment by expressing interest in the laptop's part in the procedure. She's told to lie on the narrow X-ray table and the computer is behind her head. First an ultrasound. Dear tells about seeing her second grandchild on ultrasound. Watching the little mite bouncing and jiggling around.

"He's six months old now," Dear says.

THE THINGS THEY DO TO DEAR (PART 2)

Urodynamics is the name—sticking catheters in your ureter, vagina and anus is the game.

> **anile:** *of or like a weak old woman (L. anilis from anus old woman)*
>
> —*The Macquarie Concise Dictionary*

The nurse does the preparation then the specialist takes over. "First we're going to fill your bladder with a radioactive dye." He points to a plastic container which he links to one of Dear's catheters. He undoes the stopper and the plastic pack sways gently on its chromed metal stand. Dear wonders if there's a pump or if it is just gravity propelling the fluid.

"Tell me when it becomes uncomfortable."

"Now!"

"Just a little more, Dear."

As Dear's bladder is artificially inflated she can hear the nurse clicking through the program on the computer. Bed is raised. Bed is lowered.

"Don't move, hold your breath, I'm taking some X rays." *Snap.* "Now this way, now that." Dear is lying naked from the waist down hooked up to a computer. Suddenly she's one with the machine. Security shattered when Dear looks at his full-frontal lead apron.

"Now just keep still . . ." and suddenly a motor whirrs. Bed and Dear, complete with

catheters intruding, majestically trundle to an upright position. Dear feels she's now starring in Fritz Lang's *Metropolis* and decides she's feeling pretty crook.[5] She didn't have her
feet quite flat on the upright at the end of the X-ray table and almost tips over in the turn
around. The specialist and nurse think she's going to faint and make a grab for her. She tells
them she is okay but wants to go to the toilet right now please. "No Dear, we have to take
more X rays." *Snap click. Snap click.*

"Now Dear, put your legs apart, bend your knees slightly and urinate." Dear reacts in
abject horror. "I can't—not standing up like this."

"You must."

I can't I can't you will she doesn't and so they turn on taps and talk about running
water and waterfalls and put Dear's hands into a bowl of cold water until she wets herself
standing up and bursts into tears.

"Thanks Dear."

Then the specialist takes Dear into a small room the size of a toilet with a chair just like
a small birthing bed. *Knees up Mother Brown* and he sits with his face level to Dear's fundamental orifice as her mother used to say and pokes and prods.

Dear tries to pretend she is somewhere else. "Get dressed, Dear and we'll see you same
time next week." Dear listens to the sobbing of the woman in the cubicle next door.

More tests. Dear signs the consent form and so to hospital.

7 JULY 1994

It was my fourth visit to Jamieson hospital. I didn't complain when I didn't get the private
room I'd requested a month before. I found out later it had gone to someone who had
complained. By 5.30 p.m. I was tucked into the two-bed ward listening to the quiet moans
and groans penetrating the grey curtain. Her operation had been that morning. I tried to
block out the sounds and longed for privacy. At 7 p.m. the anaesthetist arrived. We'd met
once or twice before. Stethoscope. Breath in and out. Health history. How much do you
weigh how much alcohol do you drink how often how many analgesics do you take?

He explains the procedure, says he's going to use a PCA for pain management and that
I will have control of the dosage of pethidine via an intravenous tube. He smiles and leaves.
Then the surgeon arrives. "We'll have to stop meeting like this," I try to joke. He's wearing
a navy Bermuda jacket. I ask if he enjoyed his week on the ski slopes. "Great," he said and I
hope he is well-rested and that his hands are steady, because I realise he's getting older too.
He has a kind face and thick grey wavy hair. He explains the procedure again in detail, a
vaginal hysterectomy, anterior and posterior repair, the suspension not necessary now according to the urodynamic tests, so I won't have an outside scar. He reminds me I will be
placed on a drip and have a catheter in for four days. I decide not to have the sleeping tablet he prescribes "if necessary."

"I'll see you to-morrow afternoon." I lie and listen to the nurses change shifts, staff bus-
tling around, patients using the toilet opposite. Their bodily smells mingle with food aro-
mas emanating from the kitchen. Corridor lights on all night. Night sister checks regularly
shining her torch. "Are you awake Dear—everything all right Dear?"

The woman in the next bed moans most of the night. My surgery is scheduled for 2 p.m., so just before 6 a.m. I'm given a cup of tea and a biscuit then nil by mouth. At lunch time my room companion has her first cooked meal. Food glorious food.

THE THINGS THEY DO TO DEAR (PART 3)

Sister arrives with a safety razor and removes the thinning pubic hair. "Have you used your bowels today Dear?" Dear expects a pre-surgical enema but sister says they don't do that any more. Dear, remembering pre-childbirth enemas, breathes a sigh of relief. "Have a shower, put on this gown and cap, leave your panties off, take off your rings, pop your dentures into this bowl and pop back into bed. Then we'll give you a pre-med injection after which you mustn't get out of bed." Dear hasn't slept and is anxious. The bed is clammy with protective blue plastic. The operation is delayed until 3 p.m.. Dear lies quietly contemplating the ceiling.

A male ward attendant arrives and converts the bed into a trolley. The rattling trip to theatre begins. Dear's eye is a camera watching the ceiling roll past. Swinging doors clip the side of the bed. Arrival. Eyes and masks begin to introduce themselves. "Hi, I'm Julie. I'm your theatre sister[6] today. Could you tell me your name and why you are here?" Dear is reminded of Pizza Hut and apologises for her toothless speech. "Just lift your bottom, Dear, and slide across to the operating table." Dear's eye camera stares up at the encompassing circle of metallic bright lightedness. Stainless steel instruments and bowls arrayed beside eyes and masks. "This will just be a small prick in your left hand," and Dear swirlingly slides into oblivion.

"Come on, Dear, take deep breaths, come on keep breathing, Dear. It's all over." Somehow Dear feels something is wrong. She can hear them talking about her. They are saying that every time they take the oxygen off she stops breathing. "Take deep breaths, Dear, come on now." Dear experiences a lot of little deaths but there isn't any long tunnel with someone greeting her at the end like her Aunt Anne in Parkes once said after her heart attack. Then Dear thinks about her Uncle Bill, who died of bowel cancer, sharpening the carving knife on the foot-pedalled grinding stone in the chook yard where the huge lucerne tree was. He'd spit on the stone and grind first one side of the knife then the other. She remembers her cousin Ted lopping off the head of a Rhode Island Red on the chopping block in the woodshed. The body ran around and around looking for its head and she was about eight and Ted put her head on the chopping block and said he was going to chop her head off but he didn't. She wakes up.

"Where am I?"

After the bleeding stops, Dear experiences four weeks of dryness, then ... *incontinence finally gets to you when you can feel the pad filling even when you're not jogging, sneezing or coughing . . .*

POSTSCRIPT

After the urodynamic tests, when the gynaecologist said the "suspension" part of the operation would not now be necessary, my relief outweighed the fact that I knew I had a significant problem. It seems the "favourable report" was mainly due to my heroic resistance to the command to urinate standing up while naked from the waist down and attached to three intrusive devices—an experience I found mortifying and against my every basic instinct. The test results outweighed the clinical examination, and my "narrative" and I have had to cope with the consequences.

> *The treatment of illness typically, and necessarily, involves a sort of narrative collaboration between doctor and patient. Diagnosis often relies, at least in part, on a "medical history"; the patient offers up testimony that the physician interprets according to codes and conventions of their lives. Thus physicians may both reinterpret patients' pasts and literally prescript their futures.*
>
> —*Thomas Couser*

NOTES

1. *The New Idea* and the *Women's Weekly* (which is now published monthly) are women's magazines; the *Telegraph Mirror* is a Sydney daily newspaper.
2. An over-the-counter laxative sold in the 1950s, also advertised as a pill to help weight loss.
3. Bex and Vincents were widely advertised preparations particularly targeted to women for pain and as a general "pick-me-up." The powders contained aspirin, phenacetin and caffeine (APC). By the 1960s, Australia had the highest incidence of APC-related kidney damage in the world. See Eileen Hennessey's *A Cup of Tea, a Bex and a Good Lie Down*.
4. Many of Dennis Potter's television dramas feature illness. The main character in *The Singing Detective*, like Potter himself, suffered from psoriasis. In a dream-like sequence the hospital staff are transformed and perform a song and dance number.
5. Colloquial expression "pretty crook" means to feel extremely sick.
6. The term "theatre sister" refers to an operating room nurse.

REFERENCES

"Anile." *The Macquarie Concise Dictionary.* 2nd ed. Australia: The Macquarie Library Pty Ltd, 1988.

Couser, Thomas. "The Body and Life Writing." *Encyclopedia of Life Writing: Autobiographical and Biographical Forms.* Ed. Margaretta Jolly. Vol. 1. London: Fitzroy Dearborn Publishers, 2001. 121–23.

Garrett, Catherine. "Anorexia and Theories of the Body." *Working Papers in Women's Studies: Feminist Cultural Studies Series.* Kingswood: University of Western Sydney, Nepean, 1995. 5–20.

Hennessey, Eileen. *A Cup of Tea, a Bex and a Good Lie Down.* Townsville: James Cook University, 1993.

Potter, Dennis. *The Singing Detective.* London: Faber and Faber, 1986.

QUESTIONS

1. Comment on the author's tone throughout the narrative. How would a different tone alter the reader's reading of the text?
2. Discuss how and why the author interrupts her own story.
3. Discuss the use of the term "dear," especially as it relates to the particular medical events surrounding her.

On Falling Up

⌒ Evelyn Scott ⌒

It's three a.m. in San Francisco, and my eyes fly open: *Sleep is practicing for death*. I dash to my computer, only three feet from the futon on which my husband and I sleep. How will I get it all done before I die? I must figure out a way to live forever. That should be simple, given my clear understanding of everything.

Lisa! I must call her immediately and let her in on this shattering vision, this staggering knowledge of… *all*. I am totality, whole, entirety. I am without end. Everything is Me, and I am Everything. One.

She listens patiently to my frothing claim *I am infinity*. She's compassionate. She is a psychologist, and insists that I am manic and should go to a hospital.

Now *that* harshes my mellow. "Sure, Lisa. Bye!" Without waiting for her response, I hang up and take the phone off the hook.

So much to do! The novel must come first. Before I have completed the first sentence, it is obvious to me—and will no doubt be obvious to everyone—I am beginning the world's grandest masterpiece, a work that will shatter all conceptions of reality, cast darkness from every intellectual pursuit, and define as well as create a massive artistic awakening. More metaphorical than the Bible, more revolutionary than the Declaration of Independence, and truer than *God and the New Physics*, my book shall overhaul all religion, government, and science.

Tramp jumps onto my lap. Since cats can't speak English, I say, "Bon soir, Tramp. La nuit, tous les chats sont gris." He digests this truism, smiles broadly, then scampers over to his brother asleep on the tattered sofa. He whispers in Bill Jones's ear. Bill looks dismayed; it's lost on him, a cat who is gray by day as well as by night. To clarify, I carry him to a window, open it, and place him on the ledge. I can speak to him only through Tramp, as he doesn't know French, so I will shove him into the night; he can see for himself. But our unheated efficiency is three stories above the junkies and whores strolling along lower Fillmore, so I can't simply push him over the ledge; he'd smash into the filthy pavement, be scavenged to supplement the diet that maintains the residents of the halfway house across the street. I must teach him to fly.

We've gotten a good ways into the lesson (Bill Jones is an apt student) when my husband wakes up.

"What the fuck are you doing?"

"Teaching Bill to fly."

He picks up the cat and slams the window shut. Brief gunshots from the projects around the corner punctuate his next words: "You're high. Get back to bed."

Eric's angry I woke him on a work night, so I lie down. He can't make me sleep, though. I use the time until dawn to make a mental list of everything I must do: finish the novel; resume my instruction with Bill Jones; call all my friends in Toronto, Houston, and Austin; reread the *Mahabarata*; run ten laps from the panhandle to the Pacific in Golden Gate; buy emerald jewelry; repair our Malibu Chevelle; walk across the bridge to Marin and commune with tree nymphs in Muir Woods; and get that holiday piece written by five so my boss at *The Guardian* won't yell at me again. Lying in bed is torture.

Ten years later, I can't help but smile at the memory; mania is fun, and no drug can touch its high or intensity. That's something they don't mention in the classroom. My psychopathology professor at Austin talked about "mood disturbance," and this "disturbance" could manifest as *elevated*, *expansive*, or *irritable.* By the time I went mad, I knew this criterion for a manic episode by rote. I'd flown through all of Dr. Cohen's notoriously exacting exams, and had received a solid A in Abnormal Psychology. So no one, not even Lisa, was going to tell me I was "manic" when I was just having *fun*.

Mania's fun, all right, until the cops break down the door and take you in handcuffs to a psychiatric emergency room where several large men wrestle you onto a "bed," strap down your arms and legs, and shoot you up with large quantities of Haldol and Thorazine. Then the rage sets in, then terror, and finally misery. Everyone's gone home, you take the lampshade off your head, and you suddenly realize your apartment's wrecked. And there's no way you'll ever get back your deposit.

Fun indeed, but it's hard to accomplish much and even harder to remember what you'd been trying to accomplish—before, say, you started teaching a cat to fly. What novel? Why write a novel when here's this enthralling *cat?* "Distractibility" is what *The Diagnostic and Statistical Manual of Mental Disorders* calls it. But I didn't think I was having difficulty focusing. No! I was having a delightful time focusing intensely on a great many fascinating things. Clearly I was far from manic; I was engaged, *attuned*.

Of course I noticed I wasn't sleeping, and I knew that "decreased need for sleep" is mania's flashing red light. Yet this did not apply to me since I'd discovered that sleep is intolerably dull. If I were not enlightened, maybe my insomnia would have been a symptom. Considering my latest epiphany, however, sleep was for people who had time to spare.

I did have many goals, but what ambitious American didn't? How could "increase in goal-directed activity" be a *problem?* People paid top dollar to attend motivational seminars to help them become goal-oriented. None of my goals struck me as odd or excessively strenuous, and they certainly didn't seem to fall into the incriminating category of "pleasurable activities that have a high potential for painful consequences." Investing in emeralds would have indeed ruined me—Eric and I could barely afford groceries, much less heat—but at the time, I needed gems more than shelter.

It took several months, but I came to accept that I am, as far as the American Psychiatric Association is concerned, a patient living with Bipolar I, Severe with Mood-Congruent Psychotic Features, Full Interepisode Recovery, Recurrent, with Seasonal Pattern. But I am a patient with a great deal of patience, so I am one of the lucky ones who is indeed *living* with it. (About 10 to 15 percent of us off ourselves, or "successfully complete suicide.") In fact, as long as I live, I will be living with it. Moreover, it's an illness with a bleak course. The characteristic episodes, both manic and depressive, tend to last longer and longer and occur with progressively shorter and fewer periods of "normalcy" separating them. And the depressive episodes eventually dominate. My illness is my constant companion, whatever else comes and goes. My instability is the only stable thing in my life.

But I exaggerate. It's not that reliable. The weak October light slants in at an angle, and I should feel hollow. I should be bored with everything, unmotivated even to brush my teeth, slow in thought as well as movement, incapable of holding the simplest conversation. I should want to buy guns. (During my first major depression, in 1995 and the spring of 1996, I owned a Colt .45, a nine-millimeter Beretta, and a World War I rifle.) I should be gaining weight and sleeping over twelve hours a day. But I seem, at least to myself and the psychiatrist who serves as my mirror, normal. I was last happy during fall months in 1994, before the first fracturing. Why I'm okay is anyone's guess.

My psychiatrist guesses he has finally hit upon the exact combination of medicines in just the right dosages to provide maximum therapy. Maybe he's right or maybe just self-congratulatory. At any rate, the days are getting shorter, and I don't mind. Feel good in October? Why not. Since I am, in antiquated but perhaps more descriptive terms, manic-depressive, I know how to play the game as it lies. If, in the wake of the episode that left me hospitalized, I could handle the loss of my husband, Eric, and Sheila, my best friend; if I could live through the ensuing years of alcoholism and financial ruin; and if I could conduct graduate work in psychology despite constant interruption by the very disorder I sought to understand, then surely I can be happy off-season.

I live, stay happily remarried, and maintain employment by a few sleights of hand: first, I take the pills—mood stabilizers, hypnotics, anticonvulsants, antidepressants, benzodiazepines, antipsychotics *(lithiumzolpidemvalproicacidfluoxetineclonazepamquetiapine)*—no matter what. No matter the nausea, the tremors, the forgetfulness. Addiction illness?

Whenever I meet a psychiatrist, I floor him or her with the disclosure that I have, since correctly diagnosed, taken the drugs. They complain that few of their patients take the drugs at all, and if they do, quit whenever they think they are well, only to wind up back in a hospital. "How can I convince them to take their medicine?" they want to know. "Enroll them in a good psychology program," I say.

They think I'm flippant; not every bipolar can pursue a degree in psychology. But I'm serious. The only reason I didn't wind up like every other manic-depressive who experiments with the drugs, flushes them, or overdoses on them in a frenzy of suicidal irony is because I know how they work, because by the time I got sick I already had a degree in psychology from UT Austin, a school that is bullish on the "nature" side of the "nature/nurture" debate.

I'd read about defects in the hypothalamus, abnormalities in the norepinephrine and serotonin mechanism and in the acetylcholine mechanism, and endocrine abnormalities. I had no doubt that chemicals could fix chemical problems.

But if she doesn't know how the drugs work, it's difficult to convince an artistic or literary type, a "mind-over-matter" person, that she should take medicine that makes her throw up every morning. The level at which lithium is therapeutic is often close to the level at which it is toxic. The patient information forms that accompany the prescriptions for lithium and the other drugs that complete the typical bipolar cocktail would give anyone pause. *Common side effects: vomiting, rash, headache, decreased libido, anorexia, hair loss, blurred vision, dizziness, amnesia, confusion, backache, insomnia, nightmare, anxiety.* WARNING: DO NOT OPERATE MACHINERY, DRIVE, OR PERFORM TASKS THAT ARE HAZARDOUS OR REQUIRE ALERTNESS. AVOID ALCOHOL, SALT, AND SUN EXPOSURE. TAKE WITH FOOD *(but how, if I can't hold down water?).* Few people voluntarily take these drugs, and even fewer can bring themselves to stay on them once they are recovered. No one wants to believe that the only thing sustaining her recovery is pills. *Why not quit taking them and see if I'm better?* Then in sweeps the mania, or if you aren't lucky, the depression, and it's straight to the hospital, where you aren't greeted with empathy, but with an exasperated "I told you so" or "Why, when you were doing so well?"

In today's pseudo-efficient labyrinth of HMO bureaucracy, no clinician has the patience to explain the biological etiology of bipolar disorder and why it needs to be treated with medicines like any other illness. Besides, doctors aren't teachers, and the friendly, pastel pamphlets stacked neatly about their waiting rooms aren't textbooks.

I know many brilliant bipolars who have degrees in disciplines like theater arts, and all of them are disasters. Jerome, a talented actor, prefers "self-medicating" with alcohol to taking mood stabilizers. He's covered in self-inflicted scars, most notably one from slashing his throat and another from placing his face on a hot electric stove burner ("parasuicidal behavior"). Kelly, a semi-anorexic, well-published writer, hoards her antipsychotics for recreational use (sleep). With the blasé apathy of a rattler shedding its skin, she recently threw away the coveted position of doctoral candidate at the most prestigious creative writing program in the country. Lee, an established visual artist, has (again) decided he doesn't need the drugs and has moved back in with his abusive, unemployed dad. Each of these people views the medication as an attempt to alter his or her personality. That is one way to put it. None of them believes in psychiatry.

My mother took psychiatry, like Jesus, as a given. Neither was questioned or examined. Though she knew I took a dozen pills a day, she refused to acknowledge I did that to stave off the symptoms of a disease that would outlast her—she could not see that her daughter had gotten ill and would stay that way. Her quaint, southern farm girl ways surfaced like poorly weighted corpses when she whispered about my "nervous breakdown" and stubbornly insisted I was "cured" and "all that" was in the past. *Not for me, Mother.*

So not everyone is up for a degree in psychology. My advice to doctors falls short. Maybe this suggestion doesn't: Build an office library for the patient, so she can investigate psychiatry's assertions for herself. A few copies of *The Day the Voices Stopped, Skin Game, The Quiet Room, An Unquiet Mind, Night Falls Fast, Touched with Fire, Prozac Diary, Lying,*

Welcome to My Country, *Electroboy*, and *Out of Her Mind* would be a start. The patient's only ammunition in the face of ignorance is an acquisition of vocabulary.

Besides reading such books and taking the pills, I have one final trick: I cultivate comrades in madness, friends who know mania and depression firsthand. It's not difficult; such people are drawn to me as keenly as I am to them. You have to experience a psychotic manic episode to understand it, just as you have to endure a migraine to believe that it feels like an ice pick being driven through your eye.

For example, it is impossible for most people to believe that the behavior of someone in a manic psychosis is beyond the person's, and often medication's, control. I have been called to task for things I don't remember doing, by my ex-husband and my long-gone best friend, and by many seemingly reasonable people as well. But how is it possible *not* to challenge someone to take responsibility for violence, shoplifting, drunken driving, drug abuse, and other "antisocial behaviors"? Only a peer could empathize. But stand warned: These are high-risk, high-maintenance allies. I've driven Jerome to the ER in the early morning hours several times for stitches. Kelly demands my constant support for a decision I find idiotic. When I asked Lee how his lip got busted last week, I had to feign belief in a preposterous story starring not his dad, but a street gang. Nevertheless, having like-minded companions is a matter of survival. Don't get me wrong: My psychiatrist and psychoanalyst are priceless, except for the fact they have their price.

But no matter what, mania returns—followed by guilt, embarrassment, and outright disbelief in terms of "what I did last night, and the night before." *Did I dye my hair chartreuse? How did I get these Dolce & Gabbana stilettos? And who is this man drooling on my pillowcase?* Then depression takes hold—followed by shock at how much time I wasted, how many opportunities I slept through, and how much weight I gained. *Will this bloodstain ever come out? How did I break my hand? Have I missed another final? What day is it?* The first thing I learned was that the episodes return, despite the pills, and fling me into the thrills of ecstasy and brilliance only to bury me under apathy and paralysis again and again.

Would I have it any other way? Never. I've published many articles and short stories, as well as a few essays, and I count on the energy and creativity that comes with the manias. And excepting my first depression, a seventeen-month meditation on blowing my brains out ("chronic suicidal ideation"), the depressions are mild, a modest price for the joyful productivity that balances them. Perhaps this is better for me than to feel normal day in and day out.

But perhaps that's a lie. Who wants to take so much lithium that walking into walls is always an option? Who wants a thyroid low functioning enough to render hormone "therapy" a constant consideration? Early senility, anyone? Memory loss is another thing the textbooks don't mention, and doctors will discuss it reluctantly *if* you remember to bring it up. God forbid you should even consider stopping the drugs—lithium, quetiapine, and valproic acid—that cause it. It's the liver they obsess over, as well they should. The leeches draw blood as often as once a month to check for signs of damage. And pregnancy? Maybe if you're comfortable substituting ECT (electro-convulsive therapy) for the drug regimen. But I am de facto "unfit," and my offspring would have an elevated risk (the estimates range from 1 to 24 percent) of developing bipolar I or II, major depression, cyclothemia, dysthy-

mia, anxiety disorder, or schizoaffective disorder. My college texts, concerned as they are
with the genetics of disease, discuss these familial patterns in detail, without ever suggesting how families can deal with them.

Blessed or cursed, I'm only ten years into the battle. Who is to say which of us will win?
In the maximum security psychiatric ward, where the ER psychiatrists quickly transferred
me after I slipped my skeletal wrists through the leather restraints and picked the leg shack-
les open with the one hairpin my captors missed, I saw an old woman. Most of the time
they kept her locked in her room, where she screamed endlessly. For feedings they took her
out, bound to a wheelchair. She tore at what little hair she had yet to yank from her scalp,
howled like a tortured infant at us "regular" patients, and scratched enthusiastically at the
many scars looping around the mottled skin of her scrawny neck.

It's San Francisco, but I have no idea what time it is. I think it's still 1994. Eric is gone. I
don't know what day it is, so I can't figure out when he left. He comes back over and over,
demands that I stop it, then gets a suit for the next day of mindless drafting. I don't want
him to leave. I throw his hotel key out the window. He leaves anyway. Again.

Then an extraordinary idea hits me. I squeal in amazement, though it escapes me before the police knock on the door. Someone in the building heard a scream. Am I okay? Yes,
officer, I just burned my hand. They don't bother to look at my hand. Stupid cops.

I turn on the TV. I'm watching a sketch on *Saturday Night Live* about a flirtatious young
woman and her romantic shenanigans. Apparently my brother, a D.C. political lobbyist, has
called Clinton, who in turn called Lorne Michaels only seconds before I turned on the set.
The president ordered him to have the *SNL* staff improvise a lesson. They are calling me a
slut! I'm married! The misogynist, puritanical bastards. I'll show them.

I decorate the tiny, cold apartment symbolically to demonstrate to all surveyors that I
am an adamant feminist. I place a copy of *Backlash* in the window and prop *A Vindication
of the Rights of Whores* outside my door. I do a hundred push-ups and then three sets of fifty
sit-ups to prove I am as strong as any man. Then I hold my breath for a minute-and-a-half
to show my superior self-control.

Having averted that misunderstanding, I lie on the futon perfectly still. I am dead already. We are all already dead. I smell my body rotting. The Hindu goddess Kali, deep blue,
with severed arms encircling Her waist and a garland of skulls around Her neck, dances on
the wall. I read about this manifestation just a few days ago, not in the *Mahabarata*, but in
a book on Aghora. I knew I would, now that I've died, see Her at last. I must tell everyone
of such divinity!

I call Brian in Toronto. "I want to show you something," I say. "Close your eyes." He
doesn't understand. He thinks I'm committing suicide, but I only want him to see Kali. He
hangs up, and within minutes the same cops are at the door. They got a call from Canada.
They ask me what I'm doing, and I tell them I'm trying to sleep. Can't they see how late it
is? They poke around the apartment but find only a small bag of marijuana. They ask me
questions about heroin, about guns, but I pretend to fall asleep. At last they leave. I sit bolt
upright in bed. Where is Kali? At least they didn't take the pot.

Since people can't appreciate my insight, as they aren't enlightened like me, I keep the volume on my stereo low. I play *Live Through This* incessantly because Courtney Love is a manifestation of Kali. I fill notebook after notebook with revelations. I can see all the way from Heaven's ceiling to the floor of Hell. I can see everything, everywhere, all at once. My vision astounds me. I am in complete awe of myself.

Since I am divine, I must look the part. I pin my hair up in elaborate curls. I put on a long, antique black gown, dark red lipstick, high heels, and all of my jewelry. I am hungry, but I will not eat or drink, as mortals do. I haven't eaten or drunk for many days now. This proves my holiness. I lie down again and wait for God.

But it is Eric who walks in. I realize, with great indignation and furious wrath, that he, my husband, has no right to stay out all night, night after night, doing Christ knows what. He is fundamentally wrong. He is disloyal. He has abandoned me. I have been needing him, missing him, wanting to share this exquisite experience with him, and he has been neglecting me for reasons like "I need to sleep" and "I can't miss any work." He must understand that he is wrong.

I sprint to the kitchen, grab a butcher knife, and hold it to his throat. I'm not going to cut him; I'm going to make him think. I am going to get his attention. It is a mere gesture at my righteous anger. How fortunate he must feel that I am sparing his life.

But he bolts. This time the cops come in without knocking. I'm pretending to read a magazine; these two are so easy to fool. I thought we were old friends, but they rip my beautiful gown and drag me into the freezing January air. An old black man hunched over a carved cane stops short, and I cry out to him for help. But he keeps his distance, jaw dropped at the sight of a half-naked, starving white woman getting beaten black and blue by The Man as her husband passively looks on. The cops shove me into their car while I bite and kick and shout obscenities at Eric, who stands sobbing quietly on the stairs.

"Flight of ideas" is another symptom of mania I thought I understood a couple of years before my own ideas started flying, before I lost my husband and my best friend. Whatever had struck me as so amazing that I screamed like a banshee at some ungodly hour and provoked a well-meaning neighbor into calling the police had evaporated as quickly as alcohol off hot skin by the time the knock came. Racing thoughts? Nonsense! I was simply a genius. A genius having a lot of *fun*. Only sleep-deprived medical students think they have the disease they are studying. *I* didn't have medical student's disease. I was merely thinking my profound thoughts, thoughts that I would expand on in my next feature story.

My mania had psychotic features, such as delusions concerning my brother's influence over the president and the president's deep concern with late-night sketch comedy. I've never let my analyst kick that around the office because I know what he'd say: "Evelyn, your guilt over your sexuality manifested as a persecutory delusion hinged on male authority figures, and you responded to that by attempting to display your control over your sexuality and over the sex that has exploited it." I had no guilt over my sexuality. I've always been an unapologetic libertine. And no one has ever exploited *me*. As convenient as that Freudian interpretation may be, I'd never open up and swallow. That delusion must have been a "mood-*incongruent* psychotic feature." That's what I've always told myself anyway.

The Kali hallucination, and the conviction I was dead, really creeped out the incompetent, overworked, and understaffed "team" that took me into the psychiatric emergency room. It also confused them. I'd seen a floating blue witch covered in blood and I believed I was a zombie of some kind. We all know vivid hallucinations are far more common in schizophrenia, virtually unheard-of in mania. And this "somatic delusion" of being dead was strange enough to qualify as a "bizarre" delusion, a hallmark of schizophrenia.

But, doc, you know as well as I do that elaborate visuals aren't just for schizophrenics, and you also know that "bizarre" is a matter of judgment, often culturally colored. But you didn't question yourself or me, and you didn't consider a differential diagnosis. You didn't even ask if I'd slept. The important thing was to label me in order to justify legally the cell, straps, and antipsychotics. I'm sure that was much easier for you, less time-consuming.

The criterion secondary only to "elevated, expansive, or irritable mood" is "grandiosity." That the medicine men didn't think much of my delusions of divinity further addles my lithium-saturated brain. There I was, dripping in jewels, bathed in expensive perfume, prancing around in a silk gown. All I lacked was a tiara. I told them I was God. Did they write that off as a schizophrenic delusion? Didn't they remember grandiosity is particular to mania?

They did make a fuss over the knife, and I denied everything. I was terrified I'd go to prison, but I also knew they had nothing on me. I didn't so much as scratch Eric, no one saw, and naturally my prints were all over the hilt anyway. Yes, that is the violence I spoke of. Would I have cut him? I'd like to say no, my behavior was mere histrionics. But I don't really know. I was "irritable" by then, and most would agree that he should have done something for me rather than nothing. Come on, your wife starts to make no sense, behave strangely, talk as fast as an auctioneer ("pressured speech"), and stay awake for a couple of weeks and you *ignore* it? Eric acted only when he was threatened. Unless I had pulled the knife, I suppose I would have simply swung down into a depressive episode and jumped off the roof. Maybe the gesture was in self-defense.

⸙ ⸙

After the ER, in the psychiatric ward, I am inconsolable. I throw myself repeatedly at the doors and badly bruise my shoulders. I keep telling the doctors that I am not, for the last time, hearing any voices. They speak of schizophrenia in hushed tones. They want me to participate in "occupational therapy" and refuse to believe I have a job I must return to immediately. They say I am too thin and try to make me eat, but whatever it is they force me to drink makes me puke. I cry, stare out the barred window, and imagine running wild through the city. I call Eric over and again. *Where am I? Why am I here? Did you put me here? When will they set me free? Why are my legs convulsing?*

I finally look in the mirror. Oh, no wonder they think I'm crazy; my hair is a mess. I brush it. This should clear up everything.

A young, blond doctor, still trapped in his rotations, approaches me. He talks to me for a few minutes every afternoon. "Do you hear any voices?"

"Yours."

He looks at me as if I've disappointed him, then tells me I need to stay here two more weeks and that he is arranging the paperwork. He talks about a court order, now that the seventy-two hours of police custody have passed. He asks me if that is okay. He pats me on the head like I'm his dog and moves on to a real crazy person.

For several minutes I weep in terror of surviving fourteen more days in this inexplicable torture chamber. But then I get it: The seventy-two hours have *passed*; there is no court order *yet*. I race to the nurses' desk. The blond doctor walks past me and picks up some forms. I can see him dialing the phone number. I can hear him saying my name.

"I want to sign myself out now," I say to the nurse. She turns and consults him. He slams down the phone and she urgently says something about "patient's rights." He charges out from behind the desk, points his big, ugly finger into my face, and calls *me* manipulative.

"It's you who are trying to manipulate me! I'm not trying to hold *you* hostage." Stupid pill-pusher. I sign the papers, change into my black gown, and walk out into the glorious San Francisco fog.

☙ ❧

Only to go back to the ER. The Haldol and Thorazine wear off after a day or so, and I begin causing a terrible commotion, storming through the halls of my apartment building and proclaiming the deaths of various tenants, leaning out the window and yelling into the courtyard that Buddha has come to dwell with me, removing strangers' wet undergarments from the shared washing machines and tacking them to the bulletin board in lewd formations of inverted anatomy. The landlord—a psychiatrist—soon threatens Eric with eviction if he doesn't quiet the ruckus. This time the two cops are rather gentlemanly about the procedure and ask me if I would like to get a jacket before we leave. I put on a cheap green and blue plaid pea coat, and one of them solicitously buttons it for me. They skip the cuffs and we walk to the car like childhood friends playing a familiar but boring game.

When I get to the ER, I sit quietly on a bench while the nurses process me. I'm not scared; I know they're just playing doctor. I get the impression I have been here many times before, and I will return many times again. A psychologist takes me into a private room and "counsels" me for several minutes. She contends there is something wrong with me, but admits she doesn't know what it is.

"So let me go."

They have no idea what to do with me, so they call my father in Houston. Highly sedated, I sleep in the "common room," and he arrives early the next day, looking, in his trench coat, shined shoes, and fedora, the picture of top-secret government authority. At least to me. He doesn't talk long before the doctors willingly, no doubt eagerly, hand me over to this resolute Texan. *Just get her out of our jurisdiction for the love of God.*

After we arrive in Houston, I become disenchanted with the insomnia, but the pills the San Francisco psychiatrists gave my father to administer can't touch it. Within days I am so rabidly enraged that I take to throwing bricks at the side of the house. Though I do no damage, my mother kicks me out, and as usual, my father backs her up.

I wind up staying with Sheila, my best friend, and she doesn't find my performance amusing. Though I am paying the full rent to live with her, for some reason she doesn't want me to rearrange her apartment. She orders me to mop her floors in exchange for allowing me to bear the entire cost of a duplex she has long planned to give up at the end of this month. I am insane, but she accuses me of not respecting her "boundaries." *Boundaries? Who took care of you, accompanied you to your classes at Rice University, when Michael left? On whose doorstep did you show up raving drunk, and who kept your head tilted and your esophagus clear until you came to? Who defended your hedonistic use of boys even when it meant losing friends?*

My father picks me up every day or so and takes me to Dr. Hernandez. I can't sit, so I pace about his elegant office and announce I am going to become a stripper. At our first consultation, he echoes Lisa: "You are manic. You have bipolar disorder. Do you know what that is? Here's some lithium. And here's some valproic acid, some clonazapam, and some fluoxetine. Lithium is just a salt. It will steady your mood. One in the morning, one at night. The valproic acid enhances its effect. Three at night. The clonazapam will help with the nausea. Take it morning, noon, and night. The flouxetine will lighten your affect. Don't take it until you've slept three full nights in a row. Then take one in the morning. If you start to get restless again, stop taking it and call me." He smiles and hands me the prescriptions written in an alphabet that's apparently Sanskrit.

The next consultation is not with Dr. Hernandez, but with an analyst. Dr. James has me take a simple diagnostic test, but it takes me a long time to finish because I am still hallucinating; reading is almost futile. I finish after several hours, and yes indeed, I am bipolar, manic phase. He solemnly urges me to take the pills as Dr. Hernandez advised.

Nevertheless, it's a week before I sleep, and during that time I damage irrevocably all of my relationships. Eric mails a postcard that reads, "Consider us divorced." Sheila phones from a boyfriend's and says, "I have no use for you." My father and brother are the only people who take my calls. Though I take the pills, I don't bother to see Dr. James, because I want only to win Eric over, and that is beyond Dr. James's expertise. So I start drinking whiskey at noon and smoke a pound of marijuana a month. Once a week I order a pizza.

Despite everything, after a few months in Houston, I begin working as an editor at a *TV Guide* knock-off, a supplement distributed to the newspapers around the nation that can't afford *TV Guide*. The worn carpet is flea-infested, I hate television, and my boss is a screaming demon who smells like an ashtray, but I console myself that I am "functional." I spend every weekend in bed.

In 1997 I enroll in a graduate program. At this point, I'm ravaged by whiskey and pot, and I figure taking fifteen hours a semester will force me to clean up. But as the comprehensives close in, things get weird. I can drift off, but I wake at one in the morning. For days I go through the motions despite sleep deprivation, but I eventually break down and drag myself into Dr. Hernandez's office. He reluctantly gives me some zolpidem, a hypnotic usually prescribed as a sleeping pill for no more than a week, since perpetual insomnia is extremely rare and because the drug is highly habit-forming; and some quetiapine, an antipsychotic typically reserved for schizophrenic as well as manic psychosis, largely unheard-of in the treatment of bipolars during interepisode recovery (the period of normalcy between mania and depression). He asks me if I would like to go into the hospital. *No.* He suggests I might be overstretching my limits, but I tell him everyone gets stressed over comps. Right?

In orthodox practice, zolpidem is a short-term fix for a passing problem, but I've been on it for over four years. Dr. Hernandez didn't originally think I'd need long-term quetiapine maintenance, but I responded to it so brilliantly he didn't dare take me off it. He figures it's better for me to be a zolpidem addict than to risk mania, and that it's preferable to keep me perpetually dosed with quetiapine than to allow the sheerest possibility for a psychotic break. Better Charybdis than Scylla. *Presto!* The cure.

But my life is still a bit like a novel. Everything's peaceful, but that doesn't mean a thing; disaster could be just a chapter away. But the calm still lulls me. I start to think that I'll always go on sleeping seven hours, working productively, keeping track of bills, showing up on time, making and keeping friends, and steering clear of sharp objects. I've been asymptomatic since late 1999. With each month that passes I grow more vigilant; I know I'm all the closer. As the days slip quietly by, I know they only bring me nearer to the inevitable crack, the splintering I can sometimes postpone but never evade. The quiet only whispers watch out, they're right behind you: the cuts, the bullets, the cops, the drugs, the bolted doors, the self-indulgent masochism, the joyless debauchery. My old friends are sharpening their teeth.

QUESTIONS

1. What does this narrative suggest about possible pitfalls and strategies for living with someone with manic-depression / bipolar disorder?
2. To what extent is a physician responsible for her patient with mental illness?
3. To what extent is a person with manic-depression responsible for her conduct?
4. Should people with bipolar disorder be encouraged (or forced) not to reproduce? Why or why not?

Double Trouble

⟿ Richard A. Ingram ⟿

Although the idea that psychiatry deals with the analysis of communications is not new, the view that so-called mental illnesses are idioms rather than illnesses has not been ad-equately articulated, nor have its implications been fully appreciated.

—Thomas Szasz, The Myth of Mental Illness, 145

EVER AFTER

There has been no resolution of the events I am about to relate, only further transformations. In the summer of 1995 I was informed that I had suffered a "psychotic break." This judgment has changed every aspect of my life, down to the minutest detail of daily interactions. Whenever I talk to someone who knows about my "psychiatric history," I am usually able to say that I am doing fine. But my response is often tempered by apprehension about sounding too enthusiastic, because the questioner might be led to infer that I am going "manic." Farewell to the time when it was possible to answer the question "How are you?" without hesitation. Welcome to the world of second-guessing, of seemingly inescapable mind games, of double trouble.

GOOGOLS AND GOOLIES

I had barely begun junior school before deciding that I wanted to be a mathematician. An uncluttered domain of idealized starting points and determinable end points appealed to my desire for certainty. Everything was perfectly ordered in mathematical space, and problems had definite solutions. The discipline held out the promise of a precise knowledge that was not compromised by the endless ambiguities of answers provided by adults. For more than a decade I remained convinced that mathematics stood at the pinnacle of human achievement. Later I would come to view it as a quasi-religious endeavor to transcend the body in favor of a purified, supernatural existence.

.. age nine, my ascent towards numerical heaven was interrupted by two surgical op-
.tions to correct my cryptorchism—that is, the refusal of one of my testicles to complete
its descent into the scrotum. The procedure, which is known as orchidopexy, was unsuccessful: my right testicle was removed because of the risk that it might become cancerous.
Before I left the hospital, one of the doctors decided that it would be edifying for me to be
shown my deviant pod. I gazed at the small glass cylinder, feeling puzzled about the fate
of the entombed gonad, and wondering what my life was going to be like now that I had
moved into a perpetual state of "minus one."

The medical staff reassured my parents that their son's "development" would not be affected in any way. These words of consolation were relayed to me, but I do not recall anyone
explaining why the extraction had been necessary. Neither did it occur to me, as a teenager,
to ask for an explanation, in spite of recurring dreams in which I chased after golf balls that
were buried "in the rough" or had strayed "out of bounds."

Once, during a fever, I had a terrifying vision of an enormous sphere crushing my body,
as if the prodigal ball had swollen to gigantic proportions and returned to wreak revenge
on its former host. Often I would feel a sense of incompletion that set me apart from other
children. Gradually my anxieties over being not quite male, yet not female either, gave way
to relief at not needing to conform to gender stereotypes. It was as if I could stand with
my right leg beyond the binaries that structure what most people understand as the "real
world," and look at it askance.

Admittedly, deep-seated unease about the condition of monorchia sometimes overtook me. What if the universe was a joke at my expense, in which I had been singled out as
the punch line? Might I be a pinball bouncing around the machine, a mere spectacle for
others' amusement? Perhaps no one could be trusted, not even my parents. After all, who
else was responsible for submitting me to the surgeon's knife?

To anyone who wishes to categorize these troubled thoughts as early signs of paranoia, I would advise caution. Keep in mind that there was only one other monorchid man
known to my peers, and his name rang out in playgrounds around the country to the tune
of "Colonel Bogie." The song may once have boosted the spirits of British soldiers fighting
in World War II, but it did precious little for my fragile self-esteem:

> Hitler has only got one ball
> The other is in the Albert Hall
> His mother, the dirty bugger
> Chopped it off when he was very small.

Hitler is commonly perceived to have been *less* than human. Indeed, in one of the labels
applied to him, "insane monster," there is an allusion to the hypothesis that orchidectomy
was the cause of Hitler's "madness." The expression "lone nut" retains the idea of a causal
relationship between monotesticularity and madness.

ADVOCATES OF INCOMPLETENESS

Eleven years after entering a state of oneness and/or minus oneness, I graduated from a university in the northwest of England with a degree in mathematics. I barely scraped through,

however, after failing half of the first set of final examinations.[1] A second-year course in logic had shattered my image of the mathematical method as an infallible device for proceeding from secure foundations to irrefutable knowledge. In 1931, Kurt Gödel demonstrated that this process is strictly limited due to the inevitability of arriving at undecidable statements. If the veracity of two contradictory statements that have been deduced from the same axioms is indeterminate, then the attainment of complete and coherent knowledge is jeopardized. Gödel proved that incorporating either one of the troublesome statements into the axioms in order to reestablish consistency would not prevent new outbreaks of undecidability. When two undecidable statements arise, the choice is between pursuing completion by abandoning coherence or preserving coherence by accepting incompletion. Either contradictory statements must be tolerated, or one of them must be disposed of arbitrarily. Far from serving as a model of epistemological perfection, mathematics shows that all knowledge falls prey to double trouble.

Having discovered that the hot air balloon could not rise indefinitely, I bailed overboard and began reconciling myself to life on earth.[2] A degree in the social sciences supplied me with a basic grasp of the behavior of people who were for the most part more grounded than I had been. Nevertheless, I was aware that surface stability is every bit as illusory as the Babelian towers of academic learning that are built within mathematics, the social sciences, and elsewhere. My master's degree program was organized around the work of Ernesto Laclau and Chantal Mouffe, and it was here that I chanced upon an attempt to integrate the concept of undecidability into social and political thought.

Just as Gödel develops formal logic in such a way as to demonstrate that mathematics cannot surpass certain limits to its development, so Laclau and Mouffe apply semiology—the analysis of sign systems—to the study of politics to substantiate their claim that "society" is an unattainable goal. Referring to "the social" as the field destined to fall short of the society that it aspires to be, they declare that "the social only exists . . . as an effort to construct [the] impossible object" of society (*Hegemony and Socialist Strategy,* 112). From Michel Foucault, they appropriate the concept of "discursive formations" to name the clusters that frustrate each other's expansion towards the completion and coherence of a fully realized society; the version of "society" that each strives to bring to presence is blocked by competing versions. The social, like the field of mathematics, remains riddled with absences, and could be compared to Swiss cheese, for which absences (holes) are integral to its presence. Laclau and Mouffe reserve what may be the most important term in their lexicon, "antagonism," for the ineradicable absence that haunts discursive formations that achieve any degree of presence. However, we need not mourn the essential limitation that stymies all versions of society, but instead should exploit the possibility of democratic contestation that antagonism permits. Or in the words of Leonard Cohen, "There is a crack in everything, that's how the light gets in" ("Anthem," *Stranger Music,* 373).

THE UNBEARABLE WEIGHT OF UNDECIDABILITY

Two years after publishing his proof of insurmountable undecidability, Kurt Gödel experienced a "crack-up," or a "breakdown," as an eruption of mind problems is variously described. Near the end of my first year in a doctoral program in the United States, having accomplished rather less in life than Gödel, I was compelled to admit myself "voluntarily" to a psychiatric institution.

Until this juncture, my impression of the psych discourses—psychology, psychiatry, and psychoanalysis—was that they were generally beneficent enterprises. Reading Foucault's *Madness and Civilization* had familiarized me with some of psychiatry's shady past, but I assumed that the anti-psychiatry movement of the 1960s and 1970s must have engendered positive reforms.[3] The brand of psychoanalysis that appealed to me was marketed by Slavoj Žižek, the Slovenian promoter of heavyweight theorist Jacques Lacan. Žižek highlighted "the homology between the Laclau-Mouffe concept of antagonism and the Lacanian concept of the Real" ("Beyond Discourse-Analysis," 249). In Lacanian psychoanalytic practice, the subject is guided towards a confrontation with its constitutive *lack* in a pivotal interlude of "subjective destitution."[4] The Lacanian subject is what is left over when everything it believes itself to be is taken away, that is, when it is reduced to nothing but the desire to be someone or something.[5]

PISS POOR TREATMENT

For several hours, I have been locked inside a cold cell that contains only a blue mattress and a coarse blanket. I tried banging on the door when I started wanting to go to the washroom, but no one paid any attention. Eventually I had no choice but to urinate on the floor. At least it has given me a *solution* for my severe dehydration. I crawl on all fours, edging closer to the pool of yellow liquid. Overcoming my revulsion, I begin to lap it up. Have I fallen through to the underworld?

THE PERILS OF CONFESSION

More disgusting than this spectacle is how the hospital staff would have interpreted it: "The patient was observed consuming his own waste. He is clearly in the grips of a psychotic hallucination." In modern medicine, "anamnesis" refers to the history of early symptoms, whether recounted by the ill person or recorded by the physician. But the self-descriptions of psychiatrized people are routinely dismissed, leaving psychiatrists and their underlings to invent narratives that are unconstrained by any obligation to overlap with the perspectives of patients. Foucault's *Discipline and Punish* depicts the incessant techniques of documentation that allow institutions to turn every individual into "a case which at one and the same time constitutes an object for a branch of knowledge and a hold for a branch of power" (191). Hospitals, like prisons, are disciplinary spaces in which biographics organize and direct activities of surveillance and judgment. No longer reserved for the heroic adventures of the privileged few, the biographical genre has expanded, subdivided, and multiplied into vast repositories for exhaustive information on the masses. When authority figures are writing a life story without even bothering to consult the protagonist, the obvious response is to struggle to gain the position of narrator. Unfortunately, confessional memoirs have a tendency to reinforce the regimes that they set out to contest. The insights imparted by these texts can easily serve to broaden the range of medical, psychiatric, and penal knowledge without posing a serious threat to existing power relations. Perhaps it is better to arrest the progress of existing narratives by interrupting them with multiple complications, to render them confused, to deflect them from their righteous paths, to fragment them.

POSTMODERNISTS ANONYMOUS

Best known as an engineering school, my fifth university seemed an unlikely venue for a hotbed of postmodernist theory. Adrift in the American Midwest, I doubt that it could be bestowed with a more appropriate alternate moniker than the French word that is its near-homonym and near-anagram: *perdu*, lost. Having been encouraged to move on from the political science department of a Canadian university that was not receptive to my questioning of disciplinary boundaries, I was delighted by the prospect of settling into a more hospitable milieu. In intellectual terms, the change of scene freed me from the role of spokesperson and scapegoat for a homogenized postmodernism that I had enacted at my previous institution. Instead I could enter a swirl of cross-fertilizing postmodernist varieties.

The "lost university" is located on the western shore, or left bank, of the Wabash River, and most of its students live in the twin towns of West Lafayette and Lafayette. When a heat wave hit the Midwest in July 1995,[6] this terrain presented me with an opportunity to stage my distress at having lived for almost two decades without any explanation for my orchidectomy, as if the geographical landscape itself was re-awakening the trauma of my childhood operations.

My hyperreal performance assumed the form of an epic perambulation and embodied meditation that lasted over twelve hours. Wandering back and forth across the bridges connecting the east and west sections of a split conurbation, I became disoriented and experienced temporary left-right vision reversal. Having walked throughout the night, recovered my sight, and regained my sense of direction, I visited two police stations, one on each side of the river. Confused by an apparent division in the "Law of the Father,"[7] I was possessed by fear and fascination over the implications of logics of reversal that had been vigorously explored in class discussions. Riding a wave of pleasure and pain, I finally crashed against the rocks of power-knowledge. Tagged as a "danger to myself and others," I was reeled in by the psych cops.

THE UNDECIDABILITY OF HEALTH AND ILLNESS

A few months before landing at the local loony bin, I was reveling in intellectual debates of exhilarating intensity. Such was their momentum that, alone in my cell, with a major tranquilizer coursing through my veins, I continued to puzzle over how it could be that my favorite professor at the "lost university" found the egoist philosophy of Max Stirner so appealing.[8] What I was sure about was that during the class in which the professor had prescribed the achievement of *ataraxia*—a calm, undisturbed disposition—he had not intended that it be attained through neuroleptic injection.

One of the key texts in this professor's course during the spring term had been Derrida's essay "Plato's Pharmacy." In Derrida's reading of Plato's *Phaedrus*, undecidability spreads through the disciplines, unleashed by the multivalence of the term *pharmakon*. Whether the word is being used to describe the effects of writing on memory, of filiation on writing, or of philosophy on well-being, it signifies not only medicine, remedy, and cure, but also poison. Derrida goes on to investigate another multivalent term that, despite being absent from the *Phaedrus*, nevertheless exerts an influence over its dialogues: *pharmakos*.

In addition to meaning wizard, sorcerer, or poisoner, the word *pharmakos* connotes a scapegoat. According to this scenario, organs are expelled from bodies, and bodies from cities, because they are held to be poisonous. It now becomes evident just how many life experiences were condensed into my delirious ramble along the streets of West Lafayette and Lafayette; and as a penalty for revisiting my operations by traversing the two towns, I was about to be deprived of my liberty, and almost of my life.

Derrida reminds us of the fate of the scapegoats of ancient Greek culture: "In general, the *pharmakoi* were put to death." However, because they were seen as corrupting elements within an otherwise healthy social body, the primary purpose of this ritual was to prevent them from reproducing: "Death occurred most often as a secondary effect of an energetic fustigation aimed first at the genital organs. Once the *pharmakoi* were *cut off* from the space of the city, the blows were designed to chase away or draw out the evil from their bodies" (130–132; my emphasis).

Pumped full of a drug that was contraindicated for people suffering from dehydration, I was fortunate not to die in that Indiana cell.[9] It is possible that drinking urine, a substance that is usually placed more on the side of poison than the side of cure, saved my life. What almost killed me was a medical system in which care of the body and care of the mind are *cut off* from each other, a system in which physicians neglect the psychological impact of the removal of a sexual organ, and psychiatrists ignore the history of the body.

"Why did you walk all night and long into the next day?" one of the psychiatrists asked. "It felt like a test," I replied. They decided that I must be a paranoid schizophrenic and subjected me to their "anti-psychotic" poisons. "What were you thinking about at the time?" they wanted to know. "My childhood operations." If the connection between a "test" and a "testis" ever crossed their minds, they did not let it deflect them from indoctrinating me into their belief that schizophrenia is a genetic condition, a hereditary defect, and perhaps a reason to discourage "patients" from reproducing.[10] Etymologically, the words "schizophrenia" and "castration" are related via the Greek verb, *keazein*, to split. A deeper understanding of the diagnostic term with which they were labeling me might have helped the psychiatrists to grasp that they were as out of touch with my reality as I was with theirs.

As soon as I was released from hospital, I stopped taking their poisons. Able to think clearly once more, I questioned my parents and learned that the removal of my testicle had been a preemptive measure necessitated by the risk of cancer. It took me more than eight years to piece the puzzle together in the form of this essay, but I know that I will spend many more trying to overcome the impact of the Cartesian division between medicine for the body and psychiatric "treatment" for the mind.

AFTER WORDS: BEYOND DISCOURSE ANALYSIS

The term psychotic has historically received a number of differ-
ent definitions, none of which has achieved universal acceptance.
The narrowest definition of psychotic is restricted to delusions or
prominent hallucinations, with the hallucinations occurring in
the absence of insight into their pathological nature. A slightly less
restrictive definition would also include prominent hallucinations
that the individual realizes are hallucinatory experiences. Broader
still is a definition that includes other positive symptoms of Schizo-
phrenia (i.e., disorganized speech, grossly distorted or catatonic
behavior). . . . The term has also previously been defined as a "loss
of ego boundaries" or a "gross impairment in reality testing."
—American Psychiatric Association, DSM-IV-TR 297

There is . . . a war between the odd and the even.
—Leonard Cohen, "There Is a War," Stranger Music, 202

Psychosis is diagnosed when a psychiatrist perceives that someone is no longer communi-
cating according to the standards of a shared reality. In this relationship, the power to determine what qualifies as "reality" resides entirely with the psychiatrist.[11] Yet when individuals
reenact the traumatic events of their lives, forgotten experiences tend to surface in fragments.
I have tried to show that jumbled speech and behavior need not be pathological, that alternative forms of expression may be contained within apparent incoherence, and hence that,
in Szasz's words, "so-called mental illnesses" may be "idioms rather than illnesses."

Following my two operations, my body did not hold together, or cohere, as did the
bodies of most other boys my age. This corporeal incoherence may have spurred my flight
into mathematics, a realm that held out the promise of absolute coherence. My identification with this discipline supplied me with a distinct view of the world. When I discovered
Gödel, the picture dissolved before my eyes. Living through the collapse of what I believed
to be the most solid reality gave me a glimpse of a simple fact that psychiatry has not been
prepared to admit: there are many realities.[12]

As a monotesticular child, I was made to feel not just peculiar, but potentially threatening in my difference. I was an oddity, oddness personified, out on a limb with Adolf Hitler.
I hoped that learning about feminism might save me from becoming a tyrant, and began
with Germaine Greer's *The Female Eunuch*, which seemed like an appropriate text for a
teenage semi-eunuch to read. My abnormal body appeared to set me apart from the general
population, as well as positioning me somewhere between "male" and "female." Mathematics offered a secure link to a shared reality at a time when my world was veering away from
common knowledge, until it revealed the fallibility of all systems of thought.

For Laclau and Mouffe, there is a shared reality only to the extent that one discourse
successfully occludes its rivals. Moreover, the ongoing struggles between discourses disclose

the fact that "reality" is never any more than an effect, a construction that is always in the process of being deconstructed: "Any objectivity . . . is merely a crystallized myth" ("New Reflections," 61). Laclau has proposed the concept of "mythical space" for the metaphorical representations that are suggested as alternatives to the dominant discourse. Yet he is careful to distance himself from "irrationalism":

> In speaking of "mythical spaces" and their possible transformation into imaginary horizons, it is important to point out that we are not referring to anything that is essentially "primitive" and whose re-emergence in contemporary societies would constitute an outbreak of irrationalism. On the contrary, myth is constitutive of any possible society. (67)

The fear of being associated with madness becomes even more evident in Laclau's ensuing proclamation:

> A society from which myth was radically excluded would be either an entirely "spatial" and "objective" society—where any dislocation had been banished, like the model for the operation of a perfect machine—or one in which dislocation lacked any space for representation and transcendence. In other words, the cemetery or the lunatic asylum. (67)

Once we have arrived at the view that "reality" is an effect, is there any basis for distinguishing between the rational and the irrational, the normal and the psychotic? What justification can there be for the psych wars that keep people confined in psych wards? Is it not time to abandon the dangerous prejudice that life without sanity is equivalent to death?

NOTES

1. In this three-year degree program, the first set of final examinations was administered in the second year.
2. With the publication of the *Tractatus Logico-Philosophicus* in 1922, Ludwig Wittgenstein believed that he had established the presence of logical structure in the world. After a seven-year hiatus, he resumed his investigations into language, developing a more sophisticated understanding of its workings. This transition is recounted to the dying Wittgenstein by his friend, the economist John Maynard Keynes, in the film *Wittgenstein:*

> Let me tell you a little story. There was once a young man who dreamed of reducing the world to pure logic. Because he was a very clever young man, he actually managed to do it. And when he'd finished his work, he stood back and admired it. It was beautiful. A world purged of imperfection and indeterminacy. Countless acres of gleaming ice stretching to the horizon. So the clever young man looked around the world he had created, and decided to explore it. He took one step forward and fell flat on his back. You see, he had forgotten about friction. The ice was smooth and level and stainless, but you couldn't walk there. So the clever young man sat down and wept bitter tears. But as he grew into a wise old man, he came to understand that roughness and ambiguity aren't imperfections. They're what make the world turn. He wanted to run and dance. And the words and things scattered upon this

ground were all battered and tarnished and ambiguous, and the wise old man saw that that was the way things were. But something in him was still homesick for the ice, where everything was radiant and absolute and relentless. Though he had come to like the idea of the rough ground, he couldn't bring himself to live there. So now he was marooned between earth and ice, at home in neither. And this was the cause of all his grief. ("Wittgenstein: The Derek Jarman Film" 142)

3. Robert Whitaker's *Mad in America: Bad Science, Bad Medicine, and the Enduring Mistreatment of the Mentally Ill* (Cambridge, MA: Perseus, 2002) suggests that my experiences of psychiatrization in the United States remain all too common.

4. Žižek makes this distinction between subjectivization and subjective destitution: "'Subjectivization'. . . consists in the purely formal gesture of symbolic conversion by means of which the subject integrates into [its] symbolic universe—turns into part and parcel of [its] life-narrative, provides with meaning—the meaningless contingency of [its] destiny. In clear contrast, 'subjective destitution' involves the opposite gesture: at the end of the psychoanalytic cure, the analysand has to suspend the urge to symbolize/internalize, to interpret, to search for 'deeper meaning'; [she] has to accept that the traumatic encounters which traced out the itinerary of [her] life were utterly contingent and indifferent, that they bear no 'deeper message'" (*The Indivisible Remainder*, 94; gendering amended).

5. In a sentence that establishes the homology of "antagonism" and "the Real," Žižek shows how "trauma" is a synonym of these terms: "The Lacanian notion of the subject aims precisely at the experience of 'pure' antagonism as self-hindering, self-blockage, this internal limit preventing the symbolic field from realizing its full identity: the stake of the entire process of subjectivation, of assuming different subject-positions, is ultimately to enable us to avoid this traumatic experience" (Žižek, "Beyond Discourse-Analysis," 253).

6. This event is referred to in Persimmon Blackbridge's novel *Prozac Highway*, and emphasis is placed on the threat that it posed to people diagnosed with psychiatric conditions: "In America it's summer, 200 people died from the heat in Chicago over the weekend. Most at risk are those with medical conditions, including the 'mentally ill'" (176).

7. The police epitomize the Law of the Father: they impose a patrilineal order by serving as a place of prohibition. The doubling effect of two adjacent towns, each with its own police force, suggested that there might be inconsistencies in the patrilineal order, depending on which side of the Wabash River one lived. Another reminder, perhaps, of the different ways that the two sides of my body, left and right, had been treated nineteen years earlier, for reasons that I was still struggling to grasp.

8. We had been reading extracts from Max Stirner's *The Ego and Its Own.*.

9. "Neuroleptics can produce a condition called neuroleptic malignant syndrome, which can be fatal. This is an extreme toxic reaction occurring in a small number of people who take these drugs. It closely resembles a disease called lethargic encephalitis, characterized by fever, sweating, unstable cardiovascular signs and in severe cases coma and death" (Irit Shimrat, *Call Me Crazy*, 6).

10. On hearing this story, my psychotherapist wryly observed that contemporary psychiatrists lack a sense of the poetic.

11. Pierre Klossowski describes psychiatrists as "the surveyors of the unconscious who . . . control the more or less variable range of the reality principle, to which the person who thinks or acts would bear witness" (*Nietzsche and the Vicious Circle*, xviii).

12. Michel Foucault discusses the concept of the "limit-experience" in the interview "How an 'Experience-Book' Is Born": "experience according to Nietzsche, Blanchot, and Bataille has . . . the task of 'tearing' the subject from itself in such a way that it is no longer the subject as such, or that it is completely 'other' than itself so that it may arrive at its annihilation, its dissociation" (31). He adds: "It is this de-subjectifying undertaking, the idea of a 'limit-experience' that tears the subject from itself, which is the fundamental lesson that I've learned from these authors" (31–32).

REFERENCES

American Psychiatric Association. *DSM-IV-TR*. Washington, DC: American Psychiatric Association, 2000.

Blackbridge, Persimmon. *Prozac Highway*. Vancouver, BC: Press Gang, 1997.

Cohen, Leonard. *Stranger Music: Selected Poems and Songs*. Toronto: McClelland and Stewart, 1993.

Derrida, Jacques. "Plato's Pharmacy." *Dissemination*. Trans. Barbara Johnson. Chicago: University of Chicago Press, 1981.

Foucault, Michel. *Discipline and Punish: The Birth of the Prison*. Trans. Alan Sheridan. 2nd ed. New York: Vintage Books, 1995.

———. "How an 'Experience-Book' Is Born." *Remarks on Marx: Conversations with Duccio Trombadori*. Trans. R. James Goldstein and James Cascaito. New York: Semiotext(e), 1991. 25–42.

———. *Madness and Civilization: A History of Insanity in the Age of Reason*. Trans. Richard Howard. London: Routledge, 1971.

Greer, Germaine. *The Female Eunuch*. London: Paladin, 1971.

Jarman, Derek. "Wittgenstein: The Derek Jarman Film." *Wittgenstein*. London: British Film Institute, 1993.

Klossowski, Pierre. *Nietzsche and the Vicious Circle*. Trans. Daniel W. Smith. London: Athlone Press, 1997.

Laclau, Ernesto, and Chantal Mouffe. *Hegemony and Socialist Strategy: Towards a Radical Democratic Politics*. Trans. Winston Moore and Paul Cammack. London: Verso, 1985.

Laclau, Ernesto. "New Reflections on the Revolution of Our Time." Trans. Jon Barnes. In *New Reflections on the Revolution of Our Time*. Ed. Ernesto Laclau. London: Verso, 1990. 3–85.

Millett, Kate. *The Loony-Bin Trip*. New York: Simon and Schuster, 1990.

Shimrat, Irit. *Call Me Crazy: Stories from the Mad Movement*. Vancouver, BC: Press Gang, 1997.

Stirner, Max. *The Ego and Its Own*. Cambridge: Cambridge University Press, 1995.

Szasz, Thomas S. *The Myth of Mental Illness: Foundations of a Theory of Personal Conduct*. 2nd ed. New York: Harper, 1974.

Whitaker, Robert. *Mad in America: Bad Science, Bad Medicine, and the Enduring Mistreatment of the Mentally Ill*. Cambridge, MA: Perseus, 2002.

Wittgenstein, Ludwig. *Tractatus Logico-Philosophicus*. Trans. C. K. Ogden. New York: Routledge, 1992.

Žižek, Slavoj. "Beyond Discourse-Analysis." *New Reflections on the Revolution of Our Time*. Ed. Ernesto Laclau. London: Verso, 1990. 249–60.

———. *The Indivisible Remainder: An Essay on Schelling and Related Matters*. London: Verso, 1989.

QUESTIONS

1. In what ways does the structure of this narrative resist the value of coherence? Does such resistance serve a valid purpose? for whom and under what conditions?
2. What meanings does the title carry in this essay?
3. Who or what gives psychiatrists power? How does this power compare with and differ from that of the police or courts of law? What rights does one have if s/he is pronounced "psychotic"?
4. What are the implications of the mind-body split in healthcare?

Climbing Mountains

☞ MICHAEL EDMOND DONNELLY ☜

In the spring of 1998, I was preparing to return to my favorite sport, mountain climbing. It had been over twenty years since I had actively climbed, in which time I had completed law school, started to practice law, and with my wife, Mary Frances Kingsley, who is also an attorney, started to raise our family of Katherine, now age 19, and Peter, now age 15. In that earlier time, I had been a mountain-climbing instructor for Outward Bound and had climbed the Rockies of Colorado, the Smokies of North Carolina, and the Tetons of Wyoming. Mary Frances and the children had given me a great Christmas gift, a course in technical rock climbing that I would begin in late spring. I knew that the equipment and techniques had changed during my time away from the sport. The kink-ridden gold line rope that we used in the 1960s had been replaced by the super-smooth Perlon and synthetic ropes of the 1990s; but more than that, I knew that I had to get back in shape to keep up with a crew of active twenty-year-old climbers. To do that, my training of choice was long-distance running and jumping rope. My equipment of choice was a fine eight-foot-long rawhide Everlast jump rope with wooden handles and built-in ball-bearing swivels.

As I started to run and, in particular, jump rope, a persistent pain developed in my upper back. I attributed this pain to muscle strain from jumping rope and thought a break from the jump rope would allow me to heal. However, when neither the rest nor doses of Extra-Strength Tylenol and mugs of hot tea with brown sugar helped my back improve, I sought relief by sleeping on our living room floor.

Around this time, I made an appointment with physicians at a local sports medicine clinic, intending to secure relief for the pain in my back. After a number of sessions with doctors from the clinic telling me that this was only a muscle pull and nothing else, I had had it. I made arrangements for a thoracic MRI. Ever the lawyer, I directed that the MRI results be sent not just to the sports clinic, but also to my primary physician, a friend of some years.

The phone call that morning from my primary physician was troubling. The MRI revealed either a serious infection or some sort of a tumor on T7 of my spine. I remember walking out of the house that morning and having a rather blunt discussion with God and my deceased father and father-in-law, telling them about the results and reminding them that they had better start helping and helping now.

Court that morning seemed to drag by as I prepared for another meeting with the doctors at sports medicine. The advice of my primary physician and other lawyer friends was simply, in no uncertain terms, to demand action on that day. The doctors' advice just to go home and deal with this all on another day came as no surprise.

The humor in this situation comes back to me as I write this article. I stood in the sports medicine examining room in my best black wing tips, more or less enshrouded in a green paper johnny that failed to cover my exposed backside. As I stood there in this outfit, I asked the doctor if he had read the MRI report. I noted that I was aware of what was in the report and that he was damn well not going to just send me home. I had just "made a scene" over getting correct medical care and the world had stopped spinning. For a moment, I could picture the hospital security officers being summoned and their less-than-ceremonious arrest of me in my black wing tips and green paper johnny for disturbing the peace and trespassing on hospital grounds. I could also picture my arraignment back at the courthouse; that truly was a possibility to ponder.

The wheels of reason fortunately kicked back into operation. Justice was served and I was not arrested, though I did prevail. With newfound determination, I marched my doctor and me upstairs to the cancer unit and the chief of oncology announcing that I had "arrived to be admitted." Clearly, one should never argue with a man wearing only black wing tips and a green johnny, and the wise chief of oncology agreed, promptly admitting me.

At this point, events started to progress quickly. Shortly after my admission, my wife, daughter, and I met with an excellent radiologist who gave me some very difficult news: the mass on my spine had invaded or was constricting the neural column of my spine. If untreated, this presented a serious risk of paralysis from about the neck down. We later learned that my physicians had engaged in a spirited debate over treatment, ultimately agreeing to recommend prompt radiation to shrink the mass and steroid treatment to reduce the swelling and nerve constriction. My wife and I now mulled over the options. When procedures failed to capture cells from the mass on my back for analysis toward a diagnosis, we agreed to the radiation and steroid treatment. I am convinced that the doctors' good decision on this procedure prevented certain paralysis. In this decision, and in all others, my wife, who kept a spiral notebook of all of our meetings with the doctors, became a vital advocate for my cure. I cannot overemphasize the importance of having another person available to support a patient in this kind of situation. As a lawyer, Mary Frances would politely, but firmly, ask questions about drug dosages, test procedures, and a hundred other factors of treatment that I was unable to ask, as I was either in bed or too tired to think of them. It quickly became clear that Mary Frances's keen questioning, cheerful disposition, and notebook were having a significant effect on my treatment process. People in the hospital were alert to explaining what they proposed in treatment and, at this stage, diagnosis. The fact that we were both lawyers was not missed. Let me also note that, in my judgment, we were careful not to misuse our professional positions; we were merely aware that our professions made a difference in how information was presented to us.

My legal training came to be of greatest value when I had been in the hospital for several days. During this period, no diagnosis had been made and the doctors started to talk about discharging me without diagnosis. At this point, we called a meeting of all the medical team, which had grown in number, since I was a hard case to figure out. In the meeting, I made it clear that (A) I was not leaving the hospital until we had a diagnosis and (B) that we needed all the staff to work together to reach a diagnosis. The meeting was more like a business meeting, with Mary Frances asking oncologists and radiologists questions and taking notes, while I reminded everyone that there had been some confusion before in Sports Medicine, and that this was not going to happen again. I put on my crazy game face, whereas Mary Frances was professional and welcoming. It worked. I stayed in the hospital and a new series of tests and a medical case conference were to be held. The intervention of a senior hospital staff member who was a friend of mine calmed the hospital staff and helped to resolve this conflict in a positive way. In hindsight, this was our most important moment, as it focused the medical team toward rethinking the diagnosis and convinced my wife and me that we were not helpless at this time; we could be active participants in my care. Our legal training shaped our handling of that meeting, and our responses were consistent with our styles in handling cases in our respective practices. We fell back on our training as lawyers educated in critical analysis, negotiation skills, and advocacy for our position, and all of these skills worked for us.

Shortly after this general meeting with us, the physicians met again as planned. At that meeting a suggestion was made to explore the possibility that the tumor might be secondary, related to testicular cancer. A test was quickly ordered and conducted by a gifted technician who told me that he prayed for God's help in heightening his perception before each test. His work revealed my diagnosis was indeed testicular cancer. We had turned a corner but we now faced a very uncertain future of treatment and a less than reassuring survival rate for this advanced stage of cancer.

As the treatment began—radiation, a partial orchiectomy (a removal of one cancerous testicle), and chemotherapy—I was thrilled to be returning home. I was frightened, but family, friends, and faith started to give us hope.

It was then that it happened: I went into severe steroid psychosis.

I knew something was afoot when I started to obsess about people intending to kill me and to worry that breaking glass from windows and tabletops could kill me. I really started to scare myself and Mary Frances when I told her that I would have to walk around our car three times to make sure that we didn't crash on our way back to the hospital. It was clear that I needed to return to the hospital. One of my fondest memories from my readmission to the hospital, though not at the time, was the observation made by one of the amazing nurses who so gently cared for me during the steroid reaction. Several years after the reaction, I met her and she told me that the day I came into the hospital, my hair was all ruffled and standing on end and that I was engaged in some obsessive, repetitive behavior, walking around mumbling some strange, internal gibberish to myself. I laughed when she told me that she and the other nurses could not believe that I was a lawyer. They were convinced that I was a bagman. I commented that in my experience, it was a very, very fine line between these two fields.

I still remember that feeling from the steroids, with their power to wipe away all logical thought and literally drive a person mad. I now keep that experience in mind when I prosecute drug cases or propose treatment as part of a disposition in a drug case.

When I consider the treatment experience of that year, I am pleased that I can laugh about so much, but I still remember the terror and loss of control. I am convinced that my legal training played a crucial role in my ability to negotiate my care and in actually getting better. So did my teaching.

Teaching has always been my second profession—after being a lawyer—and my first intellectual love. Through a line of academic positions from college professor to medical and law school professor, I have been blessed in being able to balance my work as a trial attorney with my love of teaching. It was, therefore, no surprise that when I was diagnosed with cancer, I would turn to my teaching as a support and consolation through some very difficult days.

Early in my treatment with chemotherapy, I had one of those special experiences characteristic of some cancer patients: a sense that if I worked hard enough, I could just push my way through this illness and return to teaching. With great care and kindness, the administration of Assumption College, where I had taught for years, agreed to help me hold my seminar on "Children and Violence" in my home. This lifted my spirits. I was going to resume teaching, and it was going to happen in my family room. We live on a cape, in the small New England town of Paxton, Massachusetts, with stone walls and acres of trees behind our home. I pictured my students sitting, drinking cups of tea, and eating cookies with me, as we discussed the latest literature on youth murders—a truly charming image. Sadly, this idyllic situation was not to happen. I was just too tired and I had overestimated my energy level. The thought of conducting a three-hour seminar, when all I really wanted to do was sleep, brought me back to the reality of my illness. However, the thought of teaching kept my mind focused and active. Even if my body would not let me carry through this effort, the fact that I could still think and plan my future classes served as a great comfort. I would adjust to the reality of the disease, but not give up the hope for another day's work.

As the summer moved ahead, with weeks of recovery from the chemotherapy, I moved to my wife's family's summer home, in Sunapee, New Hampshire, where I could rest and regain my strength. The provost and my friend from Worcester Polytechnic Institute, Lance Schacterly, wisely suggested that I might like to work on a rewrite of my book *The Use of Scientific Evidence in Service to Children in American Courts*. This suggestion was perfect, because I could do my writing on the porch at the cottage on Lake Sunapee between naps and cups of tea. I took up the suggestion and moved quickly through the chapters, taking breaks to read things that I enjoyed from the town library that my family brought to me. I felt whole and productive with this addition, which was a gift in the midst of the illness.

During my recovery, I also enjoyed conversations and collaborations with other faculty members. While undergoing treatment, I had read Dr. Herbert Benson's book *Timeless Healing*, an exploration of the impact of spirituality in healing. Friends from my undergraduate university, Wesleyan, had learned that I was reading Benson, and they contacted him, as a fellow Wesleyan graduate, and suggested that I might benefit from a phone call. One morning, while I was reading his book, Dr. Benson, a cardiologist at Harvard Medical School, called me. I had majored in religion at Wesleyan, and our conversation about his book was absolutely riveting. We talked about faith as an unexpected factor in the healing process, about his work concerning the so-called "placebo process," and about the promise of my achieving a cure for my cancer. Our conversation felt as though I were talking in a faculty lounge with a fellow colleague about a new idea, while at the same time placing me into a reassuring consultation with a kind and gifted physician.

Faith itself was critical to my recovery. On the day I first learned I had cancer, I spoke to God, my deceased father and my deceased father-in-law as members of the Communion of Saints—urging them, as Abraham urged God when he petitioned God to spare the city of Sodom from destruction, to bring about my salvation and to do it quickly. Like Abraham, I was deeply respectful to God; but also like Abraham, I was not afraid to argue aggressively for my life and for my family. This pleading with God was similar to what I do as a lawyer. From that first day and throughout my recovery and final cure, my faith and my legal training were like two straight, strong railroad tracks that led me forward in the direction I needed to go. Law and faith worked hand-in-hand as one force to secure my healing and recovery.

I have changed as a person and as an attorney through the experience of that year. I am happier about what I can do for people as a lawyer, because I remember what it was like to be out of control, afraid of dying, or just plain sick from the chemotherapy. Things happen in ways that just can't be predicted. But remembering what carried me through difficulties like cancer—family, friends, faith, and profession—can be great sources of strength.

EPILOGUE

The sweat came running down my face and the surge of the field moved me slowly forward. My Superman tee-shirt and shorts, both gifts from my children, were, as I later learned, picked up by Boston TV and broadcast so that a friend watching me from home could see them. I was fifty years old and, for the third time, I was running the Boston Marathon. This was part of the "more time" I had wanted when I first learned that I had cancer. It became my challenge. As I headed to the finish line that April afternoon in my Superman tee-shirt—having discarded my shorts in Wellesley to the shock of some ladies who were reassured to see that I had a second pair of shorts underneath—I saw my wife and children in the crowd at the finish yelling and crying for me. The announcer boomed out to cheers over the loudspeaker, "Ladies and Gentlemen, would you welcome to the finish line Superman … able to leap tall buildings in a single bound …" (then he paused and said) "… well, maybe not today …" (I was finishing, but exhausted) "… but still, we welcome Superman to Boston …"

Every six months, I take a day off for myself. I dress in a jacket and slacks, and I head off to Boston for the day. I spend the day with a copy of the *New York Times* and a good book, which I enjoy slowly reading along with a drink.

After about a quart of a special liquid, I climb on my back, into an MRI machine. Beautiful clouds and a blue sky are painted on the ceiling, beyond the machine. The technicians are friendly and helpful as they tell me alternately to hold my breath then blow it out as the MRI scans my body looking for a return of my cancer.

When my scan is over, I leave quickly, usually to get a quick bowl of soup, since I have not been able to eat for about twelve hours, then walk out of the hospital and up Longwood

Avenue to the Museum of Fine Arts. My parents used to take me to this museum when I was a little boy, and I love this part of my day. I tell my friends that I am going to Boston for a "Ten Thousand Mile Checkup," but I am really going to the museum to see paintings.

This past week, I spent an hour in a large room of paintings by Monet and Renoir. The best part of the day was the chance to see *Fruit Displayed on a Stand*, by Gustave Caillebotte. It was cold in Boston that day, and the wind blew down Longwood Avenue with a vengeance. However, in front of Caillebotte's painting, I was warm and relaxed. The fruit in the picture are laid out on clean white tissue paper. I like the blueberries and figs best, but the oranges are also wonderfully round and ripe. Maybe the best parts of his painting are the dark green leaves at the top of the stand of fruit. These leaves are so deep and earthy they are almost black. They make me feel rich and easy in their lushness; they make me feel healthy and alive. The beauty and richness of the color in Caillebotte's painting serve as my talisman for overcoming cancer and for staying cancer-free. And so, when it is time to leave and go back to see my friend and oncologist to get the result of my test, I am relaxed and warm. I make this day a good day, a good day for me.

QUESTIONS

1. What actions on the part of the author enabled him to take control of his own health care?
2. Discuss the differences between primary and iatrogenic illness in this particular story. How might the differences be significant?
3. How do family and faith function in the author's healing?

A Calculus of Advocacy
A Patient, Positionality, and Chronic Illness

☞ JANE E. SCHULTZ ☜

A serious and unforeseen illness in 2000 and 2001 taught me that recovery was far more than a series of physical and psychological steps one undergoes to feel better. The illness forced me to accept a shattered self and remake a self—a journey whose protean metaphors helped me confront and embrace an alien identity until I could absorb it into a new framework.[1] The imagery of volcanology provides a useful analogy for the process of deep immersion that medical subjects undergo when their humanity takes new forms. Much of the work of transformation takes place underground, within the body and within the psyche, but it does not begin on its own. Medical subjects reestablish their connection to the world through self-examination and a conscious willingness to regard the sick self. In this narrative I show how the rough ride of self-examination led me to advocacy. I had to become my own advocate in order to heal.[2]

The concept of the examined life is familiar to most academics. Liberal arts training in philosophy, history, language, and literature engages students in an examination of the human condition, but no training prepares us, as Elaine Scarry has noted, for a sustained encounter with pain and sickness.[3] The essential linguistic unrepresentability of physical suffering sent me on a search for a new rhetoric of self-examination—one in which my old model of self-reliance gave way to a model of dependence. What initially felt like a compromise—asking for help even to sit up—was in fact an early assertion of advocacy. If I could consider seeking help as a rhetorical act, then it moved from the realm of compromise to that of assertion. As I probed the sources of my alienating infirmity, I began to comprehend that my dependence, far from being an occasion for humiliation, required me to put my self at the center of my illness as a subject, not its object.[4]

The patient's subjectivity and not the practitioner's absorbs my attention here: the states of mind and body that sick people pass through on their way to recovery of the self. Historically speaking, conceptualizing the patient as a subject with voice is a relatively recent development, and it is no coincidence that the emergence of illness narratives has corresponded with interest in patient advocacy.[5] "Advocacy," as I use the term, rests on the principles of acknowledgment and assertion: In order to achieve advocacy in our own behalf, we must acknowledge a sick self—a psychologically painful acceptance of physical incapacity that requires us to confront the possibility of death. Acknowledgment prompted me to hit the books. I wanted to learn about the scientific origins and cultural history of my disease. I wanted to know who else had it and whether other sufferers had written about it.[6] Acquiring information, not just from books but from a wide array of sources, allowed me to participate in decisions made about my treatment. Implicit in this second piece of the advocacy equation is the patient's role as collaborator with medical practitioners—an assignment that many hospitals now understand as integral to healing. As Rita Charon, an MD-Ph.D. specialist in narrative medicine, has put it, "the doctor and the patient co-author the story of an illness."[7] The doctor-patient collaboration resembles a hospital with multiple lab sites, where the patient moves from test to test and reinterprets the narrative of illness in light of new findings. Today patients and doctors may enhance collaborations electronically, but what they find may help or hinder the recovery of self, and by extension the goal of advocacy, depending on the quality of the sources.[8]

To identify the self as sick requires an act of distancing. An individual acknowledges illness as a compromised self. The process of identification with this unfamiliar self takes place at precisely the moment we lack the physical ability to enable the realization. When illness proceeds gradually, it may be easier for us to accept a new self because we are transformed by imperceptible degrees. However, when onset is sudden, acknowledgment may be fraught with denial. In either case, the psychological work of surrendering a self to illness occurs during a period of vulnerability when, in the context of Western medicine, medicalization takes place.[9] A medicalized body—a patient absorbed by the apparatus of the health-care system—has relinquished subjectivity, often unwittingly. Thus, surrendering the self, unlike its linguistic attribution of agency, may amount to a kind of institutional body snatching, where the patient wakes up from exploratory surgery and sees an intubated Other on the gurney.

I was fortunate to come to the realization that snatching my body back would remake my subjectivity. The struggle to wrest my self from practitioners intent on treating my body created a *calculus* of advocacy—a dynamic set in motion initially by deference to my doctors' medical knowledge. Over the course of six months, as I amassed knowledge about my condition and gained the ability to articulate its manifestation in me, I threw off the subordination implicit in these relationships and began to see myself for the active healer I was. Such a calculus never really proceeds in isolation, though the patient may initially perceive it that way.[10] The calculus varies according to changes in the players or the institutions that order patients' conduct. Cancer patients in Kansas City found this to be the case when a profit-motivated pharmacologist diluted their chemotherapy.[11] But much less dramatic examples, like those of the surgeon who dismisses the patient's medical insights or the patient who lacks the vitality or support network to access pertinent information, may also reroute the calculus. In my own case, my status as a single parent isolated me in ways that made recovery more protracted.

My work on advocacy is both academic and autobiographical. Historical study of nineteenth-century hospital systems and the *dramatis personae* of those institutions have informed my scholarly life of late. In a recent project, I suggested that the patient's body became a symbolic site of conflict between nurses and surgeons engaged in professional turf battles.[12] When in 2000 I was diagnosed with pseudomyxoma peritonei (PMP), an abdominal cancer of the peritoneum, I lost the tidy perspective of the patient as a kind of pawn in a medical chess game and was immediately absorbed in the internal struggle of self that I have outlined above. Immersed in pain, nausea, and a mental fog about the survivability of the disease, I became intimately familiar with the patient's positionality, which radicalized my understanding of advocacy. I make no claim to universality in this pathography because each of us experiences illness differently. It might even be argued that one need not experience illness to grasp the metaphysics of being ill. Still, my own journey as patient-with-cancer left me with the conviction that sick people, and those with chronic illnesses in particular, serve themselves best from positions of advocacy. I might not have arrived there had I not gone there myself.

In the spring of 2000 I was in Cambridge, England, on sabbatical from Indiana University-Purdue University-Indianapolis, where I am an English professor. During an unusually rainy March in East Anglia—one of the few regions of England that enjoys dryer weather than most—I developed a respiratory illness that confounded physicians at the Newnham Walk Surgery. Dr. Swan, who met me in an office that doubled as his examination room, commented over his reading glasses that lots of visiting Americans had presented with these symptoms in the past month. Because English doctors are reluctant to use antibiotics, Dr. Swan waved me away, optimistic that my symptoms would dissipate on their own. If I were not better in six weeks, he would prescribe antibiotics. Six weeks later I returned, debilitated from coughing and lack of sleep and increasingly unable to walk my eight-year-old daughter the mile and a half to school. Confident in my medical ethnocentrism that amoxycillin would make me well again, I almost ran to the village chemist to fill the prescription. No improvement three weeks later: continued fatigue, cough intact, difficulty breathing, and thick phlegm. This was beginning to look more like a virus than an infection. Dr. Swan now hypothesized that I might have "seasonal asthma" and started me on steroids. These made me manic but did not clear my lungs. By the time I returned to Indiana late in the summer, the symptoms were not as acute and I had learned to live with them.

Swept up in the whirlwind of a new school year, I sought no further help. I felt tolerably well and considered any debility to be age-related (I was 46). I did schedule a routine gynecological exam because I had not had one in over eighteen months. Before my departure to England, my insurance company had informed me that routine checkups were covered only once annually. Though it had been more than eleven months since my previous checkup, a caseworker told me, despite my explanation that I would be out of the country for nearly a year, that I would have to wait until I returned in the fall of 2000. In September my gynecologist, Dr. Wanabebe, detected a nine-centimeter mass as she palpated my abdomen. Such masses, she noted, often turned out to be fibroids, causing little more than discomfort. Still she ordered an ultrasound the following month to get a better look. I was eating and exercising regularly; surely nothing could be the matter.

When the technician who performed the ultrasound left the room and returned with the gynecologist on duty, I still was not alarmed. When I asked her what she saw, she stonewalled: "I will have your doctor call you." Dr. Wanabebe phoned me two hours later with news that the mass would need to be biopsied. "Tell your chair that you need to take off the rest of the semester," she announced. The mass was floating near an ovary, but she could not be sure whether the reproductive organs were implicated. The mass was not hard, which was "a good sign," but surgery would provide a direct look, allowing her to rule out a malignancy. A needle biopsy (much less intrusive than full abdominal surgery) was not possible because the puncture of what might be a malignant mass would spread cancerous cells throughout my peritoneum. "O.K.," I remember thinking, "this is inconvenient, but I could hardly feel this good if it were something that bad." I found colleagues to teach my remaining class sessions, made arrangements for my daughter to spend my days of hospitalization at her father's house, and fielded questions from my anxious septuagenarian parents. Near retirement and no longer carrying major malpractice insurance, Dr. Wanabebe asked Dr. Pistil, chair of the obstetrics and gynecology department at the Indiana University School of Medicine, to perform the surgery.[13] She confided *sotto voce* that he was the best gynecological surgeon IU had and that if it were her body, she would choose Dr. Pistil.

After a brief consultation concerning what Dr. Pistil anticipated would be a 45-minute operation, the date was set for November 20—three weeks later. I went back to the business of grading papers, reading Hawthorne, and finding somebody to look after my ancient cat. I felt more anxious about what clothing to bring to the hospital than I did about the impending surgery; it was my habit of mind not to dwell on what I could not alter. I asked my mother to come from St. Louis to look after me until I could fend for myself. We entered the hospital on that late fall day an hour before sunrise. By 7:30 a.m., two nurses in pink scrubs walked with me into the operating room where two surgical nurses in blue scrubs bedded me down on the table and "tucked me in" with freshly warmed towels. I appreciated walking into the OR on my own power—no wheel chairs for the ambulatory patient here! Even before the anesthesiologist arrived, I was moving into the twilight land of relaxation, aware that my fate was now in the hands of Dr. Pistil and his team.

When I woke up more than four hours later, my first thought was, "If I need to die now, it is all right." I was in unimaginable pain and had no idea, of course, how much time had actually passed. Nor did I know that Dr. Pistil had removed my appendix, ovaries, uterus, and over a foot of intestines in those hours. Though I was not conscious of the facts for many days, my doctors had discovered a peritoneal cancer that had begun in my appendix and had seeded my intestinal cavity with small mucinous tumors. I had pseudomyxoma peritonei—a diagnosis made scarcely more than a hundred times annually in the United States.[14] As I came to understand later, Dr. Pistil's swift diagnosis saved me considerable grief.[15] I was fortunate that my local hospital was a tertiary-care facility and a teaching institution; as a faculty member, I was a privileged client, and my privilege related directly to the speed and accuracy of the diagnosis.

In a mental and physical purgatory for two days, I was aware that something had gone wrong, but I could not perceive what. Later I learned that in her funk my mother, usually a pillar of strength, could not locate the car in the parking lot that first night. Had I been able with out-of-body omniscience to witness this, I would have better understood the serious-ness of the case. But no one in my midst used the word "cancer," and I did not hear anyone utter the words "pseudomyxoma peritonei" until the third day. With a gastric tube, IV lines, pumps, and catheters, I was wheeled, jingling, from the ICU to the gynecology ward. I was now conscious of having lost organs and I felt sorrow at the prospect of my compromised self. On day 4, I began to understand that I had a condition about which little was known. Family and friends were searching websites to unlock its mysteries. Around the clock, my days consisted of sweating through nightgowns (the product of post-hysterectomy hormonal havoc); having my temperature, pulse, and blood pressure taken; surviving the pulsations of the compression cuffs on my legs; having my abdominal catheter flushed with heparin, an anticoagulant; enduring daily blood draws in light of the high fevers I was spiking; hit-ting the morphine pump for intermittent relief; and listening to the incessant beeping of my IV monitors—or so it seemed—whenever the saline bags ran dry.

On post-operative day 7, Dr. Pistil prescribed a series of intraperitoneal chemothera-pies. He had launched this plan during the surgery by installing a Tenckhoff catheter in my abdomen. The prospect of chemotherapy was perplexing (did I have cancer?), but given the fog I was in, I could not have declined treatment. Even if Dr. Pistil had been able to ask me whether he could proceed with the catheterization, I could not have responded. I was a dependent without the capacity to think critically. I received 100 milligrams of cisplatin—a drug that does not go gentle into sensitive tissues like the peritoneum.[16] Within ten minutes I vomited up the first bites of solid food I had had in over a week. In subsequent infusions that winter and spring, I took anti-nausea drugs intravenously before the cisplatin, which gave me three "good" hours before the severe nausea set in. The cisplatin inalterably dam-aged my kidneys (elevated creatinine) and my hearing (tinnitus) and produced edema in my hands and feet.[17] Though I had scrutinized the hospital handout on side effects of cis-platin, I had not thought to ask about the cumulative effects of this drug or its long-term impact on other organs. I was released from the hospital twelve days after surgery and five days after chemotherapy, barely able to hoist myself upstairs to my bedroom. Despite the presence of my mother and a friend, I felt like a fledgling pushed out of the nest.

I began a residence of six months in bed, punctuated only by trips to the bathroom to flush my catheter with heparin, to the oncology building for successive chemo infusions, and on rare occasions, across the street to my campus office. In time I sent my mother and my friend home (their distress was making me feel worse), so I now spent most of the time between infusions by myself. I stumbled around to care for my daughter, but my stiff upper lip did not fool her. I tried a succession of nausea drugs—seven in all—but nothing worked. Dr. Pistil had warned me that I would feel tired and perhaps unable to go to the office for a couple of days during each three-week cycle. No one told me that nausea would rule my life 24/7, and that with successive infusions, the accumulation of cisplatin in my system would make the nausea worse. No one had prepared me for the awful metallic taste or chemical smell I would experience every time I inhaled. No one had prepared me for the cold shock of the daily heparin cleansing of my abdominal catheter, like a snowball in the guts, or for the rawness of skin that would develop where the catheter pierced my belly. Without put-ting too fine a point on it, there were days when all I could stomach were a half-cup of water and a half-cup of broth.[18] I could not read, I could not sleep; twenty-minute catnaps alone spared me from continual consciousness of nausea.

Before I left the hospital, it began to dawn on me that I had cancer. My parents had not yet used the word, but why, I wondered, had chemotherapy been prescribed for me?[19] A sense of betrayal and anxiety seized me; the anxiety was a higher order of affliction than nausea because it spurred me to action. An uncertain prognosis meant that my survival was tenuous. Through a depression so thick it might have been cut with a scalpel, I believed that my only chance was to learn everything I could about the disease. In a follow-up appointment, Dr. Pistil explained why he had prescribed such a strenuous course of chemotherapy. My health had always been excellent and he believed he had caught the disease at an early stage; after "debulking,"[20] or excising as much tumor as he could find, he wanted to follow surgery with a prophylactic washing of the peritoneum via chemotherapy. This seemed like a good plan to me after the fact, especially since I knew that Dr. Pistil, who had seldom encountered pseudomyxoma during his surgical career, would do his medical homework.[21]

My 77-year-old father also did his homework. He sent me every article he could find related to pseudomyxoma, though I would not read them for about three months—unwilling (and I think unable) in my nausea to digest anything at all.[22] He had found a website about the disease sponsored by Dr. Honeycutt, a surgeon who specialized in a fourteen-hour procedure to remove all unessential organs in the peritoneum. With the object of discouraging the spread of tumors, Dr. Honeycutt proposed removing the umbilicus, the colon, any diseased portion of the intestines, the appendix, the gallbladder, the reproductive tract, and the peritoneum itself. When I mentioned Dr. Honeycutt's surgery to Dr. Pistil, he rolled his eyes and asked whether I had been reading Dr. Honeycutt's website. Apparently Dr. Pistil had been surfing the web also. Explaining that Dr. Honeycutt's procedure was at the radical end of the surgical spectrum, Dr. Pistil encouraged me to find out more. Even in my physical and psychic distress—conditions that make us more and more remote from others—I sensed his displeasure. Three months after the initial chemotherapy, I made an appointment to see Dr. Honeycutt in Washington, D.C. It was all I could do to board a plane; I was unable even to carry my briefcase. My brother and my friend journeyed from Connecticut and Michigan to help me sort out the consultation with Dr. Honeycutt and to plot a course of action. After waiting nearly three hours to see the eminent surgeon, he examined me and scheduled me for "cytoreductive" surgery five months later, when I would have finished the regime of cisplatin. He recommended in the face of this daunting surgery that I get myself in top physical form by starting a program of weightlifting.

Presumably to save time, Dr. Honeycutt made his dictation as I sat in his examination room. By the time he was finished, tears were falling quietly down my cheeks. His statistical projections of PMP patients' survival odds were grim; a certain percentage did not survive the operation. Many others developed life-threatening complications in its aftermath. In my debilitated state, it sounded as if he were saying that I would surely die if I did not have the surgery and that I might still die even if I did. Though I have always been a resisting reader, I felt too weak to dispute this (death) sentence. Fearful for my life, I was able only to hear that statistically the odds were against me and that any alternative interpretation of my case was impossible. I would simply have to steel myself for the trauma ahead. When Dr. Honeycutt finally looked up from his dictaphone, he asked me what was the matter. When I told him that I was not ready to die, he said, "Oh, but you have a very good chance because your disease has not progressed that far." I left the office in a daze and spent the whole night wondering how I could accomplish the *psychological* work leading up to this surgical ordeal. The physical work of enduring chemotherapy had already brought me to my knees. I felt that there was nothing left in my psychic reserves for a protracted physical struggle.[23]

When I mentioned the scheduled surgery to Dr. Pistil, he did what he could to discourage me, even going so far as to ask me how I would like living with a colostomy bag at my side. I responded that I had little choice if I wanted to be alive in ten years to see my daughter graduate from high school. Dr. Honeycutt believed that the disease killed every one eventually and that his prophylaxis arrested its spread, giving people at least ten more years to live. As he intoned in his dictation, "Unfortunately, if the cytoreduction is not complete, we do not have any patients who survive ten years."[24] I had to begin preparing myself for the six months of recovery this operation would require, not to mention the three- to six-week hospitalization in a city far from my home. All the while, I saw Dr. Pistil's furrowed brow in my mind: he had been uneasy about specialists with websites trolling for patients with excellent chances of survival. He had even observed in our conversations that when a patient enters a surgeon's office for consultation, there's a 90 percent chance that the patient will schedule surgery. Though I did not see why at the time, I later concluded that surgeons improve their survival rates, and their professional reputations, by operating on patients like me: in good physical shape before onset, obedient, and motivated to follow a medical regimen to the letter.

The surgery and hospitalization that Dr. Honeycutt was proposing would cost between $250,000 and $500,000; the more virulent the spread of the tumors and the more severe the complications, the more costly the procedure would be. As a long-time faculty member with what I believed to be adequate university health insurance, I erroneously assumed that IU Health Care would cover a medically necessary surgery. I learned upon further investigation that only 50 percent of any procedure contracted out of network would be covered. I could choose a doctor within the Indiana University system to treat me, or I could incur a debt I would never be able to repay. I appealed the decision to the insurance provider to no avail. They replied that they would happily assign a local doctor to my case. Never mind that no local gastroenterologist or oncologist specialized in the treatment of PMP and that fewer than ten doctors in the United States treated it.[25] The injustice of the insurance provider's position added immeasurably to the stress under which I already labored. Not only did I have to consent to an operation that might kill me and would surely derail me professionally, but I would lose my house and the few assets I had been able to accrue.

My visit to Dr. Honeycutt yielded one other significant development: A former patient of his was constructing a website to provide information about PMP physicians to patients and their caregivers. Though the site did not presume to supplant the physician, it did offer a list of specialists and helped connect patients (PMP "pals") with one another. As soon as I could sit at a computer for ten minutes, I devoured this website; it was the first satisfying meal I had had in nearly four months. Through it I became aware of the larger constellation of practitioners, clinical trials at the NIH, differing methods of treatment, and patients' unique narratives. The sheer weight of personal testimony made it possible for me to see my own case in the context of others'—the perspective I had lacked when I saw Dr. Honeycutt—and thus to realize that I had options for handling subsequent surgeries. The website propelled me beyond the stage of identification with a sick self into a more proactive frame of mind—a process that I contend is an integral piece of the advocacy puzzle. The information I sought and found there rescued me from isolation, but it also needed to be understood and interpreted as a text. I later processed the rhetorical architecture of the site and realized that, despite its support-network function, it was a money-making proposition for the patient who had created it.[26] The site's posting of death notices had the unanticipated consequence of narrowing my vision of possible outcomes. There was 44-year-old Cheryl Chaykowski of Ontario, who had died two years after her diagnosis and was "dearly missed" by her husband and two school-age daughters. Tina Pelley, a 49-year-old geologist from San Jose, had "enjoyed running marathons, gardening, [and] rescuing and caring for a variety of pets." Then there was Ken Marshall, aged 54, the owner of an excavation business in Shingle Springs, California, who "chose never to complain and always spoke well of others."[27] I found myself bound by a rhetoric whose point was to forestall death instead of to invite alternatives to its dark closure.

Armed with addresses of two specialists in Texas, I made appointments to get other opinions about how to proceed with my case. On two days in May, I saw Dr. Ladywood at Houston's palatial M. D. Anderson Cancer Center, and Dr. Murray at the University of Texas medical branch in Fort Worth. Both doctors independently advised me that further treatment was not critical at this juncture; that it would be more prudent to scan the tumors every three months, since they appeared to be growing slowly. The encounter summaries from these visits presented me new interpretive challenges. Each offered a familiar template in terms of its demographic situating of the patient, its description of her current complaint, the results of physical examination, and finally suggestions for treatment. But there was not much else on which all three doctors agreed, even on something as minor as my academic specialty (which one of the surgeons noted erroneously as history). Here were three stories about me, and all of them without endings. It was my job to sift out the meaning in each of these prognostications: to decide which narrative seemed to parallel most closely my sense of the illness and thereby to determine which treatment plan augured the most satisfactory closure. In effect, I had to decide which of these stories was *my* story. I include the three encounter summaries at the end of this piece to demonstrate the interpretive challenge I faced. I had to familiarize myself with the medical lexicon relevant to my case, I had to sort through the risks and odds for survival implicit in each proposed course of treatment, and I had to weigh the relative persuasiveness of each practitioner's voice. As I look back on the summaries now, they seem less puzzling than they did when I was engaged in deciding my medical fate. However, their technical language even now conveys the clinical detachment, the ideal of objectivity that made it so difficult for me to attach myself to one of them. In other words, no one voice spoke to me as more real or promising than either of the others, which would have made it easier for me to choose. Instead I had to look for motifs and resonance—places where I noticed concurrence of opinion and places where the scripts departed from one another. Most of all, I had to resist the scripting of me that the summaries proposed.

It was not clear whether Drs. Ladywood and Murray believed that the radical surgery proposed by Dr. Honeycutt was premature. In the space between conversation and written summary, they had impressed me with caution, but I had left their offices without any sense of the risk I would be taking by postponing Dr. Honeycutt's surgery. Dr. Ladywood wrote that he "favor[ed] observation," that I "had time," that mine was "not an urgent or emergent decision to be made," yet he also suggested laparoscopy to take a closer look at tissues not crisply enough represented in scans.[28] If I wanted to arrest the spread more aggressively, he would do an exploratory surgery with the possibility of "perfusion," a new protocol in which cancerous tissues were continuously bathed over the course of several days in a variety of heated chemotherapies. His thirty-two-page description of the procedure and the follow-up armed me with knowledge of the worst possible outcome; it also cast into doubt how wise it was to wait.

Dr. Murray also hedged. He recommended further study of the tissue specimen because its biology had been "only incompletely characterized" with the tumor markers for CEA, CA19.9, and C125. He advised testing for additional markers—"Ki-67, Cox-2, ploidy, and thymidylate"—in the hope of determining the "biologic propensity" of the tumors. That is, Dr. Murray believed that through a more complete histologic examination of the biopsied material, he would be able to predict with more certainty the likelihood of the tumors' return. His summary noted, "I told the patient that she certainly is at high risk for recurrence, although it is not clear that the risk is necessarily 100 percent. Nevertheless, I would regard it as high."[29] Dr. Murray's wish to do further lab work seemed like a good idea to me, but would it take more time than I had available before Dr. Honeycutt's surgery? Would I be able to postpone the surgery with Dr. Honeycutt if I had not heard from Dr. Murray's office by late June? How would I be able to make a decision about cytoreductive surgery if Dr. Murray's findings proved less conclusive than I had hoped? These questions pressed upon me as I contemplated Dr. Murray's assessment of the case.

Even though I visited the Moncrieff Diagnostic Center in Fort Worth the day after I had given my medical history to Dr. Ladywood, Dr. Murray managed to elicit one further piece of crucial information: I remembered that in 1992 when my daughter was born, Dr. Wanabebe had observed during the Caesarian section a "mysterious yellow goo" all over the peritoneal cavity. Anesthetized from the waist down, I asked her jokingly whether this was simply postpartum fat. She responded that she had no good idea what the substance was or whether it was related to my pregnancy. This dialogue from nine years earlier, coupled with the fact that Dr. Murray was already working with a diagnosis, pathology reports, and a patient history constructed by two other physicians, allowed him (and me) to expand the narrative of my illness. It now appeared that these mucinous tumors had been with me for at least nine years and that they were growing slowly. After all, Dr. Wanabebe had closed up the Caesarian incision without any protest in the ensuing years from the mysterious yellow goo. In the course of his exam, Dr. Murray also asked me why I had submitted to chemotherapy. I confess I was dumbfounded by this question because I assumed that when tumors were present, chemotherapy could arrest their spread. Dr. Murray implied that in light of tumor markers that were well within the normal range,[30] the prescription of cisplatin might have needlessly subjected me to months of nauseous suffering. Here was a doctor who saw PMP patients day in and day out, implying that I ought to have questioned my surgeon's treatment plan. Whether I was more incensed by Dr. Murray's impertinence or by the growing sense that I had been duped, I cannot tell. Had I been an unwitting cog in the machinery of the oncology industry? Had I been dosed with pernicious chemicals as a matter of course?[31]

Each of my doctors had provided essential information that redirected the calculus of advocacy. Instead of considering each encounter individually, I now had to interpret the interwoven text of their opinions. Dr. Honeycutt's belief that PMP was always fatal shocked me into researching medical journals, which in turn forced me to engage in acts of interpretation that would serve my emerging advocacy. Dr. Pistil had urged me to reconsider Dr. Honeycutt's cytoreductive surgery and to seek other opinions. His insistence that I regard other possible treatments required me to become a decision-maker and an agent in my own destiny—the very push I needed to come to terms with a new subjectivity. Dr. Ladywood—a man with whom I felt immediate kinship because he was my age and at my professional rank—volunteered that there was no need to rush into a surgery when the tumors could be monitored for growth and that I ought to see what "his buddy," Dr. Murray in Fort Worth, had to say before I took any action at all. Dr. Murray, like a medical *enfant terrible*, made me angry by suggesting that the months of nausea and debility had been in vain and that I might have declined the chemotherapeutic regimen of misery. Whether he intended it or not, Dr. Murray's adversarial questions provided some of the best medicine I got: They jump-started my sense of righteous indignation and led me to see that only *I* could act in my own best interest. There was simply too much at stake to leave the decision-making to any one of the surgeons. I want to emphasize that I was not searching for a doctor to tell me what I wanted to hear; this was not a consumer transaction. Instead I had to think of the interactions with these four doctors as textual portions of a larger narrative that I myself was writing—a sort of modern-day palimpsest whose meanings I had to uncover by slowly rubbing away the confusing signs of individual texts superimposed upon one another.

After absorbing the full significance of Dr. Murray's recommendations and his agreement with Dr. Ladywood that indications for surgery were inconclusive, I channeled the anger in what seemed at the time the most positive direction I could: I wrote to Dr. Honeycutt in Washington and canceled the cytoreductive surgery, now only six weeks away. Before Dr. Murray proceeded with the additional tumor markers and despite his caution that "it [was] prudent to maintain surveillance with scanning and tumor markers," I believed I now had enough information to challenge Dr. Honeycutt's interpretation of my disease and to advocate for myself. The lightness I felt at the prospect of this decision taught me what an oppressive weight it had been on me for three months, like a psychological tumor pressing against my cerebral cortex. My act of advocacy was tantamount to a symbolic act of surgery, where I had weighed and measured a potential malignancy and, after much study of the literature and hands-on interaction with other surgeons, had devised a way of excising the part that presented with gross morbidity.

Although more might be said about my steps and missteps in choosing a less invasive procedure to monitor my disease, I would like to offer some distillation of these experiences. I have been making sense of illness, of course, through narrative, and narratives may be therapeutic in the sense that they impose order and coherence on a chaotic sequence of events. Intruding a framework on our own disorder offers us the opportunity to remake, literally to re-member, our subjectivity. This, I would argue, is the central discursive sign of advocacy. At the same time, there is much that narrative cannot do, and we need to be clear about this. I perceive an essential dishonesty in representing through narrative events that so fundamentally defy order. Making sense of pain, nausea, or physical discomfort requires us, as Elaine Scarry has noted, to narrativize the non-narrative.[32] But re-rendering the chaos cannot proceed through conventional narrative; it is one of the failures of words, I suppose. Even the scripting of the encounter summaries misleads in the sense that they did not elicit from me a scripted response, which, in the context of U.S. medical practice, would have led me to "swallow the medicine" of enduring that harsh cytoreductive surgery and surrendering a return to physical normalcy perhaps forever.

Despite my conviction that achieving advocacy was a positive trajectory, my reassembling the fragments of a shattered self does not culminate in triumph or heroism. For one thing, the chronic nature of pseudomyxoma peritonei makes the reconstitution of self a work-in-progress. I face repeated surgeries if and when the tumors reestablish a mucinous/mutinous hold on my peritoneum. The prospect of additional surgeries requires me to stay abreast of changes in the scientific as well as institutional character of medicine. How will advances in PMP research affect its treatment and in turn its public visibility? How will increasingly virtual technologies of delivery affect my continuing course of treatment? Will new technologies supercede the CT scans that now monitor PMP? How will the gradual decline in health insurance coverage affect any future surgical interventions? Will I continue with the specialists I have already seen, or will my understanding and lived experience of the bodily signs of the disease urge me to seek out other practitioners? If canceling the cytoreductive surgery was the point of origin for my own advocacy, then seeking answers to ongoing questions and generating new questions form the body of advocacy. Understanding the place of advocacy in recovery of self puts me in a stronger position should setbacks occur. In this sense, I strive for the power to *interpret* my evolving narrative rather than closure.

As recent work with videotaped patient narratives suggests, the work of assembling a story of illness may be as illuminating for patients as for those who listen to their chief complaints.[33] For patients, they provide a mechanism for the recovery of self and a launching pad for the advocacy integral to managing chronic disease. More generally, the aggregation of such narratives provides a support function to seekers of information; they constitute a "pedagogy of the dispossessed," where through reading about experiences that resemble their own, patients regain entry to an ordered life and, by implication, contest their isolation.[34] We have yet to explore fully how narratives may alter the etiological landscape of a disease or whether physicians will use them toward this end. Clinical trials gather narrative information, but their objective has traditionally been to read the physical text of the body: to make statistical comparison of symptoms and to document how varying the protocol produces different physical results. A critical reappraisal of the role of narrative in medicine could ultimately affect research methods. Of even more consequence to those of us with chronic diseases is how the advocacy reclaimed through narrative will influence more broadly the practice of medicine in the future. Will physicians and hospital administrators seek a more complex understanding of the linkages between advocacy and healing (a cue they might take from the nursing profession)? And how will practitioners institute systemic changes that place advocacy alongside the physical and medicinal therapies for healing the body? How will patient-advocates insist on what is in essence a reconceptualization of a medical paradigm that has valorized science too often at the expense of individual will?

This narrative provides at least some evidence that the forging of a new medical paradigm is already underway. As medical subjects become ever more involved in representing the signs of their illnesses, our knowledge about the utility of patient-directed narrative will also evolve. There are inevitably places in illness that defy linguistic representation, but by undertaking a regimen of representation, by insisting that we as medical subjects sort out our unique experiences through the construction of narrative, we at once discover ways to depend less upon our physicians and to take more responsibility for our own healing. It may be, as Arthur Frank has observed, "that more is involved in [the patient's] experience than the medical story can tell."[35] Yet in striving to tell, we contribute to the cultural story of medicine and we may just make ourselves well.

NOTES

1. Anne Hunsaker Hawkins has written that "the task of the author of a pathography is not only to describe this disordering process but also to restore to reality its lost coherence and to discover or create, a meaning that can bind it together again." I see my recovery process in these terms. See Hawkins, *Reconstructing Illness: Studies in Pathography* (West Lafayette, Ind.: Purdue University Press, 1999), 2–3.

2. Behind this premise lies the assumption that illness is figured in the intersection between medicine and culture. David B. Morris has examined this concept at length, and sees a distinction between "disease," a purely scientific term, and "illness," the cultural manifestation of disease. See Morris, *Illness and Culture in the Postmodern Age* (Berkeley: University of California Press, 1998), 1–3. Diane Price Herndl provides these definitions: "A disease is usually understood as a physiological process; illness, on the other hand, is the individual or the social experience of the disease." See Herndl, "Critical Condition: Writing About Illness, Bodies, Culture," *American Literary History* 10:4 (Winter 1998): 778.

3. See Elaine Scarry, *The Body in Pain: The Making and Unmaking of the World* (New York: Oxford University Press, 1985), 3–11.

4. Herndl observes a cultural shift with regard to being ill that resonates with my own experience of it: Instead of thinking of ourselves as patients under siege by germs that we must fight, we instead imagine illness ontologically, as an inevitable state of being. See Herndl, 783. See also Frank, *The Wounded Storyteller Body, Illness, and Ethics* (Chicago: University of Chicago Press, 1995), 6.

5. Hawkins notes that pathographies are unusual before 1950. See Hawkins, 3. Recent media coverage of the patient's role in advocacy also serves to foreground this issue. See, for example, "Healthy Exchange/Communicate with Doctor for Better Care, Compassion,"

Indianapolis Star, 7 March 2004, p. J2; and an advertisement that reads, "There are 126 schools in the country that teach you how to be a physician but not one for how to be a patient," in *USA Weekend*, 31 October 2004, pp. 16–17.

6. My experience with acknowledgment corresponds with Arthur Frank's description of "the disciplined body," whose goal is control. See Frank, 41–42.

7. On the need for collaboration, see Rita Charon, "Doctor-Patient/ Reader-Writer: Learning to Find the Text," *Soundings: An Interdisciplinary Journal* 72:1 (Spring 1989): 138; and Michael Balint, *The Doctor, His Patient and the Illness* (New York: International University Press, 1957), quoted in Charon. See also "Stories in Medicine," 28 October 2003, National Public Radio, <http://www.npr.org>.

8. Recent work by Paul Helft has suggested that among patients who are using the Internet to seek information and support, some have been intimidated by the quantity of information to sort through, while others have left physicians altogether out of the decision-making process. See Paul Helft et al., "American Oncologists' Views of Internet Use by Cancer Patients: A Mail Survey of American Society of Clinical Oncology Members," *Journal of Clinical Oncology* 21:5 (March 2003): 945–46.

9. Claudine Herzlich and Janine Pierret discuss the transformation in Western societies from illness as a collective phenomenon because of contagion to an individualized experience. Medicalization has been one result of this transformation. See Herlich and Pierret, *Illness and Self in Society* (Baltimore: Johns Hopkins University Press, 1987), 49–52.

10. There are those who would argue that the medical-technological complex creates an environment where physicians cannot be well-meaning. See, for example, Wendell Berry, *Life Is a Miracle: An Essay Against Modern Superstition* (Washington, D.C.: Counterpoint, 2000), 17–18.

11. See coverage of Kansas City pharmacologist Robert R. Courtney in August 2001 numbers of *The New York Times*.

12. See my *Women at the Front: Hospital Workers in Civil War America* (Chapel Hill: University of North Carolina Press, 2004).

13. Note that I have changed all the doctors' names.

14. An ophthalmologist friend wrote me to say that while she was doing a surgery residency, she had come across one patient with the disease, which was quite a curiosity for the physicians at the University of Iowa medical center. For a general outline of pseudomyxoma peritonei (PMP), see *Stedman's Medical Dictionary;* and *Current Diagnosis in Gastroenterology*, 2nd edition, 2003, which describes the disease as "a rare clinical condition characterized by copious amounts of gelatinous fluid and benign tumors that eventually fill the peritoneal cavity." PMP is also known more popularly as "jelly-belly syndrome."

15. Pseudomyxoma patients are frequently misdiagnosed because the condition is so rare. Physicians often believe the disease to be a gynecological abnormality in women. Men often present with hernias. Because of misdiagnosis, crucial time may be lost, which sometimes wreaks havoc on the outcome. See *Current Diagnosis in Gastroenterology*, 2nd edition, 2003.

16. Robert Lipsyte's pathography about his diagnosis with testicular cancer makes reference to cisplatin as the "toxic drug" of choice for treating stage III testicular cancers. See

Lipsyte, *In the Country of Illness: Comfort and Advice for the Journey* (New York: Alfred Knopf, 1998), 30. See also Atul Guwande's comments about the misery of nausea with regard to cancer patients in *Complications: A Surgeon's Notes on an Imperfect Science* (New York: Picador, 2000), 133.

17. My ears began ringing the day after I ingested the first round of cisplatin. Tinnitis is a common side effect of cisplatin, as are numbness and tingling in the hands and feet. My fine and large motor capacities were all compromised by the drug's effect on my circulatory system. Fortunately, the drug was not delivered intravenously, which would have caused me to lose my long hair.

18. My reality resembled that of Emma Thompson's character, Vivian Bearing, in *Wit*. Vivian is an English professor who develops cervical cancer. The film does not sanitize Bearing's nausea. In one scene, she vomits water, there being no food in her stomach—for me, an especially evocative scene. Mike Nichols, *Wit* (New York: HBO Home Video, 2001), videorecording.

19. I knew little about cancer at this point, except that those on chemotherapy "had it." I later learned that cisplatin, or "platinum," as some oncologists call it, is routinely prescribed for lung, testicular, and colon cancer patients.

20. This is a term used by James W. Smith et al. in "Pseudomyxoma Peritonei of Appendiceal Origin," Memorial Sloan-Kettering Cancer Center, New York, 24 October 1991.

21. This amounted to his finding the most recent literature on PMP and sharing it with me when I asked for it. See Robert T. L. Long, J. S. Spratt, Jr., and Edmund Dowling, "Pseudomyxoma Peritonei: New Concepts in Management with a Report of Seventeen Patients," *The American Journal of Surgery* 117 (February 1969): 162–69; and James W. Smith et al., "Pseudomyxoma,"pp. 396–401.

22. Paul Helft notes that avoiding the problem is one way that many patients initially cope with the trauma of a long-term and possibly terminal illness. See Helft, "Hunting for Mushrooms: Patients, the Internet, and the Changing Doctor-Patient Relationship." Presented to the Seminar in Ethics and Humanities, Indiana University School of Medicine, 10 April 2003.

23. Barbara Ehrenreich has attested that she "seem[ed] to lose [her] capacity for self-defense" and thus advocacy in her account of surviving the consumerist base of the American breast cancer industry. See "Welcome to Cancerland," *Harper's Magazine*, November 2001, p. 45.

24. See Washington Hospital Center encounter summary at the end of this essay.

25. The local oncologist assigned to follow my case, in conjunction with the insurance provider's directive, specializes in the treatment of testicular cancer. This doctor has seen the disease during his career, but makes no claim to having specialized knowledge about its treatment.

26. The site advertised a newsletter and asked patients and families to make contributions to cover the costs of printing and postage. It is not clear if Gabriella Graham derives a salary from these contributions. One of the primary functions of <http://pmppals.org> is to ask members to send postcards and notes of condolence to convalescents and families of the deceased.

27. See *PMP Pals Newsletter*, January 2001, Spring 2001, and Fall 2001. Compiled by Gabriella Graham.
28. See M. D. Anderson Cancer Center encounter summary at the end of this essay.
29. See Moncrieff Diagnostic Center encounter summary at the end of this essay.
30. The tumor markers used in tracking pseudomyxoma peritonei are CA19.9, CEA, and C125.
31. In her reading of the medical cultures of the United States, Great Britain, France, and Germany, Lynn Payer observes that American doctors are more inclined to treat with strong medicines to address their patients' symptoms. See especially the chapter entitled "Great Britain: Economy, Empiricism, and Keeping the Upper Lip Stiff," in *Medicine and Culture: Varieties of Treatment in the United States, England, West Germany, and France* (New York: Henry Holt, 1996), 101–23.
32. See Scarry.
33. See Karen Christopher, "Using Patient Videos to Understand Better the Illness Experience"; and Sue Ziebland, "DIPEX Narratives: A Resource for Collaborative Research"— presentations made at the Second Global Conference on Making Sense of Health, Illness, and Disease, 14 to 17 July 2003, St. Hilda's College, Oxford University, UK.
34. The "pedagogy of the dispossessed" is a play on words of Paulo Freire's *Pedagogy of the Oppressed* (1972).
35. Frank, 6–7.

REFERENCES

Balint, Michael. *The Doctor, His Patient and the Illness*. New York: International University Press, 1957. Quoted in Rita Charon, "Doctor-Patient/ Reader-Writer: Learning to Find the Text." *Soundings: An Interdisciplinary Journal* 72:1 (Spring 1989): 137–52.

Berry, Wendell. *Life Is a Miracle: An Essay Against Modern Superstition*. Washington, DC: Counterpoint, 2000.

Charon, Rita. "Doctor-Patient/ Reader-Writer: Learning to Find the Text." *Soundings: An Interdisciplinary Journal* 72:1 (Spring 1989): 137–52.

Current Diagnosis in Gastroenterology. 2nd edition, 2003.

Ehrenreich, Barbara. "Welcome to Cancerland." *Harper's Magazine*, November 2001, pp. 43–53.

Frank, Arthur. *The Wounded Storyteller: Body, Illness, and Ethics*. Chicago: Univ. of Chicago Press, 1995.

Guwande, Atul. *Complications: A Surgeon's Notes on an Imperfect Science*. New York: Picador, 2000.

Hawkins, Anne Hunsaker. *Reconstructing Illness: Studies in Pathography*. West Lafayette, Ind.: Purdue University Press, 1999.

Helft, Paul. "Hunting for Mushrooms: Patients, the Internet, and the Changing Doctor-Patient Relationship." Working paper presented to the Seminar on Medical Ethics and Humanities, Indiana University School of Medicine, 10 April 2003.

Helft, Paul, Fay Hlubocky, and Christopher K. Daugherty. "American Oncologists' Views of Internet Use by Cancer Patients: A Mail Survey of American Society of Clinical Oncology Members." *Journal of Clinical Oncology* 21:5 (March 2003): 945–46.

Herndl, Diane Price. "Critical Condition: Writing about Illness, Bodies, Culture." *American Literary History* 10:4 (Winter 1998): 771–85.

Herlich, Claudine, and Janine Pierret. *Illness and Self in Society.* Baltimore: Johns Hopkins University Press, 1987.

Lipsyte, Robert. *In the Country of Illness: Comfort and Advice for the Journey.* New York: Alfred Knopf, 1998.

Long, Robert T. L., J. S. Spratt, Jr., and Edmund Dowling. "Pseudomyxoma Peritonei: New Concepts in Management with a Report of Seventeen Patients." *The American Journal of Surgery* 117 (February 1969): 162–69.

Morris, David B. *Illness and Culture in the Postmodern Age.* Berkeley: University of California Press, 1998.

Nichols, Mike. *Wit.* New York: HBO Home Video, 2001. Videorecording.

Payer, Lynn. *Medicine and Culture: Varieties of Treatment in the United States, England, West Germany, and France.* New York: Henry Holt, 1996.

Scarry, Elaine. *The Body in Pain: The Making and Unmaking of the World.* New York: Oxford University Press, 1985.

Schultz, Jane E. *Women at the Front: Hospital Workers in Civil War America.* Chapel Hill: University of North Carolina Press, 2004.

Smith, James W., et al. "Pseudomyxoma Peritonei of Appendiceal Origin." Publication of Memorial Sloan-Kettering Cancer Center, New York, October 24, 1991, pp. 396–401.

QUESTIONS

1. How is advocacy defined in this essay? The author suggests that developing advocacy as a patient is best understood as a rhetoric. What does she mean by this, and what aspects of persuasion are rooted in the concept of advocacy?

2. What aspects of this narrative are the most poignant, frightening, amusing, and mundane? Even though pathographies are nonfictional, does the author use any fictional techniques in her representation of events that occurred in the past? How does she use voice and suspense to draw the reader into her story?

3. What particular problems and conflicts result from the rarity of being diagnosed with pseudomyxoma peritonei? Are there any advantages, as the author sees it, from contracting a rare cancer?

4. How do the author's interactions with physicians change over the course of her illness? In what sense might we view her encounters with physicians as collaborations? How does she make the transition from *reactive* to *proactive* behavior?

WASHINGTON HOSPITAL CENTER

CANCER INSTITUTE
ENCOUNTER SUMMARY

PATIENT: SCHULTZ, JANE ELLEN
DATE OF VISIT: 02/26/01
MEDICAL RECORD NO.: 233 2241

NOTE: Please indicate that this encounter summary is dictated
in the presence of the patient, her brother, and a friend.

HISTORY OF PRESENT ILLNESS: First Cancer Institute visit for,
this 47-year-old woman who comes in with the chief complaint
of mucinous spread of an appendiceal tumor throughout the
abdomen and pelvis.

The patient was completely asymptomatic. She went to her GYN
who noted an ovarian mass on the right side. An ultrasound
was performed. She was taken to the operating room where
mucinous tumor was found throughout the pelvis. This was
removed and irrigated extensively. The patient underwent a
supracervical hysterectomy and bilateral salpingo-oophorectomy. She also underwent a right ileocolectomy with stapled
anastomosis.

The pathology report showed an appendiceal neoplasm of "low
malignant potential". Also there were epithelial cells found
at numerous sites within the abdomen and pelvis within the
mucoid material. The pathologist comments that the appendix
contained a mucinous cyst adenoma of low malignant potential.
He thought that the disease was compatible with pseudomyxoma
peritonei and thought the lesion was identical to the adenomucinosis described by Ranet.

The patient had a Tenckhoff catheter inserted and she has now
had several cycles of intraperitoneal cisplatinum. Except for
weakness, she seems to be tolerating this chemotherapy well.

PAST MEDICAL HISTORY: No allergies to medicines. No asthma,
heart disease, or other serious illnesses.

REVIEW OF SYSTEMS: unremarkable.

FAMILY HISTORY: Her father and mother both have some hyper-
tension. Her father is alive at age 77 and mother at 75. She
has an older brother and younger sister who are living and
well.

PHYSICAL EXAMINATION: Well-appearing woman in no acute distress. Nodes including Virchow's node negative. Chest clear
to P&A. Heart: No murmur. Breasts not examined. Abdomen:
Well-healed Pfannenstiel incision. Vaginal examination. Nul-

liparous cervix without masses. Rectal examination: No masses
in the cul-de-sac. No stool recovered for Hemoccult testing.
Extremities unremarkable.

In summary, this is a 47-year-old woman who has known pseudomyxoma peritonei syndrome with primary tumor known to be in
the appendix. The pathologist thinks this is a borderline-
type malignancy of low malignant potential and compatible
with adenomucinosis.

I have to preface my comments to this patient by saying I can
never predict how an individual patient will do. All I can do
is provide her with the information that we have regarding
approximately 600 patients with mucinous appendiceal tumors
and carcinomatosis.

The results of treatment are completely dependent in our experience on a complete removal of the tumor surgically. After
the tumor is removed surgically, the skin edges are tented up
on a selfretaining retractor and the abdomen is washed for 90
minutes in a chemotherapy agent called mitomycin-C. In the
early postoperative period an additional drug called 5-fluoro-
uracil is utilized. If further treatments are indicated, this
would come about as a result of lymph nodes being positive in
some part of the specimen. Usually this is the extent of the
treatment.

If this is indeed adenomucinosis and a complete removal of
tumor is possible, then the patient's likelihood of being
alive and well at ten years is 85%. Unfortunately if the
cytoreduction is not complete, we do not have any patients
who survive ten years.

These extensive treatments have a cost. The likelihood of
dying as a result of the procedure is 2%. That means one
patient out of 50 dies as a result of these aggressive surgical procedures. The complication rate is also high. One out
of three patients has a serious complication. The complications are pulmonary embolus, pancreatitis, bowel fistula, and
intra-abdominal infection. The hospitalization without a complication is usually about three weeks. With a complication,
it can be six weeks or even longer.

This patient already had a right colectomy. By CT scan she
has fluid down in the pelvis and this means she will probably
need a limited left colectomy, removal of her residual cervix, and complete stripping of the pelvic peritoneum with the
procedure. It is possible that she would need an ostomy probably a temporary ostomy as a result of this surgery. I would
suggest the need for a temporary ostomy to be about 30%. The
likelihood of a permanent ostomy would be less than that,
maybe at around 10%.

I agree with the treatments that the patient is having at this point in time. She is having intraperitoneal cisplatinum chemotherapy. We need to make sure that this chemotherapy is discontinued at least six weeks prior to any surgical intervention because a full course of chemotherapy would be given at the time of the cytoreductive surgery.

Special mention should be made about her Pfannenstiel incision. We would not reexcise the Pfannenstiel incision for this procedure. Rather we would make a vertical incision, removing the umbilicus. With CT scan follow up over the next several years the high index of suspicion for recurrence in the Pfannenstiel incision must be maintained. There would be a high likelihood of localized tumor recurrence at this site. This does not interfere with her overall prognosis but is bothersome in that sometimes a second surgical procedure is necessary.

Following this dictation, the patient and her associates were given an opportunity to ask any questions that they wished and I did my best to answer them.

THE UNIVERSITY OF TEXAS
MD ANDERSON CANCER CENTER

Primary Medical Evaluation Date: 05/24/2001
Patient Name: SCHULTZ, JANE E.
MR#: 047-76-61
DOB: 02/12/1954

CHIEF COMPLAINT: Pseudomyxoma peritonei.

HISTORY OF PRESENT ILLNESS: Ms. Schultz is a 47-year-old
white female from Indiana who reports a diagnosis of pseudomyxoma peritonei, diagnosed late last year. On routine
pelvic examination she was noted to have a mass. Ultrasound
showed a complex structure and surgery was recommended. At
the time of operation on 11/14/01 the patient was noted to
have a significant amount of mucin. This was sent for frozen section. The surgery included resection of the ileum
and right colon, supracervical hysterectomy and bilateral salpingo-oophorectomy, appendectomy, omental washing,
and Tenckhoff catheter placement. The pathology showed the
appendiceal lumen to be occupied by mucinous tumor, having
the feature of a low malignant potential tumor. There were
superficial deposits of mucin on multiple surfaces, including both ovaries and both fallopian tubes and the small and
large intestinal serosal surfaces. It should also be noted
that the omentum was adherent to the colon in the right
lower quadrant and only this segment was removed. The mucoid
substance showed dissecting mucin with reactive fibrosis,
containing atypical mucinous epithelium. Postoperatively the
patient received intraperitoneal cisplatin × 5 between 11/00
and 03/01. She had the Tenckhoff catheter removed shortly
after her last treatment.

Currently the patient reports that she is feeling well overall. She reports that she had significant side effects from
the cisplatin, including nausea and vomiting, headaches, hand
and foot pain and swelling, and ringing in the ears. The
patient reports that the nausea as well as the headaches have
since resolved. She continues to have hot, numb and swol-
len-feeling hands and feet. She reports that she is somewhat
clumsy as a result of this. She still describes a ringing in
her ears. The patient reports no problems with urination. She
reports bowel movements each day without pain or straining.
She does have occasional bright red blood per rectum and has
not had endoscopy. The patient denies any urinary complaints
at this time, specifically no dysuria, frequency, or hematu-
ria. She does describe an increased creatinine since on cisplatin.

ALLERGIES: No known drug allergies.

Current medications include:
1. Zoloft 50 mg 1 p.o. q.d.
2. Vitamin C 50 mg 1 p.o. q.d.
3. Centrum multivitamin 1 p.o. q.d.
4. Calcium 500 mg 1 p.o. q.d.
5. Climara, unknown dosage, 1 p.o. q.d.

No aspirin or anti-inflammatory medications.

PAST MEDICAL HISTORY: Situational depression, otherwise negative. The patient specifically denies heart, lung, liver or
kidney problems, seizures, diabetes, transfusions or hepatitis.

PAST SURGICAL HISTORY:
1. Cesarean section in 02/92.
2. Right arthroscopic knee surgery in 05/99.
3. Surgery as noted above in 11/00.

SOCIAL HISTORY: The patient lives in Indiana. She is an English professor at Indiana University. She is in clinic today
with her mother and father. She drinks less than 1 serving of
alcohol per week. Tobacco and recreational drugs are never.

FAMILY HISTORY: There is family history of cancer in a maternal grandfather with stomach cancer diagnosed and deceased at
age 47.

PHYSICAL EXAMINATION: Temperature is 36.7, pulse 64, respira-
tions 16, blood pressure 157/75, height 160.2 cm, and weight
60.5 kg. HEENT: Head is atraumatic. Eyes: Corrective eye wear
is worn. EOMI/PERRLA. TMs are pearly bilaterally. Oropharynx
shows no ulcerations. Nares are patent. Neck is supple with
no thyromegaly and no adenopathy, including no submandibular,
occipital, supraclavicular or infraclavicular adenopathy. The
axillae are without adenopathy. Breast examination was performed. The breasts are symmetrical with no dominate or discrete masses, and no nipple retraction or discharge. Lungs
are clear to auscultation in anterior, posterior, and lateral
lung fields. Cardiovascular is regular rate and rhythm without
murmur, ru[n], or gallop. Abdomen reveals an extended Pfannenstiel incision as well as two small incisions in the right
mid abdomen, consistent with catheter placement and removal.
The abdomen is soft, nontender, and nondistended. There is
no hepatosplenomegaly, no abdominal masses, and no ingui-
nal adenopathy. Rectal examination was performed. It showed
no external lesions. Sphincter tone is moderate. There is a
small amount of stool within the rectal vault. It was tested,
and it was guaiac-negative. Extremities reveal good distal
pulses, no edema, no cyanosis, and no mass. Muscle strength is
5/5, bilateral upper and lower extremities. Range of motion is
full, bilateral upper and lower extremities. Neurologic examination shows cranial nerves II-XII to be grossly intact.

DIAGNOSTIC TESTING:
1. Outside pathology, reportedly submitted to M. D. Anderson
Cancer Center on Tuesday, not yet logged in.
2. Outside CT scan of the chest, abdomen, and pelvis performed on 05/14/01 was reviewed in clinic today by Dr. It
was reviewed with the patient and her family members and
explained. As well, a previous CT scan from February was
reviewed. Dr. reported that the quality of the scan was significantly limited by the fact that there was no IV contrast
and overall poor clarity. There is an area in the right lower
quadrant with a questionable abnormality; although, it could
be consistent with postoperative change.

The most recent creatinine from our records from March is
2.3. For review of outside pathology and operative report,
please see HPI.

IMPRESSION: Ms. Schultz is a 47-year-old white female with
a history of pseudomyxoma peritonei, with superficial deposits of mucin on multiple surfaces, including both ovaries,
fallopian tubes, and the small and large intestinal serosal surface. There is also a positive abdominal washing with
abundant extracellular mucin consistent with PMP. Please note
that on review of the outside operative report, there was
no evidence of disease outside of that area, specifically no
involvement of the liver or diaphragm and no intra-abdominal
deposits. The patient has no overt evidence of disease on CT
today; however, it is a significantly limited study.

RECOMMENDATIONS AND PLAN: Dr. spent over 1 hour today discussing the pathology and treatment options. He did explain
in detail that he recommended that she seek several opinions
regarding treatment. The patient reports that she has already
seen Dr. and is interested in other names that Dr. has to
offer. He explained that what treatment she chooses and where
she decides to have follow-up care should be based on her
comfort level. The treatment options that Dr. addressed specifically with the patient included:

1. Laparoscopy for assessment of overt disease.

2. IPHP. Dr. did explain that if at the time of perfusion
there was no evidence of overt disease, he would not recommend the perfusion. He did explain that mitomycin would be
the agent of choice. He did explain that the perfusion could
be a significantly toxic procedure, necessitating a stay in
the ICU for at least 3 days and at least 3 months of postoperative follow-up before feeling well. He reported potential
side effects including renal toxicity, which is an increased
risk in this patient who already has poor kidney function.

3. The third option is for observation. Dr. does recommend a
baseline MRI to be performed, as the CT is going to be lim-

ited in this patient where contrast cannot be used. He recommends that this MRI be performed in the next 2-3 weeks.

Dr. also explained that the patient has time; this is not an
urgent or emergent decision to be made. She was given an educational handout today on perfusion.
Of the three choices given, Dr. would favor observation due
to three reasons:
1. Poor kidney function.
2. The fact that the pathology showed acellular mucin.
3. Because there was no evidence of disease outside of the
right lower quadrant.

The patient thanked Dr. for his time. She does plan to get an
opinion by Dr. in the Dallas-Fort Worth area. She has asked
that we forward her pathology slides on to him once review
has been completed here. The patient was sent with her outside scans.

This patient was seen and examined with Dr. who participated
in all aspects of her care. He reviewed the history and outside records, examined the abdomen, reviewed the outside CTs,
formulated the impression and plan, and explained it to the
patient.

ADDENDUM:
The patient brought laboratory data from 05/14/01 that
includes a CA 125 of 20, CA 19-9 less than 10, and a CEA that
is 0.7

ADDENDUM: This is an addendum to Angie McIntosh's note of the
same date. Please see her note for complete past medical history, social history, family history, review of systems and
complete physical examination.

HISTORY OF PRESENT ILLNESS: Briefly, the patient is a 46-year-
old white female who is a professor [of] English literature
from Indiana University with a history of pseudomyxoma peritonei, diagnosed in 11/00. According to the patient and her
parents, her symptomatology actually began at least a year
ago with symptoms of abdominal bloating while she was a visiting scholar at Cambridge University in England. She underwent an exploratory laparotomy, supracervical hysterectomy,
bilateral salpingo-oophorectomy and right hemicolectomy in
11/00. She had a catheter placed and received intraperitoneal
cisplatin therapy, 5 cycles since then. She finished therapy
in 03/01. She has had significant toxicity from this including significant hearing loss according to the patient as well
as paresthesias of the hands and feet and evidence of renal
failure. Her creatinine last available is 2.3. She presents
with a CT scan from the outside which is of suboptimal quality for 2 reasons; one is the lack of IV contrast material,
and the second is the quality of the scanning; however, there

is nothing grossly obvious on this set of film. Her tumor
markers are also within normal limits.

PHYSICAL EXAMINATION: She has no evidence of supraclavicular
adenopathy. There are no palpable abdominal masses or organomegaly. She has a healed extended Pfannenstiel incision.
Again, there is no organomegaly or palpable abdominal masses.

ASSESSMENT AND PLAN: I discussed at length with the patient
and her parents for roughly an hour her disease and its management. She is scheduled to go see Dr. shortly and Dr.
shortly after that. I outlined for her 3 options:
1. Observation.
2. Exploration with the possibility of perfusion.
3. Laparoscopy with further treatment planned [sic] based on
laparoscopic findings.

I also recommended that we obtain an MRI of the abdomen to
attempt to evaluate her disease status with this. After
extensive consultation, my final recommendation would be for
her to undergo observation as certainly with this renal failure, she would be at increased risk with peritoneal perfusion. She has had obvious significant symptomatology from her
previous treatment, and I believe that there is a chance,
given that this is acellular mucin and no obvious evidence
of disease outside of the lower abdomen, that she may do
well without a perfusion. We discussed all of these things
at length, and she will see Dr. and then we will also have
her pathology reviewed here once the slides are into the system and then we will discuss with her pending that report. In
addition, as mentioned above, the patient will have an MRI
of the abdomen to further evaluate for any evidence of peritoneal disease. This has all been discussed with the patient
and her parents again, and they appear to fully understand
and agree with this plan of action.

THE UNIVERSITY Of TEXAS SOUTHWESTERN MEDICAL CENTER
AT DALLAS

MONCRIEF DIAGNOSTlC CENTER

CONSULTATION

DATE: 05/25/01
PATIENT: JANE SCHULTZ
CLINIC #: 72555719

The patient is referred for a second opinion consultation for
her known diagnosis of pseudomyxoma peritonei. The patient
has brought operative, pathology, and office records as well
as copies of her scans from May and February, which I have
seen and also reviewed with the patient. Pathology is currently being reviewed at M.D. Anderson. I will summarize the
details for our records.

HISTORY: The patient is a 47-year-old woman. She is a professor of history and lives in Indianapolis. The patient went
for a routine gynecologic examination in September of 2000.
Her examining physician found an adnexal mass and recommended ultrasound, which confirmed the presence of a pelvic
mass, which was worrisome. The patient tells me that in retrospect, she had been having some abdominal bloating and some
vague additional symptoms predating this over the past year.
On 11/14/00, the patient underwent exploration and a large
amount of mucoid material was found in the lower abdomen and
pelvis. She underwent a TAH, BSO, and right hemicolectomy.
She had a grossly abnormal appendix. A Tenckhoff catheter was
placed at that time. The subsequent pathology reviewed in
Indiana was felt to be consistent with a mucinous neoplasm of
the appendix with low malignant potential (adenomucinosis).
The patient subsequently received five courses of intraperitoneal Cisplatin 100 mg per meter squared. She had considerable morbidity associated with this treatment. She also has
persistent neurologic side effects (changes in sensation in
hands and feet). She also has diminished kidney function and
a recent creatinine was still elevated. For that reason, she
did not have IV contrast with the CT scans. She has also suffered tinnitus. She has had weight loss, fatigue, and loss or
appetite associated with this, which is now improved. Similarly, shortness of breath as well as gastrointestinal symptoms including nausea, vomiting, diarrhea, and blood in the
stool, all of which are improved.

The patient brought up an interesting point during our interview. She says that in 1992, at the time of her C-section,
her obstetrician had noted "gooey, yellow stuff" in the
abdominal cavity at the time of the C-section. She was uncertain what to make of this.

REVIEW OF SYSTEMS: The patient has numbness in the feet and

hands as noted above. She has persistent problems with renal function related to the platinum.

PAST SURGICAL HISTORY: C-section in 1992, arthroscopic knee surgery in 1999.

SOCIAL HISTORY: The patient is divorced and has a 9-year-old daughter. She is an English professor. The patient is a non-smoker and non-drinker.

FAMILY HISTORY: She has no family history of cancer.

PHYSICAL EXAMINATION: On examination, the patient is accompanied by her parents. She is well nourished and appears fit. She is 5'3" and her weight is 132½ pounds. Blood pressure is 148/84. Pulse is 68. The patient has no cervical supraclavicular or axillary adenopathy. Breasts are moderate in size, lumpy, and bumpy compatible with fibrocystic change. She has normal breath sounds. She has normal heart sounds.

Examination of the abdomen reveals a non-distended abdomen. She has a well healed, lower abdominal incision, which extends up bilaterally towards the ASIS. She has two, well healed, transverse incisions in the lateral aspect of the right mid abdomen status post Tenckhoff catheter removal. Palpation reveals no mass at the base of the umbilicus. She has no palpable masses in the abdomen. She has no evidence of ascites. There is no abdominal tenderness or fullness. She has no deep or superficial groin adenopathy. Rectal examination reveals no perianal pathology. She has normal sphincter tone. The cervix is palpable anteriorly and is mobile. There is no fixation scarring or tumor shelf. There is no fluid palpable in the lower pelvis. The stool is negative for occult blood. Extremities are warm, and dry with palpable, distal, peripheral pulses.

LAB AND X-RAY: I have looked at the recent CT scan, which shows a little bit of fluid lateral to the cecum in the gutter on the right hand side. I see no evidence of scalloping around the liver or of obvious mucin accumulations. The patient is status post removal of the Tenckhoff catheter. She is status post hysterectomy and right colon resection.

Tumor markers were not done prior to her surgery but the most recent tumor markers specifically CA 125, CA 19-9, and CEA are well within normal limits. CA 19-9 is immeasurable. CA 125 is 20 and the CEA is 0.7.

The outside pathology as noted above was interpreted as showing an appendiceal primary. The patient had multiple deposits of mucin, largely acellular. The gross features are consistent with findings, which are currently called adenomucinosis.

IMPRESSION: The patient is status post both surgical treatment and IP chemotherapy for a pseudomyxoma peritonei likely
of appendiceal origin diagnosed in November/2000. From the
operative report, it sounds as if all gross visible disease
was removed. There was no evidence of disease in the upper
abdomen. It is curious that the patient was noted to have
abnormal material in her abdomen back in 1992 at the time of
her C-section. The current pathology on the appendix shows
clearly an appendiceal neoplasm, which has the features consistent with this as an etiology and the appendiceal is
thickened but no point of penetration of the appendiceal wall
was recognized. It is curious to speculate whether this tumor
has in fact been present over that time period. That would
certainly be consistent with a benign variant of pseudomyxoma
peritonei.

I had a long discussion with the patient about appendiceal
neoplasms in general and more specifically about pseudomyxoma
peritonei. We discussed benign, borderline, and malignant
forms and some of the differences.

I told the patient that she certainly is at high risk for
recurrence although it is not clear that that risk is necessarily 100%. Nevertheless, I would regard it as high. To me,
the issues are several. First, recurrence is a possibility.
Second, the biology of the tumor is only incompletely characterized in my opinion, but [sic] histologic examination.
We have been looking at additional tumor markers and I think
that they are valuable in making some kind of a judgment
about the biologic propensity. We have found differences in
behavior that are not clearly accounted for by the biologic
definitions particularly that of adenomucinosis.

For that reason, I am recommending that blocks be obtained
from the tumor material. We would be requesting additional
markers including Ki-67, Cox-2, ploidy, and thymidylate syn-
thase.

I spent approximately two hours in face to face conversation
discussion with the patient and her parents reviewing pseudomyxoma peritonei in considerable detail and the specific features in this case.

RECOMMENDATIONS:
1. I am recommending that we obtain the blocks and do additional staining. In some cases this can give us insight into
whether we are dealing with a more aggressive neoplasm than
is apparent by histologic examination or criteria. This can
also yield additional, useful information, which may have
bearing on future treatment.
2. It is possible, but no means clear, that the tumor may
have been present as long ago as 1992. If that is the case,
then we are indeed looking at attenuated biology and this

should have some impact on considerations and recommendations for treatment.

3. I have recommended that she continue to have CT scanning. We currently use this as our test of choice recognizing its limitations and the fact that it always underestimates any disease. I also would also recommend ongoing surveillance with the tumor markers, specifically the CEA, CA 19-9, and CA 125. The scanning empiric [sic] but I would recommend three to six month intervals for the first two years and approximately six months thereafter.

4. I also feel that it would be worth considering a re-staging laparoscopy at some time in the next six to 12 months.

5. With respect to intervention, I am not recommending any operative treatment at the present time. I would like to see the definition of the tumor they noted above. Certainly for a tumor with more aggressive characteristics, I would be recommending intervention with very aggressive cytoreduction and heated intraperitoneal chemotherapy. For more attenuated tumor, there is certainly the risk for recurrence. I think in that incidence, it would be reasonable to consider a laparoscopic examination. In either case, it is prudent to maintain surveillance with scanning and tumor markers. I have emphasized that it is important to recognize the risk for recurrence with whatever form of biology that we are looking at. It is not likely that an early, asymptomatic recurrence is going to require much more or less in terms of surgery than if surgery was performed now or in the near future. However, I did emphasize that waiting until disease is bulky or symptomatic runs a very high risk of treatment failure. At the present time, the patient has an excellent performance status. She has no clinical evidence of disease by tumor markers. The changes on the CT scan we see currently are just as likely to be associated with the recent IP chemotherapy, which has been discontinued.

6. At the present time, and unless there is evidence to present it to suggest we are dealing with a malignant variant, I see no role currently for systemic chemotherapy. There is no proven role for intraperitoneal chemotherapy at the present time. If the patient has persistent disease which is below the visible limits of markers and CT scanning, then treatment before a major recurrence should be associated with excellent outcome.

7. In view of the fact that the patient has been recently diagnosed with an appendiceal neoplasm, I am recommending that she should have colonoscopic screening.

White Coat Syndrome

⌒ Rebecca A. Pope ⌒

I don't go to the doctor very often—or at least not to the MD who, my insurance card tells me, is my "primary care physician." When I want a check-up, I visit Dr. Hu, OMD (Doctor of Oriental Medicine), Licensed Acupuncturist. She takes my pulses—I hardly feel her finely trained fingertips at three places on each of my wrists—looks at the color and shape of my tongue, and, with her needles and herbs, has fixed all the miscellaneous maladies I've brought to her and even a few, like "low kidney chi," that I didn't know I had. Fixing the low kidney chi had the added and unexpected benefit of doing wonders for my PMS and SAD. So much for the placebo effect. Dr. Hu doesn't promise miracle cures. Like a good malt scotch, the bitter herbs are an acquired taste. They work slowly. I am patient, a good patient, for Dr. Hu.

When I, as I occasionally do, fear that I am suffering from something serious and horrible that might require treatments more high-tech and invasive than Chinese herbs, I put off visiting the internist for a while—which is often restorative in itself. If procrastination doesn't cure me, I reluctantly make an appointment. The last time I went in, they couldn't find my file. It was probably so thin, flaccid and full of dust that an efficient clerk decided that I was inactive (which in a way is true) and consigned my file to basement storage with the thick and well-leaved files of the former and the dead.

Four female internists, a physician's assistant and a nurse practitioner all see patients in this office. I noticed on my last visit that only the nurses, phlebotomists and clerks wear white coats. I suspect this is an attempt to be politically progressive. I think of Dr. Hu's office; she wears a white coat, as do the slight and smiling man who boils the herbs and takes out the needles and Cathy, who sits behind the desk with the appointment book and teaches Qigong with Dr. Hu, whose real name can't possibly be Cathy. Dr. Hu's office is a democracy of white coats.

"We haven't seen you for a while," says the physician's assistant, a woman I have never

---

An abridged version of this essay is part of the collection *Stories of Illness and Healing*, ed. Marsha Hurst and Sayantani DasGupta (Kent, Ohio: Kent State University Press, forthcoming 2007). The essay here appears with the permission of Kent State University Press.

met. She wears a bright purple shirt, grey trousers and a stethoscope. Not yet 50, she is entirely gray. I like that she doesn't feel compelled to dye it.

"I think the last time was three years ago. Stress fracture in my ankle. Too much running." I offer little else. I don't come in for regular check-ups. I am not a good patient.

She takes my blood pressure. 180 over 110. "Your blood pressure is really high."

"White Coat Syndrome. It's usually about 110 over 70."

⌒ ⌒

I had hardly unpacked in Bethesda with my new life and new partner when the call from Chicago came. What my mother had for months been claiming was a bleeding hemorrhoid turned out to be the malignancy we had all been trying to deny. Surgery in a few days. I offered to fly home. "No, we can handle it," my father said.

"She was really lucky," the surgeon pronounced afterwards; "the tumor was low, which inhibited metastasis. Everything looks fine, but she should have a course of radiation just to be safe. In case there are any stray cells." We exhaled; only a few wandering cells, and they could easily be mopped up with a little radiation. Of course the colostomy bag was unlucky, but there was a general air of reprieve and relief in which my mother, determined, as they say, "put it all behind" her (a rather unfortunate phrase considering the circumstances), and participated. Without complaint she learned to manage the colostomy. She took the radiation treatments. We didn't think to question that recommendation; it came, after all, from the man in the white coat, and we were all amateurs at cancer then. She was compliant; she was a good sport; she kept her pain and fear and frustration to herself, which, I suppose, was lucky for the rest of us.

Of course the seven weeks of radiation burned her and made her sick, no doubt sicker than she allowed her children to see. But soon she regained her physical strength; and as the number of checkups and tests which pronounced her "clean" accumulated, we began to regain our faith in her body and in her continued presence. After five years without recurrence, she became a statistical "survivor" and we celebrated. How close she had come; how lucky we were. Time to forget.

Two years later the pain returned. She had a hard time sitting. Probably scar tissue, the doctor said. The pain got worse. The MRI wasn't clear. Into the hospital for a biopsy. It took a few days to get the results: "good news, it's benign." The tightness of our shoulders, our heads, our stomachs—tightness we hadn't been conscious of—began to dissolve. We could celebrate again, even if she was still in pain. The next day another call: "We're really sorry; we don't know how this could have happened. There's been a mistake; it's malignant."

More appointments and consultations. More men in white coats. They were confident they could get it out. More surgery. My father, brother and sister waited at the hospital ("No, you don't need to come," my father said again). I waited by the phone. This time the surgeon came out of the operating suite early, too early. He brought them to a small, windowless room—the kind of room that is supposed to insure privacy and confidentiality but is really about shielding other waiting families from someone else's bad luck. He shut the door. My father knew. "Sorry. The tumor is resting against her backbone. And up against the sciatic nerve. We couldn't get it. She's probably got a year, maybe a year and a half." Later, one of the other doctors said that this new tumor was probably caused by the mop-up radiation after the first surgery, the radiation done "just to be safe." The doctors put a few radiation needles directly into the tumor before they closed, but that was all they could do because— and this was news to us—she had used up her life-time allowance of exposure earlier. The maximum exposure guidelines are necessary, of course, because too much radiation can give you cancer. Too much radiation can kill you.

My father forbade the doctors to tell my mother that she had twelve to eighteen months. Perhaps this was denial, perhaps a sense that no one, even someone in a white coat, can ever really know when someone else will die. Patients surprise. Perhaps he knew of those studies that suggest that people who are put on the clock die by the clock because they are so invested in being good patients. But then she didn't really need to be told. She knew that an inoperable tumor next to her backbone was serious trouble.

A major post-op infection added to her suffering and the general misery, and with a few days off for Thanksgiving, I flew to Chicago to stay with her in the hospital and give my father a break. In times of catastrophe, we fall back on what we know. The family academic, I know reading and research. I bought some books about alternative treatments and nutrition protocols for cancer and read them on the plane. I learned enough in a few hours to be appalled at what the hospital kitchen gave a cancer patient for Thanksgiving dinner and to bring her organic yogurt with live cultures to replace the good bacteria that her superantibiotics destroyed. When I pulled out some yogurt during a visit from the hospital's infection control specialist and explained why, he looked a little startled, as if I wasn't supposed to know anything about infections or antibiotics or the breaking of the surgical field.

Meanwhile, my father took her records to the University of Chicago; maybe they had some cutting-edge technological miracle to offer. The move miffed my mother's oncologist. His sense that his judgment shouldn't be supplemented or questioned, that my mother was somehow his property, miffed me. What the doctors at the eminent U of C Medical Center could offer was a grotesque operation that would hollow out the lower half of her abdomen and leave her in a wheelchair with even more tubes and bags. She would be a literal bag lady, all sterile plastic and encased in steel. My mother rejected their futuristic medicine that seemed, well, medieval.

When I returned east the next week, I taught my classes on automatic pilot and cut my office hours to a minimum. My students hardly minded that I was only half there, and I decided not to think about what that might mean. I read everything I could get my hands on; some of it was quackery and junk. All of the people I talked to were kind and generous with their knowledge and experience, although some were a little "out there" for my comfort. But I was surprised by how much good research on cancer and nutrition was out there. You'd never know it talking to a conventional oncologist; in all the years of treating her, none of my mother's doctors had mentioned diet. I came up with a nutrition and supplement plan that corresponded to most of the more credible work that I had read. It was not a program for the faint of heart or for the devotee of Domino's pizza: an organic whole foods vegetarian diet supplemented with a little salmon. Lots of soy and garlic and greens. All very worthy, but lacking in the high fat and sugar that the standard American diet teaches us to associate with gastronomic pleasure, a lesson my mother had learned all too well. The supplement regimen was vast and expensive (although cheap in comparison to radiation or chemo). It ranged from high doses of vitamin C and selenium to more exotic substances like Cat's Claw and maitake mushrooms and germanium. Her insurance, of course, covered none of it. She took fistfuls of pills four times a day, nearly a hundred in all. Every Saturday night, after my mother went to sleep, my father sat down with all the bottles in front of him—they completely covered the kitchen table—and counted out a week's worth of each and put them in little trays. Once his fingers grew quick and nimble, the task took two hours. He has an accounting degree but never became an accountant; bean counter, pill counter, we offered to buy him an eyeshade.

In many ways it is easier to think of enduring all kinds of horrible treatments, treatments which will have an end, than to change permanently the bedrock habits of our lives. We are what we eat—not just in the sense that what we eat affects our health and size but that what we eat in many ways defines and constructs us socially and politically. The hardest part for Mom was the no-sugar rule. Like people, tumors love sugar and grow fat and happy on it, and she was the sort of person who, on opening a restaurant menu, looked first at the desserts. I found a recipe in a Moosewood cookbook for an apple cake—all whole wheat flour and sweetened with maple syrup, not much fat. It didn't look like much, but it tasted remarkably good and seemed to palliate her craving for sweets. I knew she'd never bake it herself—whenever my father talked about buying a new house my mother said that she would only go through the trouble of moving if the house was kitchen-free—so I baked one for her once a month or so. It took most of a morning to make; and between organic ingredients and overnight delivery, the little cake cost a week's pocket money. But it seemed a small price to keep her from the temptations of tiramisu.

I give Mom credit for going along with such a drastic change in her eating and living. I know that she sometimes departed from the script—"cheating," as she called it—as if this way of eating were an imposition and I the nutrition police. Like most of us, her taste for whole grains had been practically obliterated by fast and processed foods. She assumed that good-for-you meant bad-tasting, an attitude only exacerbated by the "eat to live, don't live to eat" school of nutrition.

A believer in "mind over body," my mother was convinced that she would get well. She had once injured herself so severely while working out that my father had to carry her into the doctor's office. Diagnosis: a hernia; prescription: immediate surgery. "What if I refuse?" she asked. "The tear will get bigger and your internal organs will end up outside the muscles rather than in," was the frightful prediction. "Let me think about it," my mother said. She had my father lift her up, bring her home and ensconce her on the couch in the family room. We thought she was nuts. Settled there, she spent a few days picturing her muscles knitting themselves back together. She was walking again in a week. We had always known she was stubborn, but after that feat, no one doubted the power of her will. So this time she did visualization exercises every day and cultivated the positive "love yourself" attitude that all the feel-good cancer books recommend. I lamented the dualism of her paradigm, which seemed to encourage thinking about the ailing body as a hostile foreign country that must be subdued and conquered, but how can a cancer patient not on some level feel that the body has betrayed the self and must be made obedient again?

And what woman who grows up in this culture manages to escape seeing her body, with its flesh and curves, as the enemy? Like her, I decided to concentrate on the positive and feel lucky that she was active and confident of her recovery, even if I, her overeducated daughter, didn't like the metaphor.

Like Dr. Hu's herbs, these methods of building the immune system take time. After about four months, though, her pain was nearly gone. At five months, the test that tracked the cancer in her body registered 0.1. Since 5.0 usually signals remission, this result seemed miraculous. Not bad for someone the white coats had written off. Relief, reprieve, we celebrated again.

The oncologist called her his "miracle patient."

He must have meant this literally because he never evinced the least bit of interest in her regimen. Perhaps his was not an inquiring mind. Perhaps he thought that no effort counted unless he directed it. (I once saw a surgeon on a television talk show, a grieving and chastened man whose wife, suffering from severe post-partum depression, had committed suicide. He had no idea that the condition could cause such catastrophe. "I was a surgeon," he said, "I figured that if I didn't know about something it wasn't worth knowing about." I don't want to generalize here, but his tone seemed to imply that this is just how most doctors think). The oncologist's lack of interest worried me, and I urged my parents to find another doctor. I gave them the name of an oncologist who uses both conventional and alternative, especially nutritional, approaches to treat cancer. My mother saw him a few times but didn't really like him and besides, she was weary of doctors. When he mentioned special (and expensive) tests and analyses that their insurance wouldn't cover, my father began to feel suspicious. They returned to the man-without-curiosity.

Just as things were going, in his own words, miraculously well, the oncologist suggested that my mother try some chemotherapy. "I'd give it a 15% chance of wiping it out entirely," he said. I was appalled when my parents told me of his suggestion, and sick and panicked at the thought of it. I reminded them that chemo destroys the immune system, that to take it would put all the gains at risk. But I knew that I couldn't lobby too loudly. What if she felt coerced by me, skipped the drugs and died anyway? Besides, I told myself, everyone has the right to make decisions about such grave matters without pressure.

My mother was pathologically impatient. Her father abandoned the family when she was five. Her mother would threaten suicide and then leave the children alone for hours. A childhood filled with extraordinarily stressful waiting. Once, when I was a child and too young to understand this, she became incredibly agitated and then disintegrated into tears while waiting for the washing machine repairman. Patience, in matters long and small, came hard. She readily agreed to the chemo—the doctor had recommended it, and he should know, after all. And if the cancer was truly gone, she could go back to Lou Malnatti's pizza and tiramisu.

The doctor prescribed a course of 5FU. I later learned that people in the cancer business sometimes refer to this drug as "Five Feet Under." I'm not sure if the phrase implies that the drug is so toxic that it can make you feel like you're dying, or that the drug is so ineffective that it won't save you from dying or, most likely, that the drug will kill you more often than not. (I often wonder if the obituaries "complications from cancer" refers primarily to death-by-chemo).

The drug trashed her immune system, as I feared. She lost her appetite and was too sick to take the supplements. The tumor came roaring back—her test numbers climbed to 15—and so did the pain. When it was clear that the treatment hadn't worked and that my mother was sicker than ever, the oncologist shrugged his shoulders and said, "Actually, I've never seen it work in a case like this, but it was worth a try."

When I tell this story people sometimes say that surely the physician should be sued for something. For what, I wonder: being unable to let a good thing alone? I paraphrase for them a passage from *Harrison's Principles of Internal Medicine*, a weighty two-volume canonical text of thousands of pages. I quote here from the third page of the 14th edition: "in those cases which do not lend themselves to easy solutions or for which no effective treatment is available, a feeling on the part of the patient that the physician is doing all that is possible is one of the most important therapeutic measures that can be provided."

The longer you linger over this passage the more stunning it becomes. It so casually licenses overtreatment. And there's the breathtaking arrogance of it. The physician, not the patient, is and always must be the active and powerful agent in the drama of illness. Finally, it seems to acknowledge the value of the placebo effect, which in other circumstances conventional medicine has roundly scorned. (Vitamins and herbs to treat cancer? Pure quackery. The placebo effect.) Here scientific medicine endorses the very "superstition" from which it claimed to save us. If all else fails, try the power of the white coat and the pointless treatment that you know won't work.

Perhaps cancer invites overtreatment and pointless treatment more than other illnesses. We have been engaged in a "war on cancer" since the Nixon administration. We die of cancer "after a long battle." War licenses extreme and aggressive and often hasty action. In times of war we are less critical of leaders and generals, more willing to go along with what they say must be done, feel greater pressure to fall in with the party line. We are more likely, in our fear, to mistake the propaganda for sound and credible argument, the horrific for the reasonable. We let profiteers masquerade as patriots. We tell ourselves that we can't really concern ourselves about collateral damage.

And of course in a few months she died. An ugly and painful and excruciating death. The tumor pushed mercilessly against her sciatic nerve, and all the morphine—in pills, patches, and IV pouches—hardly took the edge off. She weighed less than a hundred pounds by then, but enough Ativan to down an elephant only rarely produced relaxation and the relief of sleep. Perhaps because she was a goner, the oncologist stopped returning my father's phone calls; Dad was left to guess at how much morphine he could give his wife of nearly fifty years without killing her. Finally the tumor grew so large that the blood in her legs could barely return to her chest to be pumped again. They swelled to three times their normal size and dripped so much fluid that she was constantly soaked—weeping they call it. When you pressed your fingers into those big boggy legs, the indentations remained. Her toes began to blacken. She died by inches.

Cancer is insidious; you can think that it's dead, and like a vampire it returns to renew the parasitic feasting that leaves the patient bereft of flesh. I don't know for certain that Mom would be alive today if she had refused that chemotherapy. I do know that she died sooner because of it. I don't know if the seven weeks of radiation caught those stray cells, but it certainly didn't keep her safe from anything. A few weeks after my mother's death, my father began to wonder why he hadn't been told at the time of her first surgery that the radiation treatments would use up her lifetime allowance. The trained accountant became suspicious. "Did she really need all that radiation, or was that more about keeping the machines, which must be paid for, busy and billing?" he asked one of the people at the hospital who had treated Mom. He got an awkward smile and shrug in response.

I've become interested in the private language of oncology. In the lingo of the lesion, when a patient stops responding to treatment, he or she is "refractory." (Doctors also call the tumor "refractory" when it stops responding to drugs, but this rhetorical equation of patient and disease is another essay.) When chemotherapy fails to put the patient into remission, he or she has "failed chemotherapy." Language so hostile to the patient, so protective of the physician's authority, language so eager to blame the patient and exonerate medicine. What do they say when the treatment kills the patient? "Collateral damage"?

℘ ℘

I told the physician's assistant a shorter version (she was, after all, on the managed-care clock) of this story as partial explanation of my raised blood pressure and my air of I'd-rather-be-anywhere-else, -even-the-dentist. She listened sympathetically, and her empathy was welcome. But I think in the end this narrative was to her like the stories of so many disease-of-the-week movies and pulpy sentimental novels: a sad story about the suffering of one person and the consequences of cancer on those who loved her—consequences like a daughter's stress in the doctor's office. It was a private story. It wasn't a story about the politics of medicine or the economics of illness or the assumptions of the cancer establishment. Perhaps she filled in the gaps of my narrative with the conventions to which those books and movies have schooled us and imagined a mother who grows more noble as her body declines, children who happily give up old resentments and lovingly bond anew with parents and each other, good coming out of suffering and healing triumphing over death. She probably didn't imagine Mom's acid jesting in the last week that the only doctor she was willing to see was Dr. Kevorkian.

Because I wasn't sure that she got it, I told the physician's assistant another story— my own (although it's a very common one), a story I think of as the comic subplot to my mother's tragedy. A few years before my mother became sick the second time, I let a doctor talk me into having a baseline mammogram. There was a shadow on the film but the radiologist thought it probably wasn't cancer. Watch it for a while, he said, which meant trudging to the doctor's office for an exam every three months and trying to ignore the chronic low-grade anxiety that I might be walking around with breast cancer. After nine months, the doctor ordered another mammogram and I dutifully complied. The lump was larger now, and the radiologist said again the he was pretty sure (they'll never say certain, of course) that it was benign, but that I might want to have it out within the next six months just to be safe. When my internist got the report a few days later, she called and said that I had to have it out immediately. But the radiologist said it looked benign, I protested. Oh, it could be cancer, could very well be cancer, she said. Hysteria can be contagious, and I caught hers. The surgeon I consulted a few days later looked at the film and said, probably a benign fibroadenoma, but you should have it out just to be safe. So I let him take it out and it was of course benign (for which I am very grateful), and there were no lasting side effects except that I didn't feel nearly as confident in my body and I couldn't bring myself to touch my breasts for several years and I developed the sense that I had better be careful when someone in a white coat starts talking about doing something just to be safe. I certainly don't have the peace of mind they all promised when I think about all that radiation—at least six, maybe eight X rays—over the course of that medical adventure.

These days I'm a medical refractory. The physician's assistant wanted to bring me back into the fold of patients herded along from test to test and specialist to specialist. This is, I recognize, what she understands good, and safe, medicine to be. Overdue for a pap, she said, and I'd like to refer you to someone to talk about a colonoscopy. Given our culture's cancer hysteria (and I'm not implying here that some of that worry is not well-founded, but I also recognize that some of it is generated by a cancer industry more interested in detection and high-cost treatment than prevention), she expected me to comply. Why wouldn't I, why shouldn't I, now that I had a family history of cancer? Instead, I was ungrateful and resistant. I'm not even close to 50, I said. At least do the fecal occult blood test, she persevered. But I take a lot of vitamin C and eat a high-fiber diet; I'll false positive, and besides, up to 90% of the positives on that test can be false, I said. She sighed. She felt some nodularity in my breast. Mammogram, she prescribed. I'm premenstrual, I said. "Come back in two weeks."

I didn't feel the lumps after my period, so I didn't go back, in part because she and I have such vastly different notions of what it means to take good care of yourself. She thinks it's about submitting to regular medical surveillance, and I think it's about exercising and eating organic and polluting the environment as little as possible. She wasn't interested in the way constant testing for cancer and other ills reduces the patient to a disease-waiting-to-happen or in the consequences of that construction for the patient. ("I guess since I can no longer have children, all I can have is cancer," a friend summarized a recent visit to the doctor). She wasn't curious about the dangers of overtreatment that can result from all the screening (overtreatment that, even a recent pro-mammogram study acknowledged, leads to increased mortality). She didn't want to discuss the values of preventive medicine that is less about prevention than detection. Cancer exists; we can test for it; it's only sensible to submit because then you can feel safe: this seemed to be her line of reasoning. And if you have it, we can cure it if we catch it early (which is not true for certain kinds of breast cancer, but medical professionals won't tell you that, either). It was black-and-white for her. White witches and wizards, white hats, white coats, the good guys of fantasy and myth. Their goodness is always self-evident and unquestionable and without serious side effects.

It turned out that there wasn't much wrong with me the day I saw the physician's assistant, just a stage 3 panic and a hemorrhoid, probably the consequence of bad form while lifting weights. She gave me a prescription, which I dutifully filled. It cost $20, after the insurance discount of $40, and made me feel like I had a bad hangover. It didn't work. I went back to Dr. Hu, who prescribed a $3 ointment (available at your local Chinese grocery) that smelled like Chinatown and felt good—and did the job.

Last week I read about a newly published study on white coat syndrome: people whose blood pressures spike in the doctor's office are at higher risk of heart attacks. I suspect (these articles are often frustratingly, even misleadingly vague) the study concluded that white coat syndrome is a symptom of blood pressure that tends to spike in response to stress—and such an irrational, even hysterical, stress at that; after all, it's not rational to have a fight-or-flight response in the doctor's office. But perhaps fight-or-flight is a reasonable response to the white coat. An alternative conclusion from the data might be that reducing the risk of white coat syndrome is as simple as avoiding the white coats.

QUESTIONS

1. Discuss the author's advocacy of alternative medicine and nutrition as presented in this essay. What are the advantages to such an approach? the disadvantages?
2. Discuss the politics and the metaphor of the "war on cancer."
3. How does the author's perspective impact how she understands and how she tells the story of her mother's illness?

AIDS in Academe

A Story of Silence, Struggle and Success

⌒ CHRIS BELL ⌒

[handwritten: I = present/regular = Past present]

I never thought I'd be doing this. I can't imagine anyone having to do it. It's such a bizarre concept: to stand in front of the students in my class and inform them I will no longer be their instructor. And to do so while concealing the fact that my departure is the result of a decision that was made for me, not by me. Yet here I am about to do just that.

[handwritten margin note: Bravery, stigma]

 I walk into the classroom with my supervisor, who unobtrusively settles herself in a seat off to one side. The students have fallen silent. They know something unusual is transpiring. I take my position in front of them, equally silent for the moment. I cannot muster the strength to convey what must be said. Abruptly, I decide to share an approximation of the truth. My voice cracks as I state, "You're probably wondering why another graduate instructor led our last two class sessions. Well, there's a fairly good reason. I've had a lot on my mind since I saw you a week ago. I found out I am HIV-positive." Although I would rather not pause, I do so briefly [handwritten: illness stigma] *in response to the students' shocked expressions. Their reactions make it all the more difficult to reveal the lie I am about to tell. My tongue trips while racing through the following words: "Don't worry about me. I'll be fine. But in order to get to that point, I need to take some time for myself. And so I have decided to relinquish my teaching duties for the remainder of the semester. This is Dr. Leonard,* the codirector of Composition. She's going to talk to you about what happens next and who your new instructor will be. Thank you for allowing me the chance to get to know you. I wish you nothing but the best."*

 Without looking at the students, I nod in Dr. Leonard's direction and careen through the doorway. There is a boisterous assortment of coeds in the hallway, their presence preventing me from breaking down just yet. It is only after I have stormed into an empty classroom down the hall, shut the door, and turned out the lights that I allow myself to collapse on the floor, crying bitterly.

 I enrolled in graduate school because it seemed like a reasonable thing to do. Midway through my senior year in college, one of my favorite professors asked me what I planned to do after graduation. My inclination was simply to make it through *that* year and then spontaneously turn my attention to the next matter, but I realized there was something appealing about pragmatism. Accordingly, when my professor suggested I apply to his graduate institution, I took his advice and, shortly thereafter, received an admission letter as well as a prestigious university fellowship.

I enjoyed graduate school that first semester. Perhaps it was the newness of it all. Or maybe it was the small class sizes and individualized attention that appealed to me. In any event, I liked it and felt privileged to be in the environment. But my level of contentment diminished measurably at the beginning of the second semester. Too many of my seminars were devoted to literary theory and its practitioners. I mean, really, who cares what Derrida thought about (insert literary "classic" of choice here)?! Why couldn't we just revel in the text, I wondered. In her recollection of her graduate experience at Yale, renowned scholar Jane Tompkins observes:

> People were afraid to show who they really were, and most of all they were afraid to show what had drawn them to study literature in the first place. It was love that had brought us there, students and professors alike, but to listen to us talk you would never have known it. The love didn't have a conjugation or a declension; it couldn't be articulated as a theory or contained in a body of information. It wasn't intellectual—that was the shameful thing,—though it had an intellectual dimension. Being amorphous, tremulous, pulsing, it was completely vulnerable. So we all hid it as best we could, and quite successfully most of the time. (78–79)

As an individual schooled in the New Criticism model of literary theory, Tompkins grew frustrated with the focus of her graduate seminars, which warned her away, above all else, from the "affective fallacy," the concept of "confusing a literary work with its effects" on the reader (83). Tompkins's frustration is similar to my own feelings of resistance toward literary theory and its overwhelming insistence on concealing the love of literature I reveled in. Although I didn't have a referent for the sensation Tompkins identifies, I suffered from this disconcerted feeling throughout my second semester. I simply could not grasp the point of discussing, for example, critical race theory in Ralph Ellison's *Invisible Man* until we had unpacked the racist emasculation black men endure, *what Ellison painstakingly underscores in the novel*. Because I couldn't relate to my seminars, I began to tune out the professors and other students, contemplating instead which body part I might have pierced. On many occasions, I didn't attend class at all, opting to read and reread the assigned texts in an autodidactic effort to glean the knowledge I was not getting in class.

My saving grace throughout all of this was the freshman composition class I taught twice a week. I particularly enjoyed the autonomy of the class, the fact that I was allowed to choose the paper topics and course theme. My class was organized around the theme of protest. The students read and wrote about historical figures and protesters such as Nelson Mandela, Rosa Parks and AIDS activist Larry Kramer. Throughout the semester, I emphasized to my students the importance of finding and enhancing their voice, their own unique way of articulating their ideas about the world we live in. The students seemed to value this concept, liberally expressing their satisfaction in their end-of-semester course evaluations.

I began the subsequent semester, my third, at a bit of a crossroads. I loved teaching but loathed my seminars. The latter seemed particularly ill-suited to my sensibilities and contributed greatly to the waning of my lifelong love of literature. Nonetheless, I did enough to get by and even began considering Ph.D. programs in English. I did so not because I wanted to continue in my disillusioned capacity, but because I had told others that I would undertake doctoral study and thought it best for me to follow through. I existed in a trance-like state—that is, until Billy Vance died. *promises?*

Billy was a graduate student in the English Department. Although we were not enrolled in the same classes, we occasionally passed each other in the hallways. In the middle of my third semester, I learned that Billy was dying from AIDS. That reality was devastating for me. I could not believe that someone in such close proximity could be infected with AIDS. It just didn't seem "real."

Mere days after I learned of Billy's AIDS diagnosis came the news that he had died. In addition to reconciling myself to that fact, I was also forced to grapple with the reality that hardly anyone in the English Department seemed concerned with his passing. The silence was palpable, overwhelming. I remember standing in front of my class during this time, talking about Larry Kramer, the founder of the AIDS Coalition to Unleash Power (ACT UP). On a whim, I asked the students if they were aware that an individual on our campus had recently died from AIDS. They were as taken aback as I was, a reaction that reassured me that Billy's death, regardless of the English Department's silence, was significant. Later that evening, I spoke about Billy at a meeting of the Triangle Coalition, the university's gay, lesbian, bisexual undergraduate organization. I shared my memories of him—few that there were—along with my sense of bewilderment toward the silence in the English Department. Many of the Triangle Coalition members shared my grief, freely articulating their thoughts about our culture of AIDS. Thus, the problem, as I identified it, was situated in the English Department. Why was it that the faculty and my fellow graduate students were able to content themselves with studying and theorizing about lives but were somehow unable or unwilling to take that study and apply it to the situation at hand? I might have understood if Billy had been a graduate student at another university, or even in a different department at the same university, because the connection would not have been so evident. But that was not the case. Billy was one of us.

In thinking about my feelings toward the English Department following Billy's death, I am reminded of a sentiment cultural critic Stuart Hall conveys in an essay about cultural studies, a form of literary theory. Hall writes:

> AIDS is one of the questions which urgently brings before us our marginality as critical intellectuals in making real effects in the world. . . . Against the urgency of people dying in the streets, what in God's name is the point of cultural studies? What is the point of the study of representations, if there is no response to the question of what you say to someone who wants to know if they should take a drug and if that means they'll die two days later or a few months earlier? At that point, I think anybody who is into cultural studies seriously as an intellectual practice must feel, on their pulse, its ephemerality, its insubstantiality, how little it registers, how little we've been able to change anything or get anybody to do anything. If you don't feel that as one tension in the work that you are doing, theory has let you off the hook. (284)

Although Hall is specifically addressing cultural studies as a field of inquiry, I believe his remarks are relevant to academia as a whole. If I have understood Hall correctly, it isn't enough to theorize about how lives are lived in an academic sense; one must be willing to do something to acknowledge the inherent value of human life. That acknowledgement was sorely lacking in Billy's case.

Ultimately, Billy's death had a profound effect on me because he was the first individual I knew with AIDS. The fact that his death went virtually unheralded in the English Department was haunting, because I got the sense that his spirit remained in that space, primarily out of a justified fear of being forgotten, erased. It was almost as if he was there among us, listening for his name and not hearing it. To a large extent, Billy's death—particularly the pervasive silence following his passing—led to my break with the English Department. I completed the semester from a distance; I rarely entered the department because I wanted to avoid my professors and fellow graduate students at all costs. I didn't even attend the memorial the department cobbled together for Billy, largely because it occurred several weeks after he had died, almost as an afterthought. In lieu of taking classes during the summer term, I wrote a new syllabus for my freshman composition class, one that focused on women's issues like sexual violence, female genital mutilation and lesbian marginalization. One key difference in this revised syllabus was that I pointedly scheduled my office hours in the Women's Center, which was located across the campus from the English Department. The only time I intended to venture to the department was when I had to attend a seminar. I became nauseated at the thought of entering the building.

Several months after Billy Vance died, I took an HIV test because my doctor at the Student Health Center could not pinpoint precisely why I remained fatigued from a bout with mononucleosis. She ran a series of tests—"bloodwork," she somewhat gruesomely referred to it—including the one for HIV antibodies. As I sat in the doctor's office two weeks later awaiting my results, I thought about the work I had to do: thesis research, papers to grade, Ph.D. applications to complete, a *Canterbury Tale* to read. In the midst of my reverie, the doctor walked into the room. After we exchanged greetings, she calmly informed me the HIV antibody test had come back positive. While she proceeded with post-test counseling, I tuned her out, thinking to myself, "When I came into this room, I was already HIV-positive. Nothing has changed except my level of awareness. Therefore, I should continue with the things I have to accomplish." With that in mind, I interrupted the doctor's counsel, stating, "You know Doc, this whole HIV thing is really a bit of an inconvenience for me. I frankly don't have time to be HIV-positive right now. So I'm going to come back later when I'm ready to deal with this. How's next week looking for you?" Without giving the doctor much of an opportunity to respond, I left.

After departing the Student Health Center, I made an effort to proceed with the tasks I had planned to accomplish that evening. This was lesbian, gay, bisexual pride week at the university, and to commemorate that fact, a series of events was scheduled for the next few days. The program slated for that evening was a safer-sex seminar. Having left the Student Health Center, I strolled my little HIV-positive self into the Women's Center for this safer-sex instruction (better late than never, eh?). The first individual I spied in the room was Anna, president of the Triangle Coalition. I spontaneously approached Anna and asked her to join me in the hall. When we were alone, I informed her of my HIV diagnosis and asked if I could share this news at the Triangle Coalition meeting the following week. Anna blinked a few times in surprise, then abruptly hugged me. She said, "Yes, Chris, I think that'd be a great thing for you to do." After Anna returned to the safer-sex seminar, I walked home. I chose not to stay because the situation struck me as somewhat too surreal. Instead, I spent the evening reading the dreaded *Canterbury Tale* and watching *Law & Order*. Then, I went to sleep.

A few days later, while grading papers in the Women's Center, I was approached by JC, the editor of the school newspaper. She explained she was writing a small article about college students' attitudes toward HIV/AIDS and asked me for a quote. JC knew me as an AIDS advocate in the local community, knew that I had integrated AIDS components in my composition classes and that I had talked about Billy Vance to the Triangle Coalition. She could not, however, have known about my seroconversion. As a result, I took a deep breath and apprised JC of my recent diagnosis. She asked if I would be willing to discuss this in the newspaper. I considered this for the briefest of moments, then agreed.

Naturally, I did not want my close friends and acquaintances to read about my HIV diagnosis in the school newspaper. Thus, I spent the days between the interview with JC and the newspaper's publication informing them of my situation. One of the individuals I spoke with was Dr. Gaither, the codirector of Composition. While he expressed concern about my diagnosis, Dr. Gaither's primary focus was the effect this might have on my students. He said evocative things like, "Do you really think it's fair for them to have their instructor revealing his HIV diagnosis in the newspaper?" Suggesting I had enough to contend with, Dr. Gaither relieved me of my teaching duties for the remainder of the semester. As a show of good faith and to prove I harbored no animosity toward this decision nor the person who made it, I accompanied Dr. Leonard, the other codirector of composition, to my class in order to resign my duties. That afternoon, I stood in front of my students, struggling to find my voice so I could lie and say it was my decision to stop teaching because I needed some time off. I don't know why I lied to the students, particularly considering that that is the only lie I have told about my diagnosis. Several years later, I am still trying to reconcile myself to that choice.

I expected there to be about twenty students at the Triangle Coalition meeting that same evening. A number of individuals must have been feeling particularly "prideful" as a result of the previous week's activities, though. Imagine my surprise when I entered the room and saw at least eighty individuals gathered. I don't remember much of what I said to the assembled group in the way of revealing my HIV diagnosis. I do know I spoke from the heart. My words were evidently effective, considering eighty people hugged me in rapid succession when I finished speaking. It was incredibly empowering—so much so that I did not care what happened the next day when the newspaper was published. All that mattered to me was that the community I felt the closest to supported and accepted me.

Undeniably, the newspaper caused quite a stir on campus, partly because of JC's editorial decisions. She had, in fact, "bumped" the original cover story to highlight my diagnosis. Well, this was homecoming weekend at the university. The campus population went to the newsstands expecting to see a lead article or headline about the king and queen elections or the football game. Instead, they saw a cover story about AIDS. I am neither naïve enough nor stupid enough not to realize that some individuals likely saw the newspaper and dismissed it, claiming, "Fag got AIDS. What's the big deal?" This sentiment, however, was not conveyed to me in person. Quite the opposite: the reactions I received were enthusiastic. From the food court employee who came around the counter to embrace me before I could order my Whopper Jr., to the young African-American undergraduate who asked me to speak about HIV/AIDS to her sorority, people went out of their way to thank me for being so open about my diagnosis. Not surprisingly, the majority of my professors and fellow graduate students in the English Department said nothing.

As a triumphant aside, I must mention that every year the staff of the school newspaper selects one issue to represent that year's body of work in the American College Media Association award competition. During that year, the staff picked the issue which discussed my HIV diagnosis as their entry. Out of a field of over a few hundred submissions, that issue of the paper received several awards, including "Best of Show."

The newspaper interview was clearly a pivotal moment. I have often characterized it as the climax of the whirlwind events immediately following my HIV diagnosis. Inevitably, when climax occurs, denouement abruptly follows. In keeping with that truth, a few days after the newspaper was published, I experienced a crippling depression, rendering me virtually immobile for weeks. I didn't attend classes or do much of anything else. Instead, I pondered the ramifications of my HIV diagnosis and how my life was irrevocably altered. I emerged from this depressive funk only after I received a call from a professor who asked if I would speak about AIDS to her class. The next afternoon, I did just that. The experience was so positive, so affirming, I spent the remainder of the semester undertaking a campus speaking tour about HIV/AIDS. — what about you?

At the conclusion of the term, I attended a meeting with the codirectors of composition. They approved me to teach the following semester, but with the stipulation that I teach only with "probationary" status. They did not want a recurrence of the previous situation, wherein I stopped teaching in the middle of the semester, forcing them to scramble to find a replacement. I saw no need to point out that they were the intellegentsia who had relieved me of my teaching assignment in the first place. Instead, I resigned from the English Department and the university, forgoing both my roles of teacher and student.

When I think about my experience at the university, I am inclined to wag my head back and forth and say to myself, "What a time it was!" No twenty-three-year-old should have to endure an ordeal such as that one. Hell, no one should be subjected to that level of drama! Initially, there is the Billy Vance episode to reflect on. Sometimes I wonder if I might have overreacted after Billy died, but once I think the situation through, I know I did not. That experience led me to realize that, in our culture, AIDS is troped differently from other diseases. There is usually sympathy and support accompanying afflictions such as cancer or multiple sclerosis, but not with AIDS. The history of this disease is the history of marginalization. Persons with AIDS have always been regarded as pariahs, and that ingrained attitude of aversion does not appear to be changing.

After Billy died, after the English Department did everything it could to avoid discussing his death, I took a look around the department in an effort to gauge how disability and disease were negotiated. I considered the student who was involved in a major car accident a few years before my arrival, yet was never ostracized from the community as a result of being quadriplegic. I also considered Catherine, the deaf student, who was one of the most well-liked graduate students in the department. If an administrative assistant got a paper cut, it was highlighted in the interdepartmental newsletter. Billy died, from AIDS, and nothing happened. It should come as little surprise that by their actions the English Department, collectively, reminds me of Lily Bart's aunt, Mrs. Peniston, in Edith Wharton's *The House of Mirth*. Wharton describes this individual as having "the innocence of the school-girl who regards wickedness as a part of 'history,' and to whom it never occurs that the scandals she reads of in lesson-hours may be repeating themselves in the next street" (181). Like Mrs. Peniston, the faculty and graduate students in the English Department were so preoccupied with theorizing about lives, they were unable to pull their noses out of their books and see how those lives were lived in practice. This is unfortunate, because our global community has never been so extensive, so expansive, that we can distance ourselves from disease and death. I chose to regard Billy's death as an unheeded augury reminding us of our impermanence. As John Donne remarked, "Any man's death diminishes me, because I am involved in Mankind; And therefore never send to know for whom the bell tolls; It tolls for thee."

In addition, my own diagnosis underscored the legendary silence surrounding AIDS. The disconnect is fascinating. I was allowed to engage the students in my freshman composition class in HIV/AIDS pedagogy, but somehow, as a result of my diagnosis, I was no longer fit to teach. That decision hurt and has left me perpetually guarded about revealing my HIV-positive status to the authority figures in my life. The entire experience was, truly, a teachable moment—not only for myself but, as it turns out, for other individuals as well. On one of the rare occasions when I entered the English Department after my diagnosis, I found the following note from Lauren, a student in the class in which my teaching duties were relieved:

> When I heard the news I had no idea what to say. I was walking back to my dorm room and thought about my life. I can't say everything will be ok, because I have no idea what being HIV positive is like. It makes me think that even though college and classes are important there is so much more than just school. I know if I was told that I had HIV I would not be able to function. If it's one thing that I will take from your class it will be that strength is the key. All the women that we talked about and that you admire were strong women. Although that might not mean much now I hope it means something in the future. Your voice has always been strong. I hope that you continue to use it.

Taken by itself, the note is striking. But Lauren concluded with a postscript that I have never forgotten. She quoted an unnamed source: "I have but one voice"; and she followed that with an admonition to me: "Let your voice be heard." Lauren's note touched me because I felt she understood what I was going through and why I decided to be so open about my diagnosis.

And Lauren wasn't the only one. A few weeks after departing the university, I received a letter from the administration, telling me about Joy, an undergraduate who had read the article in the newspaper and had heard me discuss HIV/AIDS during my speaking tour around the campus. Joy was inspired by my actions and wrote a letter nominating me for the university's Human Rights Award, an honor I was pleased to receive and accept. Subsequently, since leaving graduate school, I have devoted my life to presenting programs on HIV/AIDS prevention, education and treatment to high school and college audiences across the United States and Canada. I find this undertaking fulfilling because I believe that I am making a positive impact on people's lives. Of course, I occasionally become nervous during some of these speaking engagements, but somehow, I always manage to find my voice.

By way of conclusion, I would like to highlight that I am returning to graduate school. Any day now, I anticipate receiving an acceptance letter admitting me to a different institution from the one I attended previously. I am returning because I choose to, not because I think it is expected of me. I don't feel as if I have anything to prove. Moreover, when I return, I intend to draw on my experiences at my previous graduate institution and continue to use my voice to engage the faculty, my fellow graduate students, and the students I teach in discourse about HIV/AIDS. In short, I have no qualms about the decisions I made. I am also happy that I am returning to the graduate community with this experience firmly in mind. Most of all, at this moment, I feel like a survivor.

---

* For privacy reasons, all names, save the author's, have been changed.

REFERENCES

Hall, Stuart. "Cultural Studies and Its Theoretical Legacies." In Grossberg, Lawrence et al., *Cultural Studies*. New York and London: Routledge, 1992. 277–286.

Tompkins, Jane. *A Life in School: What the Teacher Learned*. Reading: Addison-Wesley, 1996.

Wharton, Edith. *The House of Mirth*. 1905. New York: Scribner, 1995.

QUESTIONS

1. The death of his colleague was an epiphany for the author. How might the author's reaction have been different if his department had been more responsive to his colleague's death?
2. The author claims that "AIDS is troped differently from other diseases." What examples from our culture support or contradict this assertion?
3. Discuss the implications of the essay's subtitle vis-à-vis the author's enthusiastic return to graduate school. If he feels that he is changing lives by speaking publicly about HIV/AIDS, why does he choose to return to the academy—a place that is, for him, a realm of silence and struggle?
4. Discuss the politics of HIV/AIDS.

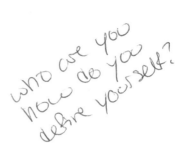

Disabled Identity in Academia
⌒ CHRISTOPHER R. SMIT ⌒

stigma

When I see my students in a nonscholarly environment, the grocery store, for example, I often sense that they are confused. As they see me groping a grapefruit, or selecting my favorite barbeque sauce from the shelf, their gaze is often one of puzzlement—Professor Smit actually goes shopping, . . . just like me? Episodes like these often remind me that the life of an academic is characterized by insularity. My students, some of my colleagues, and certainly my academic audience (i.e., those people who come to hear me give a lecture or read my essays) have no idea who I "really" am. They know me as Professor Smit, or "that guy who writes about popular music," or "the writer who deals with disability and media." This is not to say, however, that my academic identity does not include parts of the "real me." For example, my students know that I am a die-hard Chicago Cubs fan and that I find Bruce Springsteen to be one of the most influential artists of the twentieth century; my colleagues know that I am a person whose life is guided by deep belief in justice and grace; and my academic audience, I hope, knows that I am a defender of art and suspect of the word *postmodern*.

But just how much should these people, some of them complete strangers whom I will never see again, know about me? Part of "me," as you will read below, involves a physical disability. And while many people with disabilities feel comfortable allowing their own experiences of disability to play a key role in the presentations of their identity, I have always been cautious in doing so. Surely, all of us have elements of our identity which for one reason or another we would like to keep private. For me, this element has often been my experience of physical impairment. On the one hand, I can see how my sharing of personal anecdotes about disability might help other people—certainly I have done this, and have seen such results in the past. On the other hand, I am willing to keep my disability personal at times, finding the vulnerability of sharing my physical condition with others to be too much to handle.

Thus, the riddle of my career has been, and will continue to be, should my audience need to see my disability in my scholarship? Am I bound, by some unwritten, transcendent contract to include my disability status in all that I do as an academic, including teaching, speaking and writing? Are there things to be gained by making my illness an explicit ele-

271

-ment of my professional identity? In what follows, I will attempt to answer these questions by writing what is called an autoethnography. This genre uses the same principles of ethnographic writing (i.e., observation, analysis, storytelling, deduction, and theoretical exegesis, etc.), but the lens is turned back on the author rather than on another group or culture. This style of writing shifts between personal anecdotes and reflection, storytelling and analysis. Consequently, I will address the public and personal inhibitions mentioned above, writing for myself and to you, the reader, in order to explore and expound upon the identity of this particular disabled academic.

In 1994, when I was a junior in college, I was hired by a professor of special education, Tom Hoeksema, as a research assistant on a qualitative, ethnographic research project on inclusive education. Twice a week for three months, we would drive forty miles each way to visit a small middle school in western Michigan to observe and interview students with disabilities. On a typical day I would observe these students interacting with their able-bodied classmates for three to four hours, and then have more formal, tape-recorded discussions with them in a small office. As I reflect on this experience today, our work seems exciting, purposeful, and important, aiming, as it did, to analyze the interactions between disabled and nondisabled students and to offer an inside look at the highly debated inclusive education movement. At the time, however, my mind and passions were elsewhere. My research assistantship paid well and provided a good line on my resume, yet it failed to convince me that I was meant to be a special education teacher or researcher. I had recently declared a major in film studies, and cinema was my passion.

In an odd sort of way, though, this experience eventually led me to an academic career in media studies. During our long car rides, Hoeksema and I would discuss films we had seen recently and argue about what cinema had to offer culture. We would discuss, quite heatedly at times, whether cinema needed to reflect society with mirrored images. Were the images of cinema somehow chained to reality, or were they free to mingle between authentic and artistic expression? I often argued for the latter, stating that cinema was an art form, able to represent its own reality; a good film, as I saw it, offered its audience a new vision of the world, a lens of alternate meanings. By mid-semester, we were both agreeing on this definition of cinematic art, and were eager to try out our thesis. Our conversations turned to depictions of people with disabilities in cinema.

As far as I know, Hoeksema, now a dear friend and colleague of mine, did not intentionally hire me because of my disability. He had also hired two other, nondisabled students to assist him in his project. This said, however, my opinions about issues of disability were often solicited in our meetings. The assumption was that my own experience of physical disability gave me an authority on all things disabled. As a young person, this trust and confidence in what I had to say was a real identity booster, a confidence builder. And I was always glad to share my thoughts as an "expert" on the disabled experience, especially when there were disabled children involved. I assumed, incorrectly, that I could better articulate their experiences for them because "I had been where they are now." For the first time in my life, actually, I had tasted the power of authority. It was both liberating and intoxicating to redefine my physical impairment as a social enabler.

Yet, in my discussions with Hoeksema about cinema and disability, I was unwilling to let this new-found rhetorical authority of disabled identity guide my words; I was a serious film student, an identity that I felt was more salient to any discussions involving cinema. Hoeksema asked what a guy like me, a wheelchair user, thought of a film like *My Left Foot*, in which the lead character also used a wheelchair for mobility. I was outraged by these inquiries.

"What the hell does my disability have to do with this? I gauge the film by my intellectual training in a discipline, not by my disability," I argued, deeply offended because of my youthful exuberance and ignorant pride.

"How can you *not* consider your disability in your opinions of disability films?" he responded.

"Well, I just don't. I am a film student, not a disability student."

At the time, I didn't understand this conundrum, nor do I claim to fully understand it today. These were my first experiences with identity struggle, something most college juniors and seniors grapple with during this time of life. Who am I, what should I be, what can I be, what do I want to be? My own physical disability seemed to complicate the answers to these questions even more. Being disabled had, during this semester, both empowered and disempowered me. It had granted me authority with my fellow researchers in one situation and, as I saw it, discredited my knowledge of film in another. I was torn between two identities, only one of which included a clear connection to the physical state of my body. The film-thinker identity relied on my mind. My identity seemed paradoxical to me, a source of frustration. I felt a decision had to be made.

The quandary I faced during this part of my life is one that arguably plagues most people with disabilities, academics or not. Grappling with disabled identity is actually a phenomenon peculiar to the late twentieth century. Historically, having a disability has been a source of shame in the United States. In the early 1800s, for example, disability was often cast as a spiritual failing, the ill-effect of a family's perceived ungodly behavior (Longmore, *Uncovering*, 42). God made man in His own image, an image of perfection both in soul and body. Therefore, bodily difference was a sign of spiritual difference, an emblem of a failure to meet the creator's hopes for creation. Physical disabilities like cerebral palsy and what we know today as polio or ALS were, in effect, death sentences for children. Killed or left to die, people with disabilities from this unfortunate era did not have the opportunity to ponder identity (Albrecht et al., 4). They rarely survived long enough to do so.

Post-Civil War America found people with disabilities surviving longer because of advances in medicine and technology, and many disability studies scholars and historians point to this period as the beginnings of the medical model of disability (Longmore, "Uncovering"; Longmore and Umansky, *New Disability History*; Stiker, *History of Disability*). Instead of claiming that disability is an abhorrent embodiment of demonic possession, the medical model looks mainly at the medical—and thus physical—experience of physical and mental impairments in its definition of "disability." In other words, this model worked to individualize disability as the condition—and thus experience—of a "sick" individual, or patient. It is important to note that this model was, and is, utilized primarily by medical professionals, leaving the person with the disability uninvolved in her own articulation of identity.

It was only in the early 1980s that people with disabilities began to play a real role in their own identification. During this time, disabled advocates, inspired and instructed by the civil rights and feminist movements of the 1960s and 1970s, began to see disability as a potential political tool from which great changes could be made in the way this country treated individuals with physical and mental illness. Political groups like ADAPT began petitioning Congress, barricading (with their wheelchairs) inaccessible public buildings, and picketing public transportation systems which were not "wheelchair-friendly." Disability had finally become a source of social power, a phenomenon which held drastic consequences for the individual experience of disability (Zames and Zames Fleischer, *Disablity Rights Movement*; Longmore and Umansky, *New Disability History*; Longmore, "Uncovering"). The feeling that began to sweep over disabled Americans was that of emancipation. In 1990, President George Bush signed the Americans with Disabilities Act (ADA), legislation that called for equal employment rights and a "flat world" (accessible public buildings). President Bush called this initiative "a freeing of the slaves." Identity was finally a concept that disabled people could understand—and could own—on a personal level.

While approaching graduation from college with a film-studies major, I had made the decision not to allow my disability to define my entire identity. I had begun, in fact, to resent those individuals and institutions that demanded me to *be* disabled, fostering an almost anti-political stance in my approach to scholarship and interpersonal interactions. As an emblem of this decision, I decided to formalize my interest in disability in cinema by coteaching a three-week course on film and disability with Hoeksema, who had sparked some of my initial interest in the topic. While he would deal with the disability angle of the class, I would lecture mainly on issues of cinema history and criticism. My college had approved this project as an independent study in which I would gain practical knowledge of teaching in college, a vocation I had decided to pursue in graduate school beginning the next fall.

In the first week of class, the inevitable happened. During a discussion of the film *The Water Dance*, an independent film that portrays the lives of quadriplegics going through rehabilitation, a student raised her hand and asked me the question.

"Does the film seem accurate to you? You know, I mean, . . . does it seem fair, realistic based on your own experiences of, well, you know?"

I was caught off guard by this question, and to this day I am not quite sure why. Perhaps it was because I was so determined to be perceived in this class as a film scholar (though not yet a scholar) that I had blinded myself to my own physical presence in the classroom. No matter how much I had told myself that my worth in this classroom—in the world for that matter—was going to be based on my intellect and *not* my physical condition, I would never be able to completely rid myself of disability. And this student's question had driven this fact home with a blazing sword. My response, as I recall it today, would be prophetic; it would become central in my academic considerations of cinema and disability, as well as other situations in my early career as a college instructor. I remember pausing for a minute, glancing over to Hoeksema, who looked on with an expression of wonder and vindication, and then back to the student, who looked a little confused and guilty. I cleared my throat and said,

"Well, let me tell you. I have been asking myself the same question these last couple of months, but in another way. I have been wondering how my own disability will play a role in my work on cinema and disability. And here is what I have come up with as a sort of answer. While growing up as a guy with muscular dystrophy might have brought me to the topic of cinematic portrayals of people with disabilities, it is not the motivation for my work. I am interested in film as art, and accordingly, things like accuracy, authenticity, and fairness don't mean that much to me."

Saying the words clarified the ideas for me. I continued.

"I am more interested in what these films express about all people, not just disabled people. Yes, viewed one way, these movies are centered on the lives of disabled people. However, they are also about people in general, aren't they? They are also about filmmaking, which means that they teach us a great deal about what makes a film beautiful, what makes it art. Consequently, I am *as* interested in the disability issues this film raises as I am interested in how the camera, lighting, editing, and scripting of the film work. Not many people writing about disability in cinema seem interested in these additional things; they just want to talk about disability issues. I want to do more than that. I want to make sure we are not missing important elements of these films as *films*."

The student heard me, but I am not sure she understood me. Honestly, I didn't quite know if I understood myself. But something important had occurred in that brief interaction. Forced to articulate this approach to cinema and disability had also forced me, for the first time, to voice my understanding of my own identity as a would-be academic. Rather than contextualize my career within my disability, I would make a conscious effort to make a name for myself through rigorous scholarship, through good teaching, through a conscious consideration of everything else in my field of study before disability issues. I would write about disability and media, disability and culture. However, I would not simply base all of my findings on my own experience. On the contrary, I was, perhaps ignorantly, determined to keep my own disability status out of my scholarly work. While my views on this would change over the years, at the time it was imperative not to let my disability define me.

In the spring of 1996, after the three-week course had ended, I attended the national conference on international cinema studies at Indiana University in Bloomington. As a senior undergraduate student, I was certainly out of place among some of the top scholars (and filmmakers) engaged in the field of film studies. Most presentations I heard went over my head, yet I was not discouraged. That weekend I met and talked to Italian film director Victor Scola. After watching his film about a disfigured woman who falls in love with a handsome man and dies heartbroken, I asked him how disability played a role in his directing and lighting. As my question was translated to him, I was delighted to see his face twist up in surprise. No one, he said, had ever picked up on that part of his film, and he was delighted that I had. I also talked to director Peter Bogdonovich about the mute character in his film *The Last Picture Show* and about his film *Mask*. And I had a chance to meet two heroes of another sort: David Bordwell and Dudley Andrew, the two major film theorists I learned the most from as an undergraduate. They both seemed interested in my aesthetic approach to disability and cinema and were glad I had applied to their Ph.D. programs.

Alongside the cultural developments of the disability rights movement, whose victory was beginning to be sealed with the signing of the ADA in 1990, was a surge of disability-centered scholarship, which became known in the academy as disability studies. Disabled scholars from a wide variety of disciplines, including literary criticism, history, geography, and communication studies, were offering academic writing based on the same political activism that had blossomed in the 1980s. While battles over health care and equal employment for people with disabilities were being fought in Congress, other battles were beginning to take shape within the walls of the academy. In her essay "Disability Studies/Not Disability Studies," Simi Linton, a disabled academic, argues for this style of activism in the following manner: "I position myself as an advocate for the creation of a robust liberal arts-based inquiry into disability and as a disabled woman with an investment in increasing the equitable participation of disabled people in society" (525). Linton and others were beginning to see scholarship as a fruitful means of continuing the cause for civil rights for all disabled people.

By the late 1990s, disability studies had taken shape in liberal arts education across America. Inclusion of disability-centered courses on several campuses; the creation of the Society for Disability Studies, a Ph.D. program at the University of Illinois in Chicago from its Department of Disability and Human Development; and a large body of publications on disability issues proved that disability studies had grown strong. As with any new academic enterprise, however, the study of disability was not conducted without its own unique set of problems and debates. Arguably, the most heated debate in disability studies had to do with the disability status of its writers. Attending to this dilemma in his seminal collection, *The Disability Studies Reader*, editor Lennard Davis explains, "The first assumption that has to be countered in arguing for disability studies is that the 'normal' or 'able' person is already full up to speed on the subject. My experience is that while most 'normals' think they understand the issue of disability, they in fact do not" (2).

Like many others, Davis argues that scholarship based on disability issues should be written primarily by people with disabilities. Two key assumptions are inherent in this declaration: that able-bodied scholars have little to say about the way disability might factor into their disciplines, and that all people with disabilities are equally politically motivated, willing to fight for the liberation of other disabled people. Consequently, disabled identity became fixed: Presumably, if one were a disabled academic, his or her experience of physical or mental impairment was political in nature; it defined the person and his or her work. Acknowledging no other plausible alternative, disability studies argued that it was the responsibility of the disabled academic to continue the fight for the civil rights of all people with disabilities.

In 1999 I was admitted into the Ph.D. program at the University of Iowa in media studies, a specialty offered by their Department of Communication Studies. One of my first courses as a graduate student was an independent study with Professor Dudley Andrew. He and I were working on an essay regarding the depiction of people with disabilities in Japanese cinema. Part of the allure of Japanese cinema for me was the lack of American political history involved in the project. At this point in my career, I had become increasingly frustrated by assumptions made about my identity thanks to the political landscape that surrounded my acceptance into the media studies program. Disability studies work within the broader context of media studies had just begun to emerge, and although my colleagues in Iowa had not all read this literature, certain assumptions were being made about its scope and agenda. Well-intentioned classmates assumed that any work I was doing was motivated by my disabled identity. In other words, the perception was that my work was disability studies work, no matter what I intended it to be. _- must be diff_

Certainly, these assumptions would change while I lived and worked in Iowa, as colleagues, students, and professors came to know me and my work better. Nevertheless, early in my graduate work, there was immense pressure to define who I was. More accurately, a great deal of my energy was spent making sure people knew who I wasn't. I quickly learned that this was easier to do interpersonally than it was as a scholar.

My writing on disability and cinema progressed during my first two years in graduate school. I remember one particularly illuminating interaction that occurred at an annual meeting of the National Communication Association. This event alerted me to the potential dangers of conducting the type of scholarship I had chosen. Tom Hoeksema and I were presenting our now-shared interpretation of cinema and disability to a small group of disability-studies academics. With a sensitive presentation, we spent forty-five minutes arguing that disability cinema should not be critiqued on the basis of political content—ironically exactly the way our audience studied films—but rather by means of aesthetics. As we wrapped things up, we sat back and hesitantly asked if there were any questions. A man in the back of the room raised his hand and asked, "How is it possible that you two, one a disabled scholar, the other an able-bodied professor of Special Education, can agree with your own thesis? It seems that your pairing up would create another, more political analysis. Yet what we just listened to doesn't manage to argue for the rights of people with disabilities at all. The whole thing just seems a little, well . . . weird." Here, again, although in different words, was the same question asked by that first student years before.

In March 1999, colleagues and I hosted the first international conference on cinema and disability at the University of Iowa. During this event, over 35 scholars, disabled and able-bodied, met to discuss the future of disability and cinema scholarship. Much progress was made that weekend, and I was able to convey my convictions that there was a great deal to be seen in these films not only about disability, but also about the human condition more generally. Several of the presentations that weekend were included in a collection I edited with my friend and colleague Anthony Enns, entitled Screening Disability: Essays on Cinema and Disability, published in 2001. _look up._

The political, cultural, and academic progress made by disability activism has been impressive. Historically, the disabled population has been regarded as a fringe identity. Physically (and thus socially) unable to assimilate into mainstream cultural norms and behaviors, people with disabilities could not count themselves as active members of American culture. Today, this marginality is erased by the presence of a new, distinctly disabled culture. Members of their own collective, the disabled Americans of today thrive in a new-found identity, one which is not only shared, but fought for, by others who look, feel, speak, and believe in things, just as they do.

The presence of the disabled culture, then, should be celebrated. However, it should not be forgotten that the creation of any distinct minority culture always carries with it certain problems. Ironically, a common critique of the disabled culture movement is that it forces a political persona onto people with disabilities who otherwise do not see themselves as political. As with my own case, many people with disabilities do not identify themselves, politically or otherwise, by the physical conditions of their bodies. Other disabled people simply do not have time or health or political activism; their efforts and attention are toward survival, not rhetoric.

Inasmuch as any person's identity is influenced by environment, upbringing, faith background, gender, class, race, etc., disability can be seen as only one component of a person's identity. There is no single Experience of Disability. By the fall of 2001, I had come to terms with the role of disability in my private and public lives—with my wife and family, and with my students and colleagues. I was no longer afraid to be, or angry about being, a guy with a disability. My body was no longer a rhetorical hindrance.

During this fall semester, I began having severe pain in the right side of my jaw, the result of, I would soon find out, a nasty wisdom tooth that needed to be removed. Complicating matters was spinal muscular atrophy, which prevented my jaw from opening more than eleven millimeters, thus making it difficult for a dentist to access my mouth well enough to extract the tooth. I went to the University of Iowa Oral Surgery Clinic for help. After several visits with surgeons it was recommended that I be put under anesthetic, which theoretically would relax my jaw. With a calm voice that did not calm me, my doctor mentioned the possibility they might need to break my jaw during the procedure. When I told them I would get a second opinion, the team assembled in the office looked disappointed. I was an exciting case for them—a disabled guy with a challenging oral issue doesn't come their way that often. I eventually found a brilliant oral surgeon who removed the tooth in ten minutes under local anesthetic.

During this time I had missed a week of classes. I explained to my "Gender, Sexuality, and Media" students that I needed to have emergency oral surgery. They watched a film while I was gone. My "Media and Disability" students, on the other hand, got a different story. We had been discussing different historical models of disability. The night before my ten-minute, no-hassle surgery, I was lecturing on the *medical model* of disability in America at the end of the nineteenth century. As I was discussing the fact that this model polarized the relationship between able-bodied healers (doctors) and disabled patients, my tooth was really flaring up. My headache had increased throughout the night and I was certain I would need to end class early. I stopped lecturing, pulled my wheelchair from behind my desk, and addressed the class informally:

"You know that I don't usually discuss my own disability in this class. The disabled authors we are reading offer us enough testimonials, I think, to get us up to speed on what it's like to be physically or mentally impaired. But tonight, because of our topic and because my head is killing me, I think you need to hear what has been going on with me these last couple of days."

And so I told them. I told them everything. They heard about the university doctors' twisted excitement about my special case (I had lectured that night about the "*spectacle* of disabled medicine"), their apparent willingness to hurt me in order to help me ("the need to cure disability at all costs"), my feelings about wanting to take care of this for the sake of me and my wife, who had been helping me for months to ease the pain ("disability guilt"), and my decision to get a second opinion ("the medical model of disability makes it clear that people with disabilities must play an active role in their own treatment").

Because I had decided to balance my disabled identity and academic focus, I was free to run my class this way. It had been my decision, not someone else's. My students learned as much as I did that night. After my tooth narrative, I opened the rest of our session up to questions and discussion, needing a break from talking with a sore mouth. As I listened to my students (only one of whom was visibly disabled) discuss their own awkward experiences with doctors, I realized what an amazing conversation this had been. No matter what body type, we were participating in a communal discussion about issues that mattered to all of us.

REFERENCES

Albrecht, Gary L., et al. *The Disability Studies Handbook.* Thousand Oaks, CA: Sage, 2001.

Davis, Lennard (Ed.). *The Disability Studies Reader.* New York: Routledge, 1997.

Dibernard, Barbara. "Teaching What I'm Not: An Able-Bodied Woman Teaches Literature by Women with Disabilities." In Katherine J. Mayberry (Ed.), *Teaching What You're Not: Identity Politics in Higher Education,* 131–54. New York: New York University Press.

Linton, Simi. "Disability Studies/Not Disability Studies." *Disability and Society* 13 (1998): 525–40.

Longmore, Paul K. "Uncovering the Hidden History of Disabled People." *Why I Burned My Book and Other Essays on Disability,* 42–64. Philadelphia: Temple University Press, 2003.

———, and Umansky, Laurie (Eds.). *The New Disability History: American Perspectives.* New York: New York University Press, 2001.

Stiker, Henri-Jacques. *A History of Disability.* Trans. William Sayers. Ann Arbor, MI: University of Michigan Press, 1999.

Zames, Frieda, and Zames Fleischer, Doris. *The Disability Rights Movement: From Charity to Confrontation.* Philadelphia: Temple University Press, 2001.

QUESTIONS

1. Discuss the author's perspective on how one's physical disability often brings expectations of political activism.
2. How might having a disability enhance or hinder one's scholarly work in the field of disability studies?
3. What is noteworthy in the brief history of disability studies this author provides?
4. Discuss the author's tone and voice in this authoethnographic essay.

Losing My Dirty Mind

⌒ ANDREA T. WAGNER ⌒

My eyes open and fixate on the cream cheese that droops from the knife blade onto the coarse brow of our kitchen carpeting. My mother's hands shake my shoulder and hip with delicate urgency. "Honey, are you all right?"

My bagel smokes in the toaster.

I struggle to sit up, to defy the horizontal pull of my involuntary fantasy: Mrs. Glick, my first-grade teacher, with a basketball, with a spatula. Mrs. Glick with long fluorescent light bulbs, with a wet golden retriever.

I work to answer my mother.
To speak, to hear. I cannot find my ears or my
Voice.
Basketball. Spatula.
Only about a third of me is present—perhaps some ribs and maybe my right foot.
Fluorescent light bulbs.
I work not to see what my mind is already seeing (wet golden retriever), what has entered my vision (spatula), without passing my eyes.

"Dirt is matter out of place."

*I am in doctors' offices. Almost immediately, chains of them. "Teenage girls," we are told, "often experience **feelings of unreality**."*

Unreality?

There are many unrealities here. My doctors' dismissive diagnoses are unreal to me still today, twenty years after being sent home with the name of a good adolescent psychologist jotted too neatly on crisp white paper. Or perhaps it is the neatness of that paper that highlights a more important "unreality": my effort to communicate, then or now, these "feelings." Because it's not really possible. These "feelings" are actually epileptic seizures that fundamentally deny me the ability to know them, much less to write them or speak them or make them in any way *crisp*.

Doctor 1 asks, "So what are your seizures like?" I tell him something, anything. He writes things down. He calls in Doctor 2, who happens to be wearing exactly the same clothes as Doctor 1. "So what are your seizures like?" he asks. So I tell him something, anything. He writes things down. "Is that like #5^^Si9)@K or is it more like 4v(7&s?" I don't know.

I have no idea what I *experienced* during that first seizure in the kitchen.

He calls in Doctor 3, who looks a little older and has a longer coat. "So what are your seizures like?" he asks and I tell him something, anything. He writes things down.

Yes, my mother found me on the floor in front of the refrigerator. Yes, I was sweating. These details are the fallout, not the eruption. They are not the seizure itself.

*"But you told me they were like #fxo(**p2," says Doctor 2, and Doctor 1 concurs.*

The seizure (Mrs. Glick, light bulbs, basketballs) must be made up.

Epilepsy is characterized by the intermittent inability of brainwaves to remain *in place*, which, of course, results in the intermittent inability of the mind and/or body to remain *in place*.

My seizures have come in a variety of shapes and sizes, some packaged in deceptively pleasant French words like "petit," others mired in the many syllables of medical-speak. But after pulling in the broad nets of naming, The Narrative of My Experience is necessarily fictional.

The three doctors pull out the results of my MRI and EEG and nod in unison. "They must feel like r299!$sp%." Before I can answer, they all smile and write things down.

Of course all narrative is fictional to some extent. Experience is always too tidily wrapped in a story.

*"Mrs. Wagner-Martin," Doctor 3 addresses my mother, who is a scholar and a doctor in her own right. "What does Andrea look like when she is having a seizure?" Doctors 1 and 2 grunt and nod at the clever new question. "iP9*mnT," my mother replies. "It is 4Ffesiz*&asi_sth," all three say definitively.*

Academia knows well the partial, complex nature of representation. It just gets a little trickier when that which is to be represented is, for example, a partial, complex seizure of the left temporal lobe: A Home of Language.

And so I am always a failure and liar. But I answer the doctors' questions and try to create for them the fantasy that they have experienced mine.

I am sitting in class—pick any college classroom with pale laminate tables and mismatched chairs—trying to listen, write, answer, learn. And probably look pretty. Or at least cool in some shoulder-padded blazer and parachute pants with more zippers than my backpack. It is the Duran Duran era. My hair, I confess, is huge.

Resigned to endure the turmoil of my interior, I hunger for a smooth exterior. I would be polished like a stone. I hound the cosmetic section of the Rite Aid. My neck, that tender joint of mind and body, is often marred with a pasty copper line. My lips are over-sticked in a false, but consistent, smile. A matte happiness. A costume of constancy I relish.

"Andrea, what do you think?" my teacher asks me, directly. I have been his savior from silence. I can always say something, usually a smart something.

I thought I could defy my disability by denying it spectators. If I looked good, no one saw my sickness. If no one saw my sickness, it did not exist.

"Ahhhh," I reach into my head. Ginsberg. Contemporary. Poem.

I applaud my body for its good behavior and feel morally superior to those with more severe seizure disorders. I could control *my body*, even when my limbs were numb, my tongue was bloody, or bizarre visions/scents/sounds overtook varying parts of my consciousness. I could *appear*.

The sweat coats my back.

It is starting again.

The process of writing this essay (?) has made me confront how deeply invested I am—and we all are—in the collective avoidance of the dirt that is disorder. I long to forecast the points I will make, to give myself and you, the audience, the comfort of an outline to follow.

"Andrea, you raised your hand. What is on your mind?"

So much, swirling: Basketball. Jenny's body blurring, contorting, a lava lamp of pink cable knit. "It seems to me," I sputter. God, please don't do this again. The strong stench of a skunk, sour, like old anger in the back of my throat. Breathe, breathe through it. Flour. Tires. The cat's clean paws. "Not. Enough. Rhyme."

I began to crave being seen. I wanted to be *seen*, even if not heard.

Like a metronome I click out the obvious.

"Okay . . . ?" The teacher exhales his disappointment. I want to drop my head in shame but I

can't. The path in my brain is flooded and I stare blankly out over the water: the rolling eyes are a river around me. "Andrea's observation is a lack of rhyme and unpredictable meter. Yes?"

Oh, yes. Very unpredictable meter.

Thinking about dirt requires us to *not* classify it into familiar patterns, to perceive and engage the chaos we have been (perhaps neurologically) trained to either organize or ignore.

Being a mannequin was a lonely endeavor. I had few *friends*, focused as I was on *admirers*. I sought ways to garner them, looking always to show off my perfect *presentation* of a healthy, happy young woman. I got hooked on fooling people. I made a game of it, stepping into every spotlight I could find.

My eyes open and then quickly close against the bright light.

I challenged myself to be there on the stage, behind the podium, or in front of the television camera. I did not dare to *think* on my feet, but I could *stand* on them—very publicly—well-rehearsed and teleprompted. I became a newscaster. I savored every second, loving—

"Oh, God," my sister-in-law trembles. Her sandals are a grainy leather. My head rolls from side to side. "Here, let me put this washcloth on your mouth." "She'll be a little dazed for a while," says a man's voice. "It's bleeding bad." I hear the ocean and roll toward it. "You've had a seizure and I called him. He's a doctor." A doctor is coming? I sit up and fumble for some make-up in my tote bag. "No, he's here." "I'm right here. I don't think lipstick is a good idea right now."

—the attention, the sexual attention, that affirmed my "normalcy."

I drop back into the sand. I am a grand mal now. My sister-in-law wedges a clean towel underneath me, wrapping it around my waist. A sarong to hide my bathing suit, wet with my urine. I am dirty, I tell her. Disgusting. The doctor gives me Valium. The sun sets on assurances that it'll be okay.

But the more I understand, the less it is okay. I spend that night vomiting myself back to life so that I can spend the next day rediscovering my body, cursing each electrocuted limb, wondering what my brain is really able to wonder. **What have I lost this time?** *Usually it's memory (short-term? long-term?) and the ability to process language (read difficult information, follow fast conversations, talk) for a while, at least several days, maybe a week, maybe forever.* **What have I lost this time?**

The next morning I wake to find the ends of things: the end of my vacation, the end of my arm, the end of my career. The on-camera job I was slated to get at CNN is as distant as my fingers. I can no longer be in the public eye because I can no longer control the rolling and gaping of my own. I am a grand mal now.

I have forgotten a good quote. Imagine something poignant.

Limp, I walk out to the pool, where I spend the morning swimming alone. My body flowing with Valium, the water is like honey against my skin. I watch myself in the reflective glass of the hotel doors along the patio—in all the doors, my contorted image is refracted and repeated. I will quit my job in New York and go back to graduate school. I will be a critic rather than a practitioner of journalism. I will be safe in graduate school, hidden by library carrels and the smooth anonymity of intellectual image.

Pulling her pages out of a faded yellow folder, I am surprised that I had ever curled up with Judith Butler's challenging writing on the performance of gender. And yet each photocopy feels like an old blanket, worn soft with the affection of use. Those ideas were very important to me. In them I found a way to understand how I was "doing," "constructing" my body/my self.

The doctor stands over the pool again and again, saying something about getting out . . . safety . . . drowning risk . . . yeah, whatever. I lick the beads of water off my lips, waxy with a tinted sun-screen. "You're the most glamorous convulsive I've ever seen," he says.

Femininity, Butler argues, is comprised of a constellation of performable behaviors—choices to cross legs, fold hands, and hold the head just so. I learned that the somewhat paradoxical *safety* I experienced trying to be desirable was derived from my culture's support of a "normalized" role for young women. It was a scripted role. And I began to question that script, now a tangible book I could shelve or leaf through. I understood, for the first time, I think, that I was performing not just stereotypical femininity, but also, to some extent, *health*.

☞ ☜

Sick bodies are filled in, glossed over, and made up in most journalistic accounts. News stories of illness are typically restitutional: they trumpet heroes who have bravely fought dire circumstances to earn their unambiguously happy endings. Only the recovered get covered in the news. A gesture of ritualization that affirms the "immortality" of personal and social bodies, the stories transform the chaotic and the "dirty" into the comprehensible and controlled. The body of the sick is "made nice" to comfort its spectators. News coverage is, in this context, more a blanket to hide illness than a means of elaborating it. As a result, most news' attention to illness is actually attention to the absence of illness, paradoxically silencing (and shaming) those who continue to contend with the lingering effects of illness long after they are proclaimed better.

Paragraphs like this covered her. Like the news stories she was critiquing, her scholarship throughout much of her doctoral training purported to make public insights about illness and disability, all the while burying them in her own life story. She made intellectual choices that allowed her to *approach yet elide* her own health concerns. She opted to study illnesses (AIDS, cancer, asthma) that she does not have, and, perhaps more significantly, she employed research methods that were the symbolic (if not neuralgic) antithesis of her epilepsy. She sought out certainty and predictability, cause and effect; she was focused on quantitative research, much to the shock of her former mentors in the arts and humanities. She saw quantitative work as an intellectual cove of "coding schemes" where conversations about "the body"—certainly the scholar's body—were out of the realm of possibility because they were out of the realm of "Objectivity." She wanted to (want to) do studies in which words like "control" and "reliability" were standard. She wanted to (want to) write in the third person, the omniscient voice, the clean, confident voice of all-knowingness, which she could construct, on paper, to conceal her *own* voice, intrinsically prone to the *partial*, the *forgotten*, the *fictional*, the *lost*.

In this way, she wrote her own restitution fairy tale into the subtext of her scholarly work. With false enthusiasm, it read: "*I am fine! My seizure disorder left me with no liabilities or advantages! My work is just like others' work because my brain is like others' brains!*" She tried desperately to make this true, performing The Scholar, complete with mystifying props like calculators and graph paper. But finally, she was simply bad at it, and in the fissures of her frustration she found the epistemic discontinuity of her work and the brain that was doing it. In an early study, for example, she tried to operationalize "confidence" as a variable in a survey of patients' feelings about medical journalism. Her goal was to construct a net of questions that captured "confidence" totally and consistently. Confidence: contentment, constancy, assuredness . . . irony filling each pause when she would spit into a cup. She had had a bad seizure the night before and the side of her mouth was still bleeding. She wondered if she needed stitches as she noticed that her work was choppy, staccatoed by her pauses to clear her mouth.

And she realized that she needed to clear my head, too.

⸙ ⸙

Hmmmm.

How to write a scene that captures my confidence in my seizure disorder? How to theorize this new comfort? How to convey the pleasure I have found in my unreliable brainwaves and my unreliable voice, trying, in its own recalcitrant way, to pour my impermanence (impertinence?) onto the page?

Perhaps this question is its own answer. Perhaps the act of asking is telling.

Before class I try to smooth my blouse flat against my reluctantly flat stomach. A brush through my hair, a blot of powder. Futile. I rehearse what I will say and who I will call on, all noted in bold fonts in long notes. I rehearse so that I am less likely to forget. I forget a lot. But often I don't know I am forgetting, as when I stand before my students and my sentence falls

  off a

       cliff, and I look over the edge, running my scarred tongue over my teeth, hoping some crumb, some word, of it is trapped there. But it seldom is. Often, it is just a word, one simple word, which pushes my problems out into the public. As when I hold up a chalk-board eraser and call it a guitar. Or a stapler. Or a peach. There is laughter and I suspect the synaptic tie between the symbol and the sign is scarred, too, and I no longer have the means to make it right. So I turn to some eager-eyed, A-student—much like myself before the onset of my epilepsy, much like myself, still, on good days—who will say, "the eraser, you mean?" And I trust her. I have to trust her. And I am glad.

Matter out of place is "dirty" only when we choose to value matter that is *in* place.

I wrote my first "convulsive text" four years ago. The idea to fragment and jumble portions of *this* essay (?) was not new. What is new, now, at its end, is my ability to admit to recycling of any sort. My early draft was replete with old anger, sour in the back of my throat, yellowing my pages. I would make my audience struggle with a textual incarnation of the discontinuity I knew so well. I would make my audience earn my story, a smattering of spare change in thick grass.

"That isn't exactly how it happened, Sis," says my mother, who has always called me "Sis." She's always called me a storyteller, too. It's her English-professor euphemism for my tendency to embellish, which is, of course, another euphemism for my tendency to lie. Or to not really know. To not really know how it happened "exactly" or to not really know how it is happening "exactly." Things—in past tense or present—are loose for me. My mother's gentle correction is unusual. Her "ohhhhs" and "wows" are the scaffolding of most of my (tall?) tales. Standing around her kitchen, I rehearse my life into tidy packages like the petits-fours hidden on the top shelf above toaster. My mother is still my audience, my consciousness for (the lingering effects of) my varying degrees of unconsciousness.

The anger is gone now and I am tempted to return to the grass metaphor in the last non-italicized section and say something like "my lawn is mowed," but, no, that would be heavy-handed, silly, and making too much of an image that does not appear in the rest of this piece. This consideration is important because it highlights the *continuity* of the rest of the piece. It is there, it's just a little cryptic at times. I have worked to instill it, to balance the chaotic and the cogent. So please take my claims to celebrate "matter out of place" with a grain of, well, dirt; these claims, too, are "unreal." These claims, too, are only partial . . . what? Partial what?

I am frothing at the mouth again
> *I am an excellent teacher, my students like me, I like them, and the library,*
> *and my computer, I just graduated in December and have had lots of ex-*
> *perience, well, relative to a lot of graduate students, academia is my family*
> *business, so to speak,*
> *or not to speak . . .*

with the dread of another little death
> *Did you read my epilepsy essay? I can actually function perfectly well, most*
> *days, like, no one would know I have any dis/abilities, oh, you probably*
> *loathe those back-slashes, too po-mo, too self-promo, I don't really use them*
> *too much, Did you read that essay, you know, **that** essay?*

spilling me out on the floor, on my back,

I'm not, you know, an exhibitionist or anything, all that body stuff, the sexual stuff, I mean, I am straight, but I don't need everybody, every man, I'm not heterosexist, to be attracted to me anymore, I used to, but not anymore, I don't even wear lipstick anymore, well, most days, I mean, today is special, this interview and all

with my neck, that tender joint of mind and body,

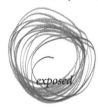

and I can write normally really well, I won the creative writing prizes when I was an undergrad, not that I always have to write creatively, I got my Ph.D. to, like, garner authority, you know, so I could write authoritatively, so my ideas would be respected, so I could be, you know, out there . . .

I now write only in the I-voice as an effort to signal and embrace the limitations and privileges of my perspective. Third person seems audacious to me. And a little boring. Its definitive statements—diagnoses of sorts—are prescriptive (proscriptive?) and can inhibit the imagination of the audience: it knows what it is *supposed* to know. Creativity stems from uncertainty: this is something I can offer, I think, staging scholarship that is akin to contemporary poetry. I hope the meter is a little unpredictable. My goal now, after my anger, after my failed attempts to be cleaned up and smoothed over, is to invite my audience to fill in my (our?) blanks, considering first what can be found in "dirty" spaces.

REFERENCES

Douglas, Mary. *Purity and Danger: An Analysis of the Concepts of Pollution and Taboo.* London: Routledge, 1966.

Butler, Judith. "Performative Acts and Gender Constitution: An Essay in Phenomenology and Feminist Theory." *Performing Feminisms: Feminist Critical Theory and Theatre*, ed. Sue-Ellen Case, 270–282. Baltimore: Johns Hopkins University Press, 1990.

QUESTIONS

1. Comment on the author's form. How does it relate to the content of the essay? Why does the author choose to jumble her story with short paragraphs and a variety of typefaces?
2. How does the author's seizure disorder shape her experience as a student, scholar, and teacher?
3. Discuss how the author casts physicians in this narrative. How do their questions impact her experience of her illness? How might the author's clinical encounters have been improved?
4. How does epilepsy influence the author's life goals, physical appearance, and sexual identity? What does this story tell us about the cultural construction of "normalcy" and the "visibility" of illness? Comment on the ways society leads us to "perform" health and illness.

Making the Impossible Possible
Imagining Alternative Experiences of Pain

⌁ Elena Levy-Navarro ⌁

> *We must keep vigilant about our discourses, the ones we pronounce as well as the one we accede to, sometimes with nothing "more" than our silence. The discourses make certain actions and phenomena possible and others impossible by making them rational or not rational.*
> —*Jesse, Nov. 20, 2002*

How does our prevailing discourse affect the way that we experience "pain"? What types of experience does our discourse make possible, or impossible, in our contemporary capitalistic American society? I use my own struggle with the pain that accompanies my chronic migraines to explore these questions, focusing especially on two very different responses to pain that I have had. First, I have internalized, to my detriment, the belief that pain is always undesirable because it impairs the normal functions of life. If I could not rid myself of it, I reasoned, I could at the very least "manage" it. Second, I have come to see pain as something that brings me closer to those around me exactly because I can no longer maintain the illusion of rational self-mastery and autonomy. I must instead admit that I am defeated and, what's more important, give way to sensations, feelings, and thoughts that I normally work very hard to control. I know in my pain that I am part of a common humanity and I feel that connection intensely in and through my very body. Only through the second response can I come to cultivate the type of transformative attachments I desire with the people I love.

For most of my life, I have played what are sometimes dangerous and certainly painful games of self-mastery. As a young woman, I reveled in anorexia, enjoying each pound lost, each missed meal, each pang of hunger, because it proved to me that I was, indeed, able to follow a regimen to its logical conclusion. Later, I imposed upon myself lengthy starvation diets, which brought with them similar pleasures of knowing that I could always subdue my body with my superior mind. Such regimens offered visible proof of superior self-mastery over what was presumed to be an ugly, offensive, resistant body. It should be no surprise that I approached the pain of my migraines with similar games.

In the beginning, I thought I could employ rational mastery over migraines to assure that I kept on going, no matter the pain I felt. Sadly, I can see this same impulse even in my very recent email correspondence with my dear friend and fellow Renaissance scholar, Jesse. I anatomize myself, diagnose myself, lay myself before him in the hope that we two together might find the means to overcome once and for all these troublesome migraines. Failing this, I reason, he will at least recognize the superiority evident in my self-mastery. He frustrates me, lovingly, with a variety of simple human responses, which I predictably find infuriating because he refuses to play my game. He offers simple expressions of sympathy—"I'm so sorry to read of your continued and intense migraines. I will have to say a special prayer for relief"—and sensible advice: "I still think you don't sleep enough, that you don't lounge enough, especially after stressful or otherwise taxing events (like our Miami trip)." Perhaps most infuriating, he celebrates the irrational states of mind that accompany my migraines: "I fear that I love the manner of thinking you fall into during your migraine episodes" or "I'm so sorry to hear of your head-ache, though, as you know, I think you think the most fascinating things in such conditions." Isn't it amazing, I think, that the thing that annoys us most is love?

I struggle as hard as I can to avoid giving way to the irrationality that accompanies migraines. Rather than spend any time experiencing the sometimes glorious states that migraines impart, I try to be as *productive* as possible. Notably, my migraines increased as I became a productive adult and took my place in the academic marketplace. Such onslaughts, I reasoned, must be met with equal and opposite force. I insisted on going to work when I experienced a migraine, even though it was overwhelmingly difficult to get through my day. If need be, I would wear dark sunglasses to class, turn off the lights, and do whatever else I could to make my time there bearable. Occasionally, I would even take my pain medication, the narcotic butalbital—only if absolutely necessary, however, since it has the effect of making it difficult for me to think. While I would have said at the time that pain was undesirable, it was obviously much more undesirable for me to be in any state of mind that I recognized as irrational and thus, from the perspective of a professional, *unproductive*. Pain must never interfere with my productivity, nor could I take any anti-pain medication that would render me unproductive. When I simply could not go to work, I worked at home. My drapes drawn, my room dark, a cold compress on my head, my head in pain, my stomach upset, my left extremities numb or tingling, I nonetheless forced myself to turn on the light next to my bed, to the lowest setting, of course. I searched the pile of books nearby for the one that I might be able to read. If I couldn't read theory, then I picked a simpler narrative; if I couldn't read that, I looked for anything I might be able to read. When I couldn't read at all, I had my husband bring me books on tapes; and when I couldn't do that, I turned on the radio. There I lay, falling in and out of consciousness, but always, always, always forcing myself to "think." When I consider now how utterly absurd this activity is, I think that I was instead performing certain rituals in an effort to keep myself from slipping away from the type of controlled consciousness that our culture values so much. To insist that I can use my will and discipline to remain productive is to align myself with those in power. I can't lose control even in the most private moments of my life because to do so, I assume, would be to lose my status as one of the professional class.

Significantly, my professional position does not account for my gripping fear of being rendered unproductive. No one is going to chuck me out on the streets if I miss a class or two; no one is going to fire me if I don't finish this or that article. Playing such games of self-mastery suggests that the point isn't productivity in an objective sense but the control that is exerted overall. Mercifully, the pain sometimes overwhelms me so completely that there isn't much else to do but to give myself over to it. At these times, my husband takes me to my primary care physician, who gives me a shot of Demerol with an anti-nausea drug that finally allows me to collapse onto my bed and rest. I've only received this shot on a few occasions because it frightens me so much. Indeed, the first time I ever got Demerol, I remember panicking as I felt it take hold of my body. As the numbing sensation grew simultaneously from both my genitals and my head, I began speaking faster and faster, sometimes giving directions to my husband, sometimes merely finishing whatever I had been saying and describing the sensations to my husband as they occurred. He spoke to me calmly, urging me just to "give in" to the sensation, to allow myself to feel for a moment the way in which the pain was subsiding from my body.

At this point, I am well aware that someone could diagnose me with some sort of psychological pathology—perhaps one of those mood disorders recently recognized as co-morbid with migraine—but surely the larger point is that these little games of mine participate in our dominant discourse. The history of migraines is a fascinating one. When my grandmother and her sisters suffered from migraines as young women, the pain was called "sick headaches" and was generally associated with the nervousness of women. Later, medicine came to speak of a "migraine personality," an achievement-oriented personality much as I am describing here. Although medicine has now discounted this idea of the "migraine personality," it emphasizes the need to look for "co-morbid conditions," many of them psychological in nature. What is insidious about this new emphasis is the way it requires the patient to subject herself to a lifelong treatment plan for both the mood disorder and the migraine.

In the pages that follow, I examine the prevailing discourse of the headache industry in order to show how it ensures that the insured remain productive workers. I do not want to be misunderstood as attacking medical practitioners, since I am well aware of the many kindnesses that I have received at the hands of many physicians and nurses. That said, even well-meaning physicians often direct their treatment more toward helping me return to work as quickly as possible rather than simply helping me feel better.

When I recently went to the emergency room for an intensely painful and debilitating migraine, the presiding physician absolutely refused to give me the Demerol that I knew I needed, because, as he told me after he asked about my profession, it would prevent me from being alert the next day. Several years before this, my primary care physician prescribed what was then a relatively new migraine-specific drug, saying that it would allow me to return to work shortly after I took it. In both cases, the physicians proved to be primarily interested in my work and productivity. They assumed that pain should be treated, but not in a way that would further impede my ability to think in a clear fashion. Indeed, the emergency room physician employed language that was morally charged to convince me that I need to be concerned primarily with my productivity. He assured me that *I wouldn't want* the Demerol after all, thereby implying that if I did want it, I must be an irresponsible professional, if not an irresponsible human being. In this catch-22, only the patient who doesn't want the pain relief is worthy of it.

Such physicians are only acting out the assumptions that dominate the prevailing discourse of the headache industry. A disease is seen as a problem when it interferes with normal function or the ability to work and be productive. One of the two tools used to evaluate the severity of headaches, the migraine disability assessment (MIDAS) focuses intensely on productivity at work. Of five questions, two are devoted to work outside the home, two to "housework," and only one to "family, social, or leisure activities" (ahsnet.org). Indeed, an offshoot of the American Headache Society, the American Council of Headache Education, lists as two of its primary goals to help the patient "achieve a pain-free state" and to "allow the sufferer to return to normal activities as quickly as possible" (achenet.org). Such goals assume that the patient must always want to return to her normal activities as quickly as possible.

Such an emphasis is mirrored in advertisements for the expensive name-brand, migraine-specific drugs. Focusing especially on overextended, young, white, working women, such commercials urge them to "Take control" and "Don't give in" in a way that places a high value on work (Maxalt). The young woman's goal should be to resume normal activities as soon as possible, no matter how taxing they are. Such advertisements gloss over real-life pressures facing these women. Ads never show the woman in danger of being fired, for instance; instead, they suggest that she *wants* to continue a seemingly fulfilling professional life. Equally importantly are such advertisements' emphases on gender expectations to manipulate the woman into feeling that she is required to return to work as soon as possible. A number of these advertisements purposefully collapse her maternal and work roles, thereby implying that she must resume her responsibilities in *both* domains without regard to her individual private needs.

One such television advertisement focuses on a nurse working in the newborn ward of a hospital. After taking her Imitrex, she is shown returning to work in a noisy, fluorescent-lit environment. In the last sequence, she beams for a photograph taken by a father in which the nurse cradles his infant. The nurse would have missed out on a glorious experience, the commercial suggests, if she had been irresponsible enough to give way to her pain. Such images encourage us to believe that only self-indulgent, even slovenly, women want to stay at home to sleep off a migraine instead of serving others.

The very same assumptions are evident in the first issue of *Headache Profiles*, pamphlets created by the American Headache Society to help train physicians and would-be physicians to diagnose and treat commonly seen headaches. Each "case vignette" begins with a quotation that is designed to encapsulate the profile of the patient. In this case, the 28-year-old kindergarten teacher, Sarah, married and with a 3-year-old son, complains, "My kids need me. I don't want to miss any more days" (Campbell, 1). This statement suggests that Sarah wants nothing more than to sacrifice herself for "her kids," presumably both her biological child and the children of her workplace. Indeed, the case study makes it clear that Sarah suffers from "infrequent but severe headaches" and so could presumably take the necessary time off work to recover (1). As a good nurturer, however, Sarah is shown as selflessly caring for "her kids" at work and at home, where they must never be inconvenienced by her. When recommending a course of treatment, the director of the "Headache Management Program" takes this supposed need of the children into account as much as she does the general well-being of Sarah. After insisting that Sarah is one of those who should be treated with migraine-specific drugs, the director suggests that the physician especially consider choosing the one that offers Sarah "a discreet, convenient way of taking medication without leaving her kindergarten classroom" (3).

Notably, productivity isn't even the primary goal here; hiding pain and feigning wellness is. In whose interest is it really for Sarah to be so obsessively discreet? Is it in the kids' interest, the school's interest, or our larger corporate culture's interest? One explanation is that children should be taught in a sanitized environment, where they never witness the pain of others, especially their caretakers. But this deprives children of the important knowledge that pain is a normal part of human life. Children could learn—as I did, for example, when I sat in a partially darkened room when my mother suffered from migraines—that their mothers don't exist only for them. Equally importantly, children could learn that they can actively help someone else—if just by remaining a bit quieter than usual. Surely, the obsession with hiding pain seems more pathological than the supposed pathology itself.

Also significant is the director's argument for prescribing more expensive migraine-specific medication instead of less expensive generic drugs, based not on their efficacy but rather on their "cost–effectiveness":

> As a busy mother and kindergarten teacher, Sarah probably cannot afford the drowsiness or reduced performance associated with many nonspecific headache medications. Despite the fact that these medications may be cheaper than newer, more targeted drugs, the "costs" in lost work time, reduced job performance and attentiveness associated with sedative medications are important to consider. Migraine is a lifelong illness which is most active during the busy middle years of a woman's life. It is therefore hard to [justify sending the message to the] patient that the way to handle [pain] is to "check out" by taking a medication that causes drowsiness or impairs function. (Campbell, *Headache Profiles*, 4)

The director seems much more concerned with profits and losses to corporations and the people Sarah is to serve than with human suffering. Corporations will save money, she argues, even if they have to bear the cost of these more expensive brand-name drugs, because they will have more efficient, productive workers. I am most disturbed in reading this to find that the director uses economic language metaphorically to describe the choices that are made by the middle-class migraineuse: Sarah can't "afford" to take narcotics because they will lead to "reduced performance." This rhetoric suggests that our lives are primarily evaluated in monetary terms.

As a final example, I examine the "bad girl" complement to Sarah. In another headache pamphlet, Jennifer is offered as an example of the dangers of drug overuse. She says, "I just need this refill, unless there's something stronger I could try" (1.3). In what follows, Jennifer is quickly brought under the supervision and surveillance of a number of medical professionals, even as the physician is urged to remind such types that they should expect lifelong treatment. Thus, in the section entitled "Communication and Compliance," the expert explains, "Many patients desire a simple diagnosis and a straightforward cure—the hope for a 'find and fix' solution—and it may take some convincing to get them to accept the concept of ongoing treatment" (5). Although Jennifer never complains of a mood disorder, she is immediately diagnosed as having "adjustment reaction with anxiety and depression" (2). The clinical psychologist to whom she is immediately referred confirms this diagnosis and adds that Jennifer has had "previous bouts of mood disturbance." She is now placed on a lifelong treatment plan, much of which consists of monitoring of her drug intake. Such patients are assumed to be irresponsible, perhaps because they expect treatment for their pain. Among the detailed advice on how to manage such a program, the expert warns repeatedly of the need of the physician to monitor and communicate clearly about the restrictions placed on her medication use. The recommendation that "instructions and limitations, written directly on the prescription, [should] emphasize to the patient (and pharmacist) your determination to closely monitor drug use" (5) indicates that physician and pharmacist act in conjunction to police Jennifer's drug use.

My own games of self-mastery obviously participate in the discourse illustrated above, especially insofar as it values productivity and rational self-control. I am no different than Sarah in my desire to subordinate myself to my job and never allow myself time to rest or think aimlessly. What differentiates me is the odd fact that the type of rational self-control I cultivate so obsessively is at odds with the type of creativity I need in order to explore alternative subjectivities, including those of the Renaissance period I study. It is primarily through my friendship with Jesse that I am free to explore. Above all, this language affects the type of experiences that are possible and impossible and thus the type of relationships we can and can't enjoy.

If the discourse of the headache industry is proscriptive, then the more flexible, occasional language of my friendship with Jesse offers an alternative way to understand and experience the pain that sometimes accompanies my migraines. Especially in our continuous email interchanges, we give voice to the most mundane pains of our bodies. As I speak to him of such seemingly negligible concerns, I experience my body differently. His descriptions of his own experiences offer me another way to speak, even as the playful questions push me to consider the dehumanizing effects of the reified medical discourse I employ. Even my most sincere expressions of concern for him can be coercive, I come to see, because I insist on imposing on his experiences a singular and inflexible view of the body and its experiences. Fortunately, he rebuffs me in ways that expose the assumptions behind my use of language. To my concern that he is depressed, Jesse responds with the simple question: "About depression and its diagnosis, what is the difference between depression and melancholy, depression and elegiac pleasure, besides the grammatical one?" Jesse draws on our shared knowledge of Renaissance poetry to suggest creative ways to experience the state I call simply "depression." Prompted by him, I imagine and experience the virtues of, for example, elegiac pleasure through our shared literary vocabulary. Even as the poet meditates upon and commemorates a deceased companion, he feels a pleasure in that mourning. How glorious, I think, to experience this sense of ennobling sadness at the parting of a friend, yet to know that this friend is always partially present in one's future. Chameleon-like, Jesse encourages a sort of imaginative exploration in which I am made aware of the provisional or constructed nature of experience. He describes my migraine in a variety of playful ways that challenge my unique experience of that phenomenon; through his language, I experience "a migraine episode," "migraines," "head-ache," "painful malaise," "dis-ease," to name just a few. His words function to deconstruct those classifications I have taken as real and natural. Introducing the hyphen into words like "head-ache" and "dis-ease," Jesse calls attention to the subjective origins of terms which are oppressive insofar as they are taken as strictly denotative. In asking myself, as I do, what the first person may have meant when she used the word "head-ache," I come to think of the term in a far different, more productive way.

In short, Jesse's language helps me attend more closely to my own bodily experiences and consider how best to describe them. Am I experiencing a single phenomenon represented by the term "migraine," or multiple phenomena? What difference would it make to think of the migraine in singular or multiple ways? In one of the more playful "literary" responses, Jesse expresses concern for my well-being by saying, "I've been wondering how your migraines have been treating you. I don't know why, but I always think of them in the plural. Somehow this makes you seem all the more besieged, though Leda certainly felt besieged enough with just one swan." His expression of sympathy calls into question my own insistence of thinking in terms of one migraine, indeed, of one pathology, migraine with aura, that strikes again and again. Finally, the entire expression is made in a playful, provisional way; indeed, his allusion draws on our common knowledge, both as scholars and individuals, to call attention to the way that my Swan, Jesse, frequently besieges me.

At other times, Jesse may offer in his expression of concern new ways to experience my migraines. He writes, "I do wish the migraine would subside or lift or dissipate or peter out or whatever it is migraines do or are experienced as doing." When I first read these words, I realized that I had never given much thought to how I conceptualize, implicitly, the way that a migraine might leave me. Jesse's gentle parody of my imbuing this phenomenon I call "migraine" with some objective power over me reveals that *it* does everything, I *nothing*. In his final phrase, "or are experienced as doing," Jesse shifts perspectives and thus suddenly undermines what has gone before. What had at first seemed objective descriptions of a migraine are now exposed as individual experiences. This shift in language suggests that the migraine has no objective importance in itself; only the individual experience of them matters.

Frequently, Jesse enters imaginatively into my detailed descriptions of pain in a way that underscores the problems inherent in them. In writing this essay, I am aware that I use language as I do to accommodate what I assume to be hostile or at least unfeeling, objective readers. Surely, they won't believe I have pain, I reason, unless I can document discreet material events that prove it. Even then, they won't care. In presuming such a reader, I force myself to offer a detached, objective view of my pain, which in turn precludes the reader from experiencing the pain with me. By contrast, in offering a description like the one that follows, I expect Jesse to respond with the sympathy I believe I deserve:

> Today, the migraine is worse than ever, so bad, in fact, that the pills I take seem to be doing nothing for it and I suspect that within moments I will be vomiting at my toilet, in a position, I must note, that will cause tremendous pain to my knee.

And, if I vomit, the pills won't be able to help me at all, and here I am without my husband available (and truly wanting to stop burdening him with what seems like endless illnesses).

To just such a description, Jesse writes, "I can't help but feel that, of course, you've written this description to be comic, even farcical. The knee, the vomiting, the pills, the migraine all together working one on top of the other—ah, life." He refuses to respond in the way that our culture demands, that *I* demand: with an expression of sympathy. Instead, he calls attention to the way that the writer imagines herself as a victim of a variety of forces outside her control, including her own body.

In another exchange, Jesse makes it clear what is at stake in our use of language. That is, he underscores the way that our narratives make certain relationships possible and others impossible. In responding honestly to what I write, he calls attention to the ways in which my language doesn't allow me to cultivate the type of sympathetic relationships I so desire. He draws on our own friendship, however, to appeal to me more directly: As your friend I would like nothing more than to feel your pain and in feeling it, feel sympathy for you; but your style precludes this. He writes:

> I don't know which attitude to allow myself to give way to concerning the hospital scene of Monday night you tacked onto your post proper. Do I give vent to the sense of charming tomfoolery I can feel the episode to be, or do I allow contempt to swell to the point of bursting in a most pathetic catharsis, which I feel the tightly associated causal actions of the mini-drama can suggest? When I think of the body of the central actor/character of the piece and the mise en scene, I only get further ambivalence of the nature I've just described. It's only when I experience the situation sympathetically that I can become alarmed and concerned about my dear friend Elena—she must be in severe distress of various sorts, I worry. But the description, somehow, does not encourage such a sympathetic reading. Surely the diction accounts for some of this, but it's also the modulation of rhythm in the prose—there's faster or more intense moments that disable possibilities to experience what's described, since the speed or intensity overwhelms the reader's experience. This then allows for the more intellectual consideration of the text, which leads to the more controlled consideration of it, which makes for unsympathetic reactions, either comic or tragic. You express yourself this way often and feel hurt or angry or violated or abused or neglected or so much else, since people are not giving you the sympathy you think you are so clearly SCREAMING for. What a fascinating case.

In reading his response, I realize the negative effects that my imaginary hostile reader has had on my language and thus on my relationships to other human beings. In my obsession to offer documentation, I don't allow my friend to experience my subjective experiences, even though my friend wants to feel such things if I would allow him. A more humane response to myself, ironically, allows for a more humane response from others—relationships built on sympathy rather than judgment. Such a stylistic change is necessary not only to extend relationships with friends I already love, but also to foster relationships with those yet unknown to me.

There have been moments, in fact, when I experience my pain very differently. In my vulnerability, I reach out to people around me as one vulnerable human being in need of another. Such relationships are not dependent on a sense of illusory superiority. In my most severe migraines, I have trouble speaking, I forget words, I misspeak, and I feel a gap widen between me and the people around me. A physician may speak—I may even understand her words as she speaks them—but I am aware that I don't understand how they fit together. At other times when I hear her speak, I know that whatever understanding I have will soon disappear. The words will mean nothing in only a few moments. Certainly, I won't remember the diagnoses she gives me or the drugs she prescribes. Perhaps because of this, I relate to these people from my body rather than from my "mind." What a relief in some ways to know that I can no longer even assert my status as a professional by demonstrating my rational mastery! I settle into a state that I would ordinarily and intolerably consider disempowered. Like the drunk, I need someone to pick me up and send me on my way, or I might just lie there, dying. Rather than feel distance between myself and others at these times, I feel intensely close to people around me. A gentle voice or touch can tell me simply that this person is there for me, one human being for another. Only in my weakness and pain can I finally abandon the illusion that I am utterly independent and utterly in control.

Such painful moments teach me that rather than try to suppress or manage my pain, I should allow myself to experience it. In doing this, I bring myself closer to those around me, whether to a presiding medical practitioner or to a good friend. I have come to see my body as the source of joy as well as pain, the source of potentially transformative experiences for myself and others. I am a vulnerable human being reaching out to others for a smooth touch, a kind word, and a little imagination.

REFERENCES

American Association for Study of Headache. *Headache Profiles* 1:1 (1990).

American Association for Study of Headache. *Headache Profiles* 1:3 (2000).

Imitrex. Advertisement. NBC. 8 Feb. 2003.

Maxalt. Advertisement. 31 Jan. 2003. <http://www.maxalt.com/rizatriptan_benzoate/maxalt/consumer/index.jsp>.

MIDAS Questionnaire. "Impact of Migraine: Measuring Disability." *American Council for Headache Education Web Site.* ACHE. 1 November 2002. <http://www.achenet.org/impact/measuring.shtml>.

"Migraine and Coexisting Conditions." *American Council for Headache Education Web Site.* ACHE. <http://www.achenet.org/news/macc.php>.

QUESTIONS

1. Comment on the relationship between illness and capitalism.
2. Discuss the ways language defines disease. To what extent do you agree with the author's ideas about altering language to alter the essence of pain?
3. What is the significance of the relationship between the author and her friend, and how does that inform her experience of illness?

Of Blood and Guts

 KIMBERLY R. MYERS 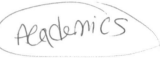 *[handwritten: Academics]*

[handwritten: can go back + reread]

It is only by putting it into words that I make it whole; this wholeness means that it has lost its power to hurt me; it gives me, perhaps because by doing so I take away the pain, a great delight to put the severed parts together.

—Virginia Woolf, from "A Sketch of the Past"

Maybe. Or maybe it will only cause me to dwell on it—what I fear, what I've lost, what I might never become. But maybe it will help me to heal or at least manage what I've been given to manage. Use the tools you have. Put your mind to work.

OCTOBER 1993

The week that changed my life. Last Friday we'd gone to see *Marvin's Room*, a play about a woman who has some sort of fatal disease. A lot of black humor . . . that I didn't find humorous. Vague misgivings as I sat there. I wore red and black, I remember, because I remember pulling off my clothes later that night after my life changed forever. 10:30 and I was tired. Friday after working all week. After the play. I went to the bathroom, and I knew something wasn't right. The toilet was filled with bright red blood. A lot of it.

Four days ago I'd eaten Mexican. The normal routine: friends getting together after seminar for some down time and to continue the conversations we'd had late that afternoon. So maybe, I'd reasoned the first time I saw the blood, maybe it was something that "didn't agree with me." And then, the next day, maybe it was hemorrhoids. But this was neither. Clearly. *[handwritten: why this structure?]*

Student health service on a Friday night. 10:45. I call and talk to a nurse, ask him if there's anything else it could be besides colon cancer. I've read the Seven Warning Signs of Cancer. Committed them to memory. He tells me yes but doesn't offer any more detail. Tells me I should be seen immediately in the morning.

Saturday morning and I can't sleep. It's pouring rain. It's fall and early morning. Pathetic fallacy, and I take it as a bad sign that the rain falls so thickly. I wait for an hour before

[handwritten: her thoughts]

the doctor sees me. She wears cowboy boots, and I like her because she is direct. She is built strong, and that gives me a kind of comfort. She sends me to the lab, where they draw five vials of blood. And then we wait. For four hours. The blood has to "settle" or something. I am too green at this point to understand the terms I would come to know all too well in the years that followed: Sed rate, BUN, albumin, CBC. One good thing: I would learn the language. I would learn more about my body than I ever thought I might.

She has coarse blond hair chopped unevenly and wears black jeans with the boots. She does a physical exam and tells me "you're a mess." After the blood work reveals nothing specific enough to tell her anything much, she sends me home and tells me to return on Monday. What will I do for that endless span of time between Saturday afternoon (the rain still pouring) and Monday morning? I can concentrate on nothing but the strange gurgling in my distal colon, at my rectum. Like constantly needing to use the bathroom. But afraid to. Can't stand the trauma of seeing that much blood. That's my LIFE there, poured out of me. I am dying.

> *Wild fear flapping madly*
> *About the tiled room*
> *Desperate to get out*

Saturday night we go into the city—just to a mall, just to get out. In the car driving there, I talk about colon cancer and plan my will. There is no humor here, no self-irony. There is only the keenest dread I've ever felt in my life, a gnawing terror. "A worm in hot ashes": no way to escape no matter how hard one wriggles. I comfort myself by saying that I have lived exactly as I have wanted to live. No regrets. No unfinished business. I sleep fitfully.

Sunday passes in a haze. I can do nothing productive. I call for the twentieth time to talk with my parents. I am keenly aware that there was a time when they could make everything okay. That time is past. This is far beyond them. Far beyond me.

If I can't control it, I decide, I will handle it with grace. Monday morning I return, determined to do the best with what I discover. I will live until I die (literally). I will not let this defeat me until it kills me. I'm at a teaching hospital. The booted doctor has asked a colleague to see me, but first I get his medical student, who takes my "patient history." A million questions, and I'm trying to figure out what each question could imply about what I might have. Not a good thing to second-guess a doctor—especially one in training. I am a strong advocate of learning, and I know this is important to him. I will be a good patient so that he can learn. He asks me very personal questions. And even though I've never been prudish or even overly private about my body, I find some of them uncomfortable. What words does one use to describe the appearance of excrement? I am asked to find the words, and I know their accuracy will factor into what comes next—the diagnosis, the prognosis. "Have you ever had anal sex?" "How many times do you go to the bathroom every day?" I do the best I can; I am as accurate as I can be, given I've never had to think about these questions before, much less tell my most intimate information to complete strangers. And I have to tell the same information to several different strangers. I ask the medical student what it could be—options other than cancer? He clearly has no idea, and I am so uncomfortable, so afraid that someone will tell me I am dying that I don't ask anymore. Not for a while.

I see a male doctor. Then the one with boots comes back. She tells me I must try to quantify the blood as accurately as I can. She hands me six clear rubber gloves like doctors use when examining patients. And popsicle sticks. I realize with a start what these items mean: they require me to play in shit. There's no pretty way to put it. It is a dirty, repulsive thing. And I must face it.

> *Hair standing on end*
> *I'm the madwoman*
> *Measuring her life*
> *In teaspoons*
> *In the first hours of morning*

I tell myself it's not too much. And then, from a different angle, six times as much appears. Like in *Catch 22:* they tell the bomber pilot he'll be okay, just flesh wounds. Then they roll him over and find half his belly blown away.

Kyrie eleison (Lord, have mercy). Please.

DEATH

I remember when I was a kid. Once I staged my own funeral. I imagined those people whose attention I wanted but never seemed to have fully: they would come and look at me and be sorry. I smile wryly at this memory. Death is often romanticized in our culture, just like suffering is. I used to consider how remarkable it was that John Keats lived only 25 years; his death at such an early age was so ineffably tragic. With time and distance and legend, it becomes Romantic. But I realize now that he watched his lifeblood erupt from his mouth every time he coughed. Watching the life inside him flow out and away. The pain of that—physical and emotional—was enormous. There is no Romance in this suffering.

LATE OCTOBER 1993

They tell me it's not cancer but inflammatory bowel disease. Could be one of two forms: ulcerative colitis or Crohn's disease. Hmmmm. Crohn's. Hearing the word only, I don't know how to spell it. I assume it's "crone's" and I wonder if having the disease means one has the wisdom of a crone, too. I don't know yet just how much wisdom this disease will bring to my life.

Both forms of IBD are categorized as "auto-immune" diseases: the body attacks itself. I read about this and infer that it's like the opposite of AIDS. My body's immune system is so strong that it attacks itself—perceives a danger that doesn't exist and attacks a phantom. Two small burnt-orange pills three times a day. So the war is being waged in two directions: my body is fighting itself, and the medicine is fighting my body, trying to stop the initial attack. No wonder I am tired all the time.

After a month, the blood is nearly gone. I am avid in what they tell me to do. I measure. I quantify. I try to feel normal, go about my work as if nothing has changed, now that I have the reprieve of a diagnosis other than cancer (which equals death in my mind). It is when I work that I am most like my old self—getting lost in the words that I handle for a living. Suddenly Wordsworth takes on a whole new kind of meaning:

> What though the radiance which was once so bright
> Be now for ever taken from my sight,
>   Though nothing can bring back the hour
> Of splendor in the grass, of glory in the flower:
>   We will grieve not, rather find
>   Strength in what remains behind. . . .

It is the culmination of my graduate career: Ph.D. comprehensive examinations. I am awfully tired these days. At night my belly howls. It, with its noises and writhings, will not let me rest. Used to work from before dawn until sometimes midnight. Lived for many years on an average of five hours of sleep per night. Now I can't make it through the day without a nap, it seems. How can I concentrate better so that I can be ready for these exams? I will handle it calmly and no one will know the difference. ~ *& appearance*

I cut off all my hair. From mid-back to above the ear, this new hair reflects the new me that I want to be: simpler, more focused. Streamlined.

I haven't seen blood for a while and go off the six pills. Energy is back, and I'm feeling blessed. But within a week the bleeding recurs and now they decide to be more "invasive." Sigmoidoscopy. A scope up my anus into the insides of me to see what they can see. Show up at the hospital on Wednesday morning. They don't tell me to bring anyone.

THE SCOPE

The room is cold and tiled in blue. It is far too big, and the lights are too harsh. Dutifully, I remove my jeans—everything—and put on the hospital gown. "Be sure to leave the ties in the back." It is cold, and I move to a corner of the cavernous room. I wrap my arms across my chest tightly—as much from fear as from cold. The person who will perform this "procedure" shares my last name. He has piercing blue eyes, and I try to establish some kind of rapport with him in the seconds before he sees more of me than has ever been seen before. He's civil. But he obviously does several of these procedures every day and can't spend too much time coaching a novice. I've been told it doesn't hurt much.

A male nurse comes to help me with the second enema in two hours—must clean me out so they can see what they need to see—and I'm grateful for his kindness. I ask him if he'd mind cleaning the toilet before I have to go in there. It's a big research hospital, and I'm concerned about germs. About everything. This disease has made me paranoid. I used to be the healthiest person on the planet—never smoked, never drank, never abused "substances," ate well, exercised. But I didn't rest enough. If only I'd . . . . If only I'd . . . . This would be the mantra of the next few years of my life. Trying to find a reason. Trying to find what was at fault in me. Not angry at God, I was nevertheless desperate to have it all make sense. If I could just understand it intellectually, then I could deal with it emotionally.

In fact, the scope didn't hurt very much. He pumped air into me to distend the colon so that he could see better. And then used water to clear a path. The pressure was bad but mercifully short-lived. But afterwards, for hours, I had sharp pain in both my belly and in my shoulder and neck. How could air escape from the intestinal tract into the chest cavity?

Test inconclusive. No real evidence of IBD, especially since I don't have a chief symptom: excruciating abdominal pain. Perhaps just a bacterial infection that's all gone now.

JUNE 1994

Bleeding worse now. This time in another city. A new doctor. The cowboy boots moved to Utah. Fitting, that. Another sigmoidoscopy. This time it comes back definite: I have inflammatory bowel disease. I go to the library to read everything I can find about the two forms. Knowledge is power.

Ulcerative colitis: ulcerations in the colon. Bleeding and diarrhea. Weight loss, joint pain, skin lesions. Liver disease? Higher risk of colon cancer because of constant cellular changes. No cure except colectomy/colostomy: removal of the colon and bringing the large intestine out through the abdominal wall to empty into a pouch. Not a very appealing "cure," but at least some *hope* of a cure.

Crohn's disease: usually affects small intestine and any part of the alimentary tract, from mouth to anus. Chronic diarrhea, low-grade fever, severe fatigue and weight loss, joint pain, inflammation of "extra-intestinal" body parts like eyes, skin. No cure. At all. Management of the disease is the optimal option.

With the cancer risk associated with UC, I go home and pray fervently for weeks that it is Crohn's disease I have and not ulcerative colitis. A *little* knowledge is a dangerous thing. I discover later that 80 percent of Crohn's patients have multiple surgeries to remove segments of intestine. The disease (always?) recurs in the part that's left.

"You should never let them do the first surgery," a person tells me. "After that, it just eats you up like cancer." I have joined a support group for people with this disease. They are my family. Although my real family and friends have been wonderfully supportive as I battle the fear and the physical symptoms, they cannot know how it feels. The people in the support group know the fears, and they have good advice about what has actually worked for them, actual people. The doctors know only the books.

And other things about Crohn's: fissures (deep cracks in the tissue around the anus) and fistulas (burrowing between body parts—colon and vagina, for instance). And the medicines used to treat these diseases: steroids like prednisone, whose side effects include mania, acute weight gain, "moonface," water retention and a "buffalo hump" in the upper back and shoulders, bone loss. Immunosuppressants, whose possible side effects include pancreatitis and hepatitis. Infused drugs that sometimes cause blood pressure to plummet during the 2.5 hours in a chair while the serum is being fed into the veins through an IV. Can that kill you? Linked to lymphoma. So what is one to do? Take a drug that will hopefully lead to a semi-normal life for a while but run the risk of developing hideously painful, *terminal* diseases? We hope to avoid all these "canon" drugs and have the six pills do the job.

MIDSUMMER 1994

Spiraling out of control. Blood and mucous. Bathroom 25–30 times a day. The minute I finish, I have to go again. So much blood. This is my body and my blood passing from me. I will die if they can't control it. I have no life, no energy. They try everything: all kinds of steroids that are "topical"—inserted rectally. They say there's less systemic absorption that way. I'm a very poor candidate for oral steroids—anatomically and temperamentally. Steroids decrease bone mass; they often lead to mania. Prednisone is the steroid of choice (*not* my choice, not chosen *for* me by the doctor working with me), and it causes insomnia, nervousness. My father's use of prednisone cost him two vertebrae and enormous pain.

Myxomatosis

Caught in the centre of a soundless field
While hot inexplicable hours go by
What trap is this? Where were its teeth concealed?
You seem to ask.
                    I make a sharp reply,
Then clean my stick. I'm glad I can't explain
Just in what jaws you were to suppurate:
You may have thought things would come right again
If you could only keep quite still and wait.
                                    —*Philip Larkin*

More scopes. Colonoscopy is very different from sigmoidoscopy; they go all the way across the transverse and then into the ascending (right side) colon, up to where it joins with the small intestine at the ileum. Can't be awake for this one; couldn't stand the pain. Three full days of fasting. Only clear liquids and nothing with red or blue or purple coloring. Not even cream in the coffee. You get pretty weak. And then drink two bottles of concentrated saline solution. Pure salt. By then, I'm so nauseated I don't know if I vomit from the empty stomach or the salt.

In the hospital I keep repeating, "Tell me about the rabbits, George." Lenny wants to hear his dream of a happy future from the man who is his best friend, the man who will murder him mercifully instead of letting him be butchered by a posse. "Tell me about the rabbits, George." Tell me there's a future I'll live to see. And that there'll be things that are comforting.

My doctor comes in wearing a yellow hospital gown. I take yellow as a happy thing, a good sign. Yellow is the favorite color of someone I love—told me it was his favorite color once because it was the color I was wearing. Benevolent Dr. J: always calm, always supportive. He is my partner in my care, asking what I think about things. Once I asked him a question he couldn't answer off the top of his head. He told me to wait a minute, disappeared, and came back with his medical book. We looked up the answer together. I knew from that minute that he would be my doctor for life.

"Myxomatosis" by Philip Larkin is reprinted from *The Less Deceived* by permission of The Marvell Press, England and Australia.

He smiles at me. The attending nurses have already told me that if they had to have a colonoscopy, Dr. J is the one they'd want doing it. A small gift they give me. I don't doubt its truth either. He smiles at me and asks if I'm ready. I smile back and hear him order the medicine be put in the IV. The next thing I know I am waking to my own moaning, and I can see a TV monitor and the scope moving through. I hear him order more medication and then I sleep again.

Kyrie ——

I am told the next day that when I woke up (you don't really wake up to a conscious state, even though you can talk), I kept asking, "Did you find cancer?" I remember this as one remembers a fun house: everything is blurry and surreal. I remember Dr. J asking how I felt, and I thought it very clever in the midst of my stupor to answer simply "shitty." Humor is the only saving grace. That and faith.

ADDISONIAN CRISIS

The topical steroids (is it *five* forms they've tried?) aren't working, so I might as well go off them. They speculate that I haven't absorbed enough to shut down my adrenal glands, so I can quit cold turkey—not taper, as I'd have to do with oral steroids. Only when I stop cold turkey, I find I am so weak that I cannot get off the couch. I wake, rest, take a shower. Then I have to sleep for two hours. I can't even sit up. I prop myself at the computer so that I can write for fifteen minutes at a time before I have to sleep again. For well over two months, I can go nowhere. For two reasons: I must be near a bathroom at all times. And I don't have the strength to walk anywhere or sit in a restaurant long enough to eat anything. I read about steroid withdrawal, and I know intuitively that I have indeed absorbed so much steroid that my own adrenal system has nearly shut down. That *can* include involuntary bodily functions like breathing. I think I'm lucky I didn't stop breathing.

SUPPORT GROUP

I'm still not getting any better, and I talk with members of my support group at our next meeting. They recommend suggesting to my doctor a combination of meds that we haven't considered yet—still avoiding oral steroids, the Dragon. We reason through this proposed protocol, and we think it is logical. There's a physician—a pediatric hematologist who got ulcerative colitis the year he retired and stopped smoking (seems that nicotine keeps UC at bay, so he often doubts his choice. Perhaps it would be better to risk lung cancer than suffer UC)—and his stamp of approval on our medical logic makes us feel easier about playing armchair doctors. I return to my doctor, who agrees it's worth a try. The new protocol designed by laymen works. It *works!*

SIX YEARS

This is how long I live a relatively normal life, now in Montana. The blood never completely stops, but I become used to it in moderation. I stay tired, but at least I can go out and eat and exercise and do my work and be with people I love. There are a couple of scary points. Like getting a gut bug in Europe. For me, that is disaster on a scale unknown to a "normal" person. I call the doctor back home, overseas. It is past closing time, but I am desperate and insist on being put directly through to the partner on call. I ask at what point I need to go to the hospital. He tells me if I pass out when I stand up, then I will need to go for a possible transfusion. I wonder how carefully they screen blood for disease in this country. I sleep for three straight days while the other members of my group continue the tour.

Traveling in general is a real trick. Absolutely imperative that one find out about the accommodations for people with this disease. Traveling through rural areas, one must also arrange for constant access to "facilities." I lead a group through Ireland, so I make sure the bus has a bathroom. And then there's packing. A month's supply of all the medicines I take requires a small suitcase all its own. And the medicine is temperature-sensitive: if it gets too cold, it will freeze and lose its efficacy; if it gets too hot, it will melt and be unusable. So it is my entire carry-on allotment.

For six years, the annual scopes are routine, stressful, but all part of this life I've inherited. I am profoundly grateful just to have this much of a normal life. And then, although I try to deny it with every ounce of my being, I know I'm headed south again.

ρ Kyrie eleison

SUMMER 2001

Wild fear madly flapping . . .

It begins in small ways—things that have happened periodically over the years: a little more blood every day. But the trend doesn't reverse itself. Constant sensation in my colon, abdomen, back. Gurgling. The minute I take a bite of anything, the process starts. I fight it. I tell myself that it will pass.

But it doesn't.

I start avoiding food. "If I just don't eat something that will aggravate it . . .," I tell myself. This leads to anorexia—not for all the reasons that people *normally* get anorexia, but because I am afraid to eat. If I don't ingest, I don't have to see the bloody effects. But that is a fallacy. Blood and mucous whatever I do; nothing really matters. I lose weight. I stop exercising because I fear that it taxes my body too much. The loss of endorphins itself makes me feel down and sickly.

BODY IMAGE

It's like hiding alcoholism: you don't want people to know because then they look at you differently, think of you as weak and doubt your competence. The irony of this disease is that you look perfectly normal; no one can tell just by looking. Oh, I might look tired and a little thin, but basically I look normal. In fact, by society's (warped) standards of beauty, I'm nearly perfect. Svelte. Only I get no satisfaction from this, knowing how it happened.

My own body has betrayed me. I know what Yeats meant:

> *What shall I do with this absurdity—*
> *O heart, O troubled heart—this caricature,*
> *Decrepit age that has been tied to me*
> *As to a dog's tail?*

I have lost 10 pounds since summer. The cosmic joke's on me. When I was younger, I worried (like most women in our culture) that I was too heavy. Now I am desperate to keep on weight, *gain* weight. But I keep losing weight. With alarm, I watch the scales go down pound by pound over the next few weeks. I weigh less than I did in high school.

In the past month, my doctor has added two new medicines, and neither has quelled the bleeding. In fact, it only increases. Day by day I calculate how much worse it has gotten. The morning is worst because it is the first—the immediate—thing I have to confront. Don't even get to wake up first. So the choices are oral steroids (which we've avoided for years for fear it will destroy me, body and soul), immunosuppressants (which make one susceptible to every kind of virus or infection going around), and the infusion drug (drop in blood pressure, lymphoma). Likely a combination of these, as the immunosuppressants don't take effect for three months.

Like J. Alfred Prufrock, *"I have measured out my life with coffee spoons."* Except now, it's in quarter cups. — blood ?

I am in the doctor's office or the hospital lab for blood work at least three days a week. I try to maintain my work, but this disease requires as much time as a whole other life. It's hard to think about anything else. I stay on the phone, trying to coordinate my doctors a continent apart. I'm convinced that having two opinions is the only way to go, and I'm glad that they concur. The benevolent doctor of the yellow gown is the one I trust more right now because I know him better, for much longer. He returns my calls after his full day at work. He does not get paid for this, and he talks to me for over an hour one afternoon. We reason through everything, and he answers questions, considers my speculations. If there are saints alive in this world, he is one.

SWALLOWING THE DRAGON

The prednisone shocks everyone, the doctors most of all. My reaction has been minimal. No insomnia, no mania, no precipitous weight gain. All I can do is thank God over and over and over. Things take on entirely new meaning and purpose, and I'm aware of just how clear things become in light of something this staggering. The simplest things that I used to take for granted seem like miracles: having the strength to get out of bed, being able to walk as the late-afternoon sun streams low over dry grass, being able to eat something besides bland chicken and mashed potatoes after four months, doing a workout for the first time in over 90 days and being able to get through most of it. The magnitude of such minor miracles overwhelms me at times. The other day as I was going to work and feeling mostly normal, I laughed out loud to think that no one would ever suspect my private demons. And I realize just how little I know about the private demons of other people. We all cover our pain so well.

CARPE DIEM

Has an entirely new meaning to me. It means being grateful for this minute at hand and not considering what tomorrow might be like. This is all I have for sure.

Having so little success with traditional Western medicine for a while, I have branched out, and now I try "imaging" and other alternative forms of therapy. The person who helps me hone my imaging technique (I've done this for years but now go to an expert) tells me to imagine a place of complete comfort and peace. I see a Friday afternoon in autumn.

Countryside, and the lane is all covered with yellow leaves. The sun is warm, and I feel the cool air against the skin of my face. I sit propped, back against a tree, and close my eyes. The person then tells me that I should imagine a "guide," something or someone who can tell me things I need to hear. I wait and wait. This doesn't come immediately, as the place did. But then I'm aware of a horse standing behind a fence across from me. He is quiet and just stands there. He looks at me, and I know that his presence is all that matters: to have some being stand there with you. In the end, all we can do is show up and *be there* for one another. I can't suspend my disbelief long enough to suppose the horse will actually speak to me. But I know the message I'm meant to hear: be patient. Look at nature, at the *cycles* of life. Things change. Trust in the change. And I look at the horse in my mind's eye, and I see how strong and beautiful his body is. He does not worry about how he feels or what might happen. When his body hurts, he simply waits until it doesn't. He is just patient, and he lives in the moment. This is my lesson, and I will learn it bit by bit. I will keep learning it.

    Kyrie—

    I feel happy right now. I am not alone. And I decide that the only choice I really have is to choose how to live my life. It's a small life, mine, but I embrace it for all its wonder,

Every Season

Every evening sky, an invitation
To trace the patterned stars
And early in July, a celebration
For freedom that is ours
And I notice You
In children's games
In those who watch them from the shade
Every drop of sun is full of fun and wonder.
You are summer.

And even when the trees have just surrendered
To the harvest time
Forfeiting their leaves in late September
And sending us inside
Still I notice You
When change begins
And I am braced for colder winds
I will offer thanks for what has been and what's to come.
You are autumn.

And everything in time and under heaven
Finally falls asleep
Wrapped in blankets white, all creation

Shivers underneath
And still I notice you
When branches crack
And in my breath on frosted glass
Even now in death, You open doors for life to enter.
You are winter.

And everything that's new has bravely surfaced
Teaching us to breathe
And what was frozen through is newly purposed
Turning all things green
So it is with You
And how You make me new
With every season's change
And so it will be
As you are re-creating me:
Summer, autumn, winter, spring.

—Nichole Nordeman

QUESTIONS

1. What does the author's style indicate about her approach to this illness?
2. What is the relationship between italicized passages and the rest of the text?
3. Notice any "gaps" in the text. What is the author not saying, and what might be its significance?
4. Comment on the qualities of the physicians the author encounters.
5. Comment on images of insects and animals that appear in the text.

Scheherazade Syndrome
Illness and Storytelling

☞ Kristin Lindgren ☜

On Christmas morning, a sudden dip in my temperature announced that I was ovulating. Every morning for over a year, before my feet touched the cold floor beside my bed, I had stuck a thermometer in my mouth and plotted my daily temperature on a piece of graph paper. If all went well, this fertility calculus produced a monthly graph showing a nicely sloping hill that suddenly dropped off. When the pencil line neared the top of the hill, it was time to "get together" with my husband, as my reproductive endocrinologist so delicately put it. Following my doctor's instructions, I cheerfully drew circles representing intercourse around the pencil points marking my daily temperature. Although my treatment for irregular ovulation involved exploratory surgery, adrenocorticosteroids, and Clomid, it all happened fairly quickly. I had moments of anger and despair, but my lapse of confidence in my body was blessedly brief. Soon I was carrying a lively, kicking creature, our little Christmas miracle. An easy and healthy pregnancy helped me to regain trust in my body's ability to do what I wanted it to do and in the power of medical knowledge to solve its problems. A trial endured, a happy ending. Everyone likes to hear my pregnancy story.

Two years later, I collapsed with a mysterious, debilitating illness. I had been exhausted for months. Because my toddler was a poor sleeper, I assumed that my fatigue was simply a response to the interrupted sleep that often accompanies parenthood. Eventually he began to sleep through the night, but then I couldn't sleep. When I did sleep, I woke up feeling as if I hadn't. I felt unwell in other ways, too: I had a chronic sore throat, a chronic low-grade fever, chronically sore lymph nodes. I wasn't terribly worried yet, just terribly tired. When I developed vertigo and began to hold on to the wall in order to walk straight, I was worried. My throat felt as if something was lodged in it, and it was difficult to swallow. I continued to produce abundant breast milk months after I had weaned my son. Should I be concerned about this? I didn't know. Everything about my body seemed odd and unfamiliar. I continued, as best I could, to teach my classes and to care for my family, but I made a second appointment with my doctor, and then a third. One afternoon after teaching, I collapsed, and I lay on my office floor trembling uncontrollably. I called my husband to tell him I was too sick to stand up, too sick to drive myself home. I could no longer ignore my symptoms or pretend that nothing was seriously wrong. My body was insisting that it had a story to tell. However, unlike my pregnancy story, this narrative has no shapely plot, no clear beginning, middle, and end. No one likes to hear my illness story.

⌒ ⌒

I was gradually losing the ability to function in my job and to care for my young child, but my doctor could find nothing wrong with me. All blood tests were normal. When I had been seriously ill for months and no one could tell me what was wrong, I longed for a diagnosis. I felt discouraged when tests for lupus and Lyme disease were negative, because it meant that I still had no answer. With no concrete clinical findings to point to, all I had was my inchoate, fragmentary story: "First I felt this, and then this, and then this . . ." But my story didn't fit into any interpretive framework familiar to my doctor. As a healthy, athletic woman in my thirties, I had seldom needed a doctor, and I hadn't chosen this one with much care. I had seen Dr. S. only twice before, once for a physical and once for an ordinary respiratory infection. He was about my age, and he made small talk about college life and graduate school. He had a habit of reciting passages verbatim from medical textbooks, and he liked to repeat maxims from his medical training: "When you hear hoofbeats, think horses, not zebras." I understood the importance of this principle to medical practice, but I had seen him several times since falling ill, and thinking horses wasn't getting us anywhere. What if I was a zebra? Increasingly, I felt that his well-rehearsed scripts left little room for diagnostic imagination. Because there was no apparent diagnostic narrative that could help him to make sense of my story, he stopped listening to it. His counter-story, which asserted that I was simply anxious and stressed and would feel fine tomorrow, began to drown out my weakening cry of "But I'm very sick, and getting sicker!"

Weary of listening to Dr. S.'s recitation of a pamphlet on sleep hygiene, I found a sleep specialist at the local university hospital. I didn't know whether my alarming inability to sleep was a cause or an effect of my illness, but I believed that sleep might hold the key to recovery. Dr. Z. told me that only interesting people had sleep disorders, so I obligingly entertained her with interesting tales of my sleeplessness. Over the course of several visits, I observed that her perception of my reliability as a narrator shaped her interpretation of my symptoms. When I presented myself as calm and competent, a fellow professional, she assured me that I had an organic sleep disorder, probably triggered by the interrupted sleep of early parenthood. When my exhaustion and increasing anxiousness about my condition made me teary-eyed as I recounted another week without sleep, she suggested that the disorder had a psychological origin. She went back and forth between these theories, depending on my state of mind. We tried two medications that had no effect on my sleep, though they left me feeling dry-mouthed and woozy. Dr. Z. told me that these medications always worked and implied that their failure to work for me was somehow my fault. On my insurance forms she checked off "adjustment disorder." There was no point in my illness at which I felt more desperate than when I realized that neither Dr. S. nor Dr. Z. could help me. Their narratives had trumped mine, and the story I was telling had failed to elicit any helpful diagnosis or treatment.

Next stop: therapist. Dr. Rachel Goldberg was a smart and compassionate woman whom I had consulted three years earlier, when I was trying to get pregnant. I was convinced that my illness had a physiological basis, but it seemed like a good idea to get a psychologist's opinion. Maybe my symptoms really *were* caused by stress or anxiety or maladjustment or being an interesting person. I tried my story one more time. Dr. Goldberg began to look more and more alarmed. She cut short our fifty minutes, saying that she was sending me to her own internist immediately. She picked up the phone and made an appointment for me. Emphatically, repeatedly, she told me that something was seriously wrong with my physical health. Clearly, she was worried. It was a relief to see that some health professional was worried.

Thus I landed in the cramped, crowded office of Dr. Bonnie Ashby. Everyone else in the waiting room was over seventy, and most of them were in pretty bad shape. I had been ill for about six months now, and I didn't have much faith in doctors of any stripe. Dr. Ashby spent an hour with me, asking me question after question. She approached my case like a detective, unearthing evidence, narrowing the field of suspects. She listened intently, furiously scribbling notes in her tiny, meticulous handwriting. Her questioning never overwhelmed my narrative; it was carefully designed to elicit the parts of my story that would be useful to her. I recognized some of the methods of literary criticism in her toolkit—close reading, attention to the seemingly marginal aspects of a story, careful construction of argument and counter-argument—and I could see that she was an astute listener and interpreter.

I provided my fragmentary story; she built on and around it, piecing the fragments together in a way that could make some sense of it. I trusted her with these fragments; I felt that her several pages of notes represented a collaborative project. Dr. Ashby clearly relished differential diagnosis, and she had the confidence and clinical experience to operate on hunches. My previous bloodwork ruled out Epstein-Barr, but one of her several working hypotheses was that I had a viral syndrome of some sort, and she suspected cytomegalovirus, or CMV. She had seen unusual cases of CMV before. At the end of our first appointment she looked me in the eye and said in her no-nonsense, gravelly voice, "We may never get to the bottom of this, but we're going to try."

Dr. Ashby explained that although she believed all my symptoms were linked, she needed to run tests related to each symptom individually. In the following weeks, I had an MRI scan of my brain, an echocardiogram, a twenty-four-hour cardiac holter monitor test, a neurological examination, a barium swallow test, and lots of blood work. The echocardiogram found a mitral valve prolapse, a relatively common cardiac problem, but in general the tests were reassuring. The neurologist wrote a two-page report, and I remember being oddly pleased, reading it, that he didn't describe me as the difficult patient I had come to believe I was. His language was neutral and professional:

> Mrs. Lindgren is a 35-year-old right-handed non-smoker who was previously employed as an English professor until she had to discontinue work because of her ongoing problem of chronic fatigue, insomnia, and daytime hypersomnolence. . .
> . Examination demonstrates the patient to be a pleasant woman in no distress. . . .
> it is reassuring that the MRI shows no pituitary tumor and there is no bitemporal hemianopsia to suggest a developing tumor. Nevertheless, microadenoma could be

present and it might be reasonable to check a prolactin level in the future if questions remain in that regard. . . . Thank you for letting me participate in the care of this interesting patient.

I paused skeptically for a moment at the word "interesting," then decided that he meant my medical history was interesting, not that I was an interesting person.

When Dr. Ashby sent me copies of my blood work and other test results, the test for CMV was circled and highlighted in red ink. Next to it she wrote, "This is the culprit! Give me a call." CMV is a garden-variety virus in the herpes family. Like its relative the varicella-zoster virus, which causes chicken pox and shingles, it generally produces more serious illness in adults than in children. My antibody titers were sky-high and indicated a currently active infection. While my case was severe and didn't explain all of my symptoms, Dr. Ashby felt confident I would recover in six to eight weeks. But I didn't recover. Months later, I consulted an infectious diseases specialist, who said he had never in his career seen such persistently high CMV titers in someone who had no apparent reason to be immune-compromised. My diagnosis became cloudier: was the infection the primary problem, or was there an underlying immune disorder that enabled the infection to flourish?

Ultimately I was diagnosed with a "syndrome"—post-viral syndrome, which is akin to chronic fatigue and immune dysfunction syndrome (CFIDS) and myalgic encephalomyelitis (ME)—rather than with a "disease." This syndrome is still poorly understood, but it is known to involve the neuroendocrine and immune systems. Current research suggests that symptoms may be caused not by the virus itself but by a dysregulated immune system that overreacts to a viral intruder. Many researchers and clinicians believe it results from a complex interaction of viral infection or toxic exposure, stress or injury, and genetic predisposition. Because a syndrome is defined by an aggregate of signs and symptoms rather than by one specific clinical finding, its diagnosis depends almost entirely on the patient's ability to tell a story about her body. This narrative is then interpreted by the doctor, transformed into a diagnosis and a case history. Once I had a diagnosis I thought my storytelling was over, but it was just beginning. Chronic illness demands that you tell your body's story over and over. I began to feel like the Arabian princess Scheherazade, who was compelled to construct a new narrative every night to save her life. Endlessly deferring closure, she grafted each evening's story onto the tale that preceded it.

꧁ ꧂

About ten months after I first collapsed with this illness, I recovered. I was able to go on walks again, to take care of my son, who was now nearly three, to get up in the morning with some confidence that I would make it through the day. My recovery lasted six weeks. It was followed by a relapse that lasted well over a year. The first months of relapse were hellish, in some ways worse than the initial episode of illness, not only because of my crushed hopes for recovery but also because the symptoms were now unremitting. Day after day, night after night, I felt unspeakably awful. For some of this time, I was literally too sick to speak. Forming words took far too much energy. And I could find no words for how I felt. The pain and malaise in my body were not localized; I couldn't point to a limb or a muscle and say, "it hurts here." My entire body was in crisis. I've never had a migraine, but I lived in

a world similar to that described by people who suffer from migraines: sunlight was painful, sounds were painful, any sensory information from the external world interacted painfully with my body. Fatigue is often understood as the absence of energy, but I experienced
fatigue as the presence of overwhelming, body-wracking exhaustion.

As I emerged from this relapse, I gradually began to function again. I was able to walk
up and down the stairs a couple of times a day. I felt grateful for any small thing I could do
with my son. Eventually I was able to drive short distances. Then I could take a short walk
outdoors. But the path to recovery was not linear. Although I never had another relapse of
this severity, I continued to oscillate between relapse and partial recovery. I learned to pace
myself carefully and take regular rest breaks during the day. Able to sleep again, I found I
needed nine or ten hours of sleep each night. I learned by experience that I was most vulnerable to relapse on the first day or two of my period, so I was especially careful at that
time of the month.

Always athletic, I was accustomed to swimming a mile with ease, to hiking and cross-
country skiing. Now I discovered that physical exertion, especially aerobic exercise, often
made me sick and sometimes triggered a relapse. The physiology of this problem is still
poorly understood, but "exercise intolerance" or "post-exertional malaise" is a hallmark of
my illness. I learned to walk slowly, and to swim even more slowly, making sure I never got
to the point of breathing hard. When I did too much, I would begin to feel symptoms of
a relapse several hours later, sometimes as much as a day later. Often, after a slightly active
day, I would wake up in the middle of the night with the odd sensation of a motor whir-
ring inside me, a motor I couldn't turn off. My insomnia would return for a few days, or
a few weeks. My sore throat and slight fever would return, my lymph nodes would throb,
walking up and down stairs would again become difficult. Recovery, when it came, did not
mean a return to my former state of robust health, to the body I had known for thirty-five
years. Recovery meant learning to live in my new body, whose abilities and limitations are
wholly different.

⌒ ⌒

Unlike the stereotypical academic who lives in her head, I had always embraced and delighted
in my physicality. I liked being embodied, and my body had rarely been a problem to me.
I come from sturdy Scandinavian stock, and I took my physical robustness for granted. At
the same time, I was not unacquainted with illness. My brother had developed schizophrenia at nineteen. At fourteen, I had surgery for a bone tumor that swelled my lower left leg
to twice its normal size. The tumor was benign, an osteochondroma, but we didn't know
this until several days after the surgery. During the days of waiting for the biopsy report, I
made a list of all my eighth-grade friends, and paired each one with an experience I then
hoped to have in my life—having a child, climbing Mt. Rainier, building my own house in
the woods, becoming a famous pianist, reading all the books in the world. I willed each of
these experiences to one of my friends in the event that I didn't live to have them myself.
After making this grand gesture, I felt satisfied and very, very generous. I had bequeathed
each gift with a certain genius, I thought, to the most appropriate person. I don't believe I
ever told my friends, later, of my unusual bequests; girls of fourteen are not eager to talk

about dying. But creating this list allowed me to feel secretly magnanimous and able to shape others' fates precisely when I felt so little control over my own.

After spending a summer on crutches while my leg healed, I returned to playing soccer and swimming laps. I never built my own house or became a pianist, but I've had two children, climbed many mountains, and read an awful lot of books. Although I still have a long snakelike scar and a patch of numbness that runs down my calf, this experience receded into distant memory until I became ill at thirty-five. Then I was compelled once again to recognize my limited ability to control my future. As a white, middle-class woman, I had found it surprisingly easy to believe that my life was determined largely by choices I made. Growing up in the age of feminism, I had thoroughly absorbed the lesson that anatomy is not destiny. Yet suddenly my body seemed to be the only thing that mattered, the thing without whose consent and cooperation nothing else was possible. My body had a mind of its own.

With illness came the end of the illusion that I am sole author of my fate, fashioning my life's narrative through acts of will and conscious choices. It became difficult to make any long-term plans, even plans for the next day, because I never knew what my body would be capable of doing. I lived entirely in the moment. The story I tell about my illness is also a story of the moment. It has no teleology; it fits into no larger narrative pattern. It tells what is happening right now.

⌒ ⌒

I began to write because in illness it was the only work I could do. Sometimes I could write a sentence in the morning, maybe another in the afternoon. Once, determined to write a letter for a colleague who was up for promotion, I wrote a full page in a day, but I was then so exhausted that I couldn't read it back to myself; the words bounced around on the page and I could no longer form them into coherent phrases and clauses. Unable to write anything for professional purposes, I decided simply to record, as best I could, my experience of illness. Now, several years later, it's difficult for me to read these fragments of writing, which are mostly in the form of undated journal-like reflections—undated, I think, because I had lost all sense of the passage of time—and to remember how it felt to be so sick. I still live with chronic illness, but I am rarely so ill that I am confined to my bed. I am able to care for my children and to work part-time. Illness has become integrated into the rest of life. I've pieced together some of my writing from earlier years, years when I was learning how to be sick.

⌒ ⌒

I am resolved to put some of my experience of illness into words, but frustrated by my inability to string together more than two or three sentences at a time. Perhaps short snippets of writing reflect my state of mind and body more truthfully than seamless paragraphs.

Space and time, the coordinates by which we plot our lives, become strangely altered by illness. I now inhabit an Alice in Wonderland world, one in which things shrink and expand without warning and the rules are difficult to discern.

Space contracts to the dimensions of my bedroom. When I am too sick to read, I meditate on the architectural details of the room and the slowly changing seasons outside the window. Time expands. I live in great pools of time that are not demarcated or structured in any way. When I can't sleep, day blurs into night.

In illness, I find that the smallest detail of the natural world offers pleasure sufficient for the day. The procession of winter birds at our birdfeeder entertains me for hours. A snowstorm amazes and delights me. The first snowdrops to bloom seem a miracle of endurance.

Illness is as demanding as an infant, and as unpredictable. It's hard to get it on a schedule. I picture this disease as squalling, red-faced, wakeful. What does it want? What can I do that will make it calm down? I take comfort in talking with a friend who is caring for a newborn. Like mine, her life has lost all pattern and predictability, and she is perpetually exhausted. For a few weeks I have companionship of a sort. But her baby begins to sleep, and she moves on to normal life.

Having a child, I was welcomed into the world of parenthood, and my new status was recognized by rituals, gifts, advice, and a proliferation of books that coach us through every stage of the process and answer every imaginable question. Having an illness, I am welcomed by no one, given no useful advice or books that map a path. While a short-term illness or surgery has a certain ritual attached to it—hospital visits, cards, flowers—a mysterious, long-term illness leaves everyone feeling awkward and uncomfortable, unsure of how to respond. There are no commonly understood rules of etiquette, no midwives to help you breathe and push.

In the last year and a half, I have become a medicalized object of inquiry, a specimen, a self constituted by antibody titers and insurance claim forms. One of the challenges of disabling illness is to retain a sense of self that is not reduced to a diagnostic label or a recitation of symptoms, a challenge made more difficult by the loss of familiar professional and social identities. Unable to do any of the things that normally would give me a sense of accomplishment and forward movement, I sometimes feel that nothing is happening, that I am moving in no direction. What does it mean to move forward when you are lying in bed? Perhaps the greatest difficulty of chronic illness—of my illness, at least—is facing diminished expectations, diminished possibilities, without feeling diminished as a person. Life can no longer be lived on a grand scale. Limitations I didn't expect to confront until old age are abruptly, rudely staring me down. The challenge is to be inventive within these limits. Living with illness is like writing a sonnet; the structure is confining, yet working within it can yield surprising beauty and ingenious solutions. But just as I think I am learning to live creatively within the confines of a sonnet, the rules change. Suddenly it is a villanelle.

☜ ☞

Time warp. My friends work out at the gym, become pregnant, begin new jobs, travel to Istanbul. They have news. I fear that I may awaken, like Rip van Winkle, into a world I no longer recognize.

People my age find my illness incomprehensible and frightening. I try to take an interest in their lives, their problems, but there is no longer much common ground. Because I and many of my friends spent long years in graduate school, our thirties have been a time of beginnings: first babies, first jobs, first homes. In our mid- or late thirties, we are embarking on a stage of life that most of our parents began in their twenties. And yet so many parts of my life seem to be ending. At exactly the time of life I imagined would be my productive and reproductive years, I can produce nothing.

The Lower Merion Coalition for the Elderly called today to ask whether we could volunteer to drive the disabled elderly to their doctor's appointments. Alex, frayed and exhausted, told them that he was trying to care for a seriously ill wife and a three-year-old and he couldn't possibly take care of anyone else. The caller kindly offered his services to us, saying that their volunteers could drive me to my doctor's appointments. More and more I seem to be grouped with the geriatrics.

Sitting in my doctor's waiting room, I hear one elderly woman tell another that she has recently given up driving. Her friend confides that she too is no longer able to drive and catalogues other friends who now depend on van services and younger relatives for transportation. "Me too, me too," I want to say. I feel a kinship with these women that I seldom feel anymore with friends my age. Unable to drive because of my unpredictable episodes of dizziness and disequilibrium, as well as the exhaustion that makes me unable to process several pieces of information simultaneously—a crucial skill at a busy intersection—I now rely on my indefatigable 70-year-old mother-in-law to drive me to the doctor. Shouldn't I be driving her to the doctor? Everything seems to be upside down.

☜ ☞

Anders wakes up at 7:30. I haven't slept. I start another day nauseous from exhaustion, hands trembling, body achy and rebellious. Anders, now three, is home from preschool and full of energy for the new day. He wants to go to the zoo or to the Franklin Institute, which he pronounces carefully and precisely. "Mommy, let's go to the Fran-kah-lin In-sti-toot!" I give him many reasons, reasonable reasons, why we need to have a quiet day at home. I scrupulously avoid saying that we can't go there because I'm feeling sick. He needs to match will against will with a healthy, strong adult. But he wears me down, he persists, he protests until my head is throbbing. Finally I say it: "We can't go because Mommy is too sick." "Oh," he says, coming close to hug me and pat my face, "I will take care of you." This boy has learned to care by being cared for, learned his sweet affectionate ways by being pumped with affection. I welcome his sweetness, but I'm saddened, and worried, that at three he has to take care of his mother.

On Halloween night I walked my son from house to house in our neighborhood. My little pump-

kin was wide-eyed as he filled his backpack with forbidden candy. I have always enjoyed the carnivalesque nature of Halloween, the opportunity to play out a fantasy. This year, the persona I desired above all was that of the "normal mother," taking normal pleasure in her child's encounter with the world of dress-up. Instead, I felt that the scariest creature out and about that night was me. Suffering from vertigo, I had trouble keeping the sidewalk under my feet and the moonless Halloween sky above my head. Twice I sat down abruptly on the sidewalk to keep myself from keeling over. The ghosts and goblins streaming down the street contributed to my feeling that I inhabit a frightening, off-kilter world.

Anders and I have become champion snugglers. There's a lot we can do together lying in bed: books, puzzles, drawing. I can't run around and kick a soccer ball, but I can play quietly with him. I can be emotionally present. His favorite activity right now is a board game called Snail's Pace Race. An apt metaphor for life with illness.

On a good day I decide to make a trip to the grocery store. I manage to negotiate the long aisles, the sensory irritants of light and noise and other people's perfumes. Standing in line at checkout, I'm feeling pleased about my overflowing cart of organic vegetables and multigrain breads. And then I feel it: the quick, frightening ebb of energy. I must assess the situation quickly, before I am too exhausted to think. How long is the line? How fast is the checkout person? Can I make it to the car, have someone else load the groceries, and still have enough energy to drive home? Calculating rapidly, I ditch my cart full of food and head for the car. I make it home, take refuge on the couch—but we still have no groceries in the house. For the next few months my mother-in-law does our food shopping.

Last month I felt well enough to take a short hike in Maine with Anders—a hike that a four-year-old could do. Gradually we reached the top of a small peak. After enjoying our view, we started down again, carefully picking our way over stones and roots. At the bottom of the trail I felt so exuberant that I briefly broke into a run. The hike, slow and deliberate, had been fine, but the run, fast and impulsive, was a mistake. I knew it immediately. I felt the sensation of pressure and constriction in my chest that sometimes signals to me that I've done too much. My hands, and then my whole body, began to tremble, and I sat down to drink from my water bottle. By evening I knew that I had triggered a major relapse, and I felt punished for my hubris and exuberance, my fleeting physical expression of joy.

Dr. Ashby unfailingly tells me that I will get well, have another child, begin to write and teach again. Sometimes I believe her; sometimes I imagine she has been reading up on psychoneuroimmunology and is experimenting on me to see whether false optimism can produce miracles in otherwise hopeless cases. How much recovery to hope for? That's the big question. As I begin to recover, I must carefully calibrate the instrument of hope. Too much hope, and I set myself up for crushing disappointment. Too little, and I invite despair.

Alex and I have been agonizing for months—no, years—about whether to have another child. I no longer have an active CMV infection, which would cause serious problems if transmitted to a developing fetus. My health seems stable. Rather, my illness seems stable. I'm approaching forty. I had difficulty getting pregnant even when I was young and healthy. Because there's no research on post-viral syndromes and pregnancy, I've been conducting my own research project: collecting anecdotal evidence from women across the country, women with illnesses similar to mine who have had babies. I have no research data or statistical studies; all I have to go on are stories. We reviewed these stories with Dr. Ashby. She said, "Go forth and reproduce."

Elias was born today, August 19, two months after my fortieth birthday. A difficult labor. A beautiful, healthy baby.

Normally, I don't feel the need to narrate my life, probably because it conforms to culturally available narratives. While my lived experience is much richer and more complex than these narratives would suggest, I can sum up my life in a way that is widely understood. People generally accept the ways in which I represent myself to them. Not so with illness. It's hard to tell a coherent story about it. Postmodern theorists aside, our culture has a love affair with closure. Illness narratives are supposed to end with recovery or death, and mine has no tidy ending. Frustrated by the chronicity of her own illness, Alice James wrote in 1890 that "these doctors tell you that you will die, or *recover!* But you *don't* recover. I have been at these alternations since I was nineteen and I am neither dead nor recovered—as I am now forty-two there has surely been time for either process" (142). Structured by alternation, oscillation, and interruption, the narrative of chronic illness is hard to listen to. I try to explain that I've learned to live with chronic illness, that while some parts of my life are hard, other parts are wonderful. I tell people that illness and disability will eventually be a part of everyone's life. It's just that illness happened to me in the middle of my life, not at the beginning or the end. I've adjusted. I've discovered a rich literature of illness, a lively disability community. I haven't fully recovered, but I'm no longer waiting for recovery. I'm living my life. However I try to frame it, my experience of illness is immediately reframed and reinterpreted by the listener. Illness generates a good deal of hermeneutic energy on the part of the well.

"Well, I'm glad it's all over now." It's hard to know how to respond to this. Yes, I'm functioning again, even teaching part time, and I believe—I hope—that the worst of my illness is behind me. But most people can't tolerate the idea that it probably won't ever be all over. They're tired of this story, of its circularity, and they want it to end. Someone sends me an article about "illness behavior." The gist of the article is that people cling to illness, even when they're not really sick anymore. They've gotten used to it, and they've found they like it. They get "secondary benefits" from being ill: attention and concern, freedom from work and household tasks. Who wouldn't want to be sick?

"Have you tried acupuncture?" "Have you tried homeopathy?" "Have you tried osteopathy? Have you tried Kutapressin?" "Have you tried green algae?" "Have you tried macrobiotics?" "Have you tried intravenous vitamins?" "Have you tried graded exercise?" "Have you tried a gluten-free diet?" People ask these questions because they want me to feel better, and I appre-

ciate their care and concern. It's possible that any or all of these therapeutic modalities might modestly improve my health. But I am weary of the endless suggestions and the expectations that sometimes accompany them. I know that none of these things will cure my illness, and I don't want to spend my limited time and energy pursuing every imaginable remedy. Some people are judgmental. "If she doesn't try this," they say to themselves, "then she must not really want to get better."

"Well, you look fine." Most people say this kindly, as in, "I'm sorry you've been so sick, and I'm relieved not to see any visible signs of suffering." Others say it in a tone which suggests that looking fine must surely mitigate, if not wholly compensate for, the difficulties posed by feeling lousy. A few say it aggressively, as if to assert: "You look all right to me, so surely you can't be as sick as you say you are." I do look fine, most of the time. And I certainly understand the confusion this creates. Yet no one who spent an entire day with me could fail to note the countless ways in which I accommodate my illness, pacing myself carefully, constantly gauging my energy before I attempt a five-minute walk or a ten-minute drive. Neighbors see me taking out the trash, colleagues see me teaching class, other mothers see me picking up my son at school. They don't realize that I can seldom do all of these things in the same day. I have lived with chronic illness for several years now, but people only know this if I choose to tell them. Mostly it's easier not to.

☞ ☜

I earn my living by reading, teaching, and interpreting stories, so perhaps it is not surprising that I would seek a narrative cure. Yes, I tried many allopathic and alternative remedies. Out of wild curiosity, and because my mother-in-law insisted, I even made an appointment with a self-proclaimed spiritual healer, who asked me to recall the details of my own birth. It was a unique experience, but I decided that curiosity had its limits and the healing powers of literature were a better bet. Early in my illness, I had often been too sick to read; later I began to read obsessively, passionately. The distanced critical vision I had cultivated in graduate school, and which has remained for me an important and useful way to think about illness, gave way to a ravenous appetite for words. I craved their sounds and rhythms, their weight and heft, their clarity and ambiguity. And I needed, above all, the words and stories of those who had been seriously ill. Still too sick to work, I had no thought of teaching or writing about these illness narratives; I knew only that I urgently needed to learn what they had to teach.

Long a reader of Virginia Woolf, I discovered her essay "On Being Ill" and felt immediate companionship. I read Reynolds Price's memoir about learning to live as a self-described gimp after treatment for spinal cancer left him with paraplegia and chronic pain. I wished he would come for a month-long visit and teach me how to make a new and satisfying life in a changed body. I read Nancy Mairs's essays on living with MS. I read Judith Hooper's smart and sassy piece about living with breast cancer. For a while, these writers, and many others, became my new community. I didn't meet any of them until years later, but when I was very sick I felt they were my closest companions, the only friends who could help me to find a path through illness. Like many healthy, nondisabled people, I had imagined that life with serious illness or disability might be almost unlivable. Reading these essays, I found that such a life could indeed be difficult, but also richly textured and full of new discoveries. I realized that ill and disabled people know things that others don't. These were not tragic tales of illness, inspirational stories of overcoming disability, or narratives of an endless search for miracle cures. They were stories about living life in the midst of illness.

Eventually, these stories found their way into my professional life. The first time I taught a course on the literature of illness and disability, I reflected on what place my own story, my own body, had in the classroom. Wanting to focus on the texts at hand, I chose to remain silent on the subject of my illness. I thought hard about this: I was aware of the risk of perpetuating the silencing of disability, but I also didn't want my own story to prove distracting or to take center stage. And I didn't want to try to explain my complicated illness to my students. It was a private matter, too intimate to discuss with them. So we read other people's stories—both memoirs and literary case histories—stories about living with MS, with cancer, with AIDS, with neurological and psychiatric illness. We discussed essays by Susan Sontag, Freud, Oliver Sacks, Paul Monette, Nancy Mairs. A few weeks into the semester I found myself, quite unexpectedly, telling my brother's story. We were reading Kay Redfield Jamison's An Unquiet Mind, a memoir about living with bipolar illness, and suddenly it seemed to me both appropriate and imperative to tell my students something about my brother Hans, who lived with schizophrenia from age nineteen until his death at thirty-two. I described his vibrant paintings, classic examples of "outsider art." My students were rapt, both because schizophrenia is a fascinating, devastating illness, and because what I was doing departed radically from their experience of me as a teacher. My decision to tell a little of Hans's story did not reflect a consciously formed pedagogy but an impulse in the moment. Teaching this course, I had tried to make space for students' personal stories when they inevitably bubbled up into the discussion, but I had also tried, gently, to frame them in a critical context, to be clear that our purpose here was academic, not therapeutic. I framed Hans's story, too, presenting it as a story about illness and creativity, one that related to some of Jamison's themes. I was aware that his story was on some level a substitute story, a way of revealing my intimate connection to illness and to the course material without talking directly about my own body. Hans's story answered the question they had all been dying to ask me: "How on earth did you get interested in this stuff, anyway? Don't most English professors go in for Shakespeare and Jane Austen?"

Near the end of the semester, during an informal after-class discussion, one of my students said, "I don't think there are any sick or disabled people at this college." I was stunned. I know many students, staff, and faculty members who live with illness or disability of some kind, and because I am attuned to fairly subtle manifestations of disability, I see it everywhere I look. It was hard for me to believe that my student had spent a semester in this class and yet didn't recognize it in her immediate surroundings or understand that illness and disability, while sometimes invisible, are everywhere. Other students countered her comment, offering many of the observations I would have made myself. But I realized quickly that the most effective way to communicate to her the pervasiveness of illness—and its invisibility—would be to offer myself as an example. She was surprised, even shocked, to learn that I live with chronic illness, but she was not upset that I had not said so earlier. We had an interesting conversation about the ethics of disclosure. The accommodations I need to perform my job—a light course load, classes scheduled in the afternoon and in a room that is reasonably close to my office—don't affect my interactions in the classroom. There is no practical reason that I need to disclose my disability to my students. Yet I've come to believe that there are other important reasons to do so, not least the fostering of their understanding that illness is often invisible and that people with disabilities, appropriately accommodated, can function at least as well as anyone else. Identifying myself as a woman who lives with chronic physical illness and as the sister of a man who lived with mental illness helps them to understand that the essays and memoirs we read in class are not by or about people living in a parallel universe that never intersects with ours. They are about us, members of a college community and a shared human community. And my story does not take center stage in the classroom, as I had feared, but simply takes its place among all the other stories.

As I piece together these fragments of writing, trying to tell a version of the story of my illness, a dear friend emails me regularly with updates on her chemotherapy. Her breast cancer, in remission for more than two years, has recently metastasized to her liver. She needs to tell her body's story, to put into narrative form the feelings and experiences that a diagnosis alone can never communicate. The first thing she did after learning of her recurrence was to send a brief letter to her closest friends, beginning to narrate this next chapter of her life. I can offer her no medicines, no miracles, but I can give her something very powerful simply by saying, "Yes, tell me your story."

REFERENCE

James, Alice. *The Diary of Alice James*. Ed. Leon Edel. New York: Dodd, Mead, and Company, 1964.

QUESTIONS

1. In this essay, what role does storytelling play in diagnosis, medical decision-making, and healing?
2. What is the relationship between the patient's story and her doctors' stories? How do they compete with, corroborate, or complete one another?
3. Comment on the relationship between illness and mothering in this essay.

The Treatment

⇒ Roxana Robinson ⇐

Here is what I do each morning. As soon as I wake up, barefoot and still in my nightgown, as though I'm on the way to my lover, I go downstairs to the darkened kitchen. I'm alone in the house: my husband leaves early, my daughter is away in college. I don't bother to turn on the lights, I go straight to the refrigerator and open the door to its icy glare. From it I take out a chilled golden globe, the size of a small orange. It's made of firm and springy plastic, and solid, with some heft. The pearly outer sheathing is translucent, obscuring the glowing interior and giving it a muffled shimmer. I set the globe, with its neat coil of attached tubing, on the kitchen counter. For the next three hours it will lie there, slowly warming, so that when the fluid inside enters my vein it will not be cold and torpid but swift and potent. What's inside the radiant globe is Rocephin, a powerful antibiotic, which will cure me.

⇒ ⇐

When you are not ill, when you are well, you think about yourself in a particular way. You take being well for granted: that is who you are. You are a person like that, someone who does not have to think about her body. It is a luxury, not having to think about your body, but since you have always possessed it, you aren't aware that it's a luxury. When you think about sick people, you think of them as different from you, set apart in some unspecified way: they are Other. They are in that Other place, beyond a mysterious divide. They have become different from you, branded somehow, in a way you don't consider much. Even if you do consider it you can't get very far. Why are other people sick? Why are you not? There are no reasons, there is no logic. Things are the way they are. In some interior subliminal place you believe that you deserve your health. The person you are, it seems, deserves to be healthy, just as the person you are seems to deserve two legs, a nose. I had two legs, a nose, my health.

⇒ ⇐

Ten days ago the line was first introduced into my vein. I lay on a narrow examining table at the doctor's office, waiting while the nurse laid out her instruments. She was pleasant and perky, rather glamourous, with long blond hair and gleaming red fingernails. I lay perfectly still. I was prepared for everything, anything: nothing she did would distress me. This was the

"The Treatment" was published in *A Perfect Stranger and Other Stories*, Roxana Robinson, New York, Random House, 2005.
It is reprinted here with permission of the publisher.

initiation ceremony, the start of the healing. It was frightening, but I welcomed it, whatever terror it held. I was embracing the source of my fear. The treatment would be my salvation.

The nurse pulled up my sleeve and exposed the white skin on the inside of my elbow, the sacrificial site. She cleaned it and laid it down, bare, before the row of instruments. She took up a length of tubing, like a long transparent snake. Casually she measured this against me—from elbow to shoulder, across the top of my chest and then down to just above my heart. Here the mouth of the snake will dangle for six weeks.

When the nurse was ready to begin, she paused and looked up at my face. "You're going to feel a pinch," she warned.

I nodded. I knew that "pinch" was code for pain. The nurse looked back down, and I turned my head away. I watched the square white tiles in the ceiling while she worked, piercing my skin, violating my body. I could feel her movements. I didn't look.

"I hate when it spurts," I heard her say crossly. "Now it's all over the rug."

I said nothing, I didn't turn to look. No part of the treatment would trouble me: this is what would save me. I watched the grid of cross-hatching on the tiles while she slid the snake into the vein and sent it up the length of my upper arm, through the widening veins across the top of my chest, and down to the great thunderous vessel directly above my poor heart, deep in its hidden fastness, now invaded and violated. I said nothing. This would save me.

Taking pills three times a day means nothing. Anyone can do it; people do it all the time. There are no implications. It means only that you are correcting something, an aberration. Having a plastic tube inserted into your bloodstream, dangling over your heart, is different. This is a violation of your deepest recesses. This moves you into a darker place, more dangerous. This means you are ill, and helpless.

After three months, the oral antibiotics stopped working, and I went back to my doctor. We sat in his office, which is pleasantly cluttered in a domestic way. There's a bright hooked rug on the floor, a tall standing bookshelf, and a big ficus tree with glossy leaves in front of the window. There is no desk; Doctor Kennicott sits in a brown plaid wing chair. When he wants to write a prescription, he sets a polished wooden board across his lap.

Doctor Kennicott is a quiet man with a kindly manner, slightly bohemian. He has mournful brown eyes and shaggy greying hair and sideburns. He wears a white lab coat, khaki pants and black leather running shoes. That day he sat in the wing chair, and I sat in a smaller chair across from him.

"My neck is stiff again," I said. "I can't turn my head any further than this." And there was more: the symptoms were back. As I talked, Dr. Kennicott frowned sympathetically, his mournful eyes attentive. His elbows were set on the arms of the chair, his fingers steepled just under his chin. When I finished, Doctor Kennicott nodded slowly.

"That often happens," he announced.

This puzzled and disappointed me: then why had we used that treatment? I'd never been to a doctor who had prescribed something which, he knew, often didn't work. I'd never been to a doctor who didn't just fix what was wrong.

"Then what do we do now?" I asked.

Dr. Kennicott pushed out his lips thoughtfully. "I'd suggest moving on to intravenous antibiotics."

"No," I said at once.

I knew about intravenous, he'd mentioned it before. I didn't want it. It was too serious, too alarming. I told him it wasn't justified: I wasn't that ill. I was basically healthy, I told him. Other people have this disease and are treated for it and recover completely. That happened to my daughter, and she was treated for it at once, and now my daughter seems fine. I am basically fine, I told him.

The doctor said nothing while I explained this. He said nothing when I stopped. He sat in the wing chair, his hands steepled under his chin. He watched me quietly, waiting for me to understand. Finally I stopped and looked at him, alarm dawning.

To understand that you are seriously ill is to cross over into a different country. You are apart from other people now. Something separates you from them, something you cannot change. The realisation is like a fall from a great height. You are silenced: there is no recourse. You cannot help yourself. Your body has failed you, and you are helpless. You must change your expectations of all things. You must put yourself in the hands of the healers. They may fail.

When I understood this I fell silent. I was in a new place. Things were not as I had thought; arguing with the doctor was of little use.

This disease, like syphilis, is carried by spirochetes. There's reason to think the spirochetes have been in my bloodstream for a decade, for who knows how long. Now, it seems, these spirochetes have set up their malign outposts throughout my body. They're in the nervous system, the muscles, the connective tissue inside my joints, my spinal cord. They have stiffened my neck and my shoulders. They have turned my muscles leaden and my limbs resistant, so that when I move it feels as though I am struggling against an invisible network of tightening bonds. The spirochetes may, too, have infiltrated my deepest and most interior spaces, the tender private whorls inside my cranial basin. This idea, though, is so frightening that I don't allow myself to think about it. I don't permit myself to slide into that well of terror. I can't afford to.

The treatment also frightens me, but I can't afford that fear either. I've given myself up to this, like a postulant giving up her soul to God's. I'm allying myself with this larger power. The treatment will be my salvation. I can't afford to believe otherwise.

This morning, when the moment for the infusion arrives, I go back to the kitchen from my study. I'm dressed now, in jeans and a sweater: I work at home, getting my doctorate in Early Childhood Development. I've finished the coursework and am writing my thesis, which means that I don't have to explain to anyone why I'm now spending every morning at home, unavailable to the world, engaged in a private and fearsome activity.

At the sink I wash my hands with a liquid antimicrobial soap, a surgical scrub. It has a thin, acrid smell, and afterwards my skin feels raw and scraped. This is proper; this is part of the ritual: I am preparing myself for the chamber. My gestures now are careful and precise. From my big box of medical supplies, from my zip-locked plastic bags I take out three blunt-nosed syringes. The two white-capped ones hold saline solution, which will be injected first and last, to clean the tubing. The yellow-capped syringe holds heparin, a mild anti-coagulant. This goes in after the Rocephin, so that the blood idling in the tubing between treatments will not form clots. I lay all these things out beside the globe. The instruments are ready.

I pull up the sweater on my left arm. Clasped along my elbow is a white elastic fishnet sleeve, open-ended, that holds the apparatus tight against my skin. I slide this off, letting a translucent line of tubing uncoil downward into the air. One end of this is taped flat to my skin in a serpentine loop before it disappears into my flesh. The other end, interrupted by a small transparent junction box, ends in a blue valve. This is called a clave, and it is shaped like the head of a lizard, narrowing and blunt-nosed. I open a foil-wrapped packet holding an antiseptic swab, and its sharp alcohol odor blooms in the air, powerful and sobering. With a little bad luck, any germ I carry at this moment will be transported directly to my heart.

Carefully I swab off the flat metal surface of the clave. Holding it aloft, sterile, in one hand, with the other I unscrew a white-capped syringe. I push its threaded nose into the clave, forcing the surface downward. Inside the clave are matching grooves, and the threaded syringe screws neatly, perfectly, into the protected tunnel within the clave. On the line of tubing is a triangular cock, and I slide the line from the narrow vise-end where it has been clamped shut, to the wide end. The line to my vein is now open.

I press down on the plunger. The loaded syringe holds two and a half milliliters of saline solution. I watch the transparent solid creep down the coil until the tube vanishes within the surface of my skin, and the liquid enters my body. I can feel its cold arrival in my vein. I press the plunger slowly down until I reach the flattened air bubble at the bottom of the shaft. I unscrew the syringe and set it down. Still holding the clave in the air, I unscrew the small angel-winged cap on the Rocephin line, and set its transparent nose into the opening of the clave. Like the syringe, it fits neatly, into its tunneled grooves. This connection feels smooth and satisfying, and I feel gratified by this, as though technical perfection means the treatment will work like this, in just this beautifully engineered way.

I sit down and lean back. Now I'm connected. The valves are open, the liquid has begun its journey into my body. The golden globe is pressurised, and for the next forty minutes, it will slowly contract, forcing the Rocephin steadily into my bloodstream.

I close my eyes. My part in this is like prayer: I concentrate on what is taking place inside me, I visualise it. I see the golden tide beginning its silent warrior's surge, past the heart and through the wide channels of the great arteries, the smaller ones of the arterioles, moving deep into the interior, into the narrow waterways of the capillaries. I see the golden tide moving into a still lagoon, deep in the interior. Calm water on pale sand. The movement is visible, a low relentless surge. Along the irregular shore a long ripple breaks in a narrow line of foam. There is a sighing hiss, a small seething commotion: the spirochetes, the tiny corkscrews of the disease, are sizzling in a frenzy of death. I hear them thrashing tinily, I see the surface of the water along the shore boil and churn as they jitter. They twist and sputter as it hits them; they are dying, dying in droves, dying by the millions, at the touch of the smooth golden surge.

During my first week of the treatment I've had the predicted reactions: high fever, chills and headaches, brief wild stabbing pains in all my joints. I'm told that all of this is the result of the spirochetes dying off. I believe this is true. The infusions are the Asian hordes sweeping across the wide plains, overwhelming our enemy. I lie in bed, sick with fever, feebly triumphant.

Now the fever has stopped, and I'm better, but not well. I know I am ill. I feel as though

I'm walking carefully, on some unreliable surface, not knowing what movement might cause a sudden terrifying crack and plunge. Yesterday I took the dogs out for a walk through the woods, down to the winter-dark pond and past it, up the hillside beyond. The woods are brown and mysterious now; the trees creak ponderously in the wind, and their grey filigree tops sway silently. The narrow path was soft underfoot. Walking along it, climbing the steep slope of the hill, I felt suddenly the delicate tangling grope of the snake inside my chest, a faint dry grappling sensation, just above my heart. When it happened, my heart began to pound, panicky, shrinking from this dangerous alien presence. There was nowhere for me to go for help. It was I who gave permission for this. My brain believes it's good; it's my body that fears it. I tried to calm my heart. Above me, the tops of the trees moved slowly, swaying against the grey sky.

This Saturday morning, my husband, Mark, comes into the kitchen when I'm getting ready to infuse. He's been out in the village doing errands, and now he stands just inside the door, setting down packages. I know he sees my equipment laid out on the kitchen counter, but he keeps his eyes away from it, as though it were a naked body.

"I couldn't find the coffee you like," he says, unzipping his parka. His voice seems loud and artificial.

"That's all right," I say. "They have it at Sgaglio's. I'll get it tomorrow."

"I got everything else," he says. His eyes now fix on mine, faintly accusatory, as though I've contaminated the kitchen.

"Thanks," I say, conciliatory.

He ducks back out into the mudroom, to hang up his coat. When he comes back in, he shuts the heavy kitchen door hard.

"You're welcome," he says. Still without looking at my syringes, his dark gaze fixed on mine until it shifts to the door, he heads for his study. Mark is a philosophy professor, and his mind moves either in great wheeling arcs or little tiny circles, depending on one's point of view. I hear him sit down in his study. Alone in the kitchen I turn back to my instruments, but now the sight of them fills me with dread. They look diabolical, like something from a horror movie.

When all this is ready, I tell myself that Mark was just uncomfortable, not horrified. Or abstracted, as he often is. I call in to him in his study, my voice playful.

"I'm about to shoot up. Want to watch?" I ask hopefully. If he'll be part of this, it will less frightening, it will seem more normal. But he doesn't want to watch.

"No thanks," he calls in from his study. His voice is not playful, and after a moment I hear his door close quietly. I know he finds all this repugnant, and why should he not? Why should he have to share it with me?

He's not the only one. My friend Sarah came over one morning, and when she saw my syringes in their bags on the counter, she jumped nervously behind my back. "I don't want to look at them," she explained.

I begin to wonder if I should wear a bell, to warn normal people of my approach. I feel frightened and isolated. I can see I am alone here.

Last night, in bed, when Mark was ready to go to sleep he closed his Kierkegaard and set it on his bedside table beside the clock.

"That's it for me," he said. He took off his glasses and rubbed fiercely at the bridge of his nose, which glistened. He folded his glasses, set them on top of his book, and turned off his light.

When he turned over on his side, toward me, I was waiting for him.

"Put your arms around me," I said, and my husband did this at once, gathering me wholly against him. My face pressed close into his chest, surrounded by his comfort, I said, "Tell me I'm going to get well."

I needed to hear the words.

I felt Mark's hand on the back of my head, stroking my hair.

"You're going to get well," he said.

"Say it again," I said, pressing my face against his chest.

☞ ☜

Tonight I'm alone. Mark's away at a conference, but a visiting nurse, Ginger, is coming. It's her second visit; she came once before, early on, to change the bandages. Now she's going to change the tubes. I'm uneasy about this, as I don't know what it means. Will she pull out the whole long snake that has burrowed its way so deep into my interior? Drag it out from its secret nest above my heart? It's frightening to have it in there, but it would be frightening, too, to have it moved.

Still, I'm looking forward to seeing Ginger. I know I've done well, and I'm proud of myself. I'm looking forward to her praise: I'm a good patient. The pains are mostly gone, and both their arrival and departure are proof of my prowess. The opening where the line enters my skin is pale and healthy, not inflamed. Each morning I have performed the infusion successfully, and sent the golden tide deep into my interior. Each day, connecting the tiny spiral chambers, screwing them into the closed valves, unlocking the entrance to my veins, plugging myself into the heavy golden globe, I feel it rush silently into my bloodstream and I feel charged with victory. I feel the spirochetes failing against this magnificent onslaught, overwhelmed, undone. I know we'll be victorious, and my nurse knows it too. She is the agent of my healing. Her presence plays a part; it will make this real. She'll infuse me with hope and conviction.

Around eight o'clock, Ginger arrives. She opens the back door and bustles cheerfully into the kitchen. "Hi, there," she says, boisterously good-natured. The dogs sniff her, wagging their tails politely. "Good *dog*," she says crooningly, leaning unctuously over them and patting their heads too hard; "good *dog*." Ginger is in her early thirties, thickset, with bushy brown hair in a wild shoulder-length aura. She's wearing a knitted wool dress, a heavy sweater and dark clunky shoes. She's somehow powerful and clumsy, like a shaggy little bull.

Ginger sets down her bag and takes off her padded jacket, already talking. "I just came from an auction in Pughkeepsie," she says chattily. "It was so fun."

"Great," I say. "Did you get anything?"

"A rocker," she says emphatically, pausing to look up me, delighted I've asked. "A porch rocker. It's real old and funky. I really love it."

"Great," I say again.

I don't care what she bought, but I'm so pleased to see her that she could read aloud from the telephone book. I listen happily as she gabs, watching her take out a big plastic packet, sealed and sterile, full of small intricate objects. She spreads it on the kitchen table and I sit down. Outside it is turning dark, and we lean together under the hanging lamp. I lay my arm out on the table and roll up my sleeve. Ginger now takes off her big sweater, and tosses back her heavy mass of hair. There is a lot of her at that table: breathy, fleshy, bulky. I wish her hair were in a bun. I wish she were lean and smooth, clipped and sterile, in a white uniform.

"So, how have you been?" she asks bumptiously.

"Fine," I say with pride. "Some aches and pains in my joints, but that doesn't bother me."

Ginger shakes her head fondly. "My patients who have this, love feeling achy," she says, as though this were an endearingly foolish trait. "They think it means they're getting better."

I smile with her: I know they're right.

Ginger opens her sterile packets, ripping back adhesive strips, putting on thin gloves. I am nervous about this procedure, the hidden snake, fearful of what she is about to do. Ginger yanks off the bandage over the plastic shunt where it enters my skin. As her hands near the opening I turn rigid. She stops.

"Where does it hurt?" she asks.

"It doesn't," I say, "I'm just wary." In fact I am terrified.

"You think I'm going to pull the adhesive back against the tube," she says indulgently. "We're taught as rookies always to pull with the tube. You pull against it"— she she makes a sudden ripping gesture, as though she is about to jerk the unprotected tube from where it snakes into my skin— "you'd pull the shunt right out of your arm. Like, that is *not* therapeutic."

I say nothing, trying to calm my heartbeat. My whole system is running on alarm; my heart is pounding. That dangerous gesture, the perilous mimicking of violence, has shocked me. She now begins to do delicate things to the tube. I don't want to watch, and to distract myself I look at her face.

"Do you do this a lot?" I ask.

She told me before how grateful her patients are, and I want to hear stories of her successes. I want to hear how this disease is vanquished, how good she is at her task, how powerful and inexorable this treatment is. I am greedy for these stories, I want to count myself among this healing crowd.

Ginger looks up. "Oh, yes," she says. "I do chemotherapy all day long."

I frown: this isn't a word I want to hear. This is not a group I want to belong to.

"No," I say. "I mean do you do this, treatment for my disease, often?"

"Oh yes," Ginger says again. She bends over the tube again. Her heavy hair falls over her shoulder, hanging in a bristly thicket over the instruments. "In fact I have one patient who lives right near you. He's been on intravenous treatment for two years."

"Two years?" I say. I've been told my treatment will last six weeks.

"Yes," she says, shaking her head. "He's in terrible shape. He's had your disease for years and it wasn't treated right away. He's nearly paralysed. He's trying oxygen chamber treatments now. Nothing really seems to help him."

I say nothing. I wish she weren't bending so closely over my arm, which now lies bare and vulnerable beneath her fleshy face. The transparent tube doubles down beneath my skin and disappears. The whole region of my arm twitches with alarm, with the extremity of its exposure. If she were to do anything now, even jostle the tube accidentally, the possibilities of pain are horrifying. The possibilities are ones I cannot permit myself to think of: infection, the lethal transmission of things directly to my heart, my poor vulnerable heart, with the snake dangling its toxic head directly over its chambers. I feel as though everything now is dangerous, that our passage together through this process has become perilous. Each step now is crucial.

Ginger shakes her head again. "No, this is really a terrible disease," she says.

I cannot bear to hear what she is saying; it is dangerous for me to hear this. I say rudely, "Don't you have any better stories?" My arm, in her hands, feels exposed and frightened.

She looks up. "About this disease? No. If it isn't treated right away it's really terrible. You see, it mutates in your system."

I stare at her, appalled, willing her to stop telling me these things.

She looks earnestly at me, her huge bristling hair surrounding her face. "What happens is that the spirochetes, if they aren't treated right away, change form, so that the treatment can never catch up with the disease. Each time the doctor tries something new the form is different. The disease goes deeper and deeper into your system. This man has it in his spinal cord, and it's gone into his brain; he has neurological symptoms. Now he's going to doctors who have it themselves, to see how they're treating their own diseases."

I stare down at my arm, mesmerised with horror.

As she talks, against my will, I am picturing the spirochetes in my own system, spiralling deeper and deeper into my defenseless system, burrowing their way into my spinal fluid, sliding unstoppably into the crevices of my brain. Each word she speaks makes this real, inevitable, incontrovertible.

All my feelings of triumph, of power and victory are sliding downwards, cascading toward ruin. She is destroying everything I have accomplished. I hate the words she is saying. I hate what she is doing to me. I want to rip the tubing out of my arm. I want to tear out everything she has touched and throw it from me and order her from my house. She is casting a spell, she is cursing my body, she is destroying the health and vigor of my flesh, she is shattering my hope. She is declaring the futility of everything I am struggling to achieve, she is showing me a future of misery and despair. She is deriding my belief in the golden tide. I hate her more than I could have imagined possible.

Looking down at my arm, I say in a strained voice, "I don't think you should talk this way to your patients."

Alarmed, she looks up. "What does your doctor tell you?"

"He doesn't talk to me like this," I say, my voice choking. "And you should never talk like this to a patient."

"I'm sorry," Ginger says. She is clearly upset. "I'm a very sensitive person. I wouldn't have upset you if I had known."

"I've had this disease for ten years and it hasn't been treated," I say. I am struggling, I am desperate to keep from crying. "I don't want to hear about this."

Shaken, Ginger bends again over the tubing. She is not touching the long snake, as it turns out. She's replacing only the outer section of it, the bit that goes from the clave to the junction, but I now hate having her touch me. She is contaminating me; her touch is dangerous, poison to my body. Her touch is a curse on me. I imagine ripping everything out of my arm, flinging the transparent coils away from me onto the floor.

She works for a few seconds in silence, then starts up again. "Last time I came," she says carefully, "we talked about your daughter, remember? Who has this too, right? And was treated for it?"

How can she not have understood me? Does she imagine I want to hear this about my daughter?

"*I said I don't want to talk about this,*" I say again, emphatically.

I am now swollen, huge with wrath and despair and grief. I am outraged that she should choose to use her power over me in this way, that she should have come to me disguised as a healer, and have revealed herself instead as a black curse, an agent of doom and anguish. I want her to get out of my kitchen, out of my house, off my property. I want to sic the dogs on her. I sit in raging silence while she finishes. She pads heavily back and forth, finishing up, throwing things away. Her head is down, her face averted; she is clearly upset. I think she's crying. I don't care.

I want only to control my tears, to keep from breaking down in her presence, to achieve merely that, and in that one small thing I am victorious.

QUESTIONS

1. Comment on the author's use of words and images related to religion, war, and alienation. Why does she choose the patterns for this story?
2. Why does the author choose not to name the disease?
3. Discuss the final scene. What does it suggest about communication between patients and health-care professionals?

Panic

⮰ Ellen Samuels ⮱

In the early hours of an April morning, I am awakened by the very force of darkness, the dusk which for months has been settling over my mind. It is quiet in my room, the door closed and locked, but I open my eyes with a sudden apprehension. Quiet: the darkness thickens, and out of it a hand strikes my face. It strikes again and again as my body propels itself across the bed, bruising the wall, twisting the blanket in sharp designs. When it ends, I've been thrown to the bed frame's foot, shivering. I cannot trace this force to a will; there is no one else in the room, no answer.

⮰ ⮱

In that April after my twentieth birthday, I took myself captive—body to mind—each a hopeless apologist for the other's erratic explosions and failings, and the "self" of their union immeasurably altered. I had returned to college that spring, after six months spent caring for my cancer-stricken mother, and attempted to plunge myself again into a familiar and comforting academic world. Instead, just before the end of the semester, I unwillingly, unwittingly entered another world: the world of panic. After that first morning, the attacks came closer and closer together, often five or six times a day. I began spending most of my time in bed, afraid to risk myself in the outside world. Visiting the dormitory bathroom late at night, I would stare at my helplessly jerking reflection, my elbow flailing like a bird's wing approaching flight, and tears washing over my face. I was terrified that someone would walk in and see me; at that time, I thought more of the humiliation of discovery than of its consequence: help.

I concealed my panic for as long as possible, terrified that if I told anyone, my loss of control would become permanent: I'd be taken to a hospital and never let go. I didn't know then, as I do now, that my condition would not be classified as a "mental illness," but as a psychological disorder, the seemingly trivial distinction carrying all the weight of the us/them dichotomy. Once I was diagnosed, my doctors reassured me over and over that panic attacks were really quite common, "could happen to anyone." They never realized how this reassurance fueled my fear by showing so clearly the lurking stigma behind that fine line between "psychological" and "mental."

Clinically defined, panic attacks are an activation of the body's defense systems against a perceived attack: muscles tense, heartbeat and breathing accelerate, adrenaline floods its channels. All our ancient reflexes respond as if we are in physical danger—but the enemy is internal: a memory or fear which eats away at those boundaries of the mind which normally function, like a cell's outer layer, to keep chaos in check and the progress of life secure. What it means to me to panic is that my mind, which I had been used to considering as an entity, an edifice of many rooms but singular structure, suddenly reveals itself as a world made up of separate elements which can be excommunicated from one another. The image in my mind which represents imminent panic is a boat suddenly cast off from shore, floating slowly but irrevocably away from me. It is almost a peaceful image, and there is a part of me that feels peaceful, as my sense of connection to the world is severed and my consciousness ascends to hover in the shadowy corners of the room—even as the rest of me sinks into a depthless well, my mind dark and unpredictable, my body a trap.

I became obsessed with walls, white plaster-smooth walls, the kind I imagined lining the wards of the mental health unit. If I could surround myself with utter blankness, with the absence of sensation, then perhaps I could be free to open my eyes without fearing the assault of colors, faces, and sounds. Even the vertical cracks between cinder blocks in my dormitory walls were too much for me; I wanted to smooth down those grooves, or fill them up, equalize the surface. As the days of panic grew closer together, I would return from a class or meal in which I had behaved (as far as I could tell) completely naturally, then collapse against the door as soon as it closed behind me, crawl to my bed and roll sideways into the mattress, reaching my left hand out to the wall that was cool, hard, and unchangeable. I could smack my palm against it as hard as I wanted, and leave it unmarked; but the pain anchored me, shocked me out of confusion for a second or two. I found that if I turned off the lights and lay in my bed staring at the wall, it would merge into the placid grayness of an empty TV screen, allowing me to be empty also, to escape the fear.

I wanted a doctor to tell me what was wrong with me, but I did not want to tell a doctor what *seemed* to be wrong: that I was going insane, that I was losing my mind. I had seen my mother default on her contract with reality a few months earlier, when a combination of tumors and drugs robbed her mind of its right to rationally analyze and express the world around her, and that betrayal stayed with me—both hers and that of the doctors who failed to assist her. Though her oncologist must have seen dozens (hundreds?) of patients with significant cancer-related dementia, he could offer neither an explanation nor any advice on how to cope; though the hospital orderlies must have had experience with drug-dazed patients, they could do no better than to load her onto a wheelchair and leave her shivering and weeping in the hallway while they called for a consult; though the candy striper must have had at least *some* kind of training on working with sick people, she kept delivering green paper menus and asking my mother—who was alternately comatose, babbling, or crying— to circle her choices for lunch, please. In fact, that pale, uncheerful brunette radiated such terror on entering my mother's room that even through her ever-shrinking peephole into reality, my mother saw enough to lean over and whisper, "That little girl is scared of me."

Five months later, I was the one who was scared—of myself, and of what other people would do to me if they knew.

Now, nearly seven years later, I can write the story of those days as if I have overcome them, and almost as if I am telling of somebody else's failure, somebody else's collapse. This is the distance of time, and of writing itself. But this familiar act of distancing through language takes on a new value in this instance, because part of my experience of panic is that separation of selves which I felt with the ascension of my conscious mind to the ceiling's corners, to a shadowy region above, from which I observed my loss of control with a dispassionate, almost skeptical eye. This was not so simple or as romantic a separation as the Western ideal of the mind-body split, for I simultaneously inhabited both the mind which floated above and the mind which remained trapped in the flailing body. In the same way, a writer's mind, conscious and dispassionate, attempts to divorce itself from the past in order to recall and contain its meaning and language—even as the person writing remains intimately and excruciatingly aware that the loss cannot be fully contained.

I wrote before, during, and after the two years that I was most affected by panic disorder. I wrote poetry, journals, and letters in which I tried to understand the meaning of my experience, and also to use it in a creative sense, to treat it as a serendipitous chance to confront myself, and to change. Most of that writing is useful only as a personal record; the self-pity into which daily panic attacks often plunged me suffuses those texts. Yet, I still believe the process of writing itself was a major component of my eventual medication-free emergence from a state of "disorder." While I still have occasional panic attacks, they no longer cripple my daily life and abilities. Writing provided an outlet for the negative energy accumulated inside me, a release that in another time or place might have been attempted by bloodletting, or acupuncture, or even by the misguided removal of my "female organs"—and I can't say whether writing would be a successful therapy for anyone else afflicted with this disorder, any more than those other methods would have been successful treatments for me.

Often, after a panic attack, I would read novels to restore myself to a world of safety, a world in which words lined up on pages like houses seen from an airplane, air and vision smoothing away imperfection, disorder. I treated a book much like a bottle of pills; once opened, it was expected to do the rest. And sometimes it did—but other times I became too aware of the emptiness between words, between lines, at the edge of the page. There was too much space into which my fears could enter and dance around the edges of narrative, drawing my eyes away. Perhaps this was because I had used books in this same narcotic fashion during the summer preceding my mother's death, when I moved back into my parents' house for the first time since my eighteenth birthday—somehow aware, without being told, that my mother's illness had become terminal. After a day of my family's "business-as-usual" avoidance of the subject, I would lie in my childhood bed reading Sara Paretsky or Jane Austen to put myself to sleep. But as soon as I'd turn off the light, every fear would return, unthought possibilities drawing nearer to speech. When the darkness had thickened to a heavy lid and I could shrink no smaller beneath it, I would turn on the light, pick up the book, and focus my dazzled, blinking eyes on the white pages. Eventually, exhaustion would come and allow me to sleep. Sometimes, before that happened, I could faintly hear my mother, also awake, crying in the room next door. I did not get up, as I might have as a child, and go to her; I didn't know if I should be seeking comfort or offering it. It seemed that, by holding back, at least I risked hurting no one but myself.

When I finally consulted a psychotherapist in Cambridge, Massachusetts, six weeks after I began having panic attacks, she sent me at once to a psychiatrist, who in turn referred me to a neurologist at Beth Israel Hospital. Their concern—and confusion—stemmed from the fact that my symptoms included convulsions, which were not typical of panic attacks and might indicate an underlying neurological problem. My visit to the neurologist was darkly humorous; he was from New Zealand, and quite nonplussed by my various American feminist appurtenances. When he bent to examine my ankles, he was clearly shocked that such hairy things lurked under my floral summer skirt, and when I told him I was in a relationship with a woman, he started visibly, and then attempted to add an HIV test to the routine blood work he was ordering (I refused). Finally, he suggested that my only sign of potential epilepsy was a disproportionately large right thumb, and therefore pronounced me disease-free. Despite the half-comic nature of our encounter, I relied desperately upon the clean bill of health that doctor gave me, the innocence which it granted my body. At least disorder had not originated in me, but had been imposed upon me; my mind was not violent, but *violated*. I walked out of the hospital into the restored sanctity of my sane mind, took the train home, and spent the next two months in my bedroom, barely able to cross the hall to find food—thoroughly absolved, but entirely unhealed.

⌒ ⌒

Like its more commonly known cousin, post-traumatic stress disorder, panic disorder was first diagnosed in young soldiers engaged in combat, a response to forced persistence in the face of horror. In 1870, a British military surgeon named Myers wrote about a syndrome involving heart palpitations, dizziness, chest pain, shortness of breath, and insomnia, and labeled it "soldier's heart." Several transformations later, the disorder has been located in the head, not the heart. In the last twenty years, panic has been found to respond to a number of psychiatric medications which regulate brain chemistry; currently, anti-anxiety drugs like Xanax, and the selective serotonin reuptake inhibitors (Prozac, Zoloft, Paxil) are used to treat panic attacks, both acute and chronic. Knowing the history now, as I did not at the time, I am not surprised that all three of my "doctors"—the therapist, the psychiatrist, and the neurologist—strongly recommended these medications to me at the time of my diagnosis.

I refused them. For reasons only half-clear to me even now, I wanted to recover from panic without using pills, which I saw not so much as crutches keeping me from healing "on my own" but as invaders, adding to the population of unfamiliar and uncontrolled forces within my mind. The mention of side effects terrified me. Would these medications change my personality, smooth down the roughness which enabled me to write, to feel, to know myself? Too much had changed already; I could not accept more outside intervention. This fear was heightened by one doctor's comment that she would "let" me not take medication only because I was not suicidal, the clear implication being that if I did become suicidal, I should conceal it or be prepared to be hospitalized and forcibly medicated.

What *is* strange to me now, however, having learned about the many non-pharmaceutical treatments of panic, is how swiftly the doctors washed their hands of me once I'd voiced my refusal. The offer to prescribe exhausted their arsenals; soon, only the psycho-therapist would see me. She reluctantly agreed to help me work out my "feelings" through "conversation," since I would not treat my "disease" with "medicine." Thus I came to realize the fundamental weakness of Western psychiatric medicine: despite its remarkable success in locating, naming, and treating the chemical causes of our despair, in the course of that progress, despair ceases to be despair and becomes pathology, infection—to be eradicated, rather than understood. It would have helped, back in that summer, if I could have been shown the roots of our Western understanding of panic, its origin in those words of a Brit-ish doctor studying the Coldstream Guards: *soldier's heart*. It would have helped to think of myself, not as a victim, but as a fighter, and ultimately, as the victim of my own perceived need to keep on fighting, to save emotion for later. Eventually I did learn to understand the relationship between my panic and the days I spent caring for my mother, watching her mind and body decay, yet feeling the demands of care-taking supplant grief, refusing to cry as I touched her body—until I couldn't even cry when alone, didn't cry when I saw her dead, but merely leaned forward to adjust her pillow, having schooled myself so far in ac-ceptance of the unacceptable.

Soldiers who are badly wounded do not necessarily develop panic; it is those who *see* their fellows wounded, dismembered, impaled before their eyes, who begin to experience racing hearts, strangled breath, a sense of doom even while lying secure in their bunks. Panic is the pain of witnessing—and so is poetry—not in any romanticized sense, but as a pure distillation of the mind's need to make sense of the messages brought by the nerves, to construct a world in which those messages can exist alongside our own vulnerability. When I panicked, I certainly did not feel creative; I dreamed of breaking off my extremities like segments of bamboo, shrinking into a single thing, consciousness without the burden of being or acting.

But there was also the moment of coming out of panic, of teaching myself to live in the world again—to overcome the agoraphobia and be among people, to feel their bodies' jostle and give; also to learn to witness *myself*, to see how my muscles twitched when too many feelings became lodged inside me, and to circumvent that process before it became full-blown. It took a long time—it is still taking time, for it never quite leaves me, this pro-cess—and I might have had an easier path if I'd taken the medication. But I do not quarrel with that choice of my earlier self; I will not look back on those times and ask "What if?" I have worked so very hard to allow myself to live in the present, to be able to write this piece, and I cannot imagine reaching this point without that work—without the gradual reinven-tion of self that took place that summer and fall, marked by journal entries such as: "Today I tied my shoes. I walked up the stairs twice without falling."

When I wrote during my panic, when I wrote about my panic, I felt both righteous and ashamed. Writing maintained a thread of self, a slender but crucial integrity—but I also felt that to describe what was happening to me rendered me hysterical, hypochondriac, relevant only to myself. The specter of Gilman's woman in the wallpaper seemed very real in those moments, reflected grimly in the eyes of doctors, in the steel door of the locked psych unit I refused to enter. That I am now able to write an entire essay about this experience does not mean I've overcome the contradictions inside me; the words emerge with difficulty through a mesh of conflicting emotions, and perhaps some words do not emerge at all. But now I can see the writing—and the panic—as a part of an ongoing struggle, a fruitful battle, both inside my calamitous mind/body, and externally, with those medical and cultural forces competing to label or "cure" me. Though I remember that struggle as a time of terrible helplessness and fear, my writing reminds me that I was also defiant, and that defiance helped me to survive. Six years later, I keep taped to my bedroom mirror a fragment of a poem I wrote that summer, a simple reminder: "I will not give up the right / to wake up in my own bed, hearing only / the birds, the cars passing / these morning noises, common as breath."

QUESTIONS

1. Discuss the stigma attached to mental illness. How do the labels "mental illness" and "psychological disorder" compare?

2. Consider the widespread prescription and use of antidepression medication in contemporary society. To what extent do you agree with the author that other, non-medical therapies are equally or potentially more effective?

3. What do you think about the author's refusal to take the medication prescribed for her, and what do you make of her doctors' decision to "wash their hands of [her]" when she refuses to follow their protocol?

⤺ PART IV ⤻
MEDICINE AT THE MARGINS

Most illnesses—like the people who experience them—defy neat categorization and are thus liminal. The first three essays of this section deal with the indeterminacy of illness. With levity, Bonnie Blackwell explores how panic disorder actually serves her well and thus raises questions about whether it should be officially diagnosed and treated medically. Similarly, Mikita Brottman uses humor to examine her obsessive-compulsive disorder in the context of the quirky, repetitious behavior of others, and also reveals how damaging such diagnostic labels are when they follow the patient for life. Both Blackwell and Brottman stress the unique manifestation of their disorders and call for individualized treatment options. Through Wordsworthian "spots of time" and diary entries, Emma Burns reveals the obsessive-compulsive nature of anorexia nervosa from her perspective as both sufferer and medical student, and indicates that proper diagnosis is often tricky because behavioral changes are gradual.

The five essays in the second group address various liminalities that occur because of race, ethnicity and culture. Ruth Elizabeth Burks explores her adult son's dual marginalization because he is autistic and African American. She argues that people with disabilities should be valued as whole persons with important contributions to make not only to medical knowledge but to society in general. "Bi-queer, Black-Chinese, working class, [and] female," Wendy Marie Thompson reveals how bipolar disorder complicates her already complex identity as a non-white, non-privileged member of society. Even as she laments not having adequate language to explain herself *to* herself, she utilizes a distinctive articulate rage in her quest for self-awareness. It is not so much her identity as an African American but her relative poverty as a graduate student that disenfranchises Tracy Curtis in the world of medicine; because of her inability to afford proper health care, her inconclusive cancer remains undiagnosed and untreated. Poverty, race and language create barriers for the Chinese family of a young, virus-stricken child whose story is told by her social worker, Ting Man Tsao. The lapses in communication between physician and parent, instances of iatrogenesis, and Tsao's reflections on his own responsibilities in the case are reminiscent of

337

Anne Fadiman's *The Spirit Catches You and You Fall Down*. And Laurence Marshall Carucci explores the international politics surrounding two divergent views of typhoid fever—in America and in the Marshall Islands. While his American doctors use lab tests to divine the cause of his malady, the Islanders understand it in the context of a love potion.

Chronic and terminal illnesses create a liminality all their own; time and space no longer function in the same way. Maggie Griffin Taylor and Susan Dick describe the protraction of time and dislocation of space in their respective essays on diabetes and Guillain-Barré syndrome, and both utilize the metaphor of illness as a foreign country in their narratives. While illness takes over and suspends the normal activities and relationships of life, Dick concludes that it also has the capacity to teach the miracle of the everyday. In her two poems, Ellen Goldsmith depicts the kind of limbo that characterizes post-breast cancer remission society; she remains suspended between the comforts of childhood play and the uncertainty of the future. The final essays, by Lynda Hall and Laurie Rosenblatt, examine two people's responses to terminal illness: a sister, whose vegetative state Hall simulates with skill akin to Katherine Anne Porter's in "The Jilting of Granny Weatherall," and a breast cancer patient whose story Dr. Rosenblatt has recorded verbatim and offers as a balance to the media's preference for stories of survival. These essays mark important considerations of dependency and agency and explore unflinchingly the truth that not all people survive illness intact, if at all.

"Speak, Mild Fran"
Panic Disorder and My Perverse Devotion to a Life of Public Speaking

⌒ BONNIE BLACKWELL ⌒

One of the constant puzzles of human behavior is the number of people who, though not particularly shy, regard public speaking as the supreme form of humiliation. Surprisingly, as a painfully reticent person, I consider lecturing one of the chief pleasures of life. I enjoy public performance not because I am a natural ham—one of those dramatic sorts born without the capacity for shame, who was always the class clown, the lead in the school play, queen of the agricultural fair, and the star of her own movie, in which everyone else is merely a walk-on. On the contrary, for as long as I can remember, I have been a shame vector. As guilelessly as a velour sweatsuit lures cat hair, I leech all the embarrassment out of any room I walk into. This is especially true if I'm watching someone who refuses to be ashamed. Needless to say, the ads for Girls Gone Wild videos proliferating on late-night television are exquisite agony. MTV's Spring Break specials actually led to cancellation of my cable TV contract. The sight of a luxuriantly dimpled woman in a bikini is such a profound personal indictment to me (having never owned a bikini, much less gone out in one) that I repeat the mantra, "it's not my ass, it's not my ass," for purposes of self-hypnosis during Sir Mix-a-lot's "Baby Got Back" video and other moments of personal hell.

For a long time it seemed like I was just one of the few women in the world so perverse that I didn't relish appreciative male gazes. In high school, kindly people offered that the consolation of my 5'9", 110-pound frame was that I could be a model, but I couldn't imagine anything worse than having my image reproduced and enlarged as a way to earn my livelihood. My pet name among my high school friends was Howard Hughes, earned through my staunch refusal to go to public swimming holes or show up on yearbook photo day. I regularly score "shrinking violet" on the *Cosmopolitan* test, "Quiz: Are You a Drama Queen?" When I read *Mansfield Park*, I note that the title is an anagram for "Speak, mild Fran" and feel exhorted in turn—though to be honest, I find Fanny not "a monster of self-complacency and conceit," as Lionel Trilling did, but a bully who takes passive-aggressive behavior to an art form.

339

For the duration of my childhood and adolescence, spent among people with no fixed opinions about Fanny Price, my affliction was just known as shyness. In my hometown, the inability to interface with all kinds of folks was a kind of birth defect cruelly ill-suited to the landscape, like being what locals called "fair complected" and condemned to blister in the unrelenting West Texas sun. In high school English, I memorized Prufrock's lament, pleased to have a partner in my painful isolation. In college, I read John Berger's *Ways of Seeing* and Laura Mulvey's *Visual Pleasure in Narrative Cinema*, and had a new vocabulary for an old discomfiture: it seemed that I longed for an escape from the "to-be-looked-at-ness" of woman under patriarchy. While Prufrock had failed to enjoy his male prerogative, to refuse the burden of objectification, I was condemned by my chromosomes to live in the world of appearing rather than being. The hermetic nature of Berger's and Mulvey's totalizing paradigms confirmed the hopelessness of my situation. And those women happily shaking their moneymakers for the camera were just not smart enough to see what I had intuited from birth. It was a very gratifying theory that conflated social awkwardness with inborn feminist propensities. However, it did not explain why other feminists had a rational response to objectification and I had a somatic one. Finally, when the pharmaceutical companies started advertising on prime-time television, I acquired still other vogue words for my predicament: social anxiety disorder, panic attacks, and a deficit of happy little serotonin bubbles traveling from circle A to circle B in the brain. There was a solution, and it was chemical.

What are the perimeters of this anxiety? It's a shape-shifting disease which takes on attributes of claustrophobia, agoraphobia, uncontrollable blushing and downright social perversity. It is often very difficult for me to leave the house, especially if I have to attend a party. Weddings are particularly shaming, perhaps because I shrink from the bride's thoroughly authorized self-centeredness, her frank appreciation of her "special day." It's quite strenuous for me to make eye contact with salesclerks during routine purchases. Like the pubescent heroine in the Judy Blume novel *Are You There, God? It's Me, Margaret*, I will leave a pharmacy rather than purchase feminine products from a teenaged male clerk. Obviously, a freak like me would be drawn to some job where one can avoid the scrutiny of other people, like night-shift attendant at the local morgue. Au contraire. I am an English professor. I give lectures several times a week to students, and several times a year to colleagues at national and international conferences. How on earth can someone who can't look at another woman in a bikini turn her back to write on the board in the full knowledge that it is *my* ass that the students have an opportunity to scrutinize? How does a woman whose chronic apprehension prevented her from learning to drive before her thirtieth birthday get on a plane, fly to a strange city, and present her research to a conference gathering of professors from all over the world?

There are many fascinating variations on what it means to be struggling with illness while working in the academy. But I'm not waiting to return to my quiet academic life when I recover from an illness. Rather, everything about the academy, from deadlines to evaluations to lectures, provokes a chain reaction of psychic and somatic distress in me. When I was in college, I had a panic attack every time a paper was due. I did not have a name for what was happening to me, however. I didn't know what it was, but if pressed, I said I was "too sensitive," an unfortunate combination of procrastinator and perfectionist. I would read, research and take notes for days, drafting the paper and explicating the thorniest passages, pasting them to the bathtub as I endlessly scrubbed it. Then, like other college students, I would stay up all night staring at the computer screen waiting for divine intervention. But unlike my peers, by 3 A.M., I was invariably trapped in the bathroom by cyclical vomiting. Once my stomach was emptied of the bitter yellow bile that remains after all the nutrients are gone, I would pace the floor for hours, wringing my hands and sobbing. The paper was always done on time, and I almost always got an A, though I often had to send someone else to turn it in, since I was finally dropping off to sleep after 72 hours of wildly agitated wakefulness.

From the beginning of study week until the end of finals, I seldom slept at all, despite the fact that I was well-prepared, coasting on an A average, and not engaging in last-minute cramming. I sat at the computer with my legs crossed twice, once at the knee and once at the ankle, foot jiggling maniacally, drinking hot ephedra leaf tea, since my tender stomach could not tolerate NoDoz or Vivarin. Once the papers were finished, I raced around campus taking tests in a sleep-deprived haze. I often saw people waving in my peripheral vision, and then turned to find no one was there. Once, walking across campus after ten days without sleep, and unable to coax my papery contact lenses into bloodshot eyes, I looked up at the clock tower and said aloud, without meaning to, "It looks like origami. It's made of folded paper." To my surprise, passing students stopped to chuckle and volunteer such encouragement as "Eat some pizza, take a nap. You look like hell."

I learned from their detached bemusement what would later be confirmed by lovers, roommates, friends and colleagues: this disease is very hard to sympathize with, since panic disorder is entirely based upon a radical distortion of the scale of rational and irrational fears. The physical reaction that a sufferer has going on a blind date—liquid bowels, chronic sweating, sobbing and pleading for a reprieve—would be entirely appropriate, if only she were facing a firing squad instead of another human being also looking to make a connection based upon attraction and intimacy.

My earliest baffled observer was my college boyfriend, a devoted power-lounger who reluctantly left his soothing natural habitat of couch and bong to hold my hand, or more often, hair, during a panic attack. Once he exasperatedly said, "This anxiety that you're giving off to the walls is just the energy that you need to write the paper." It was rather perceptive, though it betrays the dismissive response of a non-panic sufferer who would just like some peace. As Michel Foucault observes in *Madness and Civilization*, the purpose of the mental health profession is to relieve the suffering of all those *around* the mentally ill person, not the patient herself, who can live for years in her private theater of dysfunction. Still, it would be years before I would have an inkling of how to harness that energy effectively, for the benefit of boyfriends or myself. Moreover, what he didn't know was that when we started dating, I used to come home from smooching in his mint '69 Dodge Charger to cry, pace, vomit, and shake. There were boys who did not have that effect on me, with whom I felt comfortable and accepted. I did not return their phone calls.

Most upset by my baffling routine was my loving roommate, a dear woman whose wedding I actually did go to (suppressing not only natural shyness but also an education in

Sedgwickian triangulation as I endorsed the union by reading an ironic Shakespearean sonnet as if it were not ironic and homoerotic at all). Her own unflappable equanimity made
it impossible for her to understand my anxieties about being judged. Whether she's broken
her own favorite china plate, ripped her car's side mirror off on the garage door, or found
a serious typo in a paper she's about to turn in, her sanguine demeanor never falters. Once,
after a binge of all-night anxiety-induced vomiting, I lay on the couch shivering under a quilt
and proofreading my paper when this roommate came home from her job as a charge clerk
on the graveyard shift at a local hospital. She took the opportunity to treat me to a Pedialyte
popsicle and a serious dressing-down: "You have to pick another vocation," she said. "You
claim you want to be a professor, and every aspect of university life makes you sick."
     She was absolutely right, but I was not for one millisecond dissuaded from my purpose.
Indeed, the fun was just beginning. I enrolled in graduate school and was assigned a teaching
assistantship. The first time I walked into a classroom where I was to lecture, I hadn't slept
for over two weeks. I paced my university campus night after night, unconcerned about the
putative rapists and murderers waiting for some frail thing to wander by with her Walkman
blaring a U2 cassette. There was nothing they could do to me that would be worse than what
I could do to myself alone in my room. An anonymous attacker could only assault my body;
I could immolate my entire personality in twenty minutes. And experience taught me that I
had to be moving or the manic energy would turn on me and I would be vomiting again.
     So when I walked into that classroom, I had dark circles under my eyes, trembling hands
and a facial tic, a jumping muscle under my left eye which still appears like an old friend at
finals week. I was also wearing lipstick and heels for the first time in my life, because this
was the first occasion where I consented, albeit reluctantly, to put myself on review. Having skipped every prom, induction ceremony and graduation in my life, and only having
been onstage as part of a 40-piece orchestra of identically dressed nerds, I had never been
the only thing for a group of people to look at, by my design. The twenty-two youngsters
I imagined were qualified to judge me as insufficient intellectually and physically yawned,
scratched themselves, and read the school newspaper while I explained an intricate argument about the Wife of Bath. Fifty minutes later, the only student who was still listening
said, "Well, what was the right answer? I said, "You have to decide for yourself." He said,
"That sucks. When do we get the right answer?"
     It sucked indeed, and yet it seemed I was hooked. The story continues in the same vein:
the week I wrote my qualifying exams, the night before my orals and dissertation defenses,
each time a new semester started, and the week before going on a job visit, I suffered sleep-
less nights, pacing, relentless self-criticism, vomiting and shaking. My precariously balanced
regimen of private self-laceration and public performance of competence collapsed when
grad school ended and it was time for me to procure a tenure-track job. The week before I
went on my first campus visit, my girlfriend Jobi decided the situation was unacceptable, not
so much for my suffering itself but for the domestic fallout from my nightly performances
of "Lady Macbeth goes on the market." My boyfriend kept running off with her boyfriend
every night. The two men were hitting the bars resolutely, perhaps because my boyfriend
(a different one than the undergrad power-lounger) was afraid to come home to me, or
perhaps because he was also experiencing anxiety about his four back-to-back campus vis-

its, which he was muting in his traditional way, with alcohol. Anyway, combined love for me and a desire to see her boyfriend after dark prompted Jobi to throw me in the car and drive to her physician's office one morning at 7. Her doctor listened to thirty seconds of my story and said, "Panic Disorder. Acute." Tylenol PM, she noted, was not going to help me sleep. Indeed, it just blunted the edges of my awareness while my panic kept me awake. Jobi's physician gave me a prescription for ten Xanax pills. She had me take one that day to go to sleep, and one for the next three days on my visit. But, she warned, "Don't come back for a refill. You have to devise a program to deal with your chronic anxiety, because Xanax is highly addictive and you cannot depend upon it to get through life." I took the pill and it was a miracle. I slept through the night and woke refreshed. I reread my job talk, and discovered that it was quite competent and did not need eighty more hours of revision before I could deliver it. I packed my bags, including my seven remaining Xanax, and went to Utah, then Texas. I cut the tiny pills into quarters and took a sliver the night before I went to sleep. I sailed through my visits and got a job.

More crucially, I had an authority's framework for what was wrong with me. I suspected I was the person the Glaxo Welcome people were talking to in the commercials that claimed, "Your life is waiting for you," but I knew that susceptible people misdiagnose themselves all the time, so it was comforting to have a physician's confirmation. Panic was what sent me to the bathroom with a rebellious gut before every class or paper. Panic kept me pacing the floor like a caged tiger. Panic caused my hands to shake like a drunk in detox; it led to concentration problems, loss of appetite, and precipitous weight loss: I average a ten-pound dip in four weeks every time I change jobs, cities, or boyfriends. Panic disorder was why I had to be not just prepared but overprepared for every single talk and lecture. My first semester in a tenure-track job, I woke every morning at precisely 2:40, unable to go back to sleep. I then walked around my apartment declaiming my completed lectures to the disinterested walls for seven hours, until it was time to go to school and give them to a class. I tried not prepping the night before, since I had seven hours of assured prep the next day, but if I did that I couldn't fall asleep at all: my sense of responsibility had to be harnessed in order to get even the meager two to three hours of sleep I was achieving.

One night, that first semester, a colleague invited me out to dinner with his wife and mother. I ordered food that I could not eat. I pushed it around on my plate and twisted napkins to conceal the shaking of my hands, while chatting amicably with my colleague's family. My colleague's mother, a fierce ninety-pound Boston Brahmin, told a captivating story about her son's expulsion from an exclusive East-coast boarding school for having sex in his room. In the tale's climactic scene, this devoted mother thoughtfully faked an epileptic seizure at her son's reckoning to distract the headmaster. It didn't work; he was expelled anyhow. I laughed at the story, and I enjoyed myself, convinced I had hoodwinked everyone present. Brahmin Mama decided to puncture my fantasy. She eyed my trembling hands with a knowledgeable gleam in her eye and said, "What are you taking for it?" After twenty years of being around people in much more intimate proximity who did not comprehend or acknowledge my panic disorder, it was quite alarming to be recognized and called on the carpet with such speed and accuracy.

I stuttered out a shaky, defensive response to her question: "Xanax, but very rarely. I've been stretching out a prescription for ten pills for over a year." She was not impressed by my testimonial of infrequent reliance upon drugs, which was intended to inspire confidence in my coping mechanisms. Instead, she leveled her formidable gaze to mine, and said, "Valium is your only man. If it was good enough for those of us who had to raise kids in the sixties, it's good enough for you." I never sought that Valium prescription, but I did purchase a bottle of diazepam from the vet for a retired racing greyhound whom I adopted around the same time. My greyhound has to be sedated during thunderstorms and long car rides, and resembles me in more ways than her own tendency to panic first and ask questions later. But that's another story. Indeed, I have virtually no recourse to pills at all. I threw out the free Zoloft sample my new physician gave me after diagnosing it as a weak substitute for Ecstasy.

The upshot of all this pharmaceutical window-shopping was that I swore off pills altogether. Instead of medicating my anxiety away, I decided to wear myself out. I run five miles a day with the greyhound (which also helped ameliorate her mimetic panic attacks). I practice yoga twice a week and meditate daily. When I feel the panic coming on, I lift weights. I take a Pilates or yoga course, since those two disciplines are particularly good for absorbing all my concentration. Getting my utterly uncoordinated body to adopt perplexing positions like Atlas, Lone Palm, and Steer is more than a good distraction; it is neurologically soothing to what one therapist called my "anxious brain chemistry." My panic attacks have receded, I can eat a meal, and I stopped calling my friends at 3 A.M. (the few I had left, that is, after years of hysterically phoning when I was beyond consolation and could only make them feel powerless). I know the panic is still there: I know I will hear from it on the doorstep of tenure; I know it will make an appearance if I start a new romance, or fly to Japan, or do anything I haven't done at least ten times before.

The classroom still looms large in my anxiety, and I often have dreams that I show up to teach naked (comforted by the thought that if I'm really smart today they won't notice), or that my voice is inaudible and I have to teach the class in semaphores and sign language. In one dream, I am trying to lecture on film to an utterly uninterested class when aging rocker David Lee Roth pushes me off the podium and delivers a fabulously informative and witty talk on tort law. The message is clear: I can't even make something as interesting as film worthwhile, while a born entertainer can breathe life into the dullest material.

Nightly wrestling with my demons, I accidentally discovered one sort of terrorist diversion in the classroom. I can get rid of my shame temporarily if I transfer it to my students. When I explain challenging narratological and linguistic concepts like the phatic function (a linguist's term for language spoken to promote social ease rather than to communicate ideas), the students' eyes glaze over and I start to feel the panic. Drawing my example for the phatic function from *American Pie* rather than *The Turn of the Screw* is a reliable dodge. I say, "The perfect illustration of the empty nature of phatic utterance is Alyson Hannigan's character, who begins every story with the formulaic locution, 'This one time, at band camp . . .' The vacuity of her phatic speech and the rising inflection of her voice convince Jim (Jason Biggs) that no information will be shared between them, so that he actually misses the highly relevant news she is trying to convey to him: that she is kinky and willing to sleep with him." The students laugh in shocked recognition, and squirm on their hard chairs in the painful realization that I have visited their world of MILFs and muffs. Fleetingly, I am the least self-conscious person in the room.

In *Beyond the Pleasure Principle,* Freud describes his grandson's fort-da game, where the child throws a ball from his crib repeatedly, compelling his mother to fetch it for him. When she gives him the longed-for toy, the child can't get rid of it fast enough or scream loudly enough to get it back instantly. In his description of the child's abandonment fears, Freud delineates how a child takes the experience of passivity and displeasure caused by separation from the mother and converts it into a situation where he feels powerful. In other words, the mother, not the ball, is the toy, and the child transforms himself from abandoned infant to commanding agent, sending his mother away on the mission of fetching the ball. This is a fair description of my unconscious response to the horrifying effects college life had on my body. A sane person would run away from university life; I decided to stay here forever, to blunt the anxieties of being seen and judged with repetition. If being graded by a professor filled me with intolerable dread, I would become the grader, converting my passivity into action. But of course, professors are still evaluated—by their peers, by their administrative superiors, and by their students.

As I look back on my favorite teachers, I notice a common denominator in the ones I remember fondly after ten or twenty years: enthusiasm for subjecting their bodies to job-related situational irony. Just as the finest hairdressers have unspectacular hair, and respected plastic surgeons have wrinkles, the best teachers are those who seem to be missing the most fundamental lesson in front of their eyes. First, there was my wonderful high school geometry teacher, who was funny, patient, and terribly allergic to chalk. Her hands would crack and bleed as she drew isosceles triangles on the board. Her solution was to buy the chubby chalks in festive colors used by little girls for their hopscotch games. She was still in pain, but the scenery seemed to better merit her suffering. In college, I had an hilarious medieval history professor who was an endless reservoir of anecdotes about the hairy-footed conquering hordes of Europe; but she really earned my respect when she assured us she had contracted bubonic plague while renovating a rat-infested house. That's dedication to one's specialization if I've ever seen it. As an eighteenth-centuryist, I would have to combine gin ruin and greensickness to approximate to her hallowed devotion.

Also in college, I had a philosophy professor so allergic to airborne allergens, especially the residue of disintegrating paper in aging volumes, that he could not venture into any of UT-Austin's numerous libraries. Naturally, he was most afflicted by a visit to the moldy Classics library, which housed all the Greek and Roman philosophical dialogues and treatises he taught. His office bore a curious resemblance to the room where a SWAT team keeps the dying E.T. for surveillance until the children help him make his escape. Floor-to-ceiling bookcases had plastic sheeting descending over them; the room appeared to await an endlessly detained painting crew. If I didn't already love him for devoting himself to objects that made him ill, this professor warmed my heart by developing chronic hiccups which lasted over eight months, and for which he eventually was hospitalized. These hiccups punctuated his lectures on ethics and final causes with incongruous whimsy. Once I went to drop off a paper in the Mylar mausoleum of his office, and clumsily offered some sympathy for his many health problems. He cheerfully presented his pet theory about his precociously feeble body: born the same day, month and year as Anna May Bullock, he was her picture of Dorian Gray, and was aging on her behalf. Bullock, better known by her stage name of

Tina Turner, was then about fifty years old. Her taut and lithe body captivated audiences from Stuttgart to San Diego, while this poor professor appeared to be held together with library paste and Stoic resignation.

I was thinking recently about my sister. She is about three years older, and we are polar opposites, and have been all our lives. She was pretty, flirtatious, at ease in her body and the world, and boy-crazy from the word go. She "developed" early, sometime around the fifth grade, and had boyfriends from the first grade until the present. I announced to my kindergarten class at age four that I would never marry, and I did not attend a single high-school dance. She was zaftig, with soft, embraceable curves; I was twitchy, not fond of physical contact, and had a figure my grandmother referred to as "six o'clock," because my dimensions were very similar to the hands of a clock pointing straight up and down. While my sister went to dances with boys, I sat at home and read *The Great Gatsby* (eighty-six times by graduation). She became a cosmetologist, I got a Ph.D. in English. But wait: she became a cosmetologist, despite her acute sensitivity to hair bleaches, dyes, and perms. Her small, graceful hands are always swollen and purple, covered in flaking eczema, despite the fact that she wears surgical gloves when treating her clients. She covers her hands with cortisone and lotion and tans them under special lamps, yet still they crack, peel, and ooze. I find her beleaguered little paws touching, because to me, they advertise the depth of her vocation, like a nun's stigmata. Clearly, something deeper is at work here. My sister and I, who have nothing in common, decided on some preconscious level that the only job for us was one that our bodies rebel against. Isn't that how we know we're falling in love? The racing pulse, the sweaty palms, the roller-coaster drop in the stomach that tells us this is no ordinary man or woman: this is the person who makes me so sick that I have to be around him or her as much as possible.

One episode of *Seinfeld* which I recently saw in syndication begins with the comedian doing a stand-up routine in a small, intimate club. Jerry begins, "Most Americans list their number one fear as public speaking, followed distantly by death." Then after a pause in which he allows that information to sink in, Jerry points out the paradox of human nature, deducing that "at a funeral, that means we would rather be the guy in the box than the one giving the eulogy." In my family, you could say we've come to terms with the fact that all humankind is always at a funeral, but we insist on giving the eulogy. Standing on the podium displaying the shameful humanity in your sweaty pitstains and shaking hands, despite the many drawbacks of that role, is at least one way of knowing you're not the poor stiff in the box.

QUESTIONS

1. How might panic disorder be analogous to other secret afflictions, like alcoholism or anorexia? Comment on the connection between the intensely somatic nature of panic (e.g., sweating, vomiting, diarrhea) and the sufferer's sense of shame.

2. Should panic disorder be considered a mental illness? At what point would it compromise the victim beyond her ability to perform her duties as a professor? What should be done at that point?

3. How would knowing about a professor's panic disorder affect your attitude and demeanor in class?

DSM-IV 300.30

⬅ Mikita Brottman ➡

1. When were you first diagnosed with obsessive-compulsive disorder?

I didn't see a psychiatrist until I was about eighteen, but I've had my "thing" ever since I can remember. I never thought it the least bit unusual; in fact, I think a lot of people have a "thing." My "thing" was that I had to touch certain objects an even number of times in order to "even things out." For example, if I accidentally knocked my hand against the side of a piece of furniture, I had to do it again, to make sure that I'd done it twice. Sometimes, if I wanted to be very safe, I'd do it three more times, so I'd done it four times altogether. It had to be an even number. I've always felt funny about odd numbers. They feel sort of unfinished to me, like a piece of music with the last note missing.

I call it a "thing" because once I saw my sister touching the wall deliberately with her hand the same way I did, and I asked her what she was doing.

"It's just one of those 'things,'" she said. "I have to do everything on both sides. Don't you have a 'thing'?"

Until then, I'd thought I was the only person with a "thing," but after talking to my sister I decided that everybody must have one. My sister's "thing," it seemed, was similar to mine, except instead of repeating gestures like I did, she had to counterbalance them by doing them on the opposite side. So if she accidentally knocked her right hand against something, she then had to touch the same object again with her left hand. It was just like my "thing," only I think my sister's might have been worse than mine, because I saw her doing it a lot.

Later, I discovered that not everybody has a "thing," but I think they're pretty common. If you have a "thing" yourself, you always notice when somebody else has one. I have a friend whose "thing" is the opposite of mine; he can't stand even numbers, and he always has to do everything three times.

When I first told a psychiatrist about my "thing," he said it stood for my desire to be in control. He called it "a talisman to ward off contingency." If I did something by accident, he explained, it felt as though I weren't really in control. But if I went back and repeated the gesture deliberately, it meant that the first time hadn't really been an accident at all. He told me that my fear of odd numbers was a fear of things being "open" and not "closed off." He said I appeared to be anxious about anything that wasn't ordered or categorized, anything that hadn't been "put away in its proper place," as he put it.

Later, as I grew older, my "thing" seemed to change and take on other forms. I went through a stage when I was about eleven when I couldn't stand open doors. I couldn't bear to be in a room if the door was open, even just a tiny little crack, even if it hadn't been pushed completely closed. Whenever anybody came in or out of a room and didn't close the door properly, I had to get up from whatever I was doing and push it to.

When I was about fifteen, I went through a stage of being unable to read anything that was written by anyone who didn't close the loops on their *o*'s and *p*'s, or didn't dot their *i*'s. I had to pick up a pen and go over what they'd written, closing their letters and adding the dots. I always had to go back over everything I'd written to make sure the loops on my letters were closed firmly. At school, I got the reputation of being a slow reader because I had to check the page numbers of the book I was reading, just to make sure they were in the right order. Sometimes I had to read certain pages two or three times, to be certain I hadn't missed anything.

A year or so later, I remember going through a stage when I couldn't be completely comfortable if I hadn't just been to the toilet, even if I didn't need to go at all. I used to go to the toilet all the time, especially if I was about to go out of the house, or if I was settling down to do anything that would take more than an hour or so. I had to make sure I wouldn't be interrupted by needing to go in the middle. I'd often go four or five times before a show I wanted to watch on television. I'd also go during the commercials, just to make sure. Most of the time, nothing came out except a pitiful little trickle, but still, I had to go just the same. Noticing that I was going to the bathroom with unusual frequency, my mother took me to the doctor, where they did some tests on my blood sugar, suspecting I might be diabetic. But according to the tests, everything was as it should be.

As I grew older, I thought less about my "thing" and never asked my sister about hers, though I'd sometimes catch her doing it from time to time. It wasn't as though my "thing" ever disappeared, though. It was more as if it grew with me and mutated into an ever-changing series of different "things," strange obsessions that possessed me from time to time, none of which seemed far enough removed from ordinary teenage behavior to seem particularly strange. For example, when I started to get serious about reading and writing—when I realized I wanted to go to college—I made up a series of superstitions to help me study. If I started having anxious thoughts about failing my exams, I'd have to hold my breath for ten seconds to counteract their negative influence. If I got less than a B on a paper, I'd have to go to sleep with my books open, so I could absorb the material through osmosis, in my dreams. Every morning, I'd submerge my face in scalding water for thirty seconds, convinced this would drive out whatever demon it was that caused my skin to glow with burning lumps of acne, a ritual that seemed more and more inadequate every day. Looking at my face each morning in the bathroom mirror, I'd be greeted by some horrifying new cluster of swollen pimples that seemed to have cropped up in the night just to mock me and my crazy routines.

2. Do you ever find yourself obsessing about dirt and germs?

I've never had to wash my hands or shower compulsively, though I've always been very tidy. I feel uncomfortable in places that are cluttered. I don't like eating in restaurants that look dirty, and I don't like using public toilets. But who does? I can't drink out of containers that somebody else has just had their mouth on, and I can't eat from someone else's spoon; but that's just ordinary hygiene.

In some ways, in fact, I'm quite the opposite of fussy. I don't mind buying clothes from thrift stores—except underwear of course—although when I shared a bedroom with my sister, we also used to share our underwear. If I'm invited to dinner at somebody's house and I notice their kitchen is dirty, I can still manage to finish my meal. I let my cat sleep in my bed with me, and sometimes I even let him lick from my ice-cream carton, which I'm sure is about as unhygienic as you can get.

Of course, cleanliness is important, but you can't take these things too seriously, or it would drive you completely over the edge. After all, if you think about it, we're surrounded by dirt and germs all the time. Even the most spotless homes are full of dust mites, and there are spiders living under everybody's furniture and in every crack in every wall. Our bodies are teeming with germs and bacteria, especially our mouths. Have you ever looked at human saliva under a microscope? And have you ever wondered what really happens to food when you put it in your mouth, and what happens to it inside your body? Just imagine, all that stuff being mashed up and mixed together, all that meat and vegetables rotting in your intestines. If you think about it, the whole process of eating and digestion is completely disgusting, but you have to try not to think about it. If you thought about things like that all the time, you'd never be able to eat anything again.

I keep my own apartment clean, and that's all. The hallway and staircase in my building are often dirty, but I try not to worry about that. You can't clean everywhere. I'm a professor now, and I lead a busy life. I don't have time to clean every day. Sometimes I'll go three or four weeks without cleaning.

Still, when I clean, I really go all the way. It will usually be some little trigger that sets me off unexpectedly—orange juice stains in the refrigerator, or hair plugging up the bathroom sink—and then there'll be no stopping me; I'll go to war. I'll climb into my overalls, tie back my hair with a duster, and gather together my army of mops, bleach, squeegees and disinfectant sprays. Then I'll go to work on the entire apartment, from top to bottom, scrubbing the kitchen floor, scouring the oven and sweeping the deck. And it won't stop there. I'll disinfect the trashcans, descale the coffeemaker, and clean all the windows, inside and out. I'll repot the plants, realign the pictures on the wall, move around the furniture, and sometimes even bathe the cat. Often, I'll go to work on my wardrobe as well, tossing out half my clothes and other things too—shoes, books, music I never listen to any more. Sometimes I don't stop until late at night, but I have to finish before I sleep; I can never go to bed at night with anything half-done. And the next morning, it's so wonderful to wake up to a fresh, clean, tidy, uncluttered apartment; it's one of the best feelings in the world.

My office at work is always neat and tidy, too. I hate being surrounded by clutter. When I'm watching *Cops* and they show the shabby, dirty home of some thief or drug dealer, it makes me so twitchy and uncomfortable I want to switch off the television set and go and clean my kitchen. Sometimes I even have to shut my eyes until the scene is over. People with their heads cut off or their guts hanging out don't bother me at all, but show me a dirty counter top and I start to hyperventilate.

I often wonder—when does an ordinary routine or a series of habits become a disorder? These things seem to happen very slowly, the way a person who has a couple of drinks after work every night gradually becomes a full-blown alcoholic. It takes years and years for things like this to develop. I know a girl with the cutest dimpled smile, but at the same time, I can tell it's a smile that is slowly on its way to revealing a small double chin. I have another friend whose unkempt looks attract all the girls, but I can see that the things that make him look so sexy today will one day make him look like a homeless person. These things happen slowly, the same way that the choices we make always become traps for us in the end.

I've always chosen to live on my own. Ever since I left home to go to college, I've always had my own apartment. Even when I've had steady, serious boyfriends, I've never moved in with them, because I'm very independent, and I've always treasured my freedom. Recently, however, I've started to realize that I'm probably no longer *capable* of living with another person, even if I really wanted to. I've become too set in my ways. And eventually, I know, the independence I consciously chose will become solitude, then loneliness, then total isolation. And the next thing I know I'll be one of those shut-ins whose corpses they find only after they've been lying alone for months, and the neighbors complain to the police about the smell.

3. Have you ever engaged in self-mutilation (cutting, hair-pulling etc.)?

I first started playing with my hair when I was studying in my bedroom at night. I used to have long, thick hair, and at first I used to just wind it around my fingers or chew on it while I was studying. Then I got into the habit of checking constantly for split ends, and, whenever I found them, pulling out the damaged hair by the root. There was something deeply satisfying about pulling out the individual hairs. I felt a little shudder of pleasure whenever I felt the bad strand being pulled tightly out of my scalp. I found myself doing it more and more often, even with hairs that weren't split. It was just a habit, almost unconscious. I think it might also have helped me to concentrate on my work. I also started tweaking the individual hairs out of my eyebrows with my fingernails and pulling out the thin hairs on my arms and legs.

At this time, I was hoping to take the Oxford entrance exam, and I was studying for at least six hours every night after school. Since I was spending so much time reading, it wasn't long before my hair-pulling started to get out of hand. At first I was aware only of the mess; there would be hairs all over my books, my desk, my bedroom floor. Then, after I'd started pulling the hair out in clumps, odd little bald patches began to appear clustered around my scalp. It looked very peculiar, but since I was only half-aware of what I was doing, it was very difficult for me to stop. When the bald patches started to get noticeable, I tried to limit myself to plucking my eyebrows, but soon I'd plucked them completely out, and went back to my hair again. When people at school started making comments, I tried to make myself conscious of what I was doing, but before I knew it my fingers would be back in my hair again, plucking away. Sometimes, if I hadn't pulled my hair all day, I'd allow myself a small treat—five minutes of uninhibited hair-pulling before I went to bed.

Eventually, my bald patches became obvious even to my mother, who made me an appointment with a psychiatrist—a gray-haired old man who made me lie on a couch—who suggested that I find something else to do with my hands when I was reading, and gave me a puzzle-cube to play with. When that didn't work, he encouraged me to take up knitting, but that was no good because I couldn't knit and read at the same time. Finally, he came up with a complicated scheme whereby every time I found myself pulling my hair, I had to touch my left foot four times as "punishment." This worked very well because it keyed into my compulsive tendencies as well as my "thing," which I'd already discussed with him. And although I probably looked rather bizarre while I was doing it, it seemed to solve the problem very well.

4. Have you ever been diagnosed with an eating disorder?

I've always been tall, with strong bones, a long body, and long, muscular arms and legs. With a body like mine, I always felt that I had to watch out for fat. I always felt that fat had its eye on me. Inside my normal-sized body, I often thought, there was a fat girl struggling desperately to get out. I felt as though I was on the verge of turning from strong and tall into "well-proportioned," and from "well-proportioned" into "full-figured," and then from "full-figured" into "hefty." And as everyone knows, it's only one small step from "hefty" to just plain fat; and then the next thing you know, you're being hauled out of your Florida condo in a fork-lift truck live on *Jerry Springer*.

I've always enjoyed my food; and when I was at school, I was far too self-conscious to go to a gym, so I had to find other ways of keeping my weight down. Almost all the girls I knew were able to make themselves vomit—we used to call it "consulting Dr. Fingers"—but I couldn't do it, no matter how hard I tried. Have you ever tried to make yourself puke? It's actually very difficult. I could never understand how everyone else seemed to manage it. My throat would ache, and my eyes would water; I never got the hang of it. I'd try to make myself throw up, fail miserably, and be in bed with a sore throat eating ice-cream for the next three days, which would make me feel even worse.

And so I'd take laxatives instead—yes, the emetic of wimps. A handful of Ex-Lax before meals would quickly turn anything I ate into stringy, foul-smelling, light-colored threads of excrement—which, at least according to my biology textbook, was the exact appearance of the stools of a weasel. I felt kind of weaselly too, for taking them, but however disgusting my habit might have been, it worked to keep the weight off. At the time I was young and naïve enough to tell my psychiatrist about my laxative use, and ever since then I've been saddled with the burden of an "eating disorder," which is utterly ridiculous, since if anything it's all about *order*, not *disorder*—about saving myself from the madness which would surely descend upon me if I were to give in to my body and give it what it wanted, which was to get fat.

Once I was put in a psychiatric hospital after suffering what they described as a "psychotic episode," and the thing I resented most about being there was the food they made me eat. The meals were carefully planned, full of fruit and vegetables, but there was just *so much food*. When they saw from my records that I'd been diagnosed with an "eating disorder," they insisted I finish everything on my tray. I couldn't believe how much I was expected to eat, every day. There was cereal, fruit and toast for breakfast, pasta and vegetables for lunch, meat and more vegetables for dinner, dessert with every meal, and a snack before bedtime. When I complained that there was far too much food for me to eat, the nurse explained that this was a balanced diet worked out by a qualified nutritionist, and it contained exactly the right amount of calories.

"The right number of calories for what?" I asked. "To become morbidly obese?"

"The right number to keep the average person in a good state of health."

"Well that's just the thing," I tried to explain. "I'm not the average person. You wouldn't believe how easily I gain weight. For example, if I eat a quarter pounder, I actually put on more than two pounds."

"You'll need to finish all your meals before we let you out of here," he replied unsympathetically. And so I let them fill me full of drugs and move me from my bed to my food tray four times a day, like a veal calf being fattened up for the slaughter. They said I had to get back to my "normal bodyweight," but nobody seemed to understand that my "normal bodyweight" was unattractive and unfashionable. I tried to explain that by forcing me to swell up like a factory-farmed chicken, they were actually running a grave risk to the stability of my mental health, but nobody seemed to see it that way. Every mealtime they reminded me that I had to eat everything on my tray before they'd let me go. I doubted they had any right to hold me longer than the seventy-two hours specified in the emergency court order, but I ate what they gave me just in case.

And putting on a little weight didn't seem nearly as bad as being kept in a locked cell. I'd refused to admit myself voluntarily, so I'd been taken there in a police car, in handcuffs. Even worse, after I got out, they sent me an enormous bill, and at the top of the bill it said, "Thank you for Choosing Johnson County Hospital."

5. Have you ever seen a therapist on a regular basis?

When I was first diagnosed, I started seeing a counselor, Christine, who worked at the psychiatric clinic. She was woman in her fifties who wore jeans, sandals, and tie-dyed T-shirts or rainbow-colored caftans. I saw her more as a friend than a counselor. We chatted about our problems; I'd tell her about the trouble I was having with my Ph.D. coursework, and she'd complain to me about her mother, who had come to live with her after having a stroke. When Christine moved to Oregon, I made her a blue ceramic dog bowl in my pottery class. After that, I had a few other counselors, but I didn't like any of them as much as I'd liked Christine; and in the end I decided I didn't really need counseling any more.

Then one day I'd read an article in the *New York Times Magazine* about the psychiatric system which said that everyone had the right to see their medical records if they asked for them. The article said you just had to write a letter to your doctor and enclose the cost of photocopying, and you could ask for any documents you wanted, as long as they had your name on them. So I'd sent off for copies of my files from the clinic.

I was shocked to see the notes Christine had made about our sessions. For example, the first time she'd met me, she'd written, "Patient appears emotionally immature, though looks much older than stated age." What nerve! She was the one who dressed like a teenager, even though she must have been pushing sixty. She'd also written things like "Patient greeted me with superficial smile; continued to address me in inappropriately familiar manner." I was mortified. Who was she to say my smile was "superficial"? How did she know I wasn't genuinely pleased to see her? Why hadn't she told me it was inappropriate for me to consider her a friend?

Even worse, they sent me a copy of my records from the time I was hospitalized; there was my name at the top, and next to "Description," somebody had written "thin, blonde, psychotic."

6. What medication are you currently taking?

My first psychiatrist put me on a large daily dose of amitriptylene; this was before the days of Prozac, Zoloft, and all the other new drugs. The amitriptylene took a long time to get used to. I'd take it before going to bed at night, after I'd finished studying; and the next morning, I'd be totally wiped out. Sometimes it would be quite impossible for me to get out of bed; I'd sleep into the middle of the afternoon. If I needed to get up for class, I'd be walking round like a zombie until lunchtime. Sometimes I'd lock myself in a stall in the girls' bathroom, sit on the toilet and fall asleep, missing my morning classes. But after a month or so I started to get accustomed to it and stopped feeling tired all the time.

When I got my first teaching position, I registered as a patient of a psychiatrist called Dr. Lincoln. One of the first things he did was to change my medication. I was down to 75mg of amitriptylene by this stage, but Dr. Lincoln brought it down even further, to 50mg, which, he said, was much easier for him to prescribe, since it was just one tablet, not the two I'd been taking before. Whenever I went to see him, he was always friendly and chatty, asking me how everything was going; but after my experience with Christine, all I wanted him to do was write my prescription and let me go.

Then one day he glanced at my file, and asked me if I was still "depressed."

"I've never really been depressed," I said.

"Good. You're feeling better?" he asked, still looking through my file.

"Just the same," I said.

Dr. Lincoln didn't seem to like this response. "You must be feeling better than when you first came in," he said. "I see here we decided to decrease your medication. You're doing fine on the new dose?"

"You decreased it because it was easier to prescribe," I said. It was obvious that he had no idea who I was, and knew nothing about my history. He might as well have been looking at my file for the very first time.

Dr. Lincoln made a triangle with his fingers, puckered his lips, and frowned at me, swiveling from side to side in his chair, as though considering something of great importance.

"It's a lower dose," he said, finally. "I wouldn't have prescribed a lower dose if I didn't think you were improving. You look much better than when you first came to see me, much less depressed. How are you doing in school?"

If I hadn't been depressed before, I certainly felt depressed then. He'd glanced at my college address and assumed I was a student, not a professor. After that, I realized something that should have been obvious to me a long time ago: most psychiatrists had so many patients that they couldn't possibly keep track of every individual they saw. As far as Dr. Lincoln was concerned, every time he saw me, it was as though he were seeing me for the first time.

I didn't mind this at all. It was a busy clinic—I'm sure he had hundreds of patients— but what I really resented were his attempts to pretend that he knew who I was. He'd take a sneaky glance at my file, then say things like, "College still going well? Classes difficult?" or

"Any more of those obsessive thoughts?" or "How's the new dosage working out?" It seemed so transparently hypocritical; I saw quite plainly that he had no memory of me, no idea of who I was, and no particular interest in my case.

This came as something as a revelation to me—the idea that nobody was really looking out for me, nobody really cared. Around the same time, and partly, perhaps, as a result of this discovery, I decided to stop taking my medication. I knew there was nothing seriously wrong with me. It was certainly true that I had some peculiar character traits, and I could be rather compulsive at times, but that wasn't a disease that needed curing; it was just my character. I was older and calmer now; I was a professor of English with an Oxford PhD. I knew I wasn't going to go back to pulling my hair out or going to the bathroom all the time. Yes, perhaps I was rather fastidious, perhaps I could be slightly fussy, but that was hardly unusual.

And the truth was, I missed my compulsions.

So I stopped taking my medication, and this helped me to learn some very interesting things about myself. For example, if I were writing an article for publication, I couldn't leave it unfinished—I had to keep working until I was happy with it, sometimes staying up three or four nights in a row until I felt it was finished. There was something exhilarating about this obsession with writing; I started publishing regularly, in increasingly prestigious journals. Sometimes, after a day of teaching, I'd spend all night working on an article and then go straight into class again the next morning. When I was full of inspiration and ideas like that, I hardly seemed to need any sleep at all. I started working out more frequently at the gym; I started teaching a seminar on Joseph Conrad in the evening. My appetite seemed to decrease dramatically; I felt taut, slim, energetic, and healthy. This, I thought, is what it really feels like to be me.

It seemed ridiculous to me then, that my particular kind of personality had been "diagnosed" by a psychiatrist and given a specific number from a manual—in my case, 300.30. If my personality fit with a specific number in a manual, I thought, then so should everybody else's; there should be as many numbers in the manual as there are people on earth. I knew that obsessive-compulsive disorder was one of the most common forms of mental illness, and I'd met plenty of other people who'd also been diagnosed with it—who shared my number from the manual—but none of them had been anything like me, even in their obsessions and compulsions.

So I stopped taking my medication, stopped going to the clinic, and stopped seeing Dr. Lincoln. I didn't even bother canceling my next appointment, and nobody called to find out what was going on—not the nurse, not the receptionist, certainly not Dr. Lincoln. My file is probably still there in his cabinet drawer, gathering dust. After that, I had no more illusions about the mental health system. Psychiatrists don't really care about you—most of them don't even remember your name—and I felt foolish and naïve for assuming otherwise. The truth, I realized, is that you have to look out for yourself. As Marlowe tells the narrator in Joseph Conrad's *Heart of Darkness,* "we live as we dream: alone."

QUESTIONS

1. Comment on the author's choice of form, style, and tone for this narrative. How do these choices impact how the reader responds to the events and issues the author discusses?

2. At what point does one's "thing" become an "illness" or "disorder," and why might the distinction be important? to whom?

3. Discuss a patient's rights to read his or her medical records. Knowing a patient has the right to read her records certainly impacts what and how information is recorded. What issues are at stake, given this knowledge?

Mirror Image

⮞ EMMA BURNS ⮜

Anorexia Nervosa—a mental disorder manifested by extreme fear of becoming obese and an aversion to food, usually occurring in young women and often resulting in life-threatening weight loss, accompanied by a disturbance in body image, hyperactivity, and amenorrhea. (Steadman's)

I can see it all so clearly now. I had just gotten home from a day at junior high school. We had discussed anorexia nervosa that day in my Personal Development and Relationships Class. I am in my parents' bedroom, standing in front of their full-length mirror. It is spring and the sun is shining in the window across the hall. I am dressed in cut-off jean shorts and a purple Cotton Ginny T-shirt with the sleeves rolled up. I look down at the scale under my feet and see that it reads 105 pounds. I am thirteen years old, and I am 5'3". As I look in the mirror, I wonder how anyone could ever see something that isn't really there. Is the brain really so powerful? My friend at school, her brain is that powerful. She just got out of the hospital last week. She only eats salads.

Is *my* brain that powerful? Maybe every time I look in the mirror this week I will try saying to myself, "You are fat. You need to lose five pounds."

It turns out, my brain was that powerful.

Although anorexia nervosa has long been recognized and well described, the etiology of the disorder is not well understood. Societal influences promoting an unrealistically thin body size and a cultural environment that associates slimness with happiness and success have been implicated in the development of anorexia nervosa. (Goldman)

I can see myself so clearly now. I'm in a motel room. It looks like most other motel rooms: two double beds covered by thick beige duvets patterned with faint brown flowers. There's a small brown night table with a reading light between the beds, a long brown dresser along the adjacent wall, with a few glasses and an ice bucket sitting on top of it. A TV cabinet stands next to the dresser. At the back of the room is a door leading to the florescent-lit bathroom. I have been relegated to the bed near the large front window, which looks out onto the motel parking lot. I'm lying on the floor with my feet up on the bed, my wavy blond hair spread out like a fan on the scratchy brown carpet beneath me.

It is the spring of 1991. I am fourteen and I'm on my grade nine class trip in Moncton, New Brunswick. We were supposed to go to the big city, Montreal, but we weren't able to find enough chaperones to go with us. Of course it doesn't really matter where we are; the most important part of the trip is the person you room with. I travel in a pack of five girls, and, unfortunately, motel rooms only hold four. I must have been out of favour the day we filled out the "Who do you want to room with?" forms, because I now find myself in the leftovers room. One of my roommates is a large girl I have been in school with since elementary, although we've never been good friends. When we were ten years old, the leader of my group of friends called her a big chunk of fudge to her face. I still feel ashamed, even if she is kind of fat.

Right now I am on the floor of the leftovers room, the spring sun shining in the window, the itchy brown carpet scratching my bare arms, the floor pushing back against my spine every time I lift my head from the floor. Fifty-seven, fifty-eight . . . I count silently as I lift my nose up to my bare knees. Almost halfway there.

About twenty minutes ago we were playing cards. I caved and accepted some Smarties from one of my roommates. She seems to have an endless supply of junk food. I took eight Smarties and placed them on the beige floral blanket. I lined them up, sorting them by colour, and slowly, deliberately I ate them—first the brown, then the orange, yellow, green, blue and finally the red. I had to finish the game of cards before I could start sit-ups as my punishment. I concentrated on how many sit-ups I would do as the game wound down. I decided on 150.

So here I am, a bit of sweat beginning to bead up on my top lip as the sun shines on me from in the window. One hundred and eight, one hundred and nine . . .

It is estimated that 1 in every 100 females, 16 to 18 years old, has anorexia nervosa (Behrman). Approximately 1 to 2% of women and 0.1% of men will meet the diagnostic criteria for bulimia nervosa some time in their lives. (Goldman)

April 3, 1993
Dear Diary:
 Not for anyone but myself, I have to lose five pounds because I really am quite fat. Since I don't have much else to make me feel good about myself, I'm gonna need to show that I have some self control. So starting tomorrow no cookies, no chocolate, no chips.
 My schedule for the week:

Monday:	lunch—cut veggies
	dinner—1 bowl cereal
Tuesday:	lunch—cut veggies
	dinner—1 bagel with cheese
Wednesday:	lunch—apple
	dinner—salad with egg
Thursday:	lunch—nothing
	dinner—Mr. Noodles

April 4, 1993
Dear Diary:
Almost!
  lunch—nothing
  supper—2 apples with cheese, 1 bowl of cereal
  Slipped up—3 cookies, 1 bite of cake. AWFUL!

May 14, 1993
Dear Emma,
  This letter is really hard for me to write because you are the best friend I have ever had. When I first moved here this year I didn't think I would ever make any friends and then I met you. We connect so well and have so much fun together it is hard to believe it. Even though you are my best friend I am not sure that I can keep spending so much time with you. I have always felt a bit insecure about the way that I looked but I know that I am not fat. I try to eat healthy and take care of myself to stay thin. But spending time with you makes me feel fat because you spend so much time talking about how fat you are. You are not fat, but I know that you think that you are. When I got to Victoria this year I felt good about myself and now I find myself thinking about my weight too much and I don't like it. I try to tell you that you are not fat, but it doesn't seem to help you. Emma, I think that you are sick and you need to get help. I have tried to tell you that you are not fat to boost your confidence, but I guess that I can't provide whatever it is that you need. I am not sure what I can do to help you more.
  I hope that you understand that spending time with you is starting to make me feel bad about myself, and I don't want that. I really love you and want us to keep being friends, but I can't talk to you about your weight any more. If you think that we can be friends and not talk about weight that would be great, but otherwise I will have to stop spending time with you to make sure I stay healthy. I hope you can understand and that you find the help that you need somewhere.
  I love you lots,
                    Kimmy

November 7, 1993
Dear Diary:
  I'm going to bed really happy for the first time all year because today I ate:
  1 cheese scone with jam ☺

February 3, 1994
Dear Diary:
  Life is going great right now. I am almost happy with myself. I've been eating well the last week. I hope I don't go ruin it. Lunch and dinner only, no snacks or binges, plus three to four workouts a week.
  It makes me pretty happy.
  Today: pizza pop, piece of bread, muffin, potato and mushrooms

In an attempt to facilitate early recognition and improve treatment, anorexia nervosa was further subclassified into two types: (1) restrictive anorexia nervosa, occurring in persons who do not regularly purge, and (2) bulimic anorexia nervosa, occurring in persons who predominantly fast but who also purge by self-induced vomiting, diet pills, hyperexercising, or other techniques. (Rome)

I can see it so clearly now. I am in twelfth grade. I am seventeen years old. We are all in the downstairs living room of my girlfriend's house. There are three big, brown couches around the room—the kind of couches that swallow you up with their large, plush cushions. The covering of the sofa feels like velvet under my hand. My legs, wrapped in blue jeans, are tucked up under me and one hand rests on the arm of the chair; the other holds a drink of rum and Coke. That's my drink, rum. I drink 151 proof because you don't have to drink as much to get drunk. Around the room are all my friends. I look around at the girls. Long silky brown hair, thin legs wrapped in blue jeans, beautiful curly brown hair, a short blue skirt showing long athletic legs, short punky brown hair, baggy blue jeans hiding thin legs. Some sit on the floor, their hands lost in the thick beige carpeting, others on the couches. Van Morison's "Brown-Eyed Girl" plays in the background. I will never be anybody's brown-eyed girl.

I move to the kitchen to pour myself another drink. I see my girlfriend sitting on the floor outside the bathroom, her knees up and head down, her long silky brown hair streaming over her legs. She looks like she has had a bit too much to drink. I haven't yet. I take my drink and walk over to see if she is OK, as she talks to me in a blurry voice and uses my nickname, which she saves for occasions like this. I realize she's not OK.

"Do you need to get sick, Katie?"

"Hmmmm."

"OK, let's go into the bathroom."

I help her stand up and we move into the bathroom. I close the thick brown door behind us, the golden handle securing the door, the small button underneath locking us in. She sits down on the cold tile floor near the toilet and I hold back her silky brown hair from her face. Everything is brown in here. The beige and brown tiled floor, the brown countertop, the beige bathtub, and the fake wooden toilet seat. I feel out of place with my blond hair, blue eyes, blue T-shirt, and blue jeans. I rest my hand on her back and I can feel the bumps of her spine through her small cotton T-shirt. Can you feel my bones through my skin? She feels so sick, but she can't puke. The time passes. I rub her back with my hand and hold her hair.

"Emby, maybe I should make myself get sick so I feel better."

She sticks her finger down her throat and I feel her body heave under my hand. Nothing comes up. She tries again and is rewarded with a gush of liquid and brown bits. I flush the toilet, but the smell still fills the air. She is breathing hard and she has tears in her eyes. Her hand lies limp over the toilet bowl. I wish it was me.

As she rests on the toilet I announce that I am not feeling well either.

"Katie, do you think I should puke too so that I don't feel so bad in the morning?"

"Hmmmm."

I move over to the beige sink and assume the position. My bare left forearm rests against the cold tile of the sink. I turn on the tap water with my right hand and let it flow. I wet my index finger and my middle finger under the water and put my head over the sink. I put my fingers deep into my throat and feel myself heave. I have even learned how to do this quietly. It sounds like a big burp, and the liquid and food flow into the sink. It is mostly liquid, since I had dinner a few hours ago. I breathe heavily, the tears stinging my eyes, running my fingers under the cool water. I try again. All liquid. My friend shifts on the floor. She stands up.

"Emby, are you OK?"

"Yeah, I just drank too much again."

I run my fingers under the water until my tears dry up. I take a few sips of the water before I turn it off. We both look at ourselves in the large mirror that spans the wall. The harsh light surrounding the mirror shows our red eyes and blotchy faces. Someone knocks on the door. I pick up my rum and Coke with my left hand and unlock the door with my right. We walk out into the laughter and music of the party. I feel better.

> *Mortality rates of 10 to 20% have been reported (with anorexia nervosa).*
> *However, because most mild cases are probably undiagnosed, true prevalence*
> *and mortality rates are not known. (Bogin)*

I can see myself so clearly now. I am a thin, nineteen-year-old university student. You'd never pick me out of a crowd. I'm coming back from a day at my summer job in downtown Halifax. I am heading to the Dalplex gym.

I walk through the main doors of Dalplex, carrying my navy blue University of Victoria backpack on my back. I walk down the flight of stairs and past the information desk. On my right I can see the Nautilus room, where all the fit people in spandex are sweating away on the stair climbers and treadmills. I carry on and follow the blue-painted hallway to the turnstiles. I pass through and head into the women's changing room. The air changes; it is warm and humid in the large, busy room. I can smell the chlorine from the pool below and hear the showers running. The florescent lights glare down from above. The first thing I see when I enter the changing room is a very large mirror. The second thing I see is a very large scale. I hear the sound of the swimmers' bare feet on the gritty brown floor and feel the change in air pressure as someone opens the door into the field house. I walk down the rows of lockers; I pass a row of yellow, a row of white, and a row of orange and finally find myself an empty yellow locker. I change into my workout clothes and head back out into the cool hallway. I walk back through the turnstiles, down the blue-painted hallway towards the information desk and into the Nautilus room.

In the Nautilus room I am greeted by a row of machines, each facing the large window that overlooks the pool. Young, fit students face forward, their Walkmans in their ears as they complete their daily workout. The piped-in radio is playing favorites of today and yesterday. I walk to the NordicTrack and pull my T-shirt away from my body before setting myself up against the plastic waist piece. I put my Walkman in my ears, adjust the tension on the arm ropes and begin my workout. I face forward and pump my legs and my arms. Sweat drips down my face like melting fat. I watch the illuminated red counter as the time ticks down and the calories tick up. Only 300 more. I finish my workout and head to the thin blue mats to stretch and do my 150 sit-ups. I then leave the room and head back down the hall to the women's dressing room.

Back at my yellow locker I change back into my street clothes. I stop only to do the "fat thigh test," which involves putting the thumbs and forefingers of my hands together and making sure that they can still easily go around my thigh. They do. My attention is drawn to two young girls passing my locker in their bathing suits. One has beautiful long brown hair and a blue bathing suit, the other short brown hair and a green bathing suit. They can't yet be thirteen; their hips, waists and chests show no signs of puberty. They pass from my view into the next row of lockers. Suddenly, through the background sounds of many voices, bare feet on the floor, and the opening and closing of doors, I can hear their voices. Their conversation cuts straight through to my ears. They must be at the large scale by the entrance. I hear one of the girls say, "Oh my God, I can't believe I have gained three pounds." The other voice proudly replies, "I have lost two pounds!" And just for a moment I can see everything so clearly.

> *Anorexia nervosa generally begins in early to late adolescence. Anorexics usually strive to perfection, setting very high standards for themselves and always feeling they have to prove their competence. A person with anorexia nervosa may feel the only control they have in their lives is in the area of food and weight. Each morning the number on their scale determines if they have succeeded or failed in their goal for thinness. In the obsessive pursuit of thinness anorexics participate in restrictive eating, compulsive exercise, abuse of laxatives, diuretics and self-induced vomiting.[1]*

In April of 2001 I told some parts of the above story to an audience of 150 people. There were six of us who told stories, all of us about different experiences. We turned down the lights of the auditorium and lit candles. Some of us were animated and made the audience laugh. Some of us spoke softly, and people strained to hear all our words. To get over my stage fright I took out my contact lenses so the audience became blurry. I felt like a bit of a liar when I told my story. Sure I had had some eating problems, but I wasn't that sick. I was never bad enough to have to go to the hospital. I wasn't even ever that thin.

October 15, 2002
Dalhousie Medical School Lecture by David J. Pilon, Ph.D.
Eating Disorders: An Overview for Physicians

I am sitting in Theater D, fifth row back, on the left-hand side of the room, listening to Dr. Pilon. The lecture theater is small; it seats about 120 and there are over 90 of us packed in there. It is hot in the room as the Indian summer sun beats down on the thick brown curtains pulled over the windows. The lights are dim; most of the brightness in the room comes from the PowerPoint overheads projected on the screen. The chairs are cramped; even my short legs notice the lack of space. We are forever complaining about getting stuck in this theater. We pay so much more tuition than all the undergraduates, surely we could at least get a room with temperature regulation and legroom. Medical students are like that. We can complain about anything, even more so now that we are in second year.

My plastic clipboard rests on my knees and my tea mug perches on the small beige desk I just pulled out of the arm of my chair. I feel oversized in the seat. Almost claustrophobic. I knew this lecture would come, and I wondered if I would feel weird. I don't.

I scratch notes on the side of photocopied slides I received and listen for any descriptions that sound familiar.

Anorexia Nervosa

1. *Refusal to maintain 'normal' body weight for age and height—less than 85% expected.*
2. *Intense fear of gaining weight or becoming fat even though under weight.*
3. *Disturbance in way body weight or shape is experienced or undue influence of body weight and shape on self-evaluation.*
4. *Absence of three consecutive menstrual cycles in females. (Pilon)*

None of that sounds like me. I never managed to lose that much weight, despite all my effort. I never got below 95 pounds, which isn't that light for someone who never made it past 5'3". I definitely had an intense fear of gaining weight and it always played a role in determining my self-worth. I never stopped having my periods, though, so clinically I was never an anorexic. It just ruled my life.

I settle into my seat and take a sip of my lukewarm tea. The room is getting warmer as the afternoon sun beats down on the curtains.

I can see it all so clearly now.

Special thanks to Linda Clarke, Facilitator of the Narrative in Medicine program at Dalhousie University, without whom this story would never have existed.

NOTE

1. Source unknown. When I was preparing this piece I spend a number of hours searching the Internet to find statistics. I came across this paragraph and I immediately associated with it. I never wrote down the source and was unable to find it again. Despite much reading I was also unable to find a paragraph to which I associated so strongly, so I kept the original paragraph in.

REFERENCES

Litt, Iris F. Chapter 112, Richard E. Behrman, Robert Liegman and Hal B. Jenson (eds.), *Nelsons Textbook of Pediatrics.* 16th ed. WB Saunders Company, 2000.

Bogin, R. M., A. J. Fletcher, and B. Chir. *The Merk Manual of Diagnosis and Therapy.* Internet Version. Merk & Co., 1999–2003, section 15, chapter 196.

Smith, Delia. Chapter 227, Russell L. Cecil, J. Claude Bennett, and Lee Goldman (eds.), *Cecil Textbook of Medicine.* 21st ed. WB Saunders Company, 2000.

Pilon, David J. Queen Elizabeth II Health Sciences Centre Eating Disorders Clinic. Dalhousie Medical School. Brain and Behavior lecture. October 2002.

Rome, E. S. "Eating Disorders". *Obstetrics and Gynecology Clinics of North America.* June 2003. 30(2):353–77.

Steadman's Medical Dictionary. 27th ed. Baltimore: Lippincott, Williams & Wilkins, 2000.

QUESTIONS

1. How does the refrain "I can see it all so clearly now" function in the narrative?
2. How do the author's journal entries from the time of her disorder convey a different sense of anorexia than her reflections after the fact?
3. Discuss the risks and benefits of the author's decision to make public her struggle with anorexia while she was in medical school.

A Brief Portrait of an Autistic
as a Young Man
⌐ Ruth Elizabeth Burks ⌐

Between me and the other world there is ever an unasked question: unasked by some through feelings of delicacy; by others through the difficulty of rightly framing it. All, nevertheless, flutter round it. . . . How does it feel to be a problem?

And yet, being a problem is a strange experience,—peculiar even for one who has never been anything else, save perhaps in babyhood and in Europe. It is in the early days of rollicking childhood that the revelation first bursts upon me, all in a day as it were . . . it dawned upon me with a certain suddenness that I was different from the others; or like, mayhap, in heart and life and longing, but shut out from their world by a vast veil.

It is a peculiar sensation, this double-consciousness, this sense of always looking at one's self through the eyes of others, of measuring one's soul by the tape of a world that looks on in amused contempt and pity. One ever feels his twoness . . .; two souls, two thoughts, two unreconciled strivings; two warring ideals in one dark body, whose dogged strength alone keeps it from being torn asunder.

—W. E. B. DuBois

Although written to describe the particular and precarious position he and other black Americans find themselves in at the turn of the last century, W.E.B. DuBois's words also perfectly portray what it is like for my son Gyasi at the turn of this century to be both African American and autistic. Through sheer circumstances of birth, Gyasi finds himself on the periphery looking in at a world whose majority is still not yet ready to embrace difference. It is a world that he, like DuBois, scrutinizes through the unique lens of a double or even triple consciousness, alternately viewing his perch as both a blessing and a curse, but a world that he, unlike DuBois, is far less eager to engage fully as the result of autism.[1]

It is this world, the world of the autistic, which I try to unveil, first by illuminating my son's thought processes through excerpts from his written language—passages that epitomize the highs and lows punctuating his life—and then through love notes that portray my son in a more true-to-life, less clinical and truncated frame.

☙ ❧

It is raining, pouring actually, but the news station has forecast rain for the entire day, so I am prepared, even though I cannot stand driving in the rain. I am on my way to Bentley College, where I am an assistant professor of English and where, this year, the Asperger's Association of New England (AANE) annual conference will occur. It is exactly noon, the time I promised my son I would meet him for lunch. To my surprise, the parking lot is almost full, and I have more difficulty parking than I ever do on weekdays when classes are in session. This is a Saturday, and for the first time, I begin to wonder about the size of the conference.

Gyasi has left the house earlier, since he wanted to attend every event at this one-day annual conference. I, on the other hand, am going for the express purpose of being there while he presents. Once inside the building where his talk will occur, I notice a display of innumerable books on autism and Asperger's syndrome. I am surprised to see so many books on the subject. Clearly, in the ten or so years since Gyasi's firm diagnosis, what had been little more than a cottage industry has become big business.

At about 12:25, large numbers of people begin ascending the adjacent staircase, and I assume correctly that the keynote speech has just ended. Again, the numbers astonish me—it seems that hundreds of people are passing—although I am not surprised that Gyasi is one of the last. He is not very aggressive and generously lets the more pushy types go first. I have moved to the side to avoid being trampled by the hordes of people streaming in, who appear both wet and famished. When I spot my son—a twenty-nine-year-old, 5'7" slender, extremely light-skinned African American man—he looks beautiful to me, so handsome and debonair in his dark brown merino wool turtleneck, double-breasted navy blue blazer, gray flannel cuffed pants, and dark brown, recently polished Clarks. When he sees me, however, the beatific smile that usually emanates from deep within him whenever we meet is absent, and I know that something is wrong. I keep asking, "What's wrong?" and he keeps replying "Nothing," until I say, "You know you can't fool me." At that point, he admits, "It's too crowded," and immediately begins to relax a little now that he has put the problem into words.

Gyasi does not like crowds, so once I realize that nothing had actually happened, I can relax too. I also know that he will get over it shortly. His chameleon-like ability to adjust to his surroundings, even when quite perturbed by them, continues to astound me. Moreover, I, too, find myself discombobulated by the size of this crowd. Both Gyasi and I have been to other autism conferences, but the majority of them were usually quite small—fifty to seventy-five people at most. This one, we later learn, hosted more than four hundred people, people whose lives in one way or another had been so profoundly affected by the autism spectrum that they traveled all the way from Connecticut, Rhode Island, New Hampshire, Vermont, and Maine in spite of the pouring rain.

Gyasi's workshop is to begin at 1:00. By the time we get to the head of the line of what once had been a sumptuous buffet, most of the spoils are gone. We both grab the last few

pieces of rare roast beef but forfeit our choice of bread. It is already 12:50, and now that
the executive dining room is completely full, we are ushered into an overflow room, which
during the week serves as the faculty dining room but is now devoid of any tablecloths,
flowers, or heat. We join another autistic man, a tall, sandy-haired young white man of
thirty-something, who spoke to us in line, and whom Gyasi knows from AANE. Neither
Christian nor Gyasi says much as they reenact the parallel play that I know Gyasi, at least,
exhibited as a very young child. With no small talk, Gyasi and Christian eat quickly and deliberately, interrupted only occasionally by my "neurotypical"—the word autistics use to
describe non-autistics like me—need to break the silence. I discover that Gyasi had mis-
calculated his time earlier, missed the free Bentley shuttle, and taken a cab. Since both of
us are on a leave of absence from our regular place of employment, I am, to say the least,
perturbed. When I try to change the subject slightly and ask Christian how he got here, he
simply says, "My mother drove me." When I then ask where she is, he responds in the same
non-inflected voice, "Around here someplace." I reflect on how alike and, at the same time,
how different autistics can be, since I find it impossible to imagine Gyasi choosing to eat
alone when I am present.

   Christian finishes his lunch first and, without any acknowledgment to us, takes his
plate and leaves. Although Gyasi's socialization skills are more advanced, I easily accept what
an outsider might otherwise construe as rudeness on Christian's part. I have been around
enough autistics to recognize their eccentric behavior for no more than what it is.

   It is now 1:15, and Gyasi is getting anxious; he will not stop checking his watch every fifteen seconds. I am sure that the conference organizers will give everyone a chance to
finish lunch, but I am wrong. The next sessions are about to begin, so Gyasi departs, and
I quickly try to finish what still amounts to a sizeable portion of food on my plate. I think
better of it, though, and join Gyasi in the conference room where his workshop, entitled
"College Transition and Students with Asperger's Syndrome," is about to take place. We
are nearly the first ones there, but in no time the room fills up, and I am glad I am able to
commandeer a seat in the front row. Gyasi's panel, it seems, is one of the more popular afternoon attractions.

   After conferring briefly with the other two members of the panel, who are engrossed
in ensuring that the laptop they have ordered for their individual presentation is working
as it should, Gyasi sits on the makeshift platform about fifteen feet away directly facing me.
Clearly conscious of his high visibility, he is becoming increasingly tense, even if he refrains
from unceasingly sliding his thumbs over his fingers and incessantly checking his watch—two
self-stimulating behaviors in which he, like other autistics, indulges frequently. The laughs
and non-verbal assents with which he first greets the start of the moderator's talk appear
less pronounced before disappearing altogether.

   The moderator, Dr. Rachel Fox[2]—who did not, despite Gyasi's phone calls and emails,
communicate with him until we were in line for lunch—is a forty-something white woman,
with short-cropped, medium brown hair and splotchy skin, wearing a herringbone blazer
and olive green pants that accentuate one of the more muted tones in her jacket. As the
clinical director of disability services at a major university and an assistant clinical professor of psychiatry at their school of medicine, Dr. Fox is certain that her presentation takes

precedence over the other two members of the panel (despite or because of their autism) and has little trouble convincing Gyasi that he should go last. Stephen Shore, president of the Asperger's Association of New England's board of directors and a doctoral student in special education, whom Dr. Fox knows well, can go first, as long as he edits his presentation sufficiently to allow her the full half-hour she requires and to leave enough time for Gyasi's fifteen minutes.

Stephen—a thirty-five-year-old white man with semi-balding, dark, straight hair—appears oblivious to the fact that the bright red crew-neck sweater he wears does not quite cover either his wrinkled white shirt or the protruding stomach that insists on hanging over the belt holding up his un-ironed, permanent press, brown khaki pants. Like most autistics I know, Steve is generous. Recognizing that time is short since the keynote speaker had started late, Stephen severely curtails the talk he had prepared to give the other two presenters a chance.

Dr. Fox is not as empathic. She desists only after fifty-five minutes of a PowerPoint presentation aimed more toward college administrators than the clinicians, teachers, adult autistics, and family members who comprise the seventy-five or so people who fill a room intended for fifty. Throughout her talk, she persists in answering questions even though the three presenters have previously agreed and informed the audience that they will not take comments or respond to queries until all are finished.

Although his hands are steady, Gyasi's voice, which keeps undulating in pitch, reveals how nervous he feels when he gets his turn at the podium, and I am unable to ascertain why. He loves to speak in front of an audience, so whenever he receives an invitation to present his academic work or to talk about his experiences as an autistic, he manages to mask the quivering in his stomach and exude complete self-confidence. I speculate that his shakiness might stem from choosing to deliver a written presentation rather than to talk extemporaneously from a rough outline, as he has done in the past. On the drive home, I learn the answer. Yes, Gyasi was worried about having enough time to finish his entire talk when Dr. Fox refused to limit hers, but his primary fear came from the audience, who, from his point of view—he was facing them—represented a socially inappropriate, unrestrained mob in their demand to have their questions answered immediately.

From my point of view—I was facing the podium—Dr. Fox was a pompous, selfish, boring asshole, clearly at fault and unable to exert the type of control expected of a seasoned moderator. Even if one could excuse the adult autistics, who, as part of their disorder, might have difficulty following the requisite social cues, they were not the only ones speaking out of turn. I am not surprised, however, by Dr. Fox's presumption that her theoretical, more academic approach takes precedent over Gyasi's more personal and experiential narrative. As an African American female scholar, I am all too familiar with how those in the center continue to suppress the voices of others whose race, gender, class, sexual orientation, or disability places them on the margins.

In the meantime, I am as nervous as Gyasi, for I experience vicariously what he experiences. During his fifteen-minute talk, I sit suspended, praying he will have time to finish and praying he will find a way to relax. Yet I cannot help laughing when the rest of the audience laughs, and, like them, I am singularly impressed with what he has to say and the way in which he says it. Even though his voice continues to fluctuate wildly at times with this atypical nervousness, which I cannot yet comprehend, he charismatically recounts his experiences with four professors—who either begrudged or granted him the accommodations he needed—while he was earning his master's of science at Simmons College Graduate School of Library and Information Science. A part of his talk, entitled "The Politics of Accommodation," I excerpt here:

The two years I spent at the Graduate School of Library and Information Science at Simmons College could easily have been a social experiment in the impact of academic accommodations on the performance of disabled students. The mediocre grades I earned when I did not have accommodations stand in perfect opposition to the stellar grades I earned once I received them. Professor Smith, who resisted my request for accommodations, was one of my professors during my first semester. In Smith's class, I not only did as poorly as a graduate student can do and remain a graduate student, but I also considered abandoning the academy all together. Fortunately, no subsequent professor blocked my ability to receive accommodations, and the non-judgmental attitude of Professor Shoemaker opened my mind to the abundance of librarianship and enabled me to flourish intellectually.

The first book I read in library school was Professor Smith's forty-plus-page syllabus. The class was Reference and Information Services, and it was one of the first steps on my road to becoming a librarian. Like Mount Everest to an aspiring rock-climber, the syllabus looked both imposing and exciting. In addition to stating such lofty goals as "Students will leave the class having developed their own philosophy of reference," the syllabus listed one hundred or so reference questions needing answers over the course of the semester, with an equal number of reference sources requiring physical examination. I remember thinking, "If I succeed in doing all this, I will have achieved badness."

Like his syllabus, Professor Smith had a commanding presence that was both intimidating and inspiring. A six-foot-tall man with snow-white hair, wire-rimmed glasses, and a tomato-red complexion, Professor Smith looked like a professor. His usual wardrobe of a sports coat, collared shirt (sometimes accentuated with a bow tie), and slacks gave him an almost ivy-league demeanor. I remember once overhearing two female students refer to him as being "Paul Newman cute." I used to think of him as a retired Viking warrior. In the classroom, Professor Smith was all charm as he entertained with anecdotes and dazzled with erudition. Outside of the classroom, he was formal and stiff, and God help you if you imposed on his personal space. I once approached Professor Smith after a class, a class in which he had been his usual open and laid-back self, only to find myself snapped at because he had already stepped out of his teaching persona.

Moreover, I had the misfortune of experiencing more of the out-of-class Smith than of the in-class Smith because of my request for academic accommodations. Convinced that my disability must be synonymous with deficiency, Professor Smith changed the parameters of an assignment when I turned out to be the only student who had done it correctly. Not knowing that a Harvard librarian who had previously trained under Smith had assisted me with the assignment, he rendered my bibliography inferior to those produced by my classmates by implementing new rules. With a similar sleight-of-hand, Smith also managed to prevent me from finishing the final exam, a test usually administered during the 9:00—11:00 a.m. class. Since my sole accommodation was extra time, I acquiesced when Smith asked me to come in at 8:00 a.m. You can imagine my surprise when he sent me on a one-hour break at 9:00 a.m., and I returned from my break only to find that I was to join in the discussion with the rest of the class who had just finished their exam.

My final year at Simmons was the highlight of my library science education. As part of a course called Bibliographic Instruction and Methods by Professor Shoemaker, I finally could combine my interests in psychology and African American studies. Shoemaker, a middle-aged, unassuming woman with white short-cropped hair, like her look-alike Angela Lansbury of the television series *Murder, She Wrote*, had lived on the sidelines of crime—she once taught sociology in a prison. The thrust of the course was on learning theory, and our major project was to design a teaching module based on the best teaching practices. I demonstrated how the *Microsoft Encarta Africana* CD-ROM proved an effective teaching tool because its multimedia features engaged multiple modalities and catered to a number of learning styles. Ironically, I had wanted to trace the history of Encarta Africana during my first semester at Simmons. Professor Smith not only nixed it, claiming my project was too contemporary to be worthy of scholarly consideration, but also disregarded the substantive data I presented showing that the *Africana: The Encyclopedia of the African and African American* was actually the culmination of a project begun by W.E.B. DuBois in 1909, leaving a ninety-year history in its wake.

Beside the conclusions I hope you draw from my anecdotes—that those with invisible disabilities can become integral members of society with appropriate accommodations—I also trust that you recognize that not everyone would benefit from such entitlements. Research has shown that non learning-disabled students reap the same rewards from receiving extra time on assignments as perfectly-sighted people gain from wearing prescription eyeglasses. In fact, utilizing accommodations that one does not need can actually be detrimental. Where the physically impacted person requires a ramp or elevator, the physically intact person is better off, health-wise, taking the stairs.

The rumblings in the hall indicate that the next group of workshops is already beginning in some of the other conference rooms, but this heterogeneous audience finds Gyasi's talk riveting; no one stirs until he is absolutely done. His "thank-you" at the end of his presentation meets thundering applause, and it is to Gyasi whom everyone flocks at the close of the session. Dr. Fox's PowerPoint presentation has become pedantic; Gyasi's particular has triumphed over her general, and I learn another lesson from Gyasi: At times, it is okay to be last.

While I wait for the crowd of people around Gyasi to disperse, I am struck by his sense of humor as well as by his double consciousness, his ability to see the disabled as others do and, at the same time, to retain a positive vision of himself. Yet these high points in his life can still occasionally be undermined by low ones, and I recall how just two weeks earlier, Gyasi viewed himself through a very different lens, as this excerpt from his "Annals of Anxiety" illustrates:

> Outburst—I do not know what happened tonight. My mom and I were having a conversation, and I suddenly exploded. The ostensible reason for why I exploded, or more accurately, the particular thing that set me off, was actually something that had occurred hours earlier. I was forty minutes late to my psychiatrist appointment, and I might as well have missed it since I was not dressed for it anyway. I was not particularly bothered; in fact, it never even occurred to me that I was not dressed appropriately for my appointment, and, in retrospect, this lapse in judgment particularly bothers me. In truth, it was obvious that I was not appropriately dressed—I had not showered, I had not shaved, and I had not combed my hair; yet, I was going to see someone who makes a living judging the mental state of others. To top it off—to add the "pours" to the expression "when it rains"—I was late to my appointment because I failed to do some very basic problem solving. My cab was late, and I kept calling the dispatcher, half planning to practice assertiveness and give her a piece of my mind, instead of walking the quarter of a mile to the Sheraton Hotel, which has cabs perpetually parked in front.
>
> When I finally got to my psychiatrist's office, I was relieved since I still had a few minutes to talk about some of the things I wanted to discuss. When my mother pulled up in front of the hospital, she confronted my state of under-dress. I was probably as shocked as my mother was, and, when she reminded me how inappropriate it was for a man to be unshaven, I wanted to vanish—her metaphor of not wiping oneself took on literal significance for me, and I felt that my face was smeared with foulness.
>
> Several hours later, I made a comment about my personal knowledge of the dangers of jumping to conclusions. My mother knew, without my saying it, that I was referring to my recent experience with members of the mental health profession judging me superficially. My mother felt compelled to revisit my earlier unkempt appearance when she saw me in front of Cambridge Hospital. She said I looked like the other derelicts and bums who tended to congregate there and that I was not only setting myself up to be maligned in the notes of my current psychiatrist, but I was also undermining his ability to ever see me as a competent employee. Worse, my failure to adapt to the fact that my cab was late gave credence to the disability coordinator's contention that I am unable to handle change.
>
> At first, I was perfectly willing to accept my mother's criticism in silence, though I was hoping she would hurry up and finish. While I was listening to my mother, I was also thinking. I know that Cambridge is a small community. I know that one should not be so outwardly motivated. I know that one must dress the part that one would like to play. I know that we live about a block away from a fleet of cabs. I know

that I screwed up—now can we end this neurotic digression and get back to our original conversation. As annoyed as I was, I knew I deserved this castigation, and I imagined it would be a constant reminder that would remain with me for a while.

Then my mother made those comments about the disability coordinator and my psychiatrist. She added that my rigidity in response to the cab being late was analogous to my reaction to a friend having stood me up last week. When the word "prioritize" issued from my mother's lips—a buzz word my current employer likes to bandy around, and one that I have come to associate with the most demeaning type of insult—I privately cursed the very pattern recognition behavior that I usually admire and strive to emulate. I was not that angry, but I was irrational. I could not express my objections succinctly, and my exacerbation raised my voice a few octaves. By the time I lowered my voice, my mother seemed to have already stopped listening—she was now going on about the neighbors, the poor sound insulation, and the police. I stormed into my room in frustration but not before pulling away from my mother, who tried to stop me, and throwing away my sandwich in response to her command that I finish my dinner. I also banged my head against my closet door.

I lay in bed tossing and turning, alternating between berating and defending myself as my mind spun in ritualistic ruminations. I have really done it now; my life is over. My vices are no worse than any one else's. It is the residue from my early misdiagnoses that makes them sting. My failures seem to contradict my successes. I am definitely not contributing my genes to evolution . . . and so on.

I do not know what set me off, or why I failed to see it coming. I have a sense that if I had seen it coming, it would not have happened. As irrational as I knew it to be, I was overwhelmed by the fatalistic feeling that I had negated all of the work I had done to make myself more flexible and to be more professional by my day's activities. Equally important, as living proof that autistics are literal and lacking in common sense, I felt I had forever lost the right to speak or write.

Written a few days after the outburst triggered by my use of the word "prioritize," the above passages reveal a third lens, a lens that suggests cognitive difference can heighten and not just impede acuity, as it both negates and supports the research that concludes autistics lack a "theory of mind." In nonprofessional language, this lack of "theory of mind," or "mind-blindness," prevents autistics from recognizing that other people do not view the world from the same exact reference point they do. If the word "prioritize" conjures up for Gyasi a host of unpleasant connotations—stereotypes that strip him of his humanity by refusing to recognize his individuality and the labels he believes he has managed to overcome—then, in using this word, I, too, contribute to his overall condemnation and render him less than human. Nevertheless, once the outburst is over and he can review the incident in his mind—or, in this case, reconstruct it on paper—he can also see how he has erroneously attributed his negative thoughts surrounding the word "prioritize" to me.

I sometimes believe these periodic expressions of "mind-blindness," which have auspiciously decreased in frequency and intensity over the years, may be a necessary catharsis, a way to release the tension generated by Gyasi's perennial attempt to negotiate this tightrope. I only hope, as Gyasi learns more appropriate and productive ways to translate the rage he must feel in trying to balance and synchronize the discordant triad he exemplifies—black, autistic, brilliant—that his outbursts will disappear altogether.

In writing this brief portrait to illuminate what it means for Gyasi to be autistic, I fear I have omitted everything that makes him special, everything, in fact, that autistics are supposed to lack and that Gyasi has in abundance: his unconditional love, his affectionate nature, his support in everything I do, his ability to accept people as they are, his love of family and tradition, his flexibility, his inquisitiveness, his external as well as internal beauty, his intelligence, his equanimity, his generosity, and his empathic regard. My portrait may end here, but my subject is just beginning. To paraphrase Toni Morrison and W. E. B. DuBois, two of Gyasi's favorite writers—who, like him, recognize the power inherent in ambiguity and double-consciousness—"This is not a story to pass on" (275), even if "dusk began at dawn" (*Dusk of Dawn*, viii).

NOTES

1. Two weeks before he turned eighteen, clinicians determined Gyasi suffered from infantile autism, a severe disorder of communication, imagination, and socialization. Since then, Asperger's syndrome, a term often used interchangeably with autism to differentiate higher-functioning individuals from lower-functioning ones, has also been attached to him, situating Gyasi even more solidly within what has come to be known as the autism spectrum.
2. To prevent casting any unnecessary aspersions, I have not only changed the moderator's name but also omitted her actual place of employment.

REFERENCES

DuBois, W. E. B. *The Souls of Black Folk.* New York: Penguin, 1989.

———. *Dusk of Dawn.* New York: Schocken Books, 1968.

Morrison, Toni. *Beloved.* New York: Knopf, 1987.

QUESTIONS

1. Whose story is this? Comment on the relationship between the mother-author's voice and her son-speaker's voice. How might this narrative be different if it were told exclusively by the son himself?
2. Comment on the author-mother's tone throughout the piece.
3. Comment on the double marginalization of race and disability.

Her Reckoning
A Young Interdisciplinary Academic Dissects the Exact Nature of Her Disease

⌒ WENDY MARIE THOMPSON ⌒

Before completing a bachelor's degree in Asian-American studies with a minor in women's studies, I had transferred schools after threatening to knuckle up with some of the white girls who lived in the dorms with me my freshman year at college. I am not the first in my family to go to college, but coming from a family with a Burmese Chinese immigrant mother who had minimal English skills and a working-class African American father who went to San Francisco City College, my attending and graduating from a four-year university was not just some minimal everyday thing.

I have to admit that although I have done much critical work deconstructing my subjectivity and tying my young, queer, black-Chinese, working-class female experience into the greater periphery of ethnic, class, and gender studies, there has hardly been any exploration of my mental affliction. Therefore, this is my first in-depth non-medical exploratory narrative of self, and my first attempt to assemble all the parts of me into one coherent autobiographical account. Please keep in mind that I have always found it difficult to write in a consistent linear fashion. Rather, I tend to weave together not only concepts, but genres as well. And although I have been "diagnosed" and have seen several different therapists and psychologists throughout my young life, my actual mental state was never really explained to me in language that I could understand.

I suppose I was born this way, just without any kind of methodology or theorems to explain my existence, my shadow living, my pain giving, my incessant depression cycles like the circling of the earth's axis on stilted, uneven legs. Spinning in an orbit of despair. *

I had always been a "special child." Not special in the sense that I rode the "special mentally retarded" school bus to school or had the teacher explain to the other students in my class to be "very kind to me" because I was physically ill. It was never something acknowledged by the people around me, and my parents figured that I would eventually "grow out of *it*."

It was my anti-social, very emotionally secluded childhood. *It* was my silent way of internalizing trauma and abuse. *It* was the way I tried to take my life at fourteen, then at fifteen after reading about self-injury in a teen fiction library book, the way I repeated it on my body for years after. *It* almost got me arrested and put into juvenile hall at sixteen after fighting my father because I wanted to run away. *It* was supposed to go away with the prescribed Zoloft that I never took, but instead sold to my then physically and sexually abusive homeless boyfriend's childhood gang friend.

But out of the hostility of life, it was discovered that, from an early age, I had talent, a gift: I could write, create pictures and otherworlds to escape to in order to save my life. I had begun drawing at the age of five amidst the long isolated years of being locked inside a house with a beat-down mother and an angry, depressed father.

In having had a lopsided childhood experience which some would call emotionally abusive and socially restrictive, I grew up without power, falling deeper into cycles of violence and dependence. But I wasn't totally incompetent; there was always an innate desire to figure out: *What is wrong with me? What can I do about it?*

Yet as I began configuring my racial self, my sexual self, my gendered self, I never realized mental illness was connected to experiences of trauma (cultural, racial, class, diasporic, environmental, social) because so often mental illness is constructed into a "white people" disease or a "rich people who have time for therapy" disease. I figured I could just spare myself the embarrassment of having contracted such an abnormality and go on with my life, as if nothing was causing me to lose sleep and appetite, to shut down for weeks, to want to leave this place and leave everything for silence, for quiet.

An undergraduate's diary entry #138: Sept/2002

Goddamn it, how hard is it to write a 10 page academic paper on comparative race relations during the post-World War II rupture when I'm having an episode! Call up my mother, scream, cry, cuss out my roommate, kick over the table, turn back three months of sober, anti-violent, depression-coping skills and cut into the fiber of my body with stainless-steel scissors, tear down the house. The paper assignment which sits on a floppy disk with only the title page and a paragraph while I try and get my mind straightened out finally gets turned in three weeks after the quarter has ended. I fix the incomplete status on my grade sheet, hold a good enough GPA to apply for graduate school, but there are three more scars spanning the length of my upper arm. My aunt suggests I find some kind of spirituality. My mother tells me to pray and go to the student health center. The student health center psychologist tells me that I should reschedule another appointment after my initial in-take evaluation. I already know everything that's wrong with me; I just lack the sophisticated psychiatric language to define myself and my condition to everybody else. A friend asks me what "it" is, how I am feeling, can I describe why I am this way. And all I can say to explain the madness that manifests itself in me is a series of cuss words and yells.

My love is not in my eyes, the two brown fragments of evidence, of a miscegenated conquest, the gift of Asian blood, my half Orient to someone else's damning Occident. Through that dark unnamed historical landmark, I bleed fast food drive-thrus and homeless shelters, I bleed bilingually, not only in English, Chinglish, Spanglish, but other subjects as well like history, science, psychology.

I am living in cultural exile. An outsider, a mixed-roots Afro-Chinese American sister. Fuck trivial measurements of authenticity held up to the phenotype of experience. I grew up in a house where we learned to suck a crab leg dry, where we learned to swallow and internally keep violence after getting hit so many times by our father, where we learned how to strip the down off a turtledove in the warm kitchen of a neighbor from Hong Kong, unashamed of the blood and torn plumage in her hands. This cultural home I was forced from caused extreme detachment from a world that sheltered me. This outside social expulsion left me dislocated, mute, and lonely.

I was led to hate being a girl at a young age due to what I felt was my father's perception that having three daughters was a useless and disappointing venture. He had always had a strong preference for sons, boys who would never give him shame, never get pregnant or fail to carry on his name. I was the odd one who cried too much, who grew fearful at loud noises, who ran and hid from danger and pain, who asked too many questions and wanted too much of the world that neither of my parents could afford.

Subsequently as a teenager, I ran away from my house when I was in high school in search of safety. I looked to the company of gangs, through men, anyone who I thought could help me transcend my afflictions, my lonesomeness. I met a boyfriend who physically and sexually abused me worse than any father-like figure would have. Our interactions consisted of various assaults in public, forced intercourse, his threats of shooting me and killing himself if I ever left.

I tried to run him over with my car.

Goddamn it you punch too many holes in walls, too many holes and I have not enough skin to patch them up with.

☞ ☜

I yearned for love from anyone, looked for explanation in an apathetic world but found nothing but emptiness. In my relationships that I sought out with random men or women I would always be the explosive one, acting out so many years of mistreatment.

In my lived everyday, I was so accustomed to trying on different skins to adapt to any given situation that I never really thought to explore myself. I was what other people said I was: a gifted girl who could grasp simple equations and concepts, memorize parts of declarations, paint a landscape, but never fully understand or divulge her true natural talents. It wasn't until graduate school that I was given things like "social construction," "multiple cultural identities," "trauma." And as I grappled with applications, I found myself still struggling with living a transitory life with no permanent roots to place or people in a society where things have borders, things have safety nets, jobs and church and craft lessons that give us a reason to get up and live every morning.

Cuts

She hurts herself. Cuts long deep
wounds from wrist to shoulder.
Someone finds out at school and
refers her to a nurse who moonlights
as the school counselor because of

budget constraints. The lady looks
at high school transcripts, records
of previous institutions attended.
"Are you having problems adjusting?
Family problems? When did this all

start? Are you at risk of suicidal
behavior?" The girl shakes her
head, unable to explain the book,
the razor, the experiment to link
the book with the razor. What did

those girls do? She knew it was
fiction. It was in the library's Young
Adult Fiction series. What did
those girls do? Take razors,
anything able to make a cut in skin.

And whenever they were pissed,
whenever the world or their stupid
parents seemed to fuck them over,
how did they do it? Hold the blade
like this? Press down like this?

Suck in the sting like this? "That's
such an urban white chick thing.
Cutting. I mean, what black girl.
Or, excuse me, mixed girl does
that shit?"

(Sleeves feel so short in the
summertime.)

Her father was yelling again.
His words an angry slab of
concrete smashing into her face.
His violence echoing through the
water of her mind while she

searched in darkness for the
porcelain dog figurine
that her mother gave her.
Little gray Scottish Terrier
smashing against the wall. Half

of his leg cutting into her
membrane, into the core of her
anger, into the fiber of her hurt
and shutting it down.

Ma finds the sheets the next
afternoon. She tells her daughter
to put on some Vaseline and to
give her the razor, and never do

it again. The girl
opens her arms like a flower,
extends them out in front of
herself and there they are all lined
up in chaos: those long thin tracks

of madness and war. Cuts for
never being popular, for always
being the ugly girl, always being
the poor girl. Cuts because she was
tired of feeling so fucking sorry.

Blood like a small fish in her mind.
"You are an Aquarian, kind of like
your father except he is an Aries.
That is why you two don't get along.
And true, he may be depressed and

bitter like you. But I never see him
cut himself."

She likes to think of
herself as some kind of small desert-
dwelling lizard. Able to regenerate
arms skin heart eyes.

Over and over and over again.

My bones bare, have no fear.

⸙   ⸙

My tiny hybrid bones, my young woman bones, peculiar and naked to the world, have no fear. They are a warrior's bones perhaps. Bones that have existed in this body for centuries, bones that fractured but never broke. Bones that bent under the weight of the world but never cracked, never splintering like old wood after being beaten down by a father, crushed physically by a boyfriend who took me in but gave me little space to breathe or exist in safety.

They were once, but these bones are no longer petrified. They are the same bones that fought and resisted, fell and hid, forgot and muted what it was that was happening, what was unable to be revealed to a public too traumatized itself to believe it.

Some say that once the mind and memory have experienced horrific trauma, they continue to circle the emotional and psychological effects over lifetimes through the bloodlines. Much like alcoholism and other inherited diseases, the pain passes through DNA strands and infuses into the internal system, rendering the person as disturbed as if it happened yesterday and as run-down as the person who survived and witnessed the pain firsthand.

There are studies documenting the survivors of genocide and de/colonization, relocation and internment, natural disasters which show that even if the experience is erased from the history books and glossed over by the rest of the world, someone's child somewhere is born with that grief and will live it like an open wound, feel it deep in her bones, deep in his mind.

I have read other stories too, reports about survivors of war and the horror of killing fields. How after witnessing such madness and atrocity, they went completely blind and, once arriving on asylum or reunification to North America, had baffled doctors who had no way to medically justify what caused this loss of sight because the irises and retinas were all healthy. There was simply a refusal to see anymore.

Conceivably a gesture towards maintaining sanity.

My skeleton reads DNA inferiority complexes

⸙   ⸙

I survive by what I see, by what I am, by who died before me and paved my road with their backs. Take living back when a racist white supremacist society prided itself for lynching my father's kind. Colored. Put it all together in a young boy's mind, and see how it trickles down. It isn't surprising that they lived in fear: my grandfather who lost his soul to alcohol abuse and repression, my father who lost his childhood to the cruelty and desolation of a punishing world and father. There were no television commercials for Prozac during their times. There was no educational awareness for coping with abuse, no suicide hotlines. And forget running to a therapist for friendly feedback.

To the father I want to say, you pushed the suggested depression roughly aside when I confronted you about the possibility of inherited illness, as if it interfered with your (proud) black male identity and place of normalcy in an America in which you struggled so hard to succeed. But this peculiar daughter of yours wasn't born from calm, and my episodes parallel all too well the kind of wall-punching personality you possess. And to the grandfather I want to say, I was never afraid of you. And I can now understand your decision to choose wine and sleep, given the options of a southern black man with demons in 1945.

But I am still dreaming.

My disposition—which never goes away but moves in phases of intensity—walks with me every day to school, goes into my academic work, exhales the same air, interacts (or not) with people, and fluctuates on a daily basis.

My mother says it's selfish to push my thoughts, my depression, my anger onto other people. But it is difficult to care. It troubles me so much and most people don't believe in my anguish anyway, so why shouldn't I push it on them? Maybe they'll get it this time. Shit, there's the constant assumption that I'm doing the freaking out on purpose, or that I have some kind of control over when it comes up in me. Always somebody telling me to just "go out more" or "be more social" or any of their other asinine suggestions that cause me to believe in my own incompetence instead of believing it is part of the trauma-related depression that makes my life and mental balance more difficult to maintain.

So I continue to struggle with issues of "passing." Passing for normal, performing the gestures of a composed, competent, young, female academic of color. Passing for privileged and entitled. Although I have chronic anxiety attacks when it comes time to present my research in front of others and despite my interdisciplinary work which pushes hard against traditional fields of scholarship, I have been told by several professors that I am the ideal student whose fiery passion for social change and thirst for knowledge are what make me so remarkable. It will be my commitment to learning that will take me far in this career, as well as my curious way of balancing a social life with academic life, they say, although they have no idea that my life has no social dimensions and that I have haphazardly staggered this far through my young life.

At this point I continue to place my existence in the scholarly (and personal) context of a gendered and racial homespace, trying to make sense of my dislocated lack of community and connection to the rest of the world. At the same time, I am fighting against killing myself because like so many other academics who have become absorbed into the many methods and theories, I have come to sleep, eat, and shit my everyday observations of race and class and nationality and cannot help a possibly unhealthy obsession with fixing myself in all of these constructs. It becomes very difficult to balance it all on my tiny blue plate.

All things to me are personal. Nothing is a matter of being politically correct. I am always defensive, always on the edge, but I refuse to get on the drugs that will only help to "control" my "instabilities" instead of erase them, opting to fight it out as I have been doing all my life. There is no shame about the way I live: a post-trauma person getting her education, fighting to get into the big intellectual house in order to tear it open, standing on her own two feet to fight back as the daughter of working-class, struggling, immigrant, semi-literate, small-time, fucked-up parents who always told her to "Use that mind, or else what good is your brain for?"

Once I told myself that I needed the validation of the world in order to be good enough. But where is the world that is good enough for me?

To exist with what we have. I reckon this is what it means to live anyway.

NOTE

*Italicized segments are excerpts from the poem "Her Reckoning" by the author.

QUESTIONS

1. How does her position as a "bi-queer, Black-Chinese, working-class female" influence the author's understanding and response to her disorder?

2. Comment on the author's overt discussion of language and silence. How do both function in connection to her disorder?

3. Why might the author have chosen a multi-genre form to convey her story of illness? How would the narrative be different if it were in another form, and what different effects might it achieve?

The Interstices of Illness
The Elasticity of Diagnostic Time

⌐ TRACY CURTIS ⌐

No one touches you if you tell people you might have cancer. That's the first thing I noticed after the initial expressions of concern. Friends who had been affectionate showed their worry from a safe distance. Although most people understand that cancer is not contagious, this knowledge does not mitigate the fear. So for a little while, no one slides into the booth next to you. No one hugs you hello. Everyone avoids saying good-bye. This behavior comes from people who can tolerate your presence. Some cannot bear to see you at all. While never saying that they are afraid, they fail to invite you out, saying later, "I thought you wouldn't be up for anything." Others look at you with a slight wince that I take to be concern. I value this caring. I just do not know what to do with it—especially when it is accompanied by an actual physical distance that reminds me of the way that junior high school kids shun one another. I felt as though people who might love me in the best of circumstances grew afraid to get too close, if not because of some contagion, then because it seems futile to hang on to someone who might not be around for much longer.

For the purposes of this piece, I say that all of this started in the summer of 2002 when a doctor told me that I might be ill. She suggested further tests to determine the cause of some abnormalities in my blood tests. The suggestion frightened me so that my behavior changed, almost immediately and probably irreversibly. I know that my transformation was prompted from at least two sources: my need to manage the threat of illness and my perceptions of people's behavior toward me shifting. It was often unclear whether my friends' responses were to the possibility of cancer among our twenty- and thirty-something group or to the behavior I adopted because I was alarmed. However, I spent a great deal of energy that fall trying to keep my composure while responding to both challenges as best I could.

The sudden and profound absence of personal contact was bad enough without having it replaced by the touch of medical staff. Kisses were replaced by sheathed thermometers, pats on the shoulder by a blood pressure cuff. Most of the time, even this contact felt distanced. It was from the intake staff, and took place before I ever entered the examination room. Unlike my previous visit to a doctor, when I suspected that I might have broken my little toe, I felt beyond healing. A medical visit in which the only contact is to take vital statistics feels hopeless. The doctor, a specialist to whom I had been referred, a pleasant woman who behaves compassionately, sat in a chair that seemed incredibly far from me as she was giving me the news that I had been dreading.

It was July 22. She said that I might need a biopsy. The first thing that anyone reading this should understand is that after a doctor says "biopsy," there are a few moments when nothing else is heard. I had been feeling out-of-sorts and worried, but cancer was not among the scenarios I predicted. After some abnormalities in my blood tests a year earlier, I had been sent for an ultrasound examination of my thyroid and ovaries. I had not been alarmed because the test is non-invasive and because the doctor told me it was strictly a precaution. In an ultrasound, the technician passes a wand which transmits a topographical image over the area to be viewed and records some videotape. The most harrowing part of that examination was not being taken in at my appointment time after drinking the vat of water required for the ovarian ultrasound. I lay on the table nearly in tears because the water had to come out somehow. The technician told me that my bladder was too full as though their instructions and delays in calling me for my appointment had nothing to do with it. The doctors, nurses, and insurance representatives had all become "they" to me. This technician was no different, though she did win points by letting me go to the bathroom before finishing the test. Other than some idle conversation about the weather, she did not say much. Technicians are not supposed to reveal results, which is understandable but unnerving. The waiting leads not only to patient distress, but also to information falling through the cracks.

In a large, university-affiliated teaching hospital, such tests take place outside the doctor's office. The doctor asks an assistant for paperwork, which is often not passed directly to the patient. The patient has to go through a checkout procedure to make follow-up appointments, get lab instructions, etc. If the patient needs tests, there are forms to carry, most often to another building. Another set of people takes the paperwork. There is more waiting. The patient spends approximately fifteen minutes with the person who is supposed to help her, but hours to fill out paperwork, shift among offices, wait for vital signs to be taken, ask billing questions, and make another appointment. The doctor, a nurse or two, and the workers in the administrative check-out office tell the patient that she will be contacted if there is a problem. No news is good news, unless the mail gets placed into my neighbor's box again or the periodic power outages kill the day's phone messages. This set-up is frustrating at best, and acceptable only when it works.

My first ultrasound showed nodules growing on my thyroid. Both were below the size at which doctors usually suggest a biopsy. At least that is what I was told a year later when the doctor referred to these test results casually. Even now, I do not know whether those guidelines are general medical ones or rules followed by that group of doctors. For that first year, no one told me the growths were there. I am not an unintelligent person. However, I study literature rather than the biological sciences. My knowledge of anatomy and medicine is limited. It did not occur to me that the medical team might decide that two growths might not be worthy of mention. The test records did use the term "nodes." But I did not see the records until that July appointment, nearly a year later, right before the doctor sent me to repeat the ultrasound immediately.

This doctor visit came ten days before my medical insurance was to expire. I had been a lecturer, teaching large and small literature classes and mentoring student research projects. Although I was scheduled to teach an upcoming summer class, my contracted lectureship was over, and my insurance coverage did not extend beyond July 31. Because I was frightened and soon to be without coverage, I wanted to schedule both the ultrasound and the biopsy right away. Scheduling a biopsy proved challenging, but I was able to walk a few blocks to another facility and wait three hours for the second ultrasound. This technician exclaimed slightly when passing the wand over the right side of my throat. I tried to see the screen. She told me to be still. I was torn between being glad she had given me some signal and wanting the relative silence of the previous test. I left the office worried.

Before sending me to the hospital for this screening, the doctor mentioned how long it takes for the ultrasound results to be returned to her and that she gets the OR only a few days each month. So I knew I had to wait for the first open OR time after the ultrasound results passed through the bureaucracy. I could pay to extend my coverage at a cost of $254 each month. My salary as a lecturer had been inhumanely low. I had so little money that I had to start cutting things out of my life. The first things to go were vision and dental insurance. Much of what I owned was old or second-hand, so selling things would not have helped. I had moved into my apartment just before a city-wide rise in rents. There was no way I could save money by finding another place. I could not think of much to eliminate. I began worrying about how I would pay for cancer. I should have told the doctor about this concern, but I had been too paralyzed by my sudden terror. I hide my feelings well. Clearly she had no idea I was afraid because instead of saying anything reassuring or helpful before sending me to the hospital, she complained about the inconveniences of scheduling. I like her. But I did not want to hear about such "inconveniences." Also, the fright was taking over. The small part of me that was aware enough to continue polite interaction felt too vulnerable to add the embarrassment of my poverty to the conversation.

Almost as soon as I left the doctor's office, I needed to tell people. That was the first sign that after a small hint of disease, I was no longer myself. Before that day, I had been trying to be more open. It was an effort. But suddenly I was disclosing at least my status and sometimes my fears to my friends in person, by telephone, over IM and email. People were surprised, concerned, and mostly supportive. But each conversation was more harrowing for me than the previous one. It felt as though my expressions of worry were building a reality and a destiny. A friend called me one evening after I was already in bed. She began the conversation by telling me about her neighbor, who had come by to ask her to feed the cats that hung around outside their back doors. The neighbor said that she would not be around anymore. When my friend asked why, the neighbor said that she had end-stage cancer and was going to use pain medication to take her life in a few days. They had been cordial neighbors at best, so my friend was shocked when her neighbor gave her the research and a draft of a novel she had been writing. She wanted someone to finish it.

Even before my worries about sickness, I sometimes found myself drowning in others' news. I am known as a good listener, but I have always had difficulty getting people to reciprocate. When I need to talk and people tell me they do not want to, my tendency is to feel their refusal as a personal rejection and to place less faith in those relationships. This damaging reaction stems from a youth filled with questions about my own worth and aggressive self-protection. I have lived my life accommodating others and trying to prevent my presence from becoming burdensome. Often, my own needs disappear. I never learned to tell people that I have been hurt by a conversation, even after it is long over. As my friend told her neighbor's story I pictured myself giving my things to virtual strangers during my last days. Although I had not had the biopsy at the time I heard the tale, I understood the impulse to give everything important to someone. I started thinking about leaving a legacy. In just a few days I had begun giving up on the hopes I had for myself. I responded to my friend with, "So did I tell you that I have to have cancer screening soon?"

She offered to accompany me to the test. A number of friends offered themselves—and in one case her husband—for transportation and support. At least one person resisted a conversation about it at all, but still offered to drive. When the day came, I thought about articles I had read which suggested that people accompanied by others got better medical care because their companions ensure the right questions are asked. I considered the possibility that having someone there might calm me. But I also thought that having someone go with me would make this test feel like more of an emergency. Neither choice was a good one. My vacillations during this process forced me to do more and more to manage my distress.

I changed. Before July, I had been given to a kind of panic that was mostly quiet and internalized. It was also undirected. This new panic had force and constantly threatened to become more public. I tried to manage it by putting my life in order. I decided which of my friends would get my journals, which my CDs. I thought my mother should have my photographs, even though she would not recognize many of the people in them. I realized that I have a lot of books and no idea who might want them. With the exception of my laptop and my nine-year-old car, everything that I might bequeath had only sentimental value. For a moment, I worried about not having any good stuff. But that quickly became secondary to what I saw as the process of my dying.

I became efficient. I applied to twice as many academic jobs as I had the year before, all the while thinking that I would not be alive to begin any position. I wrote enough to have two pieces accepted to anthologies. I cleaned my closets and got real pleasure from putting coats I would no longer wear onto two of my friends. I caught up on correspondence. For a while, I attributed this change solely to not having a job. At the time, I could both understand and say that I was frightened. Yet I could not allow myself to feel it fully. Instead, I stayed busy and allowed myself to feel in control by preparing to die and working on other things just in case death did not come when I expected.

For the record, I assumed I would die by the end of summer 2003. A year from the time I first realized that I needed the biopsy somehow seemed like the longest time the ordeal could last. I also assumed that my year-long ignorance of the nodes' existence and the doctors' failure to examine them sooner would prove fatal even though thyroid cancers are typically slow-growing. The possibility of cancer was enough to create all of this terror. This was all before I knew for sure that the biopsy was recommended. The idea of celebrating what I took to be my last birthday seemed absurd. Friends asked me what I planned or wanted. I gave everyone who asked my morbid excuse and tried my best to look upbeat and healthy. The appointment in which the doctor confirmed the need for the biopsy was two months after my July appointment, on September 17. My birthday was the twenty-first. I went to the San Diego Zoo the day before and went to dinner and dancing on the actual day. I had wanted to go to the zoo for years. Suddenly my need to go became urgent. I felt that I was running out of time. I had a hard time eating my birthday dinner.

My appetite waned significantly. I lost ten pounds or so, primarily because I could not eat enough to sustain my body weight. This being LA, people complimented me. At times I felt as though I were getting back at my body for abandoning me—by abandoning it. I would not bother feeding it. My other response, though quite inconsistent with the first, had a healthier effect. I started exercising more intensely. This was not my typical behavior. I created routines, which I usually abhor. As some people get songs stuck in their heads, I began to hear, "I need to take care of this body if I'm going to continue to use it" each time I worked out. Both responses were signs of a mental separation from my body. For a time, I could control neither reaction.

I wanted to be a better person. I felt as though the undisciplined, unaccomplished, unsettled me was not good enough to die. There was something wrong with my soul. I needed to know how to fix this problem. Because I am not a joiner, I did not start going to church. I am an academic, given to looking for answers in texts—my own and other people's. I bought books on souls. I wrote about other people's deaths. I started meditation again. I tried to figure out how karma works. These are things that are good in and of themselves. But what they allowed me to do was feel as though I were benefiting from the possibility of illness, getting better instead of worse.

Looking back, I realize that this question of health precipitated a crisis in my life. My efficiency was a kind of numbness and self-absorption. My life passed before my eyes, albeit slowly. In the grocery store, a bottle of salsa reminded me of a meal I used to make in college before I moved to California and had real Mexican food. Surprisingly, it was a good memory. Before that day, much of what I could remember about college was about my extreme shyness, relationship troubles, and a heightened awareness of my own poverty. Suddenly, small things—tastes, bits of fabric, the way someone said a certain word—brought back pleasant memories. Often the memories were non-narrative. They felt more like déjà vu or flashback, placing me momentarily somewhere else.

This kind of recollection happened more and more often. When I was alone, I welcomed it as a new diversion. The experience fascinated me so much that I would interrupt my activities for a few moments to reflect each time it occurred. Needless to say, I could not feel completely present with my friends. Although I spent more time with them deliberately, much of the experience was buffered by my thoughts and feelings. Each late-night spiral down an empty parking garage with them might be my last. With the possible exception of exasperation, garages were not supposed to evoke sentiment. At times, despite what I was doing, my death was the only thing on my mind. I knew enough not to raise it as a topic of discussion. Still, I was continually distracted from the actions at hand. My own inner world and the predicted failure of my body consumed my attention even as I put my efforts elsewhere. So entranced was I by my own thoughts that nearly each day as I got into bed, I would immediately fall into the dream from the night before. I do not think that anyone noticed how far away I had already slipped.

In one dream, I was alone in my apartment—my actual one rather than some dream creation. I sat down in my bathtub and realized that I would not have the strength to get up again. The water grew cold. I wondered whether I would die naturally, or lose my strength, slip into the water and drown. I awoke frightened and remained so throughout the day. But I kept printing and mailing applications. I thought that the dreams, the distractions, the last will and testament, the intrusive memories, the meditation and the perseverance in my work could help me become a person good enough and strong enough to die. If I figured out who I had been and changed the things about my daily life that I wanted to change, then I could feel comfortable enough to die the way I heard that George Harrison had. I wanted to be able to welcome it.

Such introspection helped me in some ways. I became more communicative about my own fears. I began to see who I was outside of my work and outside of what behavior or level of success people might expect of me. My relationships actually became more important than my job. I became much less likely to do things that I did not want to do. People told me that I appeared calmer. Their descriptions seemed accurate. I truly felt more at ease and happier. However, I did not consider the ambiguities of my responses.

A portion of my calm was due to resignation. I was not depressed; however, my behavior was consistent with depressive symptoms. Although I enjoyed much of what I did, the absence of hope for the future meant that there was no point. So many things seemed futile. I wrote furiously, even while giving up on the idea of leaving the legacy I had always imagined. I still tried to write in my journal daily. But I began censoring a few things, considering that others would soon go through the stacks of small books, each unlined, each different. The thoughts I had, especially about the two friends who would get the journals, began to merit reconsideration. I wondered how I would be seen. My dissertation was on recent autobiographical works by black women. I dissected the details ruthlessly. Suddenly the possibility that the same thing could happen to my autobiographical writing loomed large.

I came to terms with some of my isolation. Before this whole episode started, I had imagined that if I ever had a real emergency, someone in my life would care enough to drop everything for a least a while to care for me. I found myself mid-crisis without such comfort. I realized that I could handle my difficulties without such a relationship but that I did not have to handle them alone. It became clear to me who could be relied upon and who could not. I accepted the loss of friends who remained too distant. It was not easy. Still, I was buoyed by an ability that I did not know I had. My newly discovered strength came along with a need to abandon, or at least ignore, most things that concerned my future. I scrapped any hopes of a satisfying relationship, thwarting anything that seemed to have potential. It did not seem fair to saddle anyone, especially someone I did not yet know, with my dying body.

I had the biopsy on October 8. That week was my doctor's first turn in the operating room after she had determined three weeks earlier that I needed the procedure. I barely slept the night before and spent the morning waiting for it to be time to go. I wanted my mother. But she was in Ohio, blissfully unaware. I had not told her about these tests because each time I leave town after a visit, she cries. She did not sleep when I was hospitalized in LA, and her fear of flying kept her from me. This worry might kill her. And her way of constantly voicing her concern might kill me. So it was for both of our sakes that I kept this from her. In order to maintain the silence, I left the rest of my family out of the loop. Still, I wondered about my mother. She is damn-near psychic and can detect my upsets. Often, without clues, she is accurate about the source. She knows without being told when I have traveled away from my home, which is thousands of miles from her. The messages she has left me frighten my friends. Last fall, she often sensed a problem. Each time I denied that anything was wrong, I felt like a despicable liar. In my worry about what she might sense, I avoided the conversation that might have comforted me. I left without that, instead busying my mind with a to-do list.

I drove myself to the hospital because I thought I would feel less anxious that way. It was not a good idea. I had watched the weather report. It was not biopsy weather. I wore short sleeves comfortably and had a pleasant walk four or five blocks away from the hospital, where I had been able to park free. I was forty minutes early for my appointment, yet the receptionist sent me up almost immediately. The other patient was a white woman, middle-aged, blonde. We smiled at each other. Both of us, experienced patients or patient waiters, had things to read. The intake person sent me upstairs first.

The waiting room was empty. One wall was missing; plastic sheeting hung in its place. I assured myself that exposed asbestos would not be in a hospital. I busied myself with the newspaper for a while. The blonde woman came up and sat on a wall perpendicular to mine with a magazine. A black couple, a bit later in middle age than the blonde, came in with a woman whom I took to be the woman's mother. They were taking such good care of her—getting her into her seat, providing her with things to drink, just making sure she was comfortable—that I started to tear up. I wanted to be their child or wanted my family to be there to talk with these people. My family members meet other black people everywhere they go. They find places and people in common. I almost started a conversation with the couple, but I was actually too frightened—not of them, but of what was happening. When they realized that I was not waiting for someone else to return from a procedure, they smiled. I imagined that, like the medical staff and a number of people I encountered, they felt especially sorry for me. I look younger than my thirty-four years. Students are surprised when I walk to the front of the classroom. Cashiers still ask me for ID when I buy wine. In the latter cases, looking young is flattering at best, a challenge at worst. In the hospital, it makes one an object of pity.

They took the older woman in first. Then another woman entered the waiting area. They took her. Then they took the middle-aged woman. The couple left to get snacks. I was alone again. Like many people that fall, I was reading Alice Sebold's *The Lovely Bones*, a story told from the point of view of a murdered adolescent girl. I had just gotten to the part where she begins to see her family from heaven. I tried to imagine what my heaven would be if Sebold wrote it. The couple returned. Their mother returned. After retrieving her cane from the examination space, they left, saying a polite concerned good-bye to me that nearly broke my heart. At last the staff called me. The blonde woman lay in the hall on a gurney. She was in a gown. I smiled briefly but did not want to look too long, both so that she could have privacy and so that I did not become more frightened.

Three people—my doctor, a nurse or physician's assistant and an ultrasound technician who acted as a guide—were in the room with me. I did not need to undress. They never closed the door, though there may have been a curtain. I had never been stuck with a needle in my neck before that first dose of local anesthesia. It hurts; but more than that it just feels wrong. When they began the procedure, I had not gotten enough anesthetic. The result was that the first time I was stuck with the extraction needle, I thought I might faint. Maybe it's a class thing, but I find the idea of fainting entirely unacceptable. I asked to be numbed further, as numbness is perfectly appropriate. They accommodated my wishes and started again.

My doctor stuck the needle into my neck deeply four or five times, each time guided by the voice of the technician who looked at the ultrasound monitor rather than at me. With each deep insertion, she moved the needle back and forth, in an effort to puncture this thing growing inside me. Although I knew the tumor did not belong, the needle felt even more invasive. The numbing treatment did not stop me from feeling the movement that should not have been happening inside my body.

As I was preparing to go home, the doctor told me that she had additional bad news. My blood tests indicated that a separate problem we had been treating was getting worse rather than better. I worried more, then waited for her to tell me what to expect. Her cell phone rang. She talked for ten minutes or so, with someone I took to be an old friend. This interruption left me ambivalent. On the one hand, I was relieved to see my doctor as a person. On the other, I was shaken by her treatment of what was so traumatic to me as utterly routine.

Once again, the assistant told me that they would call with results. However I was advised that for this test, I should call if I did not hear within two weeks. Somehow I had not known how long it would take to get a sample analyzed or that no one looked at any part of it at the hospital immediately after the procedure. I walked away feeling deflated.

After two weeks of hellish anxiety, I was told that my test was inconclusive. The samples turned out to be mostly my own blood rather than cells from the growing mass in my neck. Apparently faulty samples are common. The only solution was to wait for the area to heal and repeat the test. I did not know until months later that too frequent intrusion causes permanent tissue damage, so I assumed the lengthy delay in scheduling the follow-up was due to crowded schedules and bureaucracy.

I thought that I could stretch my insurance for another month or two in order to repeat the test, but ultimately could not afford to continue coverage. No good jobs had materialized. By then, I was desperate enough to tell my doctor about my financial situation. I was never able to talk to her via telephone, however, so I made an appointment in January, after my insurance had lapsed. I finally had a "conversation only" appointment with my doctor, and paid a sorely-missed $64 after she had applied all of the discounts her practice group would allow. We spent the visit discussing possible avenues of treatment for the uninsured. She gave me advice on which labs to avoid because of their reputations for shoddy work and told stories of her daughter's medical tribulation while she lacked coverage. She wanted me to return for a follow-up. I do not think she fully understood how little savings non-tenure-track faculty have.

I tried the Los Angeles Free Clinic, first walking into an office that I had passed on my way to the optometrist. The waiting room was full of people who looked somber, if not sick. A friendly older gentleman asked me what I needed. I told him that I was trying to get a biopsy. He was hard of hearing. I imagined that if I spoke any louder, I would disturb the people waiting. I think that my reticence frustrated him. He directed me to the security guard. I asked him whom I could talk to about a biopsy. "What is that?" he asked. He was trying to be helpful, but he made me say "cancer" again. He directed me to another guy, who told me that I could indeed get a biopsy, but that I needed to call for an appointment. Although I was confused about why it was impossible to schedule an appointment while I was standing there, I took the sheet of paper he handed me and left. I tried to call as soon as I got outside. The line was busy several times. I needed to go to campus, so I tried again there. The next time I called was around 11 in the morning. I got someone. Only then did I understand that each day people call at 9 and vie for the few available appointments. It was Thursday. They told me that my best bet was to try the following week. Tuesday would be my first opportunity, as they were closed on Monday for Martin Luther King, Jr. Day.

The next Tuesday, I began calling at 8:50. Pushing the on button, the redial button, then the off button requires just enough concentration so that doing other things becomes nearly impossible. I called until 11:05. The woman who heard my concerns actually admonished me for not calling earlier. When I told her about the process, she seemed surprised, then sympathetic. After being on hold for another twenty minutes, I had an appointment with a general practitioner for the following week. There is no shortcut to a biopsy. I had to start the entire process again.

The clinic seemed to serve mostly women with a good number of children. Most patients were non-white, though there were few other black people there. The shared waiting room was large and open with a play area and secondary appointment desk in the center and chairs along the outside. The doctors' offices were around the perimeter. It was designed so that everyone sat close together. When doctors and nurses emerged from the examination rooms, they and the patients addressed each other personally. I was amazed that they knew one another. The distance that had been so evident in other medical facilities was absent here. I felt better.

The doctor was a pleasant black woman about my age. I imagined that in circumstances where I was not so worried, we would have a number of things in common. Instead, I felt a slight panic. I had given the intake people a copy of my medical records from the specialist. They could all see for themselves the blood test and initial biopsy results. Still, I was met with more general questions: "Do you need advice on family planning?" "Do you have any alcohol or drug problems we should talk about?" I never heard such questions when I had insurance, and since I have been without it, it feels as though I am expected to be dysfunctional. Each appointment, even if it is with a specialist, begins with these inquiries. At times, my assurances that I am not addicted or in an abusive relationship have been met with suspicion. I spend my short appointment time trying to get the caregiver to focus on my reasons for being there. I know these questions are necessary; however, they feel inappropriate considering my concerns. "No, I just want to take care of the cancer problem if I can," I replied. That got her attention. Still, I felt as though before that moment she had not paid attention to why I was there. She felt my neck but could not detect anything.

AN UPDATE

The next Free Clinic doctor had the worst bedside manner of any physician I had ever seen. In fact, I was hard-pressed to believe that he had ever held a conversation with another person. He did not examine me at all. Instead, he looked at my records, repeated the irrelevant questions about drug use and physical abuse, and said there was little he could do for me. He told me that he would put me in the queue for those tests, but said that it might take a long time. Then he told me that the wait might be so long that I could die, even with a slow-growing cancer.

I tried another route, visiting a county neighborhood clinic. I told the receptionist what the doctor at the Free Clinic had said. She told me that her clinic would not see me because even with the other doctor's warnings about my possible death, my condition was not an emergency. When I highlighted the statement about death for her again, she told me to pray. I cried on the curb for twenty minutes and considered going at my throat with a nail file. Instead, I went to the county ER. After waiting ten hours, developing a migraine, and fighting back the urges to cry and vomit, I finally had my vital signs taken by a doctor who had to fight to get me an appointment with an endocrinologist at the same clinic that had rejected me. That took three months. The administration at the hospital and the clinic kept admonishing me to keep the appointments, as though I had shown myself to be irresponsible.

The rest is too long to recount completely. My work provided no insurance. Each time I kept a clinic appointment, I spent more than four hours in the office. If I had an emergency walk-in, it took nine or ten hours to finish everything. It usually took more than an hour to get a follow-up appointment after I saw the doctor. They did not allow me to take care of this administrative business over the telephone. I saw one doctor twice. The rest were rotating interns. The clinic endocrinologists said they would refer me to the ENT clinic for the pain. This never happened. The standard of care for those without insurance seems to be to wait until things get much worse before any treatment is offered. This is not something I am imagining. At least two of the doctors I saw at the clinic said this to me. Neither how I felt, nor the six months of fever mattered. Despite my previous doctor's insistence that malignancy should be ruled out, the clinic doctors declared the biopsy unnecessary.

Someone I met in a tea shop in late 2003 recommended a women's clinic, which I tried. It was my third post-insurance effort to start this entire process again. After a month of visits there, they set up an appointment for me at Harbor UCLA Hospital. Erroneously, I assumed they had reviewed my records, which were available to them electronically, and decided to maintain my original course of treatment. They set an appointment for me—in October 2004. I found my way to the hospital, registered and went to the basement, only to find that although all appointments that day were cancelled, no one had bothered to tell me. The one administrative person I found apologized, and told me of my new appointment date—five weeks later.

During the second appointment there, they allowed me to explain my case and even brought in a senior physician. I was determined that I would not feel as weak as I had before. It hadn't occurred to me that all it would take to get them to listen a bit more attentively was to get them to call me "Dr. Curtis." The wheels moved a bit faster then. In late February 2005, nearly three years after I was told I needed a biopsy and nearly four years after the nodes were found, someone finally examined my neck with more than a squeeze. They gave me pills and told me to be careful not to touch them. When they scanned me the next day, the technician was a bit giddy. The mass on my left side was gone. The one on the right, perhaps a quarter of the size it had been. "Are you sure these were there?" she asked. "You saw them yourself?"

Believe it or not, that shock has been hard to handle too.

QUESTIONS

1. What are the major differences between health care for those who have insurance and those who do not?
2. How do the author's economic, educational, and racial status function in this essay—individually and collectively as a unit?
3. Comment on the ways in which various health-care workers communicate with the author.
4. Which actions by the author express most power?

More Than a Case

⤜ Ting Man Tsao ⤛

Your mom's heart was broken when your twin sister died.* She was only a baby. I forgot how many months old, but she was somewhere between a crawler and a toddler. Baby Ann, Baby Ann. That was her name printed on her wristband in the hospital. Your older sister had to hide all the photos of you with your twin. They did not want your mom to see any of those pictures. But what's the point? Your mom saw you every moment, and every part of you was a living reminder of Baby Ann. Ann, Ann, she called you by mistake, like in a dream.

Your mom wanted to seek justice and sue the hospital. I found a law firm reputable for medical malpractices. I accompanied her to the appointment. We were invited to a very spacious office with a spotless panoramic window overlooking the boisterous Fifth Avenue. That was the most comfortable office I had ever visited with your mom: no crying babies or groaning patients around you, like in hospital or clinic waiting rooms, nobody who mocks your strange last name when the caseworker calls you at the top of her voice in the welfare office, and no long line to test your patience. The attorney arrived on time.

He looked very smart in a wrinkle-free suit and starched collar. He browsed through the piles of medical records your mom had spent days requesting from the hospital. He didn't seem to have any trouble deciphering the doctors' and nurses' scribbles and that medical jargon I had looked up in several thick dictionaries to translate to your mom. It took him no more than ten minutes to decide not to take the case. Not because the hospital had made no errors—he emphasized that he had already found some suspicious evidence of negligence just by glancing through the pages—but because he would not get compensated enough for the hours he and his partners would need to spend on the case. It is a baby who died. He explained that a baby is worthless in legal litigation, though he said he understood your mom's pain and suffering for losing your sister. He explained that by law, his legal fees would be based solely on damages to be paid by the hospital. Clients cannot pay attorneys out of pocket even if they are rich. A baby has not worked and does not have a college degree or a professional license. The court has no basis to calculate the loss, even though the baby meant a great deal to your mom. There is unfortunately no legal gauge of emotional loss. The attorney suggested your mom try smaller law firms. They might accept cases of this sort. But your mother gave up. Your grandparents did not want to pursue. They said it would bring more trouble than closure. "It's better to have one less trouble than one more." This was the Chinese maxim your grandparents used.

As a social worker who specialized in families with developmentally disabled children at a community-based organization, I developed rapport with your mom, as I did with most of my clients through comprehensive case management. To empower multiproblem families to help themselves, I developed a "work agreement" with them that identified problems and specified goals that we would work together to attain. I coordinated the otherwise unconnected services that clients were receiving from different providers. On a regular basis, I met with families at my office or their home to provide support and monitor their progress. I also often found myself in the "field" with clients. I advocated and translated for them in clinics, hospitals, welfare offices, schools, and other places. I did the same things for your mom; she was always a cooperative, never a resistant, client. Her case was first opened not because of Baby Ann but because of you. You had a cleft palate and other health problems, including a clubfoot. I had to work with your mom to coordinate your services, communicate with medical providers and an early intervention program, apply for entitlements, and provide supportive counseling. Your mom attended the monthly socialization club, which I organized for parents who had developmentally challenged children. Your mother was on public assistance. As much as she wanted to, she could not work because she had to take care of you and your twin sister. And at that time, before Clinton changed welfare into workfare, she was not forced to work and put her children in day care.

I cannot remember exactly how your sister died. Your mom told me everything, all the details. I listened carefully, asked questions, and took notes on everything she said. The notes were so copious that I had to bring them home and type them using my Smith Corona word processor. Having majored in English, I found writing progress notes and case reports to be the easiest, most enjoyable part of social work. It took me no more than an hour to finish a ten-page case report, no more than ten minutes to finish a face-to-face contact note. I usually handwrote those notes and reports at my office. I almost always got them right the first time without drafting, without editing or revising. Yet I treated the notes about your sister's illness differently. I remember staying up all night at home to rewrite and rewrite the notes on the word processor. I proofread them carefully and double-checked every sentence before I printed out a copy for your mom's file. Upon your request, I have found the dusty data disk containing those notes that I put away with other social work materials in my basement. The original paper copy of the notes, indeed your mom's whole file, was probably destroyed by the family service agency according to its protocol. Fortunately, I've kept the data disk. The Smith Corona, which I hadn't used for years, still works, enabling me to print out a new copy of the notes. The following are the facts of your sister's case as your mother recounted them—very specific, very detailed.

Your mom said she rushed your twin sister to the emergency room on March 15 because of a rash on the front and back of your sister's body and on her face. She also had a cough and a runny nose. A nurse suspected your sister had measles, but the doctor suspected an allergy to the medication, amoxicillin, she had been taking for an ear infection. Two hours later, she was given an injection. Afterwards, she was okay for a month or so, having only a few minor colds.

April 15. Your mom said she was shocked to see your sister. The baby had saliva on her lips; her eyeballs had rolled up, and her eyelids were fluttering; she was clenching her teeth and shaking softly. Two minutes later, your sister stopped shaking. Very tired, she didn't even cry. Your mom rushed her to the ER, where a doctor took an X-ray of her chest and drew blood from her hand for a lab test. The test came back normal, but she was running a temperature of 102°F. Your mom was asked to take the baby home, and the doctor prescribed Pedia-Profen for the fever.

Your mom came from Vietnam. She spoke Cantonese, Vietnamese, and some simple English, but she was not able to deal with complicated situations that demanded difficult English. She was one of my best clients. She was very strong and sagacious and she knew what she wanted. She could be blunt, but she always asked the right question. She took good care of you and your twin sister. She told me very little about your father. Is he the same man as your older sister's father? I don't remember well. She never told me much about him. She never told you much about him. The only thing related to him she mentioned was that your older sister had a hard time filing for financial aid for college because the father or fathers had disappeared. Those forms, your mom complained, required the father's Social Security number. And your father had vanished without leaving behind any trace of the Social Security number. My supervisor did not insist I ask much, as long as your mom took good care of the twins, particularly you—as long as you and your sister were not at any risk for foster care. You had many health problems. But your mom did such a good job. She was tough and organized and knew what she was doing. She did not seem like a romantic woman. She was practical. The public assistance office, however, was nosier. They asked again, again, and again if your mom knew your father's whereabouts. They wanted to get child support from him.

April 16. Because of another series of seizures and a temperature of 101, your mother rushed your sister to the ER. According to your mom (but I was not sure), a doctor drew bone marrow for a test. The test result was not known then, but your sister was admitted to the hospital with an IV. She did not want to eat, and she stayed in the hospital for a few days. EEG was done; CAT scan was also done.

May 1. Both you and your sister were admitted to the hospital through the ER. You had pneumonia. She had a relapse of seizures. The doctor once again had to draw bone marrow. Not allowed to see the process, your mom had to wait outside. She said she saw two or three nurses rushing into the room. Your mom peeped in and saw the doctor pushing the baby into another room with more equipment. Her body turned bluish-purple, and she looked paralyzed. Your mom said two doctors started to use an instrument to pump oxygen into the baby and applied IV. A doctor told her phenobarbital was used to treat your sister's seizures.

May 2. Some sleep medication was used, but your sister's face turned red. Your mom said she alerted a nurse, who in turn called a doctor. The doctor told the nurse if the baby's face turned red again, an EEG should be done. The nurse reported that the same medication had been used before but the baby had been OK then. The doctor asked another doctor to take your sister for a CAT scan. Two days later, your baby sister's face turned red again after another dose of phenobarbital. Her temperature fluctuated between 99°F and 101°F.

Your mom did not look superstitious to me. But before your twin sister fell sick, she once said in passing that everything is determined. She said your cleft palate originated from what your father had done. When she was pregnant with both of you, he hammered some screw nails into the bedroom wall to hang an old photo. Your mom said the holes in the wall were somehow related to the crevice in your mouth. Everything had been determined before you were born. A few months after your father hung the photo, he simply disappeared and never returned. No letter, no phone call. And he was clever, your mom said. No Social Security number. Nothing was left behind but the photo, you with your cleft palate and clubfoot, and your twin sister. Your mom told me in a matter-of-fact tone. She did not sound bitter or angry. That was her life. I thought she accepted it.

My supervisor said I was not good at exploring clients' feelings. She said I was as Chinese as my clients, too reserved to talk about feelings with them. Well! Perhaps so. But I majored in literature at college and in graduate school. Literature is all about human emotions, isn't it? What else could I have done as a social worker? Ask her about your father? Ask her how she felt about him? Ask her how she felt about the cleft palate that you had? Ask her about guilt? She was not a character; I could hardly analyze her as such. She didn't want to talk about any of this, so I didn't want to pursue it. Like all of my immigrant clients, she just wanted me to help her with tasks she couldn't do on her own. And I did my job accordingly. I did it well. I made sure you were connected with service providers and your services were on the right track. I don't recall why your mom didn't call me about the severity of your sister's condition until she was about to be transferred to another medical center. But once I learned about the situation, I visited them in the second hospital to see how they were doing. I helped your mom get all the benefits she was entitled to. When you had your third surgery very early in the morning, I gave your mom my home phone number so that she could give me updates. My supervisor reprimanded me for disclosing my home phone number to your mom. She said clients should never have access to the social worker's home phone number. But that was an important matter and I knew your mom wouldn't call me unless it was absolutely necessary. I believed your mom.

May 8. Although Baby Ann had had no appetite, she was discharged. She was prescribed amoxicillin and phenobarbital.

May 12. Rash returned, now in bigger and bigger patches. Your mom was alarmed. The thermometer read 103°F. It was morning, and your mom rushed the baby to the ER. The doctor said no more amoxicillin should be given, but Tylenol instead, every four hours. Back home, in the afternoon, your sister's temperature was 105°F. Your mom called the ER and the doctor said the baby was not allergic to amoxicillin. He said the baby should be put in warm water. He said the rash should not be a cause for alarm. Your mom did what she was told. The doctor accused your mom of not giving Tylenol on time, but she insisted she did. Your mom was very precise with all the details. She told me that ten minutes before the right time to give Tylenol, she gave two drops according to instructions. Yet more rash was developing and the temperature stayed at 104°F toward the evening. At 8 p.m., your mom decided to take your sister to the ER, where the doctor prescribed Pedia-Profen and Tylenol. Before leaving the ER, the baby was given another medicine your mom pronounced as "patrin." The doctor wanted the baby to come back the following day. The temperature was around 104° F and 105° F.

May 13. Back to the ER. A doctor asked your mom why the rash had been developing that fast. The temperature was 104.3° F, so the doctor decided to hospitalize your sister. IV had to be applied, but veins were hard to find because of the rash all over her body. Her hair was shaved in order to make it easier for the physician to locate veins in her head, but to no avail. The doctors said they were going to call a surgeon to find the veins, but no surgeon ever showed up. An X-ray was taken.

Parents sometimes know better than doctors. I once worked with a couple whose newborn son had Down syndrome as well as colorectal malfunction. Before their son was born, the parents had learned from the amniocentesis that he would suffer from Down syndrome for the rest of his life. They had decided against aborting the fetus, as they had heard from their friends that their child might come back to haunt them. The couple accepted their fate; they had conceived this son purely by accident, by contraceptive failure. The mother was already over forty years of age, and the couple had two teenage children. However, when the hospital told them that their newborn needed a temporary colostomy, they no longer accepted it as their fate. They refused adamantly. The surgeon angrily called me, warning that if colostomy were delayed, the baby would die of bowel failure. And he did not hang up without expressing his impatience with me for "not understanding English." The father didn't budge though, saying that the colostomy pouch would make the baby look "abnormal." He feared that the child would be carrying the pouch forever. The tug of war between the hospital and the parents dragged on for a few days, until the hospital decided to transfer the baby to another medical center for an innovative surgery that could fix the colorectal disorder without colostomy. Yes, without colostomy, without any visible pouch that the father and mother abhorred. So which party was right? Was the hospital right? Or were the parents right?

As it turned out, the parents' instincts were better than the surgeon's original treatment plan in serving the tiny newborn. In the other medical center, the little patient received a surgery that treated his colorectal malfunction once and for all without any temporary colostomy. Both medically and ethically, the entire medical team of the first hospital owed the parents and the child an explanation about why colostomy had initially been represented as the one and only way to save the baby's life when a better alternative was available in the city.

In fact, these parents were not the only parents I helped who rejected procedures prescribed by the hospital. I had another mother who also said no to colostomy for her chronically ill baby, but he also turned out to be all right without it—even though the hospital had insisted it was the only way to save the baby's life. Doctors are always right at the moment they say something. They are right about the diagnosis at the time it is explained to patients. They want consent rather than challenge when offering treatment plans. Well! Perhaps parents know better by instinct. As for your mom, it seems she knew that Baby

Ann had more serious problems than what the doctors could find, than what they told her. Only time would tell.

May 15. Like yesterday, your sister was given phenobarbital and Benadryl. One doctor said, however, that phenobarbital should be stopped, suspecting the medicine was her allergen. Then she was transferred to the intensive care unit.

May 16. Your sister was returned to a regular room. After phenobarbital was stopped, her temperature dropped. No IV was applied from May 13 to May 16 because no surgeon showed up to find the veins. Your mom said many visiting doctors came and told the physicians in charge to apply IV. The physicians in charge explained that they had done their best, but they had failed to find the veins.

May 17. Still no IV. But something was given to the baby for a virus infection. Your mom said her rash started to disappear. She could eat and smile for the first time in many days and, unfortunately, also for the last time of her life. Her temperature was 102° F.

May 20. A doctor determined that the baby had an ear infection and an infection in the mouth. He asked if she was allergic to amoxicillin, and your mom said she was not sure and asked him to wait for your older sister for more details. Later in the day, a nurse wanted to inject ampicillin. Your mom asked the nurse to wait. Your mom said she had to explain the possibility of allergy to the doctor. The nurse took your mom to a second doctor, but he didn't want to see her. She then insisted on seeing the first doctor, but the second doctor said it was the first doctor who had prescribed ampicillin for your sister. He said that the same medication had been given to her during the last hospital stay and everything had been OK. The nurse injected ampicillin into your twin sister. She asked your mom to alert her if the rash reappeared.

May 21. Your mom saw the rash. Your sister's temperature started to mount. Your mom noticed. More and more rash. More and more rash.

May 22. Baby Ann was shaking and had a high fever. Her smile was gone. Her appetite was gone. For good.

May 23. At 4 a.m. her temperature mounted to 105.3° F. Your mom alerted the nurse and some medication was given, but by 6 a.m. it was still 104.8° F. Your mom tried to rock your sister to sleep, but at 11:30 a.m. she turned purplish black. Your mom rang for the nurse. No one came. She took the baby to the doctor's room herself, but the doctor there said it was nothing more than a reaction to the medication. He said there would soon be a test for the baby. Why not test the baby now? This is an emergency, your mom yelled. The doctor asked her to take your sister back to her room. That was all he did. Your mom cried, but she was not hysterical. She just cried.

The nurse talked to the same doctor, who repeated what he had told your mom. The nurse said your sister had been worse when she was first hospitalized. Your mom disagreed. The doctor told her he would call a dermatologist. Your mom sobbed helplessly. Another doctor told her to calm down and went away on another errand.

Your mom asked a nurse to apply medication for the rash. But the nurse said the dermatologist would not be able to see the rash if medication were applied. Your mom was even more alarmed when your sister's temperature rose to 106° F. The electronic thermometer beeped. Your mom was shocked and furious. She started to yell. A doctor ran in and tried to pacify her, but she was so frustrated that she passed out. The doctor had to grab the baby. Another doctor rushed in and transferred Baby Ann to the ICU.

When your mom came around, she called your sister's pediatrician, who was also your regular doctor. She worked for another medical center in Manhattan, where you received treatment for your cleft palate. Your pediatrician requested to speak to the doctors at your sister's hospital. The nurse was upset, arguing it was not appropriate for an outside doctor to ask their doctors to call back. Your pediatrician did not receive any return call from the hospital. That night, your twin sister was in the ICU with two nurses taking care of her. They had to record every bit of data. One of them advised your mom to go home to rest, but she declined. She had lots of strength. Imagine spending days and nights in the hospital, watching someone you love struggling for her life. I respected your mom and still do. She was really special. She was a great mother.

May 24. Two specialists came and examined Baby Ann's ears. They couldn't find anything but lots of earwax. One of them plucked the ears and examined again. He concluded the ears were OK with no infection at all. The other doctor examined and arrived at the same conclusion. Yet the baby developed a swollen tummy and had no urination. She was still running a temperature of 105.3° F. Your mom got anxious and asked a nurse why your sister's tummy was swollen. An older doctor came and touched the belly. A nurse later said there would be an X-ray of the abdomen. That night no X-ray was taken. From May 24 to 25, no IV was applied because the doctor said your sister had too much fluid.

May 25. Equally bad condition. The baby did not eat at all, and her tummy was swollen. A doctor asked your mom to hold the baby more, saying that every baby has a different condition. That night your mom talked to a doctor who told her to give your sister an ounce of water when she was thirsty. Not too much because of the swollen belly.

May 26. Swollen belly. A tube was inserted through your sister's nose to draw fluid, yellow in color, out of the abdomen. Her mouth was bleeding. Blood red. Your mom said, "Bloody mouth."

May 27. IV was applied again. Baby Ann's body was red, and she was shivering. Your mom called the doctor. No one came. A nurse said the doctor was busy. Your mom was irate, saying your sister was in the ICU. The nurse said the doctor was busy writing reports. Your mom took the baby with IV and everything attached to the doctor's office. The baby is in a serious condition, cried your mom. Who told you to come? the doctor yelled back. He ordered your mom to take the baby away. Ten minutes later, the doctor came and said there was nothing special about the baby. This is no emergency, he explained. Your mom told me the nurses nearby were shaking their heads, though they didn't say anything audible. The doctor applied IV and commented that one out of a hundred babies was that serious, that sick. Your mom shuddered at the comment.

Your mom called your pediatrician for help again. That night, your pediatrician arrived at the hospital and talked with the doctors there. She told your mom that there was a report indicating the baby had an unusually high number of white blood cells. No one in the hospital had ever informed her of that. After calling her superior, your pediatrician said your sister would be transferred to her medical center immediately. Before Baby Ann left, the doctors took an X-ray of the abdomen and drew blood. Some nurses told your mom in private that if, God forbid, something should happen to your sister, sue the hospital. They kissed your mom good luck and made her promise to let them know your sister's progress.

I remember visiting your sister after she was transferred. I saw your mom pick her up from the hospital crib. Hospital cribs are like cages. The barred sides are silvery, cold, and high. Taking your sister out of the cage, your mom held her with IV and lots of wires attached. I didn't know how she did that—holding your sister, trying to soothe her with so many tubes and wires connected. Your mom didn't look tired; she looked more spirited than I. Whenever she noticed anything unusual, she called your pediatrician. I had quite a number of clients whose children were seen by your doctor. She is very gentle, very patient with those who don't speak English, who don't know how to navigate the health-care system. She speaks basic Cantonese with an accent. But it was her understanding and patience, not her bilingualism, that set her apart from other doctors, including those who speak Chinese dialects in the huge health-care system of New York City. Sometimes she was too busy to come right away, but your mom didn't complain. Your mom understood.

June 4. The day hundreds of students and other protesters were massacred at Tiananmen Square, your twin sister died. I was at another hospital working with a client when I got the news from my supervisor over the phone.

Your mom was very emotional when she told me all these details, a few days after your sister died. You stayed at home. A relative was babysitting you. Accompanied by another relative, your mom came to my agency. I invited her to the conference room, a large room with good ventilation. I didn't use my own stuffy office, which I shared with a coworker. She shed tears, but not a whole lot. She was as brave as a mother can be. Your twin sister was the first client of mine who died. I needed support myself.

Since I was not good at discussing feelings with clients, my supervisor suggested referring your mom to a clinical social worker for grief counseling because she seemed more open-minded than most Chinese clients and would be more receptive to psychotherapy. About a month after your sister's death, I made the referral and accompanied your mom to that agency in Chinatown. The following day, I got a call from the clinical social worker. She said it was time to draw limits between the client, herself as the chief therapist, and me. She told me not to interfere with her therapy of your mom. I should not have come with the client. From then on, the therapy should be between the client and her, the therapist. Although I was the caseworker, I should stay out so that the treatment could proceed in the way it should.

I was shocked to hear that. To be sure, I was not "clinical" enough to deal with "feelings." I did not and do not possess any MSW or CSW qualification. I was an English major after all, having a passion for interdisciplinary and cultural studies, never tired of writing and reading and doing research in libraries and archives. And it was purely by chance that I became a social worker. Yet my instinct told me something was not right about all this clinical professionalism in the dissection of feelings, alienating the client like a specimen from a caseworker, a person who had been with her during the most trying period of her life. Something was wrong, but I could not put it in words—in a professional language that refuses to take into account a partnership based not on clinical psychological exploration, but on tangible, almost mundane work, day in and day out in clinics, in hospitals, in early intervention programs, in welfare offices, in the home, in livery cabs.

I talked to my supervisor and had to follow the clinical social worker's instruction. However, after a few sessions, your mom came to my office and said she had decided not to see the clinical social worker anymore. She said she cried even more, feeling even worse each time after the therapeutic "exploration" of her feelings, after being forced violently to face what she wanted to forget, to leave behind. I said it was up to her. I followed up with your case, coordinating your services. I found the law firm for your mom, but they didn't take the case and your mom didn't want to pursue it any further.

The medical center held a conference with your mom about your sister's autopsy report. I went with her and helped with translation. Your older sister went too, but her Chinese was not good enough for complicated translation. The report found that your sister had died of a rare viral infection. According to medical databases and existing records, there had only been three fatal cases of this virus in the world. To address your mom's concerns about the other hospital's negligence and malpractice, the doctors emphasized that its treatment of your sister was not responsible for her death; the culprit was the infection. My records do not have the name of that virus, but I remember your pediatrician said, in Chinese, it was like rose rash but much more deadly for certain patients. Your sister happened to be one of the few vulnerable babies in the world. I don't remember asking your mom how she felt about the autopsy report. She probably couldn't accept it. Did she believe it? It's hard to say because of her bad experience with the first hospital.

After she decided against taking any further legal actions, I stopped discussing your sister's matter with her because she didn't want to talk about it anymore. We had a lot to do about you. We had to focus on your treatment. You underwent a few more major surgeries after your sister's death. However traumatized she might have been, your mom persevered, continuing to provide you with excellent care. I remember I visited you after your fourth surgery. As she had done after your previous surgeries, your mom held you for hours non-stop to make sure you didn't bite your wound. This time your mom's eyes were sunken, but her strength remained. Your pediatrician, your surgeon, and the whole cleft palate team were impressed. I too was impressed. Your mom sang you a lullaby. It may have been meant for your twin sister. I wasn't sure. I didn't ask and quietly left the medical center. I visited your mom at home after you were discharged. She was the one who told me casually that your older sister had hidden all the photos of you and your twin sister.

Several months after your twin sister died, I closed the case. As a matter of fact, I also closed all other cases of mine that were deemed stable. I had resigned in order to pursue a Ph.D. in English. Your mom's case, as it stood, had nothing to worry me except for her grief—its deepness and her reticence. Your cleft palate had been treated, and I had made sure your follow-up services were sufficient. Since your mom didn't want any psychother-apy, my substitute had nothing else to work on with her. The case was therefore terminated. I never saw your mom again.

Seeing you all grown up and well is the best reward for my rather short social work ca-reer. Your mom's case and my other clients' cases, twenty in all, are more than "cases." They are life experiences that have humbled me and opened my eyes to the world beyond the confines of the academy. I'll never forget how your mom took care of you and your twin sister. She was resilient. And I believe you are as strong as she. On second thought, you do look like your twin sister—not very pretty, with a flat, oblong face like your mom's.

NOTE

* This story is based on a social work case. Details, names, and dates have been altered or withheld to protect client confidentiality. I dedicate the story to families, parents, and chil-dren I worked with, to my mentor Pui Wong, and my colleague Wo Yin Chan.

QUESTIONS

1. Why does the author address the story to Baby Ann's twin sister?
2. In what ways, if any, does the author's cultural, professional and educational background influence his understanding and interpretation of the circumstances and people sur-rounding Baby Ann's illness?
3. How do the daily progress notes that constitute the main plot of the story shape your understanding of Baby Ann's illness and her mother's mentality? How does the use of progress notes as a form of documentation in the human services and medical fields shape service providers' understanding of and interactions with their clients/patients?
4. Why did the mother decide to discontinue her psychotherapy following her baby's death? If you were the clinical social worker, how would you deal with the mother's resistance to your grief counseling, and how would you review your clinical practice?
5. What were the obstacles to effective communication between physicians in the first hos-pital and the mother? How might they have been handled differently?

Medical Magic and Medicinal Cure
Manipulating Meanings of Disease

⌒ LAURENCE MARSHALL CARUCCI ⌒

Upon my return from a recent trip to the Marshall Islands I was unfortunate enough to come down with typhoid fever, a disease derived from infection by *Salmonella typhosa*, a bacterial infection commonly transmitted "from feces of asymptomatic carriers or the stool or urine of patients with active disease" (*Merck,* 85). Easily contracted in tropical countries where health conditions are marginal, the condition made sense to medical authorities in Montana who treated the infection with antibiotics and, as required by law, informed health authorities in the Marshall Islands. Unfortunately, the tests that would confirm this condition were bungled by the local hospital staff. Thus, the etiology of the disease was posited on the basis of external symptoms open to a variety of interpretations. These symptoms had to bear the burden of proof for the diagnosis. Moreover, the first sets of antibiotics, both injected into my body and administered orally, did not cure the infection. Others would be administered, and seven weeks would pass before the doctor and I agreed I was "cured."

Neither my doctor nor I knew what hit me. Nonetheless, it was a condition that had to be classified and cured. This process of lending meaning and defining action involved the appropriation and use of metaphors and tropes that classified and manipulated the world at the same moment they framed the action scenarios that altered my body's physical state. The condition, which overcame me in Los Angeles, was displaced to the Marshall Islands, since typhoid's incubation period generally lasts for 8 to 14 days. Initially the victim's "temperature rises in steps over 2 to 3 days and remains elevated (usually to 39.4 to 40 C [103 to 104 F]) for another 10 to14 days [before it] begins to fall gradually at the end of the 3rd week, and reaches normal levels during the 4th week" (*Merck,* 86). In Los Angeles, I was six days from Majuro, Marshall Islands, but more distantly removed from Enewetak (by Western assessment, the most likely point of infection). The ailment was classified as "disease"; not only dis-ease, but something pestilential. In that sense, it was the type of malady that, at least until the appearance of AIDS in the late 1980s, Montanans have come to classify as atypically Western and dangerous. Indeed, one doctor and a few of my knowledgeable associates joked about "typhoid Mary" (in this case, "typhoid Larry")—a hidden carrier who might infect the entire population. ✶

These statements and actions are simultaneously medical and political. My stigmatized status, couched in veiled quips of humorous contour, ensconced concerns about contamination of our civilized lifestyle by an unsuspected invasion of disease from dangerous and dirty natives.[1] Indeed, our Western views of medical science and our interpretations of this condition were posited ᵃˢˢᵘᵐᵉᵈ as the only possible interpretation, thus legitimizing our reasons for notifying the Marshall Islands of *their* "public health problem." Placing responsibility for ✶ the containment of this pestilence on others—on primitive, uncultured beings who might infect civilization from its fringe—reiterates the way in which civilization has defined itself in opposition to the savage throughout the colonial and postcolonial age. This became clear as I communicated with members of my family of adoption in the Marshall Islands to see if any of them shared the symptoms of my malady. No one claimed to have similar complaints. I also learned from them, and from the legal representative for Enewetak, that the proclaimed Western intention to "cure the problem at its source" was not followed up with official attempts to see if others on Enewetak had contracted typhoid. Instead, the public health warning served to pronounce a position of epistemological superiority in medicine and reiterate U.S. interpretations of extant power relationships. The disease was traced not to its source but, rather, to the margins of civilization, where blame for the infection could be placed. Public recognition of the direction of the infection—from them to us—was critical. Its cure within the Marshall Islands was irrelevant. The real threat was the unannounced presence of the disease in the United States, since, as Foucault reminds us, civilization must ✶ extricate disease and abnormality from its definitional nature. The way in which these claims double as statements of power within the medical and political sphere is especially apparent inasmuch as the diagnosis could not be "confirmed" by laboratory analysis.[2] According to Shirley Lindenbaum, "Sorcery, witchcraft, and pollution are concepts individuals with so- ✶ cial power invoke to suggest that ill health and misfortune are caused by persons they wish to keep at a distance" (145).

From the U.S. perspective, typhoid was a form of pollution, and the Marshall Islands was its source. Notifying the Marshall Islands of their typhoid risk was part of an attempt to continue to control a hierarchical political relationship established during World War II and renegotiated in the Compact of Free Association, an agreement that included unilateral assistance in medical matters. The paternalistic views of the United States expressed in Article II of the agreement—"Special needs . . . in health care"—are self-evident: they are simply "recognized" as one part of the Marshall Islands' dependence on, and subservience to, the United States (Compact of Free Association, n.d.; see also Title II, Public Law 99-239 United States Statutes at Large 99th Congress, 1st Session 1985, volume 99, Part II: 99 STAT 1800–1841 Washington, D.C.: U.S. Government Printing Office, 1987). At the same time that the Compact of Free Association gives Marshall Islanders access to certain health services, it gives the United States the power to contain the dangers to its own "purity" by keeping island residents at a distance.

The theory of "natural" causation of illness provides the rationale that justifies the universal application of biomedical categories to all humans, including Marshall Islanders. After all, in the eyes of Americans, these are understood as universal physiological processes, not as cultural processes. But if the theory of natural causation is universal, so must be the application of a biomedical ethics that seeks a cure. In this ethical domain, just as in the definitional one, medicine becomes politics. My doctor felt her primary responsibility to be the curing of her patient. After all, I was paying the bill. In her view, her responsibility to Marshall Islanders was fulfilled by notifying health authorities in Montana of the potential ✱risk to Marshall Islanders. From her perspective, it was wiser to notify officials of a potential risk based on an inconclusive diagnosis than to risk a typhoid epidemic in the Marshalls. Her actions, in other words, support her belief in the universal applicability of biomedical theory. The decision to file a public health report on the basis of a conservative diagnosis represented her commitment to a concomitant sense of medical ethics.

As my health continued to suffer, my continued inquiries with people in contact with Enewetak residents indicated that there had been no medical follow-up on Enewetak. This oversight represents the lack of concern with disempowered victims on behalf of the United States and, if the message ever reached Majuro, on behalf of officials in positions of power in the Marshall Islands. These bureaucratic bungles represent the most obvious✱ way in which medical categories are manipulated as political tools to separate the pure and the polluted.

The inconclusive diagnosis not only reinforces the political nature of this posited health risk, but it also shows how diagnostic discourse helps demonstrate the legitimacy of medical categories that are, themselves, cultural constructs. In lieu of laboratory confirmation, my doctor still treated me for typhoid. To do so, substitutions were made in the diagnostic sequence that leads from "cause" to "condition" to "cure." Without bacterial evidence, the event sequence that brought typhoid to Montana was read into my travel and residence history. If *Salmonella typhosa* was present, I might have contracted it almost anywhere, but Enewetak, the most isolated and "primitive" location, was selected as the most likely site. By the time I received medical assistance, the doctor thought the risks and dangers of my condition were diminishing, yet no direct mention was made of the wider risk to Enewetak people. Health officials elsewhere would (surely) follow through to protect "their" patients. Although my doctor felt that, in time, my body would "fight this off on its own," antibiotics were administered as part of the cure. In spite of all uncertainties, the administration of a curative agent confirmed the unquestioned nature of the diagnostic sequence. It suggested that doctors "battle" disease, "discover causes," and "effect cures." Because the disease was not definitive, and the ameliorative effect of the curative agent was not certain, the ritual sequence itself confirmed the efficacy of this set of cultural constructions.[3]

· Of course, this circuitous introduction only sets us up for the alternative analysis, which, on account of its recency and my absence from the islands, I know in only the briefest way. Nonetheless, it articulates with another view of medicine, and of food, whose outlines are quite familiar to me. This is the Enewetak view as it has been related to me through conversations with students and with the Enewetak legal representative about current affairs on Enewetak.[4] In my understanding of this still-developing account, the etiology of my condition is far less problematic. Its causes and intents are equally clear and play equally important political and historical roles. By this account, my condition might be classified as "dis-ease" in one sense—an aberration from the condition of normalcy—but not at all "disease" in the pestilential sense. Instead, it is a disease born of what J. G. Frazer once called "sympathetic magic," one of the so-called non-natural or personalistic (Foster and Anderson, 54; Frazer) causes of nearly all life-threatening conditions in the Marshall Islands. In this theory of ill- ✳ ness, the line between life and death is seldom crossed as the result of what we would call natural causes. Its crossing involves a shift in social relationships, that is, an alteration in the dynamic interplay of spirit forces controlled by noncorporeal beings and manipulable, to some degree, by humans.[5] Of course, Western images of "fighting disease" evoke a battle couched in terms of the war between life and death, which also, in a historical sense, insinuates the supernatural. Even today, bibles and other religious publications are common in hospital waiting rooms, and Western religious specialists are nearby in case doctors fail in the attempt to effect a cure. Nonetheless, the boundaries between life and death are fixed, and the passage is considered unidirectional in Western society. By contrast, for Marshall ✳ Islanders, the world of the living and that of the dead overlap, and the passage between the two domains is relatively fluid. Indeed, in illness, *naninmej* (near-death), the living set foot within the world of the dead in a complementary way to the frequent wanderings of dead ancestors in the communities of the living.

In one rendering of the Enewetak version of my condition, the illness derives not from my long stay with my adoptive nieces and four babies, who, in the assessment of my female medical practitioner in Montana, must have infected me with typhoid while "washing babies' bottoms and whipping up basins of pancake batter," but from a single incident on Majuro Atoll—a well-planned welcoming party prepared in accord with proper Marshall Islands custom by the resident Enewetak women of Majuro. For this occasion, large baskets of food were distributed to the assembled passengers from Enewetak, including me. Each visitor received typical baskets of breads and rice complemented by especially large portions of chicken, beef steak, and fish. Each passenger also received the necessary drink—in this case, cola—along with a pudding-like special dessert. The feast was thus complete with required foods balanced with drinks, and with staples supplemented with special complements. The festive character of the meal was properly represented by multiple staples, and many highly ranked categories of complements. The dessert reinforced the definition of the event as a feast. I, however, did not receive a soda with the meal.

Instead, soon after the plates were distributed, Leilan, a young adoptive granddaughter of mine, grabbed my head from the rear and pressed a drinking coconut to my lips, forcing me to ingest several swallows before releasing me. I did not resist, since such pranks are common on Enewetak and since coconut liquid is, as they knew, a favored drink of mine. Later, however, after consuming the coconut and much of the food, I gave the remainder of the meal to my adoptive niece. As she devoured the chicken and rice, she quipped that "Leilan was still trying to perform magic on me."[6] At the time I laughed, since it was well known that the community had wanted me to in-marry and that Leilan, granddaughter to a high chief, had been that chief's favored companion for me. The latest incident seemed only a continuation of the metaphoric discourses in love for which islanders are so well known (see Sahlins, 1985). In retrospect, I know that my niece's message was meant more ✳ seriously, and that my Marshallese dis-ease was the result of Leilan's magic.

Love magic is not always effectively performed, but its recipient is powerless in revoking its efficacy. Once a potion is imbibed it can be counteracted with additional magic, but the "fitness of the body" will not provide resistance to the magic (the resistance metaphor is but a variety of our "war against illness" notion). For Enewetak people, the balance of life's force within the body is a representation of the balance that a person seeks and maintains vis-à-vis others in the community. If balance is lacking, it can only be resynchronized with another eminently social act, the performance of countermagic. Without such reaffirmations of the social world, a person's physical form will change, and death is the most marked of these possible changes. Both food and drink are used to renegotiate the conditions in terms of which life and death interact. In this communicative construction of life, the exchange and consumption of food is the ultimate social act. Its very presence is often associated with growth, maturity, and stability, and one who is stingy with food is the worst sort of human being. In contrast, drinks, which balance food in the hierarchy of meal construction, are mediational substances used to create and destroy social relationships, not only among the living, but between corporeal and noncorporeal beings. In my illness, coconut liquid, the prototypical drink-class substance, was the medium used to convey an ontological message and transform my state of being.

The transformative agent within the liquid of a drinking coconut may be a physical substance or an incanted charm. Often love potions include small amounts of scented perfumes that lend irresistibility to the mix, be they ingested or rubbed on the body. Coconut liquid in itself, however, is a mediating substance that lends life. As the prototypical drink in the Marshall Islands, white coconut liquid is associated with males, and particularly with male seminal fluids. Ontogenetically, sperm provides the inseminational force that causes life to take on an external manifestation in the world. It does not "create children" in the Western sense, inasmuch as the core elements of the child are infused through clan substances contributed by the women (clan identities, the core elements of person, are passed matrilineally), but it does shape the external features of the person, including quixotic aspects of demeanor (see also Weiner on Trobriand views).

Medicines resurrect the almost-dead (the literal translation of Marshallese illness: *naninmej*) by mediating the boundary between life and death. Medicines use the liquid of immature coconuts to lend life to those whose spiritual force is escaping their physical body. This process replicates that in which male semen lends the visible external characteristics to an embryo.

Both the semen and the coconut liquid may have more specific characteristics. These male substances, in other words, open a pathway that can lead in different directions depending on their precise use. If a pregnant woman restricts her sexual partners to her husband (who is classed as a male cross-cousin) or to his brothers (who are also her male cross-cousins), their seminal fluids will reinforce one another and produce a strong child. If, however, the sperm of a man from another clan comes in contact with the embryo, it will mix improperly and damage the child. Similarly, with medicine, one must finish one medical specialist's cycle of remedies, including the repayment feast, before another can be initiated. Mixing two varieties of medicine could produce an antagonistic balance.

In love magic, coconut liquid is used to open the mediational pathway between non-life and life in a way precisely parallel to the inseminational force of sperm or the life-securing force of medicinal cures, but the direction of the movement of life's force is inverted. The potion is intended to grasp a person's throat, which is where the core feelings lie. Irresistibility is the key to this process. Love potions are constructed to incorporate irresistibility, perhaps by including the attractiveness of perfume. For one with stronger magic, a head wreath might be fashioned from *wut*, an indigenous bush tree with small fragrant flowers. To attract a lover, a charm is incanted as the wreath is manufactured, and the potency of the charm, along with the beauty and scent of the flowers, is woven into the final product. This *wut* could be given to one's paramour, or the wreath could be soaked in the coconut liquid to be consumed, or it could be pounded and bits of the resulting mash combined with the liquid. For the most potent magic, the liquid of the coconut would be steeped with the wreath, and then both the wreath and the liquid would be given to the victim. In addition to the coconut, I received two head leis at the welcoming party for visitors. One was from Leilan.

What is the symptomatic picture presented by love-sickness? Standard symptoms include extreme lethargy with prolonged periods of sleeping, hot or cold flashes, no interest in food, and aimless wandering. Successful love magic first leaves its victims with the symptoms of love-sickness. Worst-case scenarios of unmitigated love magic include the successful appropriation of a person's thoughts and throat. In the former instance, a person may become "crazy" (*tano*); in the latter, a person may fly away to join a lover (*kalok*). In either case, the shrivelled shell of a person's external being remains, devoid of essential content.[7] The person is truly almost dead, and as soon as one's body disappears in death, one's entire being will be reunited with the lover's distant spirit.

In the same manner that drink-class things (*limo-*)—and drinking coconuts in particular—lend external form to the person and lead to a tenuous physical existence in the world, food-class objects (*kijo-*) ensure growth and secure well-being. Food is associated with the women's sphere, with sociality, with the commensality of village life, and with the domestic situation (indeed, women prepare almost all food secured by men). Whenever typical domestic arrangements are disrupted, food is used to communicate the situation to others. When my adoptive brother's wife left for the government center in 1983, he exhibited the classic signs of love-sickness. He would drink liquid (a male activity associated with wandering about in the bush), but he did not want to eat. Within two weeks, he had lost ten or fifteen pounds. He slept constantly. He rarely emerged from the house, but when he did, he was shrouded in a blanket, complaining of cold flashes. After a few weeks, he left the house and began wandering. Others complained that he "just walked around aimlessly," coming home at the end of each day without having accomplished anything.

Of course, to reverse Geertz's phrase, food is used not only as a model for action but as a model of it (40–42). In Bourdieu's terms, not only does food create meaning through use, but it is also used to constitute meaning from practice (83). In other words, upon learning that I was ill, Enewetak people in Majuro posited that I must be suffering from love-sickness born of successful love magic. Knowing nothing of my actual symptomatology, they presumed I was lethargic, aimless, without appetite, and suffering from hot or cold flashes. In short, their interpretation of the illness explained my symptoms as well as did the Montana physician's, and in their case, the patient was *in absentia*.

Like the Western view, the Enewetak view carries within its definitional parameters and communicative practices a set of political implications as well. With less presumptiveness than the perspective of Americans, Enewetak people also know that their interpretation is correct (less presumptive because they do not take it to be their duty to force either their medical interpretations or the underlying system of medical knowledge upon us; correct because they believe Americans know nothing about performing or counteracting magic). They thus maintain a certain smugness in the realization that if I wish my body to be returned to proper balance with the living, I must consult them for countermagic (see also Farmer, "Sending Sickness," 21). In other words, I must renegotiate my social standing within the community of living Enewetak people.

The politics of the magic crosscuts a Western division between the personal and the public. These interpretations include, but are not exhausted by, a sexual and an international politics. First, the sexual politics. It is easy for us to read sexist themes into male-female relationships in the Marshall Islands, where the female stays put while the male travels around. Male sexual needs must be cared for to maintain good health, whereas female sexual needs do not build up in the same way as does the production of sperm within a male. These fragments, however, must be understood in terms of a larger set of male-female negotiations, ✱of which they are an integral part. In a very real sense, women are the ones who control the sphere of adult social life. They control clan substance, which gives humans their core being, and that substance must be transmitted to others through birth. Not surprisingly, then, women also control the village and domestic spheres, within which social as well as physiological reproduction takes place. And since men's sexual needs must be met for personal health to be maintained, women control the intersexual dynamic in terms of which these needs are properly mitigated.

The University of Arno, popular theme of the mid-Pacific T-shirt industry, is where women's sexual skills are reputedly honed. Too easily read as a Marshallese finishing school, the traditional "school" on Laned islet, Arno Atoll, is said to date from pre-contact times. Women only lived on Laned along with invited men. The aim is said to have been to teach women the domestic skills of adulthood. Sexual techniques were the most critical of those skills. By the 1970s, their "traditional" T-shirt totem had become the giant clam shell, metaphoric of the vagina. More recent representations elsewhere in Micronesia include the helicopter, representative of a sexual technique known only to Laned women. Although it is easy to see all of these representations perpetuating a system of female oppression—a school to train women in arts that are to gratify men—this is not an indigenous rendering. Instead, stories of Laned women are tales of empowerment. The most macho of males fall victim to their own tumescence, and their claims of sexual vigor are exposed as hollow boasting in these tales. Laned represents the successful supersession of female sexual performance over the proclamations of male sexual prowess. In this universe, the moment of praxis becomes the measure of ability. For Marshall Islanders, Laned women always "win" these encounters.[8]

The importance of this material becomes apparent in the subsequent discussion. Leilan is a woman born to the daughter of the high chief of Enewetak Atoll. Her father is from Laned, and she has spent some years in residence on that islet. In the eyes of the Enewetak people, she becomes a doubly appropriate mate for me by counterpoising the matrifocal universe of Marshall Islanders to the patrifocal universe of the United States. Leilan's Laned ties, traced through her father, allow Enewetak people to construct her into an irresistible sexual mate yet, at the same moment, an indomitable one. On the other hand, Leilan's descent from the high chief of Enewetak, invoked through her mother's line, allows local residents to create an empowered image of themselves in interactions with the United States.

In the words of a former consultant who was interested in my marriage to an Enewetak woman, if I were to marry a local woman it would be good, for some day my offspring would be president. The logic here engenders an enviable set of social relationships for a tiny group of islanders on the fringes of Marshall Islands society. Since Enewetak clans are matrilineal, their system of kinship bilateral, and chiefly inheritance patrilineal, in their minds, not only would my offspring become president—high chief of the United States— but an Enewetak clan would thus become the ruling clan in America. The logic is continuous with that used by Enewetak people to describe their relationship to Marshall Islanders, residents of the Ratak and Ralik chains of islands to the east of them. In that case, they say that the Ejoa and Di Pako clans now in the Marshalls are descended from ancient Enewetak clans, which gave birth to and nurtured them. Being on the ascendent line that leads to the source of primordial, sacred power gives Enewetak a conceptual leverage that they lack in present-day political practice. Successful love magic would secure for Leilan's line a strategic position in the ongoing negotiation of interpersonal relationships with the United States. These affinal relationships necessarily represent, for Marshall Islanders, sexually negotiated and lineally instantiated positions of power.[9]

In sum, multiple readings of a single event offer a valuable opportunity to reflect upon the ways in which humans think about their worlds and act within them. Each of these interpretations makes sense in terms of certain cultural and historical contexts, not so much because they represent a set of existing structural relationships, but because, for a fleeting moment, they constitute them. My own reflections, which posit two substantially different constructions of the same reality, are not meant to suggest that this is the only sense that can be made out of differentially constituted events. Certainly one could foreground alternative paths and ignore others in much the way I have done, to construct other views. This does not make my analysis any less evocative; it just does not make it right. But then, who was right? Was it really typhoid, a Western disease, or the early manifestations of *kalok,* flight, a Marshallese form of near-death? Each hypothesis constructed a history, measured risk factors, and made judgments based on physical or clinical presentations. Although neither account was sufficient to allow its proponent to confirm positively their suspicions, each, in its own sphere, was considered true. In my own biased view, given the way I felt, both interpretations, simultaneously, must have been "true."

ACKNOWLEDGMENTS

I wish to thank Leslie B. Marshall, Lin Poyer, C. Jack Gilchrist, and two anonymous *Cultural Anthropology* reviewers for comments on earlier drafts of this article.

NOTES

A more extended version of this chapter entitled "Medical Magic and Medicinal Cure: Manipulating Meanings with Ease of Disease" appears in *Cultural Anthropology* 8(2): 157–168 (1993). The sections included herein are republished with permission.

1. Paul Farmer points out the way in which AIDS in Haiti simultaneously represents differential medical and international political discourses. At certain historical moments, rural Haitians associated "sida" (Haitian-defined AIDS) with the collapsing Duvalier regime or used it, more generally, to malign the United States. Some saw it as part of "an American plan to stem migration" ("Sending Sickness," 11–14). These counter-accusations were only part of an established Haitian understanding that U.S. residents considered Haiti to be a dangerous source of AIDS (8–10). This is not surprising, since, even within the United States, AIDS has been displaced onto internally fashioned "others"—principally homosexuals and intravenous drug users.

2. Although an extensive literature within medical anthropology explores the cultural construction of disease, the topic is not well covered in Micronesia. Leslie Marshall's and Mac Marshall's writings on alcohol, its cultural and historical patterns of use, are the most notable exception. Fr. Francis Hezel's and Donald Rubinstein's work on suicide represents another area of recent concern (see also Hezel et al.).

3. Tambiah and others have shown how performance itself lends efficacy to ritual occurrences.

4. I have since revisited the Marshall Islands several times and confirmed the general outlines of this temporally situated local view. Had the symptoms of my "illness" persisted, the explanations would have been concomitantly elaborated. Since the symptoms had subsided prior to my return, however, the incident had been transformed into an event of relatively minor consequence.

5. The entire opposition between nature and culture is our own, and although Lévi-Strauss believes the distinction to be universal, if it is, its boundaries differ markedly from what we take for granted. In this specific case, spiritual essence must separate itself from the body to set up the conditions of illness, and, in the Marshallese view, this cannot happen without social intervention on behalf of the living or the dead (those living in a non-corporeal realm). As Glick notes in regard to the Gimi of New Guinea: "Illnesses are caused by agents who . . . bring their powers to bear against their victims. Such agents may be human, 'Superhuman' . . . or nonhuman; but always they are conceived as willful beings, who act . . . in response to consciously perceived personal motives" (36).

6. Lewis discusses how food is implicated in the diagnosis of illness by the Gnau of New Guinea. As Lewis argues, food is an obvious channel for the transmission of illness, since "everyone must eat" and "food enters the body" directly (305), yet the cultural value of foods and the ways in which illness is transmitted through foods varies in significant ways. For Gnau, spirits are generally implicated in the transmission of illness principally through vegetable foods grown or provided by the patient or immediate kin (Lewis, 296–310). In the current case, the cause of illness is magical, and the magic has efficacy because it is invested with potency by spirits connected with Leilan by pathways of de-

scent, residence, and solidarity. It makes good Marshallese sense on interpersonal historical grounds, because Leilan's clan identity is the opposite of my own (thus making us potential marriage mates), and because the illness was transmitted in unusual circumstances using a common consumable out of which culturally potent magical concoctions are often made.

7. Achsah Carrier describes a series of similar spirit-displacing illnesses for the Ponam who reside in Manus province, Papua New Guinea (166–180). As on Enewetak, soul loss and other spiritual interventions among the Ponam are responsible for most serious illnesses. On the other hand, Enewetak people contend that movements of a person's spirit can be determined on the basis of physical symptoms as well as personal history, whereas for Ponam, "Illnesses sent by ghosts, spirits, ancestors or God could not be distinguished from each other or from purely physical malfunctions by examination of the body alone" (Carrier, 172).

8. The University of Arno, its representational value, and its methods of instruction are discussed in greater depth elsewhere (Carucci). Although I do not know if the Laned training school actually existed, Micronesians today talk and act in ways that make it a valuable source of cultural empowerment.

9. In separate chapters, Gilbert Herdt and Edward LiPuma show how alternative views of medicine articulate with indigenous attempts to construct empowered identities in New Guinea. As LiPuma notes for the Maring: "The use of Western medicine and the uses made of it are part of social and political strategy. Older men . . . still reject or quietly disregard Western medicine. . . . The younger generation . . . adopts the implicit strategy of embracing Western medicine in order to differentiate itself from the senior generation" (306). Although similar strategies are used in constructing differentially empowered identities for both young and old within the Marshall Islands, the case described here shows how indigenous medical theory is used as a mechanism of international empowerment by a variety of island residents, young and old.

REFERENCES

Bourdieu, Pierre. *Outline of a Theory of Practice*. Cambridge: Cambridge University Press, 1977.

Carrier, Achsah H. "The Place of Western Medicine in Ponam Theories of Health and Illness." In *A Continuing Trial of Treatment: Medical Pluralism in Papua New Guinea*. Stephen Frankel and Gilbert Lewis, eds. Dordrecht: Kluwer Academic Publishers, 1989, 155–80.

Carucci, Laurence M. "An Atoll Called Desire: Women, War and the Language of Welcome on Arno Atoll." In *Proceedings of the Montana Academy of Sciences* (1992).

Farmer, Paul. *AIDS and Accusation*. Berkeley: University of California Press, 1992.

———. "Sending Sickness: Sorcery, Politics, and Changing Concepts of AIDS in Rural Haiti." *Medical Anthropology Quarterly* 4(1): 6–27.

Foster, George M., and Barbara G. Anderson. *Medical Anthropology*. New York: Alfred A. Knopf, 1978.

Foucault, Michel. *Madness and Civilization: A History of Insanity in the Age of Reason*. New York: Pantheon, 1965.

Frazer, James G. *The Golden Bough.* New York: Macmillan, 1922.

Geertz, Clifford. "Religion as a Cultural System." In *Anthropological Approaches to the Study of Religion.* Ed. Michael Banton. London: Tavistock Publications, 1966. 1–46.

Glick, Leonard B. "Medicine as an Ethnographic Category: The Gimi of the New Guinea Highlands." *Ethnology* 6 (1967): 31–56.

Herdt, Gilbert H. "Doktas and Shamans Among the Sambia of Papua New Guinea." In *A Continuing Trial of Treatment: Medical Pluralism in Papua New Guinea.* Stephen Frankel and Gilbert Lewis, eds. Dordrecht: Kluwer Academic Publishers, 1989, 95–114.

Hezel, Francis X. "Truk Suicide Epidemic and Social Change." *Human Organization* 46(4): 283–291.

Hezel, Francis X., Donald H. Rubinstein, and Geoffrey M. White. "Culture, Youth, and Suicide in the Pacific." Honolulu: Pacific Islands Studies Program and the Center for Asian and Pacific Studies (University of Hawaii) and the Institute of Culture and Communication (East-West Center), 1985.

Lewis, Gilbert. *Knowledge of Illness in a Sepik Society.* London: Athlone Press, 1975.

Lindenbaum, Shirley. *Kuru Sorcery: Disease and Danger in the New Guinea Highlands.* Palo Alto, CA: Mayfield Publishing,1979.

LiPuma, Edward. "Modernity and Medicine Among the Maring." In *A Continuing Trial of Treatment: Medical Pluralism in Papua New Guinea.* Stephen Frankel and Gilbert Lewis, eds. Dordrecht: Kluwer Academic Publishers, 1989, 295–310.

Marshall, Mac. *Weekend Warriors: Alcohol in a Micronesian Culture.* Palo Alto, CA: Mayfield Publishing, 1979.

Marshall, Mac, and Leslie B. Marshall. *Silent Voices Speak: Women and Prohibition in Truk.* Belmont, CA: Wadsworth Publishing, 1990.

Merck Manual, The. The Merck Manual of Diagnosis and Therapy. Robert Berkow, M.D., ed. Rahway, NJ: Merck & Co., 1987.

Rubinstein, Donald H. "Epidemic Suicide Among Micronesian Adolescents." *Social Science and Medicine* 17(1): 657–665.

Sahlins, Marshall. *Islands of History.* Chicago: University of Chicago Press, 1985.

Tambiah, Stanley J. "A Performative Theory of Ritual." *Proceedings of the British Academy* 65 (1979): 113–169.

Weiner, Annette. *Women of Value, Men of Renown: New Perspectives in Trobriand Exchange.* Austin: University of Texas Press, 1976.

QUESTIONS

1. In what ways does the conceptual model of disease in the Marshall Islands differ from the biomedical model that exists in the United States and Europe?

2. Discuss folk models of disease in the United States or Europe (either in the present or past) that have features reminiscent of the Marshall Islands model.

3. In earlier generations anthropologists attempted to maintain an objective stance, which allowed them to feel that they had some control over the conditions of field research. New theories, however, see ethnographers as interacting subjects, shaped by the conditions of field research and by the groups of people with whom they are working. In

what ways is the author shaped by the circumstances in which he finds himself? What are some of the rhetorical strategies he uses to depict the sense of controlling/being controlled by the situations in which he finds himself?

4. Anthropology has long professed to be a relativist discipline, and its practitioners claim to work very hard to attempt to understand the views of others without judging them. Nevertheless, from the perspective of medical ethics it is sometimes necessary to make judgments and to choose between different interpretations and alternate courses of action. How can a reasonable framework for interpretation and action be negotiated that simultaneously values multiple perspectives and inhibits the spread of contagious disease?

Seeing Mt. Fuji

⬅ MAGGIE GRIFFIN TAYLOR ⬅

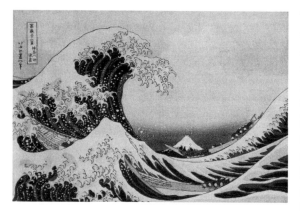

They are asking me if I am an organ donor. I say yes. They are asking me if I have a living will. I say no. The nurse seems nervous, even angry. The IV won't go in. My vein is rolling. Every time she tries to put the needle in, my arm hurts but I don't say anything. The battle is between her and my vein, and I am just an observer. I hear scratching and clicking in the background—someone is writing on a chart, and I wonder what kind of words he is using to tell my history.

They ask me if I am comfortable. They ask me if I need spiritual counseling. I say, "Who do you have? —Maybe the Dalai Lama would be good or Saint Francis." They laugh. I laugh too, but I don't really understand the joke. Everything is distorted as if I have slipped into the world of Alice in Wonderland or Gulliver. Nothing is the right size, and the cardinal directions don't make sense. I am not exactly here, but I am here. Time feels like one continuous moment that can't be broken into minutes or hours or days. There is no vantage point from which to see things objectively.

It is all sinking in now, and I know they think I am dying. Even though the room is crowded with people, I feel like I am alone in a small, fragile boat at sea on a rough day. I am not sure what I should do. There is nothing to do—just ride this moment into the next and the next as it curls out like the belly of a wave.

The IV is finally in, and the doctor says to start slamming it. The rhythm of the pump is faster than my pulse. It is loud, my arm stings, and cold fluid floats like clouds through my arm. I close my eyes and finally remember what I should do. I am supposed to look for the light. I don't see anything, but I suddenly wonder why people wait until they are dying to look for the light. Surely this light must be available for occasions besides death. I remember something Goethe wrote—Angels dwell in constant light. The devil dwells in darkness, and we dwell somewhere between. Light and dark in everything—the best we can do is lean toward the light. I begin to lean.

My husband comes into the room. He is the only one here who knows that I am not supposed to look like this. He knows I have a life beyond this room. He knows the story of each piece of jewelry piled on the bedstand. He can call my boss and tell her where I am; he can roll up my car windows, water the plants, and feed the cat. He knows what to tell our children and what not to tell my parents. He is the only comfort in this room of unfamiliar language, sharp instruments, and machines.

They tell him that I went into ketoacidosis; my organs were shutting down. Severe dehydration. Deranged body chemistry. Adrenal system did not collapse. Type I diabetes—rare for a middle-aged woman. Perhaps a genetic propensity. Likely the result of a virus. They sketch out a battle plan like the kind you see on football commentaries. T-cells, beta cells. The body turns against itself. Game over. Pancreas loses. Insulin-dependent.

A few hours later, I begin to remember what it is like to feel normal, and I don't want to be here anymore. I don't want to have diabetes. It is all a big mistake. I want to cry, but there are too many people coming in and out of the room. Nurses prick my finger for samples of blood; they check the machine feeding my arm; they dig deep for arterial blood; they write on charts. I try to be a good patient. Later the doctor on duty comes in and explains what diabetes is, and I don't comprehend much of what she says. I just know that diabetes is a bad thing. Diabetics can't eat sugar. They have to take shots. They die. She hands me some pages xeroxed from a medical textbook. One page includes a chart that shows how insulin peaks and ebbs. She explains that carbohydrates can be translated into units of insulin. She tells me that I have to time my injections so that the insulin will intercept what I eat. She asks me if I understand, and I nod, but I really don't understand. I feel certain that I could recite this information well enough to pass a multiple choice test, but I don't know how I am going to constantly calculate every factor that needs to be accounted for in order to "control" my blood sugar. It sounds a juggling act involving plates and sharp objects.

The doctor tells me that if I inject too much insulin or wait too long between injection and food intake, I will become hypoglycemic and perhaps go into a coma. If I don't inject enough insulin to match carbohydrate intake, I will become hyperglycemic and face long-term risks like renal failure, heart disease, neuropathy, amputation, and blindness. I tell her that I think it is all a big mistake and that I am going to be OK. She glances down at my chart and tells me in a calm, rational voice that my blood sugar was running at 600 when I was admitted to the hospital and that I was spilling ketones. She is sure there is no mistake. The doctor leaves and the nutritionist comes in with xeroxed sheets that explain exchanges of insulin and carbohydrates. The pages look like they came from a coloring book. There are foods that have happy faces and foods that have sad faces and pictures of plates with food translated into units of insulin.

I feel like I am sinking, and I want to go back to shore. I want to go back to the ground I used to walk on, but it isn't there anymore. All I can do now is tread water for the rest of my life. At night, I grip the bedrail like an anchor.

Three days pass, and the nurse tells me I can go home after I learn how to inject. She brings a syringe and an orange so I can practice. I tell her that I don't want to practice. I just want to get it over with. So I do the unthinkable. I put a needle into my arm. She is impressed and calls for a plate of food. I study it and try to translate it according to the pictures and graphs. The food tastes terrible, but I eat everything on my plate. I am worried about intercepting the insulin.

The next day I go home. Everything looks different, slower. I have forgotten how to use a computer. I can't remember the names of the streets in my town. I can't remember the names of my students. I can't remember words to match the things I want to say. I don't know how I am going to go back to work. I am hungry but afraid to eat the wrong thing at the wrong time. I want my brain to feel right again.

A few days later, I am standing in the grocery store trying to find something humorous about the sudden urgency to read the labels on food while my eyes are seeped in the fuzz of glucose. The optometrist says that my eyes will eventually clear, and he won't prescribe glasses just yet, so I go to Wal-Mart and buy two pairs of the strongest reading glasses available on the rack. When I stack them both on my nose at the same time, I can see well enough to read. I look in the mirror and I barely recognize my own face. I look older than I did before I got sick. Suddenly my life is divided into two epochs—before I got sick and after I got sick.

The nurse comes to my house, and I am eager for her visit. I want to tell her that my daughter is afraid to touch me because she thinks diabetes is contagious. I want to tell her that my family is afraid of needles. I want to complain about the fact that almost every food on the planet contains sugar. Instead, she takes my vital signs and records them in her book. She wants to know if I understand how to read my glucometer. She wants to review my diet. She wants to weigh me and shakes her head when she sees the digital reading—102 pounds. She can't understand how I could have missed the signs—weight loss, obsessive thirst, frequent urination. She wants to know how I let myself get to the point of ketoacidosis. She wants to call an intervention with my doctor because she thinks I have an eating disorder. She looks skeptical when I tell her that I went to the clinic twice because I thought I had diabetes, but the doctor said not to worry because I did not fit the profile. When she leaves, I cry.

Two weeks later, I go back to teaching at the university, and I "crash" in front of my class—my sugar goes too low too fast and I am suddenly incoherent. I hear myself talking, but I don't know what I am saying. I fumble for candy, but I have already missed the interception. I feel like I am drunk and drowning, and I don't know how to ask for help. I see splotches of light where faces should be, and my students leave early that day, as confused as I am. Later, when I am steady, I create a carefully choreographed parachute plan that can be quickly implemented in case I ever crash again during class. I put xeroxed copies in a red folder. It becomes the first thing I lay on my desk at the beginning of each class.

I go to a meeting at work late one afternoon and my blood sugar is running at 350, but I don't know why. My lunch is still safely tucked away in my bag, waiting for the magic moment of interception that doesn't come. My mind is slow and words that once flowed from my lips like common tap water are frozen in a sludge of glucose that won't be moved by the 6 units of insulin I injected an hour ago. I feel undignified and betrayed, and I want to scream out that life is not fair. I cannot "control" this disease. I want to tell everyone that the logical flowcharts we are examining in the meeting belong to a world that I no longer trust.

Instead, I force myself to think like Sherlock Holmes or Joe Friday. I review what I have done to make my blood sugar erratic. I exercised, injected with precision, and ate as if I were a zealot of a new religion. I can only conclude that the clean charts, crisp graphs, tidy conversion tables, and foods with happy faces do not translate into the lived version of this illness. Diabetes isn't linear, it isn't predictable, and it doesn't always play by the rules. Heraclitus once said you can never step in the same river twice. He has come the closest to mapping the land of diabetes.

Books about diabetes offer various explanations for the random patterns of the disease. Maybe I am getting sick, maybe my hormones are not balanced, or maybe I am experiencing stress. Books from the self-help section of Barnes and Noble tell me that I don't pray enough, I have unresolved issues, a secret need to be ill, or even a debt for past karma. Medical journals are less cryptic, explaining diabetes as a "histocompatibility complex (MHC) HLA region on chromosome 6p21.31." My doctor simply tells me that I am a "brittle diabetic." I feel oddly comforted by having a label for my condition and ask what it means to be a brittle diabetic. He says that it is a term used to describe diabetics whose bodies do not respond well to insulin therapy, whose patterns swing wildly and unpredictably. I tell him that diabetes feels like chaos theory—so many elements interacting in ways that defy prediction and challenge the penchant for normal science to exert *control*. He nods without interest and tells me there isn't much more he can do. Still, as he leaves the examination room, he cautions me to control my blood sugar because "the consequences are profoundly negative." I resolve to try harder.

I attend a diabetes training session where people who do not have diabetes tell me how to be one. We receive plastic bags laden with pamphlets. We receive low-fat, low-calorie, low-sugar recipes that we can share with our families. We receive a plastic bristle to check our feet in case we have lost our ability to feel sharp objects. We are cautioned to wear sensible shoes. The podiatrist suggests that we have our toenails removed to avoid amputations associated with ingrown toenails. We receive lectures about the complications of diabetes, and we recite the mantra of control. We can ask questions after the presentations, if time permits.

Months pass and I learn not to salivate at the sight of dessert but still dream about eating fruit from the trees in our yard. Sometimes the injections and exercise and healthy food work in beautiful harmony; sometimes nothing works. Sometimes I have to eat when I am not hungry; sometimes I can't eat when I am starving. Sometimes I sit at the dinner table and watch my family eat while I wait for the elusive, magical window of insulin and food interception. Often I eat alone. I check my sugar at least ten times a day, hoping to find a pattern, desperate to keep my sugar in the target range. I learn to inject on a sliding scale and discover that if I inject smaller amounts of insulin six or eight times a day, I can achieve tighter control.

My daughter suggests that someone should invent a town called Diabetesville where people with diabetes can go and be normal. We laugh when we think about glucose monitors everywhere, just like ATMs, and insulin pumps next to gas pumps and the golden arches of McDiabetes where people never ask you if "you want fries with that." The mayor of Diabetesville would pipe insulin through the air and remove sharp objects from the park so that people could go barefoot. Banks would pass out celery sticks instead of suckers. Instead of asking, "How's the weather?" we would ask, "How's your sugar?" Social gatherings, so typically punctuated with sweetened food and drink, would be different in Diabetesville, and no one would ever feel left out.

The local TV station in Diabetesville (DTV) would feature shows with characters who check their blood sugar as regularly as people check their watches. When the refrigerator door opens during the DTV soap operas, bottles of insulin would be as visible as cartons of milk, but there would be no eerie, suspenseful music to emphasize that someone had just discovered a dark, meaningful secret. During restaurant scenes, people would take out their syringes and inject right there at the table without missing a beat instead of going into the stall of the bathroom. *Wheel of Fortune* would give away insulin pumps as prizes, and *Seinfeld* would be remade to include the antics of a neighbor with diabetes. *ER* would feature diabetic doctors who dramatize the complexities of "control" in a fast-paced world. DTV's version of *Jeopardy* would include categories like "Types of Insulin" and "Famous Diabetics."

Instead of Diabetesville, people with diabetes live in an invisible land that they navigate with a modern oracle called a glucose monitor. It is a land that does not match the conventional topography of fast-food restaurants, vending machine items, appointed lunch breaks, sedentary business meetings, fear of needles, coffee and doughnuts, or cake and ice cream. To be diabetic is to skirt along the edges of common ground, aware of the ceremonial and communal aspects of food but unable to fully partake.

I avoid situations where I have little control over what and when I eat but agree to attend a dinner party with my husband. I assure him that everything will be OK and bring enough insulin to cover any food that the hostess might serve. I grapple with chicken coated in plum sauce, rice, and pasta salad, but when the exuberant hostess hands me a piece of cake called Death by Chocolate, I have to decline. She is devastated, as if I have insulted her or broken an unspoken code between women—namely to indulge together in a rich dessert. At that point, I explain that I have diabetes. She suddenly becomes sympathetic and whispers, "My aunt had diabetes." The use of past tense verbs in conversations about diabetes is very common. Nevertheless, I ask her, "What happened to your aunt?" The hostess replies quickly, as if it were simply a rhetorical question: "She died." I nod quietly as she moves on to offer Death by Chocolate to another guest.

A few months later, I manage to get an appointment to see a new doctor in town who specializes in diabetes. He analyzes my blood panel and determines that I have been misdiagnosed. He proclaims that I am a type II diabetic and recommends that I discontinue the basal insulin and take oral medication in its place. He assures me that I will eventually be able to halt all of the injections. I am ecstatic. As an act of faith, I go home and throw away my basal insulin. My glucose level goes up to 400. I call my doctor and he tells me to increase my oral medication. He thinks I am lying about my carbohydrate intake. My glucose stays at 400. He tells me to increase my oral medication. He tells me to stop obsessing about my blood sugar. I lose ten pounds and my mind begins to haze over. The doctor tells me that I have to give the medicine time to work. He decreases my prescription for test strips so that I can only check my glucose levels three times a day. He gives me a month's supply of blister packs with pills that will reduce my stress. I discover that the pills are used to treat patients who suffer from a severe form of obsessive-compulsive disorder. I throw them away.

I go to the pharmacy and tell the attendant that I need to refill my prescription for basal insulin. He checks my records and tells me that I don't have any refills left. The pharmacy will call my doctor and have the script ready tomorrow. I tell him that I accidentally broke the bottle and I need a refill now. The customer behind me says, "Give her the insulin!" The customer behind him says, "Yeah. Just give her the medicine." I have never had a fan club like this before and am grateful for their support. The pharmacist on duty notices the commotion, glances at me, goes to the shelf, and processes the prescription. She also has diabetes. Two days later, I feel fine. I never see the diabetes specialist again except at the grocery store, where he pretends that he does not know me.

Several years have passed since my diagnosis, and I have discovered that managing diabetes is like learning how to ride a bike. Instructions are useful but can never replace the experience. Words don't easily convey the myriad nuances of balance or the burdens and insights of living with such a constant companion. I make the required pilgrimages to see my doctor. A nurse at the clinic always checks my vital signs, collects vials of blood, curses under her breath at my rolling veins, and leads me into the examination room. The oral element of most visits is perfunctory. The narrative of my illness and the epic catalogue of my symptoms are secondary to the visually oriented prosthetics of biomedicine. I've learned to speak in statistics instead of stories. I have also learned how to read blood panels and to converse in a highly specialized language (replete with passive constructions and jargon). I am accustomed to metaphors that equate my body with that of a machine or that liken my disease to a military coup. I tolerate being called *a diabetic*. I patiently listen to advice about "control" and "consequences" even though I know diabetes doesn't always play by the rules laid out in medical textbooks. Similarly, my doctor tolerates my requests for referrals to an acupuncturist and patiently nods when I mention herbs, yoga, or meditation. We are like an old couple who has comfortably settled into a relationship of long-term managed care.

As I leave my doctor's office, I make a ritual stop in the lobby of the clinic to see a print entitled *The Great Wave*. It is a famous Japanese print created by Hokusai Katsushika. The print depicts several small boats struggling below the crest of a huge wave. The wave is frozen in time, and no one can know the fate of the small people poised at its belly. The wave is powerful and beautiful, with curling tendrils that frame Mt. Fuji in the background, but I know how different the wave must seem to the passengers in those tiny, fragile boats. In his attempt to present thirty-six views of Mt. Fuji, Katsushika understood that Mt. Fuji experienced from the belly of a wave is much different from Mt. Fuji viewed from an aloof distance. No single view tells the whole story. I suddenly understand the frozen beauty of the hemoglobin A1c test that my doctor has just shown me and comprehend his static picture of what I experience as an undulating sea. From my position outside of the painting, I can see a safe route around the pummel of waves and can sense which way to lean. I glance at *The Great Wave* once more on my way out of the clinic, bid goodbye to the motionless boats, and enter the flux.

QUESTIONS

1. Discuss some key differences between chronic and acute illness.
2. The author reveals complex issues of control for those with diabetes. How might knowing something of these particular challenges be beneficial to the general public?
3. How does the author reveal the difference between medical understanding and the patient's "lived experience" of an illness?

Being Ill / Being Well
Reflections on an Illness

⌒ SUSAN DICK ⌒

In the fall of 1988, I was hospitalized for ten months with an illness eventually diagnosed as a rare form of the neurological disorder Guillain-Barré syndrome. The following is an account, written three years after my return home, of my memories of that time.

When the lights of health go down[1]

My illness developed slowly. All through the late winter, spring, summer, and early autumn of 1988, its symptoms, at first only brief lapses in my ordinary well-being, grew more insistent. I began to find walking difficult; my handwriting became shaky; I slept badly and awoke fatigued. At first, I assumed these problems to be temporary and my accommodation to them was provisional. I bought a stylish walking stick, not a cane; I reduced my university teaching load from two courses to one; and I shortened the dog's walks, but promised longer ones soon.

Eventually it became clear that these haphazard arrangements would not do. Something was seriously wrong. I began to keep a journal in which I recorded my thoughts during this frightening time. The following is the first entry:

15 Oct.

Difficult to begin. My hand is stiff, for one thing, and I've done so little writing for the past two months. My idea is that it would help me to deal with this period of illness if I kept a record of my experiences of it. I've never gone through anything like this before, for one thing. In addition, my physical condition has become my preoccupation—indeed, my occupation in a sense—and writing about this may enable me to do more than brood and repeat to myself the same recurring thoughts. I need to highlight progress, because it's so slow, and, it seems, unstable.

I remember reaching a point a couple of weeks ago when I seemed to regain my sense of myself as separate from my illness. That isn't consistent, I find. When I'm out shopping, or in the office, the effort needed to do what I'm doing takes all my energy and concentration. It's hard to pay attention to other things—to speak to someone and also walk down the hall. I think this is why I seem to have more trouble walking when I'm in the office than I do at home, where there are no surprises. This just dawned on me yesterday. — discovery through writing

Another reason for writing—*I'm aware of being extremely self-centered when talking with people. Friends call to see how I am, and I give them a report, but I need to be more than my tiresome condition. Perhaps if I write it out here, I'll have less need to discuss it in detail with others.*

diff past than others

Thank goodness people are concerned. Illness is so isolating—no one can know how I feel. It was cold comfort Thursday to have Dr. H., up to now so impersonal, ask me how I felt. "I didn't think there was anything wrong," he said, "but now I can see that there is." I'm sorry that there is, of course, but I knew it and am relieved that we are now setting out to find out more.

The isolation—people have their own lives to get on with, while the sick person's life is on hold. I don't even get much reading done because I get sleepy and then nap. Also, doing anything takes more time. And illness is itself time-consuming: exercises, the bike, visits to doctors, etc.

At this point, probably like most people when they first become ill, I was deeply afraid of the unknown. My problem had not been diagnosed, so there was no way of knowing what might lie ahead. I was nostalgic for the health I had lost and incredulous—could this, whatever it was, be happening to me? Some of these feeling are reflected in my second entry:

fear in past

16 Oct.

I was close to being in tears from sheer frustration this morning. It is so hard to move, especially just after I get up. So many things I took for granted now must be done with great concentration. And I keep wondering, will this get any better? If not, how long can I go on like this?

I must guard against self-pity. It's a lovely day and I wish I could be out in it—putting the garden to bed. I think I will feel better—I felt better last Sunday than I do today.

I have a great nostalgia for the way I used to feel.

My journal shows that as I neared the point where becoming ill would change over to being ill, my world grew increasingly narrow. My attention was focused almost exclusively on the distressing symptoms eroding my ability to do ordinary things. Illness almost inevitably makes us self-centered. It takes away the play of mind and the emotional energy we need to respond to the world around us. It is preoccupying because it cannot be ignored; it is isolating because it cannot be shared.

I recall vividly the relief I felt when, in the middle of October, I finally entered the hospital. I did not dream, of course, that I would spend the next ten months there. The isolation of illness was now, in some ways, overcome. An enormous amount of activity surrounds a new patient, and this for me provided a strangely welcome distraction from the illness itself. All those doctors and nurses were so purposeful and well-intentioned. I was encouraged to hope that I would soon be well again. The problem had been acknowledged; next it would be defined, and then it would be solved.

Now I had to accommodate not only being ill, but being a patient. In *Orlando*, Virginia Woolf considers the multiplicity of selves that exist within each individual. "Everybody can multiply from his own experience," she writes, "the different terms which his different selves have made with him."[2] One self emerges to enjoy a meal with friends, another to shop for groceries, another to read a book, and so on. I find this notion of different selves having different roles within us helpful as I try to understand what occurs when one becomes seriously ill. Many of the selves that make up oneself are put aside for a while, sent on holiday, perhaps, because there is nothing for them to do. Our memories of them, like postcards from distant friends, remind us of their continuing presence elsewhere. They do not, for the moment, take an active part in our life. The routines of home, work, and play—all the activities that seemed to be central to defining one—are suspended. This narrowing of focus is not necessarily a refining or honing of oneself down to a central core (if such a things exists), however, for other selves are called into play, first by the illness, and then by being a patient.

It seems to me important to distinguish between being ill and being a patient, even though when one is hospitalized, these are experienced simultaneously. The suffering caused by illness is private, while the treatment of it is public. The sufferer views the illness from one perspective, those who attempt to treat it from quite another.

Perhaps the most frightening aspect of my illness, one in which my body seemed to be deteriorating while my mind remained clear, was to feel myself losing control. The need now to depend upon others for almost everything was in itself distressing. The terms commonly used to describe what happens to one who becomes ill—stricken with, a victim of, suffers from—stress the passivity of the person who is ill. The only English word that specifically names one who is ill, *invalid*, derives from the Latin word for "strong," *validus*, and implies that illness is a negative state, the absence of that which makes one strong and valid. And invalid is enfeebled by disease, infirm, weak, inadequate, handicapped. The word *patient, as adjective, connotes calm endurance.* As noun it means specifically one who is under a physician's care. Yet I'm sure I am not alone in having felt a strong resistance to being ill, to being patient in the face of illness, and to being a patient. A stubborn and impatient healthy self, to return to Woolf's notion, had emerged to fight this threatening descent into passive suffering.

This assertive self had to learn how to function within the protective and controlling world of the hospital. A patient is like a traveler in a strange land. New customs, a new language, and new rules must be learned. Such an adjustment to a foreign environment is challenging when one is well; being ill compounds the challenge. My days, already fragmented and controlled by illness, were now shaped by the exigencies of hospital routine, on the surface so highly organized, underneath often as unreliable as a train schedule. In this environment, trivial things—bad food, a late porter—become absurdly important. Small things matter more as the large ones move beyond one's control.

As a foreigner in this hospital world, I was a stranger to most of the people around me. The credentials I ordinarily carried to establish my identity were not, as in the real world, the work I did, the place I lived, or even the clothes I wore, but my illness—a part of myself that I, too, was only slowly coming to know. What I felt the need to guard against at this time was being defined to myself and to others solely by my illness. Friends played a crucial role in this resistance. Their visits and phone calls maintained an essential link with the familiar world. With them, I was myself, not a patient.

I am attempting to generalize here about my first month in hospital. My journal tells me little about this period, for since I had neither the energy nor the time for reflection, it became mainly a place where I listed the names of the people who came to see me. My condition steadily worsened. I could barely walk, even with the aid of a walker, and I needed oxygen with increasing frequency to supplement my breathing. The tests continued, neurologists consulted respirologists, but no diagnosis emerged. Nevertheless, as I celebrated my forty-eighth birthday within the confines of a hospital room, I remained hopeful. Any adjustments I made to hospital life were, I assumed, provisional, like those I had first made to becoming ill. This, too, would pass.

> *Teach us to care and not to care*
> *Teach us to sit still.*[3]

One morning in late November, I quite suddenly found it extremely difficult to breathe. My room quickly became a swarm of activity. The doctor in charge described to me the intubation procedure they needed to perform and then asked me if they should go ahead. Not looking forward to this, I asked him what the alternative was. "You'll die," he said, a blunt, honest answer, which I appreciated and which certainly helped me to make up my mind. As the tube was put down my throat, I thought of the suffragettes who had been force-fed in prison that way, an odd analogy that gave me some comfort. The rest of the day is a blur which I recall more as spectator than as participant. I see myself being rushed to intensive care, then being surrounded by doctors and nurses. I recall feeling neither fear nor pain, only the wish that I would not die.

My memories of the month I spent in intensive care have no chronology, just as the days there had little shape. I drifted in and out of sleep during days and nights that were almost indistinguishable. Strangely, I do not look back on this as an unhappy time. At first, I was probably too ill to feel ordinary emotions. I may also have felt that this crisis would be the prelude to recovery. I had reached bottom; now the climb toward the top could begin. There was no question now of resisting either being ill or being a patient. The two had merged and had brutally displaced my independent healthy self. Hooked up to a respirator, I was now completely dependent on it and on the people who surrounded me.

My bed faced the adjacent room, which was divided from mine by a movable glass wall. The many get-well cards I had been sent were taped to this glass, but still I could see past them to the events taking place in the next room. I was a captive audience to scenes I would much rather not have watched. Perhaps it was good to have this distraction, even though some of the silent scenes I witnessed have left indelible pictures in my memory; for what I saw often reminded me that other people had catastrophes to contend with, too.

I shall give just one example. A young man was brought into the room. I must have been told that he was brain-dead and that he was being kept alive by a machine and that the decision had been made to disconnect this. A few grieving family members or friends came in, left, and then a while later a team of doctors entered. Fortunately, someone thought to draw the curtain between our rooms at this point. When it was opened again, that scene had ended. The room was empty.

I had been unable to speak from the time the tube had been placed down my throat. A week or so after I entered intensive care, a tracheotomy was performed. This procedure, which involves making a small incision in the patient's throat and inserting a tube through which air is forced into the lungs, also robs one of the ability to speak. I had what is called a "talking trach." This has a small external tube linking the cuff of the trach to an oxygen source. When the patient covers the small opening in this external tube, oxygen is forced over the vocal chords, enabling the patient to speak. My impaired co-ordination made it difficult for me to plug the opening in the external tube, and even when I, or someone else, was able to do so, I could only say a word or two. The "talking trach" would prove to be a continuing source of frustration, for in all the months that I was dependent on one, it never worked satisfactorily.

As an alternative, I was given a child's magic slate to write on, but again, because of my impaired coordination, I could scarcely write. The small group of close friends who visited me in intensive care must have found these visits, with their one-sided conversations, very painful. I did not know then how distressed they were by my condition, for they were careful not to show it. Nor did I fully realize how very ill I was (although when one friend asked me where I kept my will, I should have caught on). Only months later, when I was home again, did I learn that for a while I had not been expected to live.

What I later heard about this period made me feel that I had become the centre of a drama of which I had little knowledge. The only written record I have of it is a series of letters a friend began writing to me before he was able to visit me in intensive care. In one of the first of these, he wrote,

> A brief note to say that J. phoned us early this morning with the news that the tracheotomy is proceeding well. During the past eight days we have been thinking how distressingly uncomfortable you must be with the large tube down your throat. It will be a great improvement for you once you become adjusted to your new condition. J. has told us that it may take a few days before you can eat normally. It is a matter of hanging-in, then, and so keep hanging-in.

I have no recollection of the large tube in my throat being a discomfort, but I do remember being relieved when it was gone and when, a few days later, I was able to eat solid food again. *—help w/ suffering*

One of the doctors in intensive care, a former student of mine, set her mind to finding a way for me to communicate. She brought in a laptop computer, but this was too technically demanding. Then she hit upon the idea of a small electric typewriter. Although I was too ill to use it then, in time the typewriter proved to be wonderfully liberating. It became the means by which I would eventually begin to recover my voice. For the moment, however, I remained virtually silent and thus more isolated than ever within my illness.

> But is there any comfort to be found?
> Man is in love and loves what vanishes,
> What more is there to say?[4]

After I had been in intensive care for nearly a month, and Christmas neared, the doctors decided to move me to a room on the floor where I had been earlier. I was still hooked up to a respirator and very ill, but my condition, though it remained undiagnosed, had apparently stabilized. Thus began the third phase of my hospital stay. The following two months, which I would spend in this room, were, both literally and figuratively, the darkest days of the year.

I shared a large three-person room with only one other patient, a woman in the bed opposite mine, also on a respirator, whom I shall call Mrs. Bax. The room hummed and beeped with our unceasing machines. Mrs. Bax appeared to be sleeping all the time. Her relatives would visit, read to her, put posters on the walls and ceiling, but I could not tell whether she ever gave them any sign of recognition. I looked forward to their visits, for although I could not speak to them, I could listen as they read aloud from the Bible or a novel. I often wondered whether she was at all aware of her condition and, if she were, how she felt about it. One of the nurses told me Mrs. Bax sometimes wept, a fact I found deeply unsettling. I could understand why I had been placed in this room, since patients on respirators require similar care, but I could not help wishing that I did not have as a roommate someone who I feared might be a mirror of my future.

My bed was placed parallel to large windows through which I had a panoramic view of the lake. I could watch the ferry come and go all day. In the early morning the lake and sky sometimes glowed a deep pink; in the evening the still-unfrozen water became a translucent blue. After spending a month in the intensive care unit, confined within a small room with windows too high for me to see out of, it was a relief to be able to look outside again at the changing scene. The beauty of it was bittersweet, however, because that familiar landscape remained so absolutely inaccessible.

I had been a visitor in intensive care. Now I felt the threat of this room becoming, as it apparently had for Mrs. Bax, a permanent residence. One doctor, with the best of motives, suggested I have a favourite piece of furniture brought in from home. Mrs. Bax had her own television set. The idea appalled me. I had no intention of setting up housekeeping here.

Progressive nerve damage had left me almost completely helpless. Although I was not paralyzed—I could move my arms and legs and, with difficulty, feed myself and brush my teeth—I could do little else. I recall staring at a banana left on my table by a friend who did not realize that I could no more peel it than I could get up and walk out of the room. This helplessness was stressful, for I had continually to remember to ensure that anything I might need be placed within reach. I was especially anxious that the call-bell be nearby, for since I could not speak, I had no other way of summoning help. When the nurses transferred me from bed to chair, I was as limp as a rag doll. If I were uncomfortable, which I frequently was because of a raging bedsore, I had to ask someone to change my position.

These visible effects of the illness, the impairment of my motor functions, were accompanied by invisible ones, for my sensory functions were also affected. This condition, which persists to the present day, is almost impossible to describe. The neurologists refer to it as "pins and needles," thinking, I suppose, of how a limb that has been asleep feels as sensation returns. But in my experience it is not really like that. The closest analogy I can find is the way my arm feels when I strike the funny bone in the elbow and a jolt of sensation, rather like an electrical current, shoots through it. It is a feeling both of numbness—a loss of normal sensation—and of the presence of an alien, abnormal sensation, a steady current that is curiously distracting and fatiguing. I had no pain from it, as some people with Guillain-Barré syndrome do, but when it was at its worst, I would awaken feeling as though a heavy blanket were pinning me to the bed.

After the seemingly routineless, cosseting atmosphere of intensive care, where a nurse was constantly nearby, the long, dull, structured days of ordinary hospital life required yet another adjustment. The days soon settled into a routine. In the morning, following breakfast and a bed-bath (because I was hooked up to the respirator, I could not have an ordinary bath or shower), an occupational therapist would put me through a series of exercises designed to improve my coordination. I put pegs in holes, moved a stack of cones from one side of the table to the other, and did other simple but, for me, immensely challenging tasks. After lunch, the physical therapist would work on strengthening my wasted muscles.

I also saw a speech therapist, who brought me a mechanical device shaped like an electric razor. When I held this against my neck and spoke, it would produce a thin mechanical voice rather like that of the movie character E.T. It was difficult to use, and not much improvement on the sounds I continued to produce with the "talking trach." This contact with the therapists, who were clearly working hard to help me in my recovery, and the stimulation of their exercises were welcome breaks in the monotony of the day.

I felt dizzy if I sat up for long, had no appetite, and found the effort of eating very tiring; so I never looked forward to mealtimes. I spent some time reading, though I could not concentrate well and had trouble holding a book or placing it in my bookholder. I passed some time listening to tapes on a Walkman, and in the evening I watched television. Certain programs may be forever associated in my mind with the hospital. The jolly theme song of *Jeopardy* still transports me right back there.

I also spent a great deal of time, or so it seemed, waiting—for a nurse or a doctor, a therapist or a meal. The works of Samuel Beckett, a master at dramatizing the condition of waiting, came often to my mind. In one essay, Beckett describes life as a continual see-saw between suffering and boredom, and this bleak assessment now took on new meaning.[5] Unable to talk or walk, shackled to a respirator and thus imprisoned within this room, totally dependent on others for all my personal and practical needs, I began to fear that this way of life might be permanent. Perhaps I never would recover the health and independence and simple joys of life that I had lost.

Urged by my family physician, during his daily visits, to accomplish something each day, no matter how small, I began to use the electric typewriter and wrote brief letters to my parents and a few close friends. One friend has spoken of the "thingliness" of these letters, meaning that they expressed my condition not only in words, but in appearance as well. Another friend likened them to the efforts of Archy, the cockroach in Don Marquis's book *archy and mehitabel*, who typed, as I did, only in lower case. For myself, the effort I made to put into words what I was experiencing was a first step in gaining some control over it. One letter, to a friend who visited regularly, expresses better than I can in retrospect my state of mind at that time. I quote it as I wrote it:

30 Jan 89

hereare some brief notes—of some of the things i'm thinking about. Written under difficult conditions and abbreviated. My physical discomfort is a pre-

occupation. The bedsore hurts and its hard for me to get positioned well in this chair. eith few distRAcTIONS I dwell on tHIS, ON MY NUMBNESS, too, a lot. i also see images of myself as i was. i try to think of the recent pastas analogous to other periods in my life. butthe problem is that this pastlife shd.. be ongoing. it's still there—i'm just cut off from it. the feeling ofBeing left out of things is overwhelming.

i also feel very alone. thhe visits of you and my other loyal friends help combat this. but i feel that noone can know what i'm going through. self-pity. the boredom, suffering, and especially fear. how bad will it get. what does the future hold. if only it were a nightmare f4omwh.i cld. Awake. but thinking in those terms like seeing death as an alternative, will do me no good.

i miss simple pleasure, like baths, walking outdoors, talking on the phone, finding humor in everyday things. i try to do that, but seem too dispirited most of the time.

i wish so much that I cld. talk. for one thing it wld. Enable me to establish better relationships with the people around me. and it wld help overcome this isolation—an ironic condition for someone surrounded by people.

well these are not cheery thoughts. i wonder if writing them down will help distance them. i want you to have them—please save them in case i'm able later to write abt this experience. i'll try to do this often. i valuyyour friendship so much.

shd i call these notes from overground?

Although I make no mention of the respirator in this letter, in many ways it dominated my life. Its rhythms were mine, its malfunctions my malfunctions. A change in air pressure, which I would feel immediately, would set off a loud beeping alarm and a nurse would come running. The machine and tubing were checked twice daily by respiratory technicians; the tracheotomy tube in my neck had to be suctioned frequently during the day and often at night, too, in order to keep it clear. I felt invaded by the machine that was keeping me alive. I do not know how long I would have been willing to live like this.

When, recently, a young woman in Quebec, identified in the newspapers only as "Nancy B," who was paralysed by Guillain-Barré syndrome and attached to a respirator for two and a half years, requested and was finally granted the right to have her respirator turned off, I understood what had led her to the point of preferring death to life. Only she could decide, I felt, when she had had enough. I had known much of the tedium, discomfort, and stress of her daily life, and could imagine her thoughts as she fought for and then won the right to die. I was awed by her courage when she finally decided that the time had come to turn the respirator off. At a certain point in an acute illness the sufferer experiences a kind of grief, goes into self-mourning. The various selves initially sent on holiday by illness now seem to have perished. During the two months I have been describing, I found myself in a kind of limbo: not wanting to live like this and, at the same time, not wanting to die. I wanted what I seemingly could not have—a resurrection of my lost selves and of the life that had created them. I recall one nurse telling me I should accept what had happened to me, so I must have made my inability to do so clear. The first stage of grief is said to be denial. What I needed to learn, and perhaps did in time, was the distinction between acceptance and acquiescence. It was necessary to move beyond grief by accepting things as they were, and yet to continue to fight for recovery. I had to find a way for my healthy self to get to work.

> *Think where man's glory most begins and ends,*
> *And say my glory was I had such friends.*[6]

The "company of friends"[7] who continued to stand by me was now more important than ever. They were the "comfort to be found" in the midst of loss. My regular visitors, like the friends and relations who sent cards and notes, played a central role in my recovery by giving love and encouragement and support. Those who visited became witnesses to, and thus shared in, what I was going through. To the medical staff, I was a patient with a serious, stubborn, still-undiagnosed illness; to my friends, I was myself, awake in a bad dream. Their persistent presence helped me to hope that I might eventually recover.

Among my earliest letters was one to a friend in Colorado who, knowing nothing of my illness, had written to ask if I could meet her at a conference. This was my reply:

> *11 jan 89*
> *thanks for your card, wish i cld. join you at the conference, but unfortunately i've been in hospital since 23 oct. respiratory problems—i've had a tracheotomy and am attached to a ventilator all the time. i also have an undiagnosed neurological disease wh. Has made me very numband played havoc with my coordination. so at the moment i can do very little for myself. even typing is an effort. i hope eventually to get back home. so you see your premonitions of illness had some truth.*
> *a wonderful group of friends visits me regularly. but its hard to be very cheerful. i miss so much the life i had.*

This letter so alarmed her that she offered to come and see me. I replied:

> *22 jan*
> *Thanks so much flowers.*
> *i was*
> *deeply touched by your offerto fly up. thats not necessary, though a very kind thought. i'd rather seeyou wheni'm better.*

The letter I wrote a month later contained some better news:

> *19 feb*
> *i seem to be feeling a bit stronger and to be maintaining the coordination needed to feed myself, type, etc., tho the numbness seems worse.what a mystery it is. i keep thinking of a line of leonard cohen's—i want the life i used to have.*

The change I made in Leonard Cohen's line—"I want the kind of work I had before"[8] is what he wrote—made it a succinct summary of my mood.

During this period, another friend, who, like my family doctor, seemed to feel I should not let all this idle time go to waste, persuaded me to agree to co-edit with him a novel by Virginia Woolf for a new collected edition of her works. He also talked me into becoming a member of the editorial committee of the new edition. And then he urged me to begin working on the annotations right away. The friend who had begun writing me daily letters while I was in intensive care had continued to do this, and he too recognized the importance of keeping me involved in the life I had known. He knew my friend was going to make this request, and he wrote:

> When he sees you on Friday to tell you that he is going to accept Blackwell's offer to edit Woolf's works and asks you to take part in the editing, you are going to accept. That's an order. Thank him and say that you will do what you can. No excuses, apologies, shilly-shallying, or modest hesitations: just accept. Of course, at the moment you can't help at all; but in a year or more when the project is launched, you may be able to help a great deal.

How could I refuse?

Initially, as they knew, I could no more annotate a novel than I could peel a banana; but having the project to think about proved to be marvelously therapeutic. Their faith in my eventual recovery, while it then seemed overly hopeful, was also important to me. Later, when I was able to work on the annotations, I felt myself meeting again one of my familiar, lost selves. Like the letters, the edition became a significant part of the process of recovery.

Although it seemed foolhardy to be doing so, I began at this time, again with the help of friends, to plan the renovations my two-story house would require if I were to return home. No one could say when, or indeed if, I would be able to do so, but planning for it helped me to resist giving in to my condition. If I could at least imagine myself functioning again in the normal world, I might eventually be able to do so. I had more hope of recovery than did some of my doctors. One told me I would never walk again, another that I would probably never come off the respirator. Yet I could not accept these predictions, especially when no diagnosis of my illness had been made. I had walked and breathed before; surely I could do so again.

> It's certain there is no fine thing
> Since Adam's fall but needs much labouring.[9]

Another turning point came when, near the end of February, I was moved to the hospital's rehabilitation unit. While I was glad to leave behind the room in which I had spent the last two months, I was also deeply apprehensive about what lay ahead. If I failed to meet the rigorous demands of the rehab unit, I would, like Mrs. Bax in the bed across from mine, be imprisoned in this room again. The doctor in charge of rehab optimistically expected me to spend six months in the unit and then return to my renovated house. Fortunately, she was correct.

The move to the rehabilitation unit comes back to me as a transition from shadows to

Rehab

light, from stasis to movement. It was the beginning of the *nostos*, the return. I was dressed in my own clothes, not a hospital gown, since being dressed thus was one of the requirements of the unit. I had moved from the ninth floor to the first, and my bed beside the windows faced a large mirror. Thus, either way I looked, I saw the wide expanse first of the white frozen lake, soon of the shimmering water. On clear afternoons, the room was filled with sunshine.

The rehab staff bristled with energy, enthusiasm, and good humour. They worked as a team, and their job was less to care for the ill than to help the convalescent recover as much mobility and independence as possible. I felt I had come into a community of healers in which I was expected to take an active part; in this encouraging atmosphere, my fear that I would not be able to do so soon began to abate.   *— help w/ suffering*

They rigged me up in a special wheelchair with a platform on the back for the respirator, and I was no longer confined to one room. Therapists had come to me before; now I was taken to them. These sessions were the central activities of the day. An occupational therapist again gave me exercises designed to improve my coordination. The physical therapists concentrated on helping me recover my ability to walk. I was fitted with plastic shoehorn braces which in time enabled me to take a few steps, using a walker for support.

The friend who was writing me daily letters commented in one, written soon after I had been moved to the rehab unit, on the physical effort this therapy was requiring:

> *March 1, 1989*
>
> *When I saw you yesterday, I knew that you were too tired for a visit. You looked very tired, and I worry now that physiotherapy may be too physically exhausting for you. . . . Still, your nurses must know what you can take and profit by. I know that in muscle-building, one must stretch the muscle painfully so that it will reheal, and reheal more strongly. Or perhaps the new routine is tiring and you may take some weeks to become adjusted.*

helped by suffering

As he predicted, I did soon begin to adjust to the new routine, and after a few weeks I found my strength and stamina increasing.

Learning to walk was possible only because I began to spend time off the respirator. I was allowed to decide for myself how much time I would spend breathing on my own, and I turned this into a sort of contest as I extended the time from a few minutes to an hour, to several hours at a time, then ultimately to the entire day. This was the most exhausting and difficult thing I did. At first, because I had to remind myself to breathe, I could think of little else. Every breath was an event. I learned how to talk by plugging the opening of the tracheotomy tube with my finger and thus began to have conversations again. Recovering the ability to speak, even in this limited fashion, was like receiving a wonderful gift.

After several months, I acquired an electric wheelchair; and since by then I was unshackled from the respirator during the daytime, I could move about on my own. I experienced some of the pleasure I had enjoyed when driving a car as I propelled myself up and down the hospital corridors and out onto the adjacent patio. Once the warm weather arrived, I ventured further, going with other patients to the park for lunch, and even, once, racing my roommate in her electric wheelchair up the steep driveway leading to the hospital's emergency entrance. For the first time during my hospital stay, I was around patients who were getting better. Now that I could talk again, I could get to know some of them and share the frustrations and the rewards of rehabilitation. —help w/ suffering

I described these changes and some others in a letter written at the end of April to my friend in Colorado:

> i'm spending most of the day not hooked up to the ventilator. this gives me more freedom to move around in my electric wheelchair and has led them to decide to replace this trach with a smaller one which should enable me to talk more normally. they'll ventilate me a different way at night. i sure hope this works. the doctors never expected me to make this sort of progress.
>
> i'm having the addition built on the back of the house. the goal is to go home in august. i'm also trying to line up attendant care and funding to pay for at least part of it. a complex business. i'd rather be sailing.
>
> yes, i have a splendid view from my room. one wall is all windows and they give me a good view of the lake. there are also a sunroom and a patio that face the lake. i enjoy watching it and, now, the seagulls, swallows, and other birds. have yet to see a seagull land in a tree.
>
> did i tell you i was elected a fellow of the royal society of canada. a nice honor and a real surprise.

I was glad to be able to tell her some good news, for a month earlier I had had quite the opposite to report:

> i have to convey the very sad news that my father died on sunday. the cancer had spr ed and he was in a lot of pain so it's good that he didn't have to suffer longer. i've talked with mother on the phone and she seems to be doing well. it's very difficult for me, as you can imagine, to be unable to be there. what can i say. i can't do anything but sit here and think. though i don't have the consolation of family and action, i do have good friends, as you know, who have been in to see me. that is certainly a help.

His death enlarges enormously the grief i already feel, I added, *for all i've lost.*

The development of my father's illness had coincided with that of my own. I spoke earlier of the ways in which illness takes us out of our ordinary lives and into an alien territory. One of the ironies of this forced journey, of course, is the fact that the life from which we are physically exiled continues to make enormous emotional demands upon us. My concern with my father's deteriorating health and its effects on my mother, whose health was also fragile, had increased the stress I was under as my own condition mysteriously worsened. In addition, we were 500 miles apart, and unable to help or see one another.

Although the spring brought the loss of my father, there were some gains at this time, too, for not long after his death my mother was able to visit me in the hospital and to see for herself that I was getting better. As I slowly recovered, some of the selves that had seemed lost to me a few months before returned. This was also part of the recovery of the familiar. Illness defamiliarizes, as our relationship with our body and with the world around us undergoes a radical change, During recuperation, I could feel these relationships changing again.

Not only was I beginning to recover lost abilities, and thus experiencing a return of old selves, I was also becoming accustomed both to the effects of my illness and to life in the hospital. I began to understand how long-term patients may come to feel at home in the hospital and uneasy when away from its protective environment. The unfamiliar had become familiar, and the new selves created in response to illness and to being a patient were now a part of me, too. The relationships among new selves and old shifted continually. When I was taken for rides by friends and visited familiar places, I felt a clash of these selves, which made me acutely aware of how far I had yet to go before I would reach a full recovery. I was like one who returns to a fondly remembered place and finds it all changed. Only in this case, the change was in me.

[handwritten margin notes: like dinner away from camp]

After excursions away from the hospital, I would return with both regret and relief to my familiar, protective room. Part of the rehabilitation process involves breaking free of the habits and expectations of the patient. The process of relinquishing independence that began when I entered the hospital had now to be reversed. This was harder than I could have imagined, both because I was still seriously disabled and because that disabling and the months I had spent being cared for by others had eroded my self-confidence. This would slowly return, however, as I learned again how to do things for myself.

Near the end of my hospital stay, my illness was finally diagnosed as a rare form of Guillain-Barré syndrome. The diagnosis was encouraging, for if one has survived the low point in this illness and has begun to recover, as I had, continuing recovery is likely. Nerves regenerate slowly, and nerve damage may remain, but at least regeneration occurs. My slow progress confirmed this.

Also during this period the tracheotomy tube was removed and a small plug put in its place (this was removed a year later). Liberated from that invasive tube, I could now talk and breathe more easily. The respirator remained a part of my life, however, for I then began to wear at night (as I continue to do now) a nose mask attached by a long tube to the respirator, which pumps room-air to supplement my breathing while I sleep. Though bothersome, this method of ventilation is a walk in the park compared to being linked to a respirator by a tracheotomy tube. The mask comes off in the morning; the tube was a permanent fixture.

Now that I was recovering, I became more involved in the practical aspects of my life. First one friend, and then another, had since November been taking care of my financial concerns with power of attorney. These concerns had become more prominent once I decided to have the addition put on the house. I then had to worry about financing not only the addition, but the special equipment and attendant care I would need to live in it. These expensive needs introduced me to a complex world of agencies and programs I had known nothing about. I was extremely fortunate to have able guidance thorough this bureaucratic maze, as well as ample insurance coverage and sufficient funds to cover my costs. I began to feel that I was directing a small business as I attempted, with much help, to organize my much altered life.

As the time for my discharge from the hospital at the end of August neared, I was eager and apprehensive at the same time. What had seemed impossible only a few months ago was about to take place. I was going home.

Distance had an extraordinary power.[10]

Anyone who has taken a long journey knows how complex homecoming can be. For a time, one lives in two worlds. The familiar world to which one has returned is seen through eyes that are still looking back to where one has been. The backward glance highlights the pleasure of the return, but it also distracts and defamiliarizes, as illness does. Only in time do the once familiar routines of daily life become habits again. My backward glance was not only toward the hospital, but also beyond that to my life before becoming ill. I found I had a double adjustment to make: first to living outside the hospital and secondly—and this was the more difficult one—to living at home with the constraining disabilities of illness.

For a while, intense pleasure at being home alternated with unanticipated bouts of unhappiness as I confronted, in this new context, the contrast between my present and my former condition. Undoubtedly, the death of my father, and that of my elderly dog, whose death in January I did not fully take in until I came home, played their parts in my unhappiness. In time, however, as the process of regaining strength and recovering lost abilities accelerated, my mood improved, and I began to feel genuinely at home again. More lost selves were coming back and reconciling with new ones.

It has taken me nearly three years to reach the point of wanting to put into writing my thoughts about being ill and about the ten months I spent in the hospital. I have been haunted by memories of those months and have often wondered how others who have undergone a traumatic experience live with its residue. One falls back on cliché: time is a great healer, or can be. Memories may not dim in time. Nor, in my experience, does the fear of becoming seriously ill again go away. But if one is fortunate enough to be restored to a happier life, new layers of memories provide a kind of cushion for the past.

My continuing recovery has also made memories of those ten months less threatening. I have shed my leg braces and walker, and only use a cane when in crowded places. The electric wheelchair is parked in the garage, along with the car, which I can drive again. The small hole in my throat, a constant inconvenience and reminder of the past, has finally been closed surgically. Its closure brought an end to a long chapter in this story.

Writing about these events, shaping them into a narrative, has been for me a way of overcoming to some degree the isolation of illness. Imaginative literature is filled with characters who speak out of a need to express and share a profound experience, and thus to bear witness to what they have been through. "...and I only am escaped alone to tell thee," say a series of survivors at the opening of Job.[11] Such literary testaments, both fictional and autobiographical, assume and celebrate the value of the individual life. Being ill taught me, as being well had never done, how committed human beings can be to helping one another. Thoughts of the efforts made by all the people who touched my life during that time, and touch it now, are bright lights that continually play against, and keep in check, the shadows cast in memory by illness and loss.

Further, I am fortunate not only to have been given so much help in my recovery, but also to have regained so many of the abilities I had for a time lost. The simple pleasures of each ordinary day are now sweetened for me immeasurably by the knowledge of what life is like when they are gone.

NOTES

This piece was originally published in *Queen's Quarterly* 99(4) (Winter 1992).

1. Virginia Woolf, "On Being Ill," *Collected Essays,* ed. Leonard Woolf (London: Chatto & Windus, 1967), vol. 4, 193.
2. Virginia Woolf, *Orlando* (London: The Hogarth Press, 1970), 277.
3. T. S. Eliot, "Ash Wednesday," *The Complete Poems and Plays* (London: Faber and Faber, 1969), 90.
4. W. B. Yeats, "Nineteen Hundred and Nineteen," *The Collected Poems* (New York: The Macmillan Company, 1956), 205.
5. Samuel Beckett, *Proust* (New York: Grove Press, 1931), 16.
6. W. B. Yeats, "The Municipal Gallery Revisited," *The Collected Poems,* 318.
7. W. B. Yeats, "Meditations in Time of Civil War," *The Collected Poems,* 204.
8. Leonard Cohen, "Joan of Arc," *Songs of Love and Hate.*
9. W. B. Yeats, "Adam's Curse," *The Collected Poems,* 78.
10. Virginia Woolf, *To the Lighthouse* (Oxford: Shakespeare Head Press, Blackwell, 1992), 159.
11. Job I: 15, 16, 17, 19.

QUESTIONS

1. How might the reader trace the effects of Guillain-Barré syndrome by reading only the author's journal entries and letters?
2. The author expresses profound gratitude for simple accommodations when she is ill. When someone is in a state of such poor health, what are the most important necessities to provide?
3. Comment on the author's tone in this essay. How does it reflect or belie her conclusions about her illness experience?

Bone Scan

ᐸ Ellen Goldsmith ᐳ

Lying on
the imaging table
with the gamma camera
moving the length of my body
first below, then above
I remember stretching out
on freshly fallen snow
in Sharon Abrams' backyard
my arms swimming
carefully up and down

Here in this room of magical instruments
various and silent as snowflakes
where I'm not allowed to move
I am again that girl whose body
pressed an empty field
with one perfect angel
after another

On the Lake

Years ago, we canoed on Lake Placid,
me in the bow, my first physical effort
after the surgery. I remember the ease
of our glide, how quietly we traveled
along the near shore, then, feeling safe,
headed out to the islands. In the middle
of the lake, with no warning, the wind
came up. Paddling hard for a long time,
my arms aching, we were held in place.
I resisted asking if we'd make it back.

QUESTIONS

1. In the first poem, what is the connection in the author's mind between her current position and making snow angels as a child?
2. The second poem can be read literally and metaphorically. How does a metaphorical reading enrich the reader's understanding of the poet's point?
3. Comment on the poet's choice of form for each poem.

Shaman

⟜ LYNDA HALL ⟜

It is rubber, a red rubber skeleton, about ten inches long, and he raps it repeatedly against the coffee table. Her lips move. Words come repeatedly. She smiles, pats his head absently, smoothes down his hair.

Shaman enters the room, majestically, nose in the air. Her hair bristles. The boy makes a lunge for her, but misses. He has obviously hurt her in the past, to get this reaction.

Shaman leaps onto my lap, settles down in the sun.

Her lips move. Let me know when you want me to go. I don't want to take up your time.

He raps the skeleton against the table again. Its rubbery body bends, makes a thud, thud.

Sun shines into the family room, on to my lap. Shaman repeatedly digs her claws contentedly into my legs through the corduroy. She purrs softly. I drift in a dream, hypnotized by the soft purr, the soft words.

"Rupert Junior, tell Auntie about the white rabbit in your play school."

Auntie. Auntie. To all my friend's children. They keep me young. Are the only measure of time, in this timeless space of mine. Play school. Grade one. Time goes so quickly. Time doesn't move at all. Her eyes flash. Her voice is soft. Time passes. She refills her wineglass. The sun makes it gleam, red, sparkling, sparkling off Shaman's grey coat. The winter sun sinks slowly. The afternoon disappears.

She sighs. "Well, I must go. And make supper. For Rupert Senior and Rupert Junior. Schedules must be kept."

But she lingers.

Shaman's eyes watch the sun flashing beams from her glass onto the carpet. The sun is warm. I feel drowsy.

Her lips move. She will be thirty-five on her next birthday. Barely had Rupert Junior in time. But it is necessary, isn't it? Wasn't it? Children. To lead a full life. Carry on.

Fragments of speech break the silence. Continuously. Christmas in Ottawa was cold, no electricity, no way to cook the turkey. But they had to go, didn't they? Rupert's parents always expect them for Christmas. They had to go, didn't they? Her eyes flash.

Shaman blinks her blue eyes open. Digs in her nails, rhythmically. Is it a dream? Her lids close again, and she is still.

She fingers her silver silk blouse. Stands up. Runs her fingers down the perfect seam in her mauve woolen slacks.

This is what I wanted, isn't it? She says. Or is it me? Or do I just see the question in her eyes?

No more sun. It is gone.

The nurse walks over to me briskly, smells of the cold outdoor air. Her hands are cold against my arm, her fingers efficiently hold my wrist. She pours a can of Ensure into the plastic bag, runs it up the chrome pole. I watch it slowly drip down into the tube, my life force.

Her shift is from five to midnight. Easy. Not much to do. Two more cans of Ensure. Two doses of Demerol. One dose of Valium. All according to schedule.

Easy. Empty my waste bags. If needed. So regulated. Take in. Give out.

She discusses the hockey game last night. The Calgary Flames lost to the Oilers three points to five. It was too good to last, that winning streak.

She puts on one of my Talking Books—*The Diviners*, by Margaret Laurence. Do I know Margaret Laurence just died, at only sixty? Then her eyes are cast down; she looks guilty, like them all. They have to watch their speech, don't they? Don't they?

She settles in front of the television with earphones on. Watches the news, and works at her petit point. It is a vest, with delicate flowers, so delicate. Every twenty minutes she comes and changes the tape. Easy. At seven o'clock she picks me up from the chair, all eighty pounds, and places me on the couch. Carefully working around all of my tubes, she tucks in a knit blanket, green and yellow. A broomstick knit blanket. The pillow is soft under my cheek. We both watch TV.

Delicate flowers grow under her fingers.

Delicate flowers blow all around us. We look down the mountainside, spring flowers covering in purple, like a blanket. She rips a piece off the loaf of Russian rye, and hands it to me, with a piece of strong yellow cheese. We sit on a log, looking down from the mountains onto Lake Geneva, so blue, shimmering below us. The wine bottle slowly empties.

An old white-bearded man passes us, bent over, leading a donkey pulling an old wooden cart overflowing with hay. Timelessness engulfs us.

We shoulder our packs and make our way back to the stop for the sky tram. The car arrives and we step in, slowly making the ascent. Two schoolchildren get on, books in hand, pigtails waving along with their excited voices. The valley rises toward us.

The bus lurches, the radio blares in German, voices are excited around us. Tears. Finally someone tells us. Three Israeli wrestlers have just been killed at the Olympic Village. Her eyes look wild, in pain. The bus is stopped at the border, our passports checked. A fellow dressed in white, dark, like an Arab, is rushed off the bus by the uniforms, into a building. He is returned two hours later, silent, and the bus rolls on.

Lucerne is neat, clean. We eat at a second-floor cozy restaurant. I hold the roast chicken leg in my fingers, and along with the other customers we watch the black and white screen, repeating the terror.

The wine doesn't make it go away.

The morning is bright. Sun gleams off the snow. Hurts my eyes. The nurse has just flung open the drapes on the French doors leading off from my bedroom. Whiskey jacks flutter around the bird feeder on my deck. Seeds fly. Shaman blinks her eyes at the sudden light. Looks at me. Looks at the whiskey jacks. Saunters out of the room, after brushing her whiskers against my ear.

The nurse plunges the Demerol into the feeder tube, after crushing it up and dissolving it in water. I feel the familiar rush of the liquid against my esophagus. I wait for the relief. It takes twenty-five minutes to work. A needle is faster. Immediate. But I don't like needles.

She pulls the top off the can of Ensure, like opening a can of nuts. The noise. She pours the liquid. Pink. So it is strawberry today. If I could taste. But the tube goes directly into my stomach.

I forget what a strawberry would taste like. It doesn't matter. Really. Really! I hear the rush of water and smell the fragrance. Herbal. She returns to the room. Throws back my covers. Takes off my gown and lifts me gently in her arms. She lowers me into the water and leaves me to soak in the hot surging suds. It feels good.

The Jacuzzi roars. Suds tickle my nose. I sneeze. I sneeze. She rushes in. Relief washes over her eyes. She cares. I guess. She cares. I know. She has had the morning shift for eight months. I miss her on her two days off. I miss her strong arms. Her caring eyes. When she isn't here, I miss her. She lays me on the bathroom table and performs her usual ritual. Dries me off. Applies the oil. Rubs me. Rotates her hands on my back. Squeezes my toes. Massages my neck.

I float. Dream. Relax. Luxuriate. My favorite time of the day. I love her hands. I don't want this time to end. I am lost. In time and space. For the time. Lost.

What? Tears? Happy or sad? You aren't ever depressed. Why now? I hear her voice. Or do I? She wipes up the tears. The metal apparatus lunges above me, the food bag hanging empty. The metal apparatus always over me, like a cross, gleaming in the sun. Tears? I don't know whether I'm sad. And I couldn't tell her if I did know.

She strums her guitar. Sings softly. Crooning. She never talks a lot. Usually sings. Varies from Joan Baez songs, the same as she sang them fifteen years ago, to Tina Turner's latest. Her memory is marvelous. She laughs, imitates Janis Joplin: "I could use some company. On this road. On this road I'm on today."

Shaman lies on my lap and purrs louder than usual. She knows I am at peace.

She says: "This is a new song. I'm playing it tonight for the first time." Her head lowered and her hair hiding her face, she sings: "When there's anger. Out of control. Hate is fire. Love is stone." Hair on the back of my neck rises. My spine tingles.

She says: "I hope I am playing what you would like. I sometimes wish you could talk. Often. I wish." I think she says that. Or maybe she said it last week. Her blonde hair falls over her shoulder, glowing in the sunlight. Her eyes are closed, as she moans out the blues. Like Melissa Etheridge, on her record. "Am I Blue?"

Screech, Screech. Screech. The mike blares. McMahon Stadium is packed. Janis Joplin grips the mike. Grates out her songs. Peers through those crazy glasses. "Me and Bobby McGee." Her thick hair flies, red in the sun. She leans on the turf beside me. Drags deeply on her cigarette.

Strums her guitar during breaks. Nudges me with her moccasin. She's on a death trip. That
one. She says. Or did she?

Janis swears, obscene: "It's 1969. And this is where it's at. There may not be a tomorrow.
There most definitely will not be another '60s."

The afternoon is hot. I sip my Coke. Sketch the girl near me, poncho raised over the nurs-
ing head of a denim-clothed baby. I'll soon be twenty. Out of university. In the world. It seems
so far away. The world. The stadium crowd roars. The crowd roars.

Flour flies in the air. Her white hands professionally crack an egg and drop it in the bowl.
She scratches her nose, leaving a white patch. Verdi's *Aida* floats through the air. Her chubby
hands flow through the air, the mock conductor, sending hunks of dough around the room.
"I love this, I love this," she chants.

Shaman eyes her suspiciously, sniffs at a piece of dough that has landed on my lap, and
then ignores it. The kitchen is cozy, warm. She prepares for her dinner party tonight. Often cooks in my kitchen while I watch. If I squint my eyes she almost looks like my mother,
chubby, flour flying. Her energy pervades the air. "Shirley MacLaine looks younger every
year. This *Out on a Limb* would interest you. Part Two is on TV tonight. You and your other
lives would just eat it up."

She laughs, scallops the edges of the dough around the pie plate, places the pie in the
oven, rips off her apron, and seats herself at the table, eyeing me as though for the first time
today. "I now have reason to believe in reincarnation myself. Believe that this isn't all."

She reaches out and straightens my head against the metal brace. "Your crazy ideas of
transitions, separation of mind and body, incorporation of our spirits in a larger whole,
everlasting life, all that. I don't know. I thought I did." She sips her iced mint tea, rubs her
forehead. "You know, this party tonight, I don't know. I really don't know. Well, anyway, it
maintains the women's network, the business contacts. Not exactly the old motherhood
and apple pie, is it?"

She laughs. "Sisterhood and apple pie." She checks the oven, sits again. The gleam of the
ice in her tea makes my stomach gurgle. How long has it been? Two and a half years since
anything has passed down my throat. The occasional chips of ice placed on my tongue do
not quite do it! I long so for a cool drink, for a hot drink, for a taste. . . .

The doctor is efficient. She is gentle. Her stethoscope is warming in her hand, then she
applies it to my chest, writes on her pad. "We might as well increase the Demerol. Why not?
Eh? Why not? And the Valium." What are friends for, after all?

There once was a mistaken notion that Pandora's box contained hope, but Pandora
knew better.

She brushes Shaman's forehead with her knuckles. "Look, can you believe that?" She
points with her elbow at the small black-and-white TV on the cupboard. A big boot steps
off the last step and onto the surface of the moon. Some things aren't meant to happen.
She says.

Or is it me? A pleasant aroma fills the air. I breathe deeply. Some things aren't meant
to happen.

I lie on the hot sand, soak up the heat. She pants beside me, propped against her surfboard. Her kinky blonde hair is plastered again her head. She laughs. The salt water dries white on my sunburnt skin. I wake up and watch the colorful parasails above, and the people dangling from the ropes. Surfing takes all my energy. I am shot after.

She comes toward me, waving two ice cream cones. Bubble gum ice cream. An obscene blue. She laughs as she licks drips of blue off her dimpled cheek. She shakes her head in refusal to a blanket-laden peddler, and kneels in the sand. "We are going to celebrate tonight!" She laughs.

A waiter just told her the president has ordered the troops out of Vietnam. She laughs. I go to the shower. Wash the sand out of my bikini bottoms, wash away the surf.

The Acapulco sunset reddens the sky as we sip margaritas on the balcony. Waiters come and go. Surfers are glowing, silhouetted in the moonlight. Tourist boats pass off-shore, laden with passengers forgetting the world back home. Forgetting. Waves crash on the shore, silver. Two surfers rush out of the water, between crests of wavers, and sink on the beach in the dark.

The waiter comes around to each table with free "green stings"—shots of straight tequila, followed by crème de menthe and 7-Up. The whole room claps as she tosses hers back.

The night shift nurse arrives at five to twelve. I hear her talk quietly to the evening nurse, and the front door close. She enters on tiptoe. I close my eyes. I sense her come close to check my breathing and hear the familiar noise of her pouring the Ensure into the bag. Then she is gone. I can't sleep. I can't sleep. I don't know why.

Tomorrow is Friday. If it is Friday it must be . . . If it is Friday it must be . . . I can't remember. I should be able to. I am so tense. Who is my regular visitor on Friday? Who takes the Friday shift from two until five, relieving the nurses? Who? Why can't I remember?

The night nurse returns. The digital clock gleams 2:30. She plunges the Demerol into the tube.

And another. Must be a sleeping pill. Yes!

Let me go. Let me go.

Drums beat. Like the pulse of my blood. Shaman stands in front of the campfire, eyes red, watching me. Smoke encircles her. Smoke rises from the fire. All is warm, until the sunset. Drums beat. Shaman floats in the rising smoke. My protector. My healer. My magical guardian spirit. I am going into the sun.

Shaman's breath is cool on my skin, softly blowing evil spirits away. I am going into the sun. Drums beat. Freeze me in a trance. In no space. In no time. Transitions. My spirit surges.

The sun drops below the horizon. Shaman purrs. A soft warm chant. I awake. Limbs numb. Shaman's grey coat glistens from the foot of the bed. Glistens in my dream.

Sun beats down on us. A hot wind blows over, straight from Africa, they say. The ruins surround us on every side. We stand and watch the archaeologists as the guide describes the current dig. Sweat drips between my breasts. Her figure is outlined in sweat against her white top and shorts, her bra-less condition drawing occasional attention from other tourists and from the workers. The site dates back to 1100 B.C. We view the tile design, created so long ago.

I stick to the seat of the tour bus. The guide has a master's degree in Greek history. This is a profession for her. She spent a year at Boston University. The tour bus stops at an isolated beach. We strip under a set of low palms, feet sinking into the sand. The guide is much darker than we are. Her black eyes gleam. Her small strips of white glare while she steps into her bikini.

We rush into the water, the warm water. The Mediterranean water seems to make us float. We swim out. Crete disappears behind us, till we return.

The shower is warm, but removes the salt water, and we once again step into soggy clothes. The man in the little hut at the beach doesn't speak English, but he pops open Cokes we choose, and points at the thermometer. It is 110°F in the shade. The guide comes back, rushes up to us.

She heard it on the radio, on the bus. The president has been killed. John Kennedy is dead. Palm trees rustle in the hot breeze. The bus bumps along.

She enters the room, but not as jaunty as usual. Her canvas bag is heavy; she thumps it down on the floor. She smiles at me weakly. Takes my hand. Now I remember. One week ago. She said: "It is over. I will do it next week."

Now I remember. She is going to do it. They told me. They would draw straws. They didn't even know if I understood. But I did. These friends of mine. Had a meeting. Had a meeting. Like so many months ago. When they had a meeting and set up my daily schedule, the nurses, the visitations, when I would get my daily massage. They had a meeting. And drew straws.

Now I know. She got the short straw.

Shaman sits on my lap, ears erect, hair bristling.

She sits before me, holds my hand. "I wish I knew what you wanted. I wish you could talk. I wish we could have done better." She drops my hand. Tears in her eyes.

She is blurry. I see her crush up four pills, mix them in water, draw the liquid into the plunger. Her hands are shaking. She places the end of the plunger in my feed tube.

She is blurry. There are tears in my eyes. I see her shoulders shaking. I see her blue eyes, blurry.

I hear.

I think I hear:

"I can't. I can't. I can't."

I don't know what I hear. I don't know what I hear.

I watch her sink to the floor, lie sobbing. Then she gets up. Her cheek is against mine, tears wet between us. She takes the plunger to the bathroom. I hear her washing it out. She comes back.

Places the Melissa Etheridge tape in the recorder. Lets it blare. She says: "I taped this last night. At the concert at the Jube. It was illegal, but I did it for you." She laughs, her head thrown back, blue eyes clear.

Sun shines into the family room, onto my lap. Shaman repeatedly digs her claws contentedly into my legs through the corduroy, brushed her moist cheek against my wrist. I drift in a dream, hypnotized by the soft purr, the soft words.

QUESTIONS

1. How does the author represent the state of mind of the ill person?
2. Comment on the literal and symbolic function of the cat Shaman.
3. Discuss the various ways time is altered for people who are ill.
4. Discuss the implications of the story's conclusion.

32 y/o Single Female with
Stage IV Breast Cancer

⌒ Laurie Rosenblatt (with Juanita Jones) ⌒

Juanita Jones was a woman of my own age. I met her when she volunteered to be interviewed for research that Victoria Alexander and I were conducting on women's perspectives of stage IV cancer. I first interviewed Juanita at the home she shared with her partner, Debbie, and two enthusiastic dogs. Juanita was a lively, angry, no-bullshit woman who didn't pull her punches when speaking about the ways in which cancer and treatment confronted her with (at times) unbearable losses, overwhelming fear, and changes/challenges to her sense of self. She refused to sanitize her experiences by making them less confusing and painful or more transcendent than they actually were.

Victoria and I took the interview with Juanita and edited it into this monologue. We have tried to preserve her voice. When Juanita approached death, she wanted her story available to help others navigate these difficult waters. She and her partner did not want this story shorn of identifying features; they wanted it to stand as a memorial to Juanita's life and character, and her manner of meeting adversity.

—Laurie Rosenblatt, MD

⌒ ⌒

I just got some test results Friday that showed that my lung and my bone metastases actually looked better than they have, except I now have a tumor in my right breast that's pretty big. And I have a spot on my liver. I didn't know it was there before, because most of the time it's been too small to know what it was. And that's the agreement I have with my oncologist; if I don't need to obsess about it, I don't really want to know.

But it has doubled in size in eight weeks, so they have me on a new therapy called gemcitabine, and I'm going to try to get into a new vaccine trial. And I guess tomorrow I'll find out whether or not they are going to remove my breast. I want it off because it looks really weird, and it's weird to know that right underneath there is this tumor growing. Plus, that would give the researchers a lot of tumor to work with in making a vaccine. So I want them to take it out because then I may be able to get a vaccine.

I can't imagine how much worse the bad news could be. You know what I mean? My liver, come on. That is not where you want it to be. Not that I want it to be anywhere, but you don't want it there. I don't know anybody who, once it has gone to their liver, has gotten better. I guess there is still part of me that thinks I am going to get better, so I guess now that part of me is like, "Wow, okay, guess I'm not going to get better."

I think I am a little depressed. All weekend I was just like, "I am really sorry, but I just have to take some Percocet." You know what I mean? I just needed to zone out. And I don't so much feel that way now. Of course I had chemotherapy yesterday, but I feel extremely tired, and just exhausted, like I could sleep for days.

And Friday I wanted to sleep, but I couldn't sleep, so I had to take something to make me sleep. Today, I don't think I would have to take anything.

And I'm supposed to be watching for shortness of breath. I don't know why they would say that because it is like telling somebody, "Don't think about red shoes." Because I'm going, "Okay, that was a good one, okay, that's okay." Like I can't stop thinking about breathing. But I'm glad I'm on chemotherapy. It was kind of tough there for a couple of weeks not having chemo. I didn't like it. I wasn't doing anything, didn't feel like I was doing anything, and the metastases were getting bigger. And they weren't really getting bigger, but I don't want to give them any chance to regroup, to get their act together.

My friend called. . . . I don't know if you were here when she called. She's an architect, and we were supposed to study and finish our degrees together, but I don't know if I can do that. I don't know if I have the strength. . . . God that's hard. I'm sure it's tantamount to going to medical school or whatever. You have to know your shit inside and out. It's mostly to stress you out. But I have been feeling a lot better about doing things that I want to do, like art, like I'm going to that drawing class. I'm just making myself do stuff, so that I don't just lay in bed because I could do that. I could just be so depressed. I don't think that's good.

Then sometimes I'm thinking, "Why am I doing this to myself?" I don't know, and I don't think I'm going to do it actually. Here's the deal. At this point in my career I can work for another architect. The only thing I need is someone to stamp my work, which is not unlike working for a firm. Many architects don't bother to get registered. So, what would it get me to get my degree? Well it would get me a certain amount of respect, but respect from whom, the billing department? No, they respect no one. Contractors? No, they don't respect anyone, especially a woman. So who do I want this for, just me? I think I can live without that because I am doing projects, and I have a kind of thing set up with a friend of mine who has the degree. And if I got really sick and couldn't continue the project, she would just take it over. So that's good. So that makes me feel like I can work, as much as I'm able to, which is important to me. So I don't know. My friend is coming here to study.

It was a goal that I always wanted to achieve, and despite all the bullshit, fuck it, I did it. Yes, that is definitely an element, but I think the bigger element is that I don't want to spend time that I could be being with Debbie, or taking the dogs for a walk. Studying physics? I like physics and everything, but no, I don't want to do that. And I don't feel bad that I don't . . . I had a really hard time these past couple months, and I don't know what resolved it actually, probably this liver thing, about feeling legitimate, like legitimate in the field of architecture, and legitimate just in a lot of ways. Because all my peers are now getting degrees, and it's about that time. And it just feels . . . it's hard for me to be happy for them. I am happy for them, but I'm jealous too.

My friend May died three weeks ago. She was like a super person, and I mean like Wonder Woman or something. She just did so much for so many people. She worked for health care for the homeless and she was a counselor, and she didn't stop working until two weeks before she died. She worked all the way—work was very important to her, her clients. They really had nobody but her. But I think I am a little more selfish than that. I want to have some of my own time. It made me sad that May worked so long, but if it made her happy that's fine. But it did make me realize that I don't want to work till the end; I don't want to do that. I'd rather go to Europe. I don't know.

After May died, my support group meetings were heavy. They wanted to break up. I'm like, "What?" I was so furious. I'm like, "Oh yeah, May dies, you all leave. What am I, chopped liver?" So it started this whole thing about staying until you die, and what does it mean when you join this group. It is for life, really. I guess I knew that that would happen. Well I knew it would happen because my therapist told me that that would happen, that something would happen in the group. There would be some radical shift. I just didn't think it would be like that. Now they are all going to leave me, great.

Everybody in the group finally decided that they would come back in January because December is a bad month because not everyone could be there. And come back in January and talk about it some more, about whether leaving was really the right thing, or bringing in new members, or what. But May had been in the group for four years. It was me and a couple other women started the group. May was one of the first members. The group took a while to shake out, to be what we wanted it to be, but now we have an excellent therapist who runs it, and I just think it would be so sad to let it go at this point in the game.

You know, I'm assuming I'm going to be the next one. But it seems to me that . . . because everyone said they had been thinking about leaving the group before May died, but they didn't want to leave it until May died because they knew May was going to die, and I'm like, "Where was I?" Because I had no clue she was going to die. I saw her every group. I don't know, maybe other people have some sense that I don't have.

All of them, except for the three of us that started the group, were thinking of leaving the group. And it's interesting, it's because they all had issues with May. And finally I said, "Hey, hello, May's dead. She's not here anymore. Don't you think it would be worthwhile to talk about the issues that we had with her." I didn't have any issues with May because I'd known her for a long time. But I do know as she got sicker and sicker, kind of like the walls went up. She had brain metastases, so sometimes she would be a little scary. Not scary, but that little filter that says, "I'm thinking this, not saying it out loud." And like that wouldn't work always. So she would say things that you would think, not say. I thought they were funny, but whatever. A lot of people took it personally.

And she was definitely the strongest member of the group emotionally. I don't think I ever saw her cry. I cried in the group every single week. It's just what I do. And she always wanted to sit beside me, and I think it's because she had emotions via me. So I didn't have any problems with her. But you would think that the fact that she is gone would make people want to kind of stick around and at least talk, instead of like running away. Like that doesn't seem like closure to me. Correct me if I'm wrong.

I think they are all afraid that they can't stay in the group . . . I know that one person especially who said that . . . that that's her big fear, that she is not going to be able to leave this group until everybody is dead because we are all heading down that road.

I mean most people are really, really sick. And so I don't know what makes us do this group. Certainly, having new members come in, to me seems like a great idea, but then I can see how that would scare them shitless. There are some really very, very ill people in this group. Sometimes I'm one of them. Sometimes this other woman is one of them. And then there is another woman who, she is in constant pain, and you can just see it. Her face is so contorted with pain, it is hard to watch. She has had ribs removed and part of her lung, and a colostomy, and just so many parts of her are out, and it has to hurt, especially the rib thing. So I don't know about bringing in new people.

⌒ ⌒

I had a pleural effusion, so I had to have that drained, and ended up in ICU because my lung collapsed, and then I stopped breathing, and they didn't know my lung collapsed, and then I puked into the little thing, and I aspirated it, it was just ugly. And it was a lot of days in the hospital. But I lost like thirty pounds; it was great. I was like, "Damn, thank God for that pleural effusion."

But seriously, I was out of it for most of it, so I don't really remember, but I do remember Debbie and my primary care doctor. I just remember waking up vaguely when I was on the breathing machine and Debbie was just crying and crying. I'm like, "Oh fuck, am I going to die or what?" But I didn't, and I got off that machine, which was pretty amazing they thought because they didn't think I would. They don't know that I took yoga. I've been doing healthy yoga for years, so I just breathed. They said you are not breathing on your own, and I was like, "Oh, all right, well I can fix that." And I just started breathing deep into my belly, then filling up the bottom of my lungs, and just really concentrated on it. And I was off of the thing in like twenty minutes, so that was good.

I think that I am lucky I didn't die. I don't know what would have happened if I didn't . . . my surgeon came in to see me, and he looked really scared. And I had this tube down my throat and I was flipping out because I didn't want this in my throat, and so I would write on his hand, "How do I get off this?" And it was kind of funny because he knew what I was doing. I'd be like spelling it out. And he was like, "You have to be able to breathe on your own, and right now you can't do that." And I said, "Okay, so how long should it take me to breathe on my own?" And he said, "Well it could take a couple of days, maybe longer." I'm thinking, "I have to have this frigging thing in my throat for that long, no thank you."

You have this huge thing going down your throat, and it just feels like there is this thing going down your throat, and they had also these things going down my nose into my stomach. That didn't feel any better, and the other thing was that they had my arms and legs tied down. And let me tell you, that's not a way you want to wake up, even if there is nothing down your throat. I just was freaking out because I didn't know why there was this thing in my mouth. You can't communicate, and I just wanted it out. I thought, "My God, they are going to kill me." And you're choking on this thing. My surgeon kept saying, "If you relax you won't choke on it." And he was right because when I started to do the breathing and I relaxed it didn't bother me so much anymore. Maybe they ought to tell people that.

When I woke up I was like, "Aren't I supposed to be in my room?" Instead I was in this fishbowl thing, and I had a great nurse, she was great, no question, but it was just horrible. I just had these like blip memories of Debbie crying. I'm like, "Oh my God." The clearest memory I had was of my surgeon telling me that I had to breathe all by myself and I said, "I can do that," and he said, "Okay." And then ten minutes later they were like, "She's breathing by herself; we can take her off the machine." And he was like, "Oh my God, no, no, leave her on for another ten minutes." I was like, "Oh my God, I have to keep this shit on for another ten minutes." But yeah, I was off in twenty minutes. He was pretty amazed; he told me that it was really amazing. It made me feel good that I had some kind of control over what was going on.

I used to think that when I was dying I would want to be so out of it that I really wouldn't experience it. But I don't think that I want that anymore. I just want enough to take the edge off so I'm not freaking out. I think that's what I want. I certainly don't want it to be in a hospital.

After this last episode, I signed a DNI/DNR order and I had a will done out. I could have died—like seriously, that was a reality. Before, I never thought I would die. I said I was going to do a DNR when I went in for my bone marrow transplant, but at that point, I wasn't necessarily feeling like . . . I didn't want a DNR. I wanted to be R'd and I'd . . . you know what I mean? I was like, "Pull out all the stops; I don't want to die." But not that I don't . . . geez, this had made me wonder, if I did that "do not intubate" thing, if I had that thing before, would they have intubated me? That's scary because I think they should have intubated me.

I said that I did not want . . . I filled out all the paperwork so that I would not be resuscitated or intubated if . . . Well every time I go into the hospital they talk to me about that now, and I guess they talk to everyone about that. What I want to say to them is, "Look, if it's obvious that I'm going to die anyway, then obviously don't resuscitate me, but if there is a snowball's chance in hell that I might live, I want that chance." How can you say that?

What made me make the decision was when I got off the intubator and everybody told me how horrible it was and how scared they were, I thought, "Fuck, I could die, I could go into the operating room and not come out. I don't think that ever occurred to me before." Like I always thought I'd die. I don't know what I thought it would be, but I didn't think it would involve being in a hospital, or some snafu that happened, and whatever. So I guess realizing that made me think that I might not always be in control. Frankly, I don't know how you could tell somebody that, how you could say, without scaring the holy shit out of them, "Okay, you are going to have this operation; you could die." That doesn't work. I think that if somebody would have presented it to me in a way that made it feel like I would be more in control, because that's my thing, I would have been like, "Oh yeah, I'm all over that." Because there may be a time when whoever is there to make a decision for me does not have my best interest in mind. I don't know who that would be, but it could happen, so that also played a part in me doing the DNR things when I did. Because my parents were suddenly very involved and I thought, "I don't want them making any decisions about my health care because I don't trust them." Not that I don't trust them with my life, but I don't trust them to make an informed decision because they're not very savvy people, with all due respect. They are kind of like, they are jewelers, what the fuck do they know? They know a lot about jewelry, but they don't know a lot about this.

I have to say, when I was in getting my bone marrow transplant, they gave me this little packet when I got into the room, and I was all sterilized and everything. And it had all these things about being neutropenic and all this other kind of crap, and then there was a health-care proxy, and the forms to fill out for those kinds of things. And then I imagine you have to send it to your lawyer because I can't imagine if you just sign a piece of paper and it's okay, but whatever. Anyway, I looked at it and I thought, "I can't deal with this," but nobody talked to me about it. Maybe people don't think about it, especially people who like to be in control. It's more than being high. It's worse than that. You are so out of control. It's terrifying because at that point, I don't think your mind is really working for you. It's not working for you at all.

It's very interesting, most people experience themselves as their mind, not their body; it's so weird, but it's true. I think the first time I really felt like I was all one piece is after I had my mastectomy. I realized that I'm in my body, that I am my body, and it was the weirdest. I had to sit down. I was like, "Holy shit." I think I felt that more and more over time in this whole ordeal, but that was really the first time I ever felt that, that I realized my body had more of a say than maybe I wanted to give it credit for. I think it was the pain. It was very painful, and it was sad. It was sad to lose a piece of your body, a piece of my body, and it wasn't just because it was a breast, but it was a part of my body. A lot of people would say, "Well it's just your breast." What kind of cockamamie comment that is, I don't know. I would just think about, "Oh, it was there, now it's not." Like where did it go? I called up my surgeon and said, "What did you do with it?" And she was like, "Well, we froze it." And I was like, "Oh, I was going to say because if you were going to throw it away, I'd want it." I was thinking I would have a little burial for it in the backyard, but I just wanted to make sure that they didn't throw it away. I'm still sad about it, and I'm probably going to have to have this one taken out. At least I'll be symmetrical, but it isn't easy.

Yeah. It's sad.

I don't want to talk anymore.

QUESTIONS

1. Discuss the speaker's tone and its effect on the reader. Why does Rosenblatt record the words of her patient instead of telling the story herself?

2. Given the impulse of the support group to dissolve, discuss the relative benefits and drawbacks of such groups.

3. How does this narrative reflect or contradict stories of illness that one might expect in the media?

Seasons

a found poem after an encounter in the Diagnostic Pavilion

I rolled my patient gently over to her left side
And after unfastening her bra I
Placed my hand over her
Nipple and felt the thrust of her
Heart. "Oh dear" she said,
Feeling my hand riding a wave that was
Connected to an ebb and flow
In her chest, "What is that?"
"It's your heart," I said.
  "Oh dear."
That was Monday, and I stand here
Bent over her and now it is Saturday
Summer will soon be over
And already the jasmine will not flower
She is fast asleep
Her wig askew
And I worry that the seasons will
Drop away if I withdraw my hand &— *keep doing something (be active)*

—*Abraham Verghese*

Contributors

Henry Abramovitch is a clinical psychologist, medical anthropologist and Jungian analyst who teaches in the Department of Behavioral Science, Sackler School of Medicine, Tel Aviv University. He is President of Israel Institute of Jungian Psychology and past President of the Israeli Anthropological Association, as well as a published poet. He is a native of Montreal, Canada, where he went to look after his father during his illness, but for the past three decades has lived with his family in Jerusalem, Israel.

Moya Lynn Alfonso, MSPH is a currently a doctoral candidate in Educational Measurement and Research, University of South Florida, College of Education, and a staff member of the Methods and Evaluation Unit of the Florida Prevention Research Center, specializing in community-based prevention marketing, research, and evaluation. Her professional interests include community and family health, adolescent behavioral health, social marketing, and community-based research. Since writing this piece, her sister, Liza Lowery Massey, was diagnosed with invasive breast cancer at age 39. Courage, chemotherapy, radiation, and the prayers and support of her friends and family have helped Liza survive her battle with breast cancer. More recently Moya's 31-year-old best friend, Tracie Merritt Carver, was diagnosed with invasive, chemotherapy-resistant breast cancer. Although it has hurt to witness the pain and suffering these wonderful women have gone through in their battles with cancer, it has been a blessing to witness such strength and grace. They have taught Moya the importance of living in the moment—not in the past or future.

Chris Bell holds a B.A. in English from Central Missouri State University. As his essay indicates, he returned to (a different) graduate school, the University of Illinois at Chicago, where he received an M.A. in Rhetoric. Chris presently divides his time between England and Poland. In England, he is a Ph.D. student at Nottingham Trent University where his work examines cultural responses to AIDS. In Poland, he researches disability access and representation at the museum spaces of Auschwitz and Birkenau, and teaches cultural studies classes at the Warsaw School of Social Psychology. He is completing a monograph titled *Searching for Some Peace of Mind: Notes from a Black Gay HIV+ Survivor*.

Susanna Black is a pseudonym for a physician who practices medicine and teaches at a major university.

Bonnie Blackwell is a native of Amarillo, Texas and grew up in a non-academic, working-class family. While earning her B.A. and M.A. from the University of Texas at Austin and a Ph.D. from Cornell University, she collected most of the anecdotes which appear in her personal narrative, though she did not receive her diagnosis of panic disorder until 1998, just as she was finishing her dissertation. She is currently an Associate Professor of English at Texas Christian University in Fort Worth Texas, where she serves as director of graduate studies. She teaches poetry, the British novel, film adaptation, satire, and literary and feminist theory at all levels. She has published on a variety of topics in the journals *Genders*, *Women's Studies*, *Literature and Medicine*, among others, and is currently completing a book called *Immodest Proposals: The Crisis of Sex, Dating, and Motherhood in Eighteenth-Century Britain and Ireland*.

Mikita Brottman has a D.Phil. from Oxford University, and is currently Professor of Language, Literature and Culture at the Maryland Institute College of Art, in Baltimore. Her field of interest is the pathological and apocalyptic impulse in contemporary culture. Her work has appeared in both academic and alternative publications, including *New Literary History*, *The Chronicle of Higher Education*, *Bad Subjects*, *Film Quarterly*, *Headpress*, and elsewhere. Her books include *High Theory, Low Culture*, *Funny Peculiar*, and *Car Crash Culture* (ed.). Formerly a Fellow of Baltimore Washington Institute for Psychoanalysis, she is currently completing a Psy.D.

Ruth Elizabeth Burks received her Ph.D. in English Literature from UCLA, and her MA and BA from the University of California, at Berkeley, where she graduated Phi Beta Kappa and with honors in the major. Dr. Burks also attended the American Film Institute as a Screenwriting Fellow, and, more recently, earned an Ed.M from the Harvard Graduate School of Education, with a concentration in administration, planning, and social policy. Dr. Burks's previous publications include "Intimations of Invisibility: Black Women and Contemporary Hollywood Cinema" in *Mediated Messages and African-American Culture: Contemporary Issues*; "Back to the Future: *Forrest Gump* and *The Birth of a Nation*" in the *Harvard BlackLetter Law Journal*; and "*Gone With the Wind*: Black and White in Technicolor" in the *Quarterly Review of Film and Video*. Dr. Burks is currently at work on two full-length manuscripts: a monograph on the representation of African American women in Hollywood film and a more extensive portrait of her son as an African American autistic male.

Emma Burns, M.D., completed her undergraduate degree in Biochemistry at the University of Victoria in British Columbia and then returned to the East Coast to complete medical school. During medical school she took a year away from her training to live and volunteer in Narok, Kenya with teenaged Maasai women. She graduated medical school in 2006 and began a residency training program in Pediatrics in Halifax, Nova Scotia. Emma wrote this piece as a medical student at Dalhousie University. Throughout her medical degree Emma was involved in the Narrative in Medicine Program at Dalhousie and worked to incorporate the verbal skill of storytelling into the clinical learning and practice of medicine. She performed stories touching on issues such as the desensitization of medical students, student-patient, student-doctor and patient-doctor relationships, and the risk of losing one's humanity through the study of medicine. Work on written stories developed from an interest in oral narrative, and she continues to write and publish as her medical experiences and training continue. Emma's other published work can be found in the May 2004 issue of the *Canadian Medical Association Journal.*

Barbara J. Campbell, a Ph.D. candidate in English at the University of Connecticut, is completing her dissertation on representations of labor in the American academic novel. Her additional research and writing interests include Medical Humanities, Disability Studies, and the construction and interpretation of women's illness. She holds certificates in Women's Studies from UConn and in labor organizing and grievance handling through the AFL-CIO. She has taught American Literature and Freshman Composition and has served as an editorial assistant for the journal *LIT: Literature Interpretation Theory.* A frequent guest lecturer on women's health issues, her review of Ann Folwell Stanford's *Bodies in a Broken World: Women Novelists of Color and the Politics of Medicine* was published in the journal *MELUS (Multi-Ethnic Literature of the United States).*

Laurence Marshall Carucci is Professor of anthropology at Montana State University, where he has been a member of the faculty since 1985. He holds a B.A. in anthropology from Colorado State University, and a M.A. and Ph.D. from The University of Chicago. Carucci has conducted extensive research with members of the Enewetak community and with other Marshall Islanders since 1976. He has published numerous books and articles on the Marshall Islands and the Pacific, including *Nuclear Nativity: Rituals of Renewal and Empowerment in the Marshall Islands, In Anxious Anticipation of the Uneven Fruits of Kwajalein Atoll, The Typhoon of War: Micronesian Experiences of the Pacific War* (with Lin Poyer and Suzanne Falgout), and *Oceania: An Introduction to the Cultures and Identities of Pacific Islanders,* (with Pamela J. Stewart, Andrew Strathern, Lin Poyer, Richard Feinberg, and Cluny MacPherson). He has worked closely with members of the Enewetak community as they seek compensation for damages to their atoll as a result of nuclear testing, and works with several Northern Marshall Islands communities in their attempt to deal with medical problems that have resulted from their shared nuclear legacy.

Hilary Clark is Associate Professor in the Department of English, University of Saskatchewan. She teaches critical theory, life writing, and modern literature (particularly poetry). She has published on Melanie Klein's unpublished life writing, and has co-edited with Joseph Adamson *Scenes of Shame: Psychoanalysis, Shame, and Writing.* A chapter on depression narratives is forthcoming in *Unfitting Stories: Narrative Approaches to Disease, Disability, and Trauma* (Wilfrid Laurier Press), and a chapter on teaching depression and women's life writing will appear in *Teaching Life Writing* (forthcoming, MLA Publications). Her edited volume *Depression and Narrative: Telling the Dark* is forthcoming from SUNY Press. She has published three volumes of poetry, the latest being *The Dwelling of Weather.*

Tracy Curtis is alive and well in Los Angeles, California. She is currently working on a monograph on visual culture's influence on African American women's autobiography and a new media project on people's views of themselves and their work. Although painful and frustrating, the experiences detailed here have left her with an ability to appreciate all of life's details.

Susan Dick, Ph.D. completed her B.A. at Western Michigan University and her M.A. and Ph.D. at Northwestern University. She retired from the Department of English at Queen's University in Kingston, Ontario in June 2006. She has published editions of several works by Virginia Woolf, including *The Complete Shorter Fiction*. She is a member of the editorial board of the Shakespeare Head Press Edition of Virginia Woolf and of The Royal Society of Canada. She has traveled in Europe, Japan, and India, and has spent time doing research in England and Ireland. Now she enjoys gardening, reading, doing needlepoint, and entertaining her small, boisterous dog.

Michael Edmond Donnelly has served as a prosecutor for over twenty-five years in Worcester, Massachusetts and as a law school professor specializing in children's law for over twenty years at Western New England College School of Law in Springfield, Massachusetts. He is a former mountain-climbing instructor for the North Carolina Outward Bound School, a three-time runner in the Boston Marathon, completing his third marathon after undergoing treatment for testicular cancer. Mr. Donnelly is an Old Boy of the Gordonstoun School in Elgin, Scotland and was named a Kentucky Colonel for his service to the people of Kentucky in a child abuse case. He was the recipient of the Recognition Award from the Black Alumni council of Wesleyan University, his alma mater, as well as the University Service Award for "steadfast support of higher education for high school students in and around the Worcester area—especially for students of color." Michael lives in Paxton, Massachusetts with his wife, Mary Frances Kingsley, herself a lawyer and professor, and their two children, Katherine and Peter. Mr. Donnelly credits his wife and children for his survival and recovery from cancer.

Fulvia Dunham is a pseudonym for an Associate Professor of English in Montréal, Québec. She specializes in literature of the modernist period.

Ellen Goldsmith, Professor Emeritus, recently retired from the English Department at New York City College of Technology/CUNY. She founded and directed the Center for Intergenerational and co-author of *Family Reading: An Intergenerational Approach to Literacy* (New Readers Press) and *Reading Starts With Us* (Scholastic). For her family literacy work, she was named Scholar on Campus. Her poetry has been published in numerous magazines. *No Pine Tree in This Forest Is Perfect*, twenty-four poems narrating her experiences with breast cancer, won the Hudson Valley Writers' Center 1997 chapbook contest. She resides in Cushing, Maine.

Lynda Hall, Ph.D. teaches in the Faculty of Communications and Culture and the Faculty of Humanities at the University of Calgary. Her research, which focuses on autobiographical writings by women of color, has been published in *a/b: Autobiographical Studies; Ariel: A Review of International English Literature; Callaloo: A Journal of Afro-American and African Arts and Letters; International Journal of Sexuality and Gender Studies; Journal of Dramatic Theory and Criticism;* and *Postmodern Culture.* Hall edited *Telling Moments: Lesbian Autobiographical Short Stories*, a Lambda Literary Award Finalist for 2004. She also edited *Lesbian*

Self-Writing: The Embodiment of Experience, a collection of essays by seventeen writers who discuss their writing "process" in relation to the "self." In her introduction, Hall coined the term "ameliorography" to suggest how "many authors powerfully enact a healing of the past through writing and taking the agency of self-expression. They bring together the past and the present in order to re-negotiate experiences and integrate the past into present selves-in-process." Creative endeavors (writing, painting, music) are increasingly recognized by health care professionals as a means of relief and escape from current experiences for patients and health-care givers, as well as a strategic method to preserve memories and look to the future. "Shaman" is a revision of a short story that was published in *The Calgary Herald Sunday Magazine*, July 26 1987, as part of a short story contest that received 532 submissions.

Anne Hunsaker Hawkins is Professor of Humanities and Director of The Doctors Kienle Center for Humanistic Medicine at Penn State's College of Medicine. Hawkins was the first to publish essays about a subgenre of autobiography that she calls "pathography"—narratives by patients about their experiences of illness and treatment. In 1993 she published a book-length study of these narratives called *Reconstructing Illness: Studies in Pathography*, which came out in a second edition in 1999. Subsequent books include *Time to Go: Three Plays on Death and Dying* in 1995, edited with James O. Ballard; *Teaching Literature and Medicine*; a collection in the MLA's Options for Teaching series that she edited with Marilyn McEntyre in 2000, and *A Small Good Thing: Stories of Children with HIV and Those Who Care for Them*, also published in 2000, which was the result of several years' experience as a participant-observer in a pediatric HIV clinic. In 2002 Hawkins developed the idea of an NEH Summer Institute that would combine clinic and classroom, offering participants opportunities to see what patient care is like in a tertiary care hospital as well as providing lectures, readings and discussion about medicine and the humanities. She directed this Institute, called "Medicine, Literature and Culture," with Susan Squier. Subsequently, participants were invited to contribute essays to a collection that would reflect the aims of the Institute: the result was two volumes of the *Journal of the Medical Humanities*, edited by Hawkins.

Seamus Heaney won the Nobel Prize in Literature in 1995.

Tami L. Higdon is a native of North Carolina, and an ordained minister and Board Certified Chaplain in the Association of Professional Chaplains. From 1989 to 2005, she served as a Staff Chaplain in the Department of Pastoral Services at Shands Hospital at the University of Florida in Gainesville. In July 2005, Rev. Higdon accepted the exciting challenge of starting a professional chaplaincy program at North Florida Regional Medical Center, also in Gainesville. Rev. Higdon is a magna cum laude graduate of Wake Forest University in Winston-Salem, NC. She received her Master of Divinity degree from Southwestern Baptist Theological Seminary in 1985, completed her Clinical Pastoral Education training at Baptist Medical Center in Columbia, SC, and earned Master of Education and Education Specialist degrees in Mental Health Counseling from the University of Florida. Rev. Higdon enjoys her three cats, reading, traveling, hiking the Great Smoky Mountains, and is an avid Gator fan.

Rebecca Hogan is Professor of English and Women's Studies at the University of Wisconsin-Whitewater. She is co-editor, with Joseph Hogan and Emily Hipchen, of the scholarly journal *a/b: Auto/Biography Studies*. She is author of the frequently cited article "Engendered Autobiographies: The Diary as a Feminine Form" as well as several pieces on cross-cultural and mental illness memoirs co-authored with Joseph Hogan. Together they have given numerous conference papers on these topics, and are currently at work on a book about the agency of the subject in cross-cultural and mental illness autobiographies.

Richard A. Ingram is a Post-Doctoral Research Fellow in Disability Studies in the Department of Theatre, Film and Creative Writing at the University of British Columbia. His doctoral dissertation, "Troubled Being and Being Troubled: Subjectivity in the Light of Problems of the Mind," examines societal demands for conformity to narrative. His essay "Double Trouble" is part of a critique of the "order of making sense." Richard has articles published in the online journals *CTheory* and *Nasty: Academia at Its Brattiest*, and essays in *Interdisciplinary Perspectives on Health, Illness and Disease* and *Unfitting Stories: Narrative Approaches to Disease, Disability and Trauma*. Since graduating with a Ph.D. in Interdisciplinary Studies in May 2005, Richard has been more actively involved in the local psychiatric survivor movement in Vancouver, BC. He believes in creating the conditions for more people to come out as psychiatric survivors, and to join the struggle against practices that too often ensure we do not survive psychiatrization.

Barbara J. Jago, Ph.D. is Program Coordinator and Associate Professor of Communication Arts at the University of New Hampshire at Manchester. She teaches and conducts autoethnographic research in relational communication, with an emphasis on storytelling, identity, and emotion. Dr. Jago is working on a book about depression.

Lisa Katz, poet, translator and independent scholar, was born in New York and lives in Jerusalem, where she teaches literary translation and creative writing at Hebrew University. Katz is a three-time Pushcart Prize nominee, and her poems are forthcoming in *A Sea of Voices: An Anthology of Israeli Women's Poetry* edited by the Chilean-American writer Marjorie Agosin. *Reconstruction*, funded in part by the Tel Aviv Foundation for the Arts, includes a Hebrew translation of the breast cancer poems excerpted in *Illness in the Academy*. She serves as co-editor of the Israeli domain of the *Poetry International Web* (PIW), a European project for world poetry in translation http://israel.poetryinternational.org and translation coordinator of the Jerusalem International Poetry Festival. Her collection of translations of the Israeli poet Agi Mishol, *Look There*, was published in 2006, and her most recent article, on the work of Sylvia Plath, appears in *European Contributions to American Studies*. She is the mother of two children and underwent a mastectomy in 1997.

Sharon D. King, scholar, translator, writer, and actress, holds a Ph.D. in Comparative Literature from UCLA and is an Associate at the UCLA Center for Medieval and Renaissance Studies. Recent publications include the scholarly works *City Tragedy on the Renaissance Stage in France, Spain, and England* and "Early Modern Theatre for a Postmodern Audience," and the science fiction story "Quiescent." She has numerous translations to her credit, including

J. Prevost's 1584 *Clever and Pleasant Inventions, Part One*, the first book on sleight-of-hand magic in French, and *The Phantom Church and Other Stories from Romania*, an anthology of twentieth-century fiction. She has translated and performed early modern comedies with her own acting troupe, Les Enfans Sans Abri, since 1988. Her original play *Pale Pink Punch* won competition for performance in the Los Angeles-based Can Play Festival (September–November, 2005). Dr. King has served as researcher for the Getty Research Institute. She is working on her second short film, *Plant Life*.

Elena Levy-Navarro is an Associate Professor of English at the University of Wisconsin-Whitewater. In her forthcoming book, *The Culture of Obesity in Early and Late Modernity* and in a variety of published essays, she explores the way that language shapes our modern reality. Such studies, like the essay in this volume, are designed to help us imagine alternatives to what seems so irreducibly real to us and thus to promote alternative types of experiences. In so doing, she hopes to promote different forms of relationships between people now too often estranged from one another. She shares with the women from her mother's family—a hardworking, Midwestern lot—the tendency to experience what were once known as sick head-aches, now known as migraines.

Kristin Lindgren teaches courses in literature, writing, and disability studies at Haverford College. She is co-editor of *Signs and Voices: Language, Arts, and Identity in the Deaf Community* and is completing a study of fictional and autobiographical accounts of illness and disability entitled *Bodies in Trouble: Feminism, Narrative, and Disability*. She lives near Philadelphia with her husband and two sons.

Rae Luckie lives at Kiama in Australia. Working as a free-lance writing mentor and editor for the last ten years, she has facilitated memoir writing workshops in rural and metropolitan communities throughout NSW and Victoria. In 2006, Rae was awarded a Ph.D. in the theory and practice of women's autobiographical writing from the University of Western Sydney. She has worked on a number of community projects and is interested in the preservation of family life stories and the interstices of life writing, life review and writing as therapy. Rae also teaches part-time at the University of Wollongong's Shoalhaven Campus in the fields of English, Cultural Studies and Education. Her autobiographical stories have been published in *Best Australian Stories 2004, More Stories from the Shed, No Thanks or Regrets* and *Second Degree Tampering*. She won the 2001 Queen of Crime award for a story that had previously been short-listed in the international Stephen King *On Writing* competition.

Michael J. Meyer, adjunct professor of English at DePaul and Northeastern Illinois Universities in Chicago, is the present bibliographer for Steinbeck studies, having published *The Hayashi Steinbeck Bibliography (1982–1996)* in 1998. In addition to his bibliographic work, Meyer's essays have appeared in the *Steinbeck Quarterly, Steinbeck Review*, and *Steinbeck Newsletter*, and he has contributed chapters to numerous monographs and books. He served as editor for *Cain Sign: The Betrayal of Brotherhood in the Works of John Steinbeck* and is Vice-President of the New John Steinbeck Society of America and co-editor of *The Steinbeck Encyclopaedia* (2006). Since 1994, Meyer has been an editor for Rodopi Press's series Perspectives in Modern Literature, and Rodopi recently named him senior editor of its new series entitled *Dialogues*, where classic canonical texts are examined on the basis of controversial issues. He is presently at work on a book which will review the critical reception of Steinbeck's *Of Mice and Men* and on a new bibliography of Steinbeck, which will be published in 2007.

Susannah B. Mintz, Associate Professor of English at Skidmore College in Saratoga Springs, NY, is the author of *Threshold Poetics: Milton and Intersubjectivity* and *Unruly Bodies: Life Writing by Women with Disabilities*. Her work on women's life-writing and disability has been published in *A/B: Auto/Biography Studies*, *biography*, the journal of the National Women's Studies Association, and *Prose Studies*. Recent personal essays have appeared in *Cimarron* and *Under the Sun*.

Kimberly R. Myers, Ph.D. is Associate Professor in the Department of Humanities at Penn State College of Medicine. Recent essays include "Coming Out: Considering the Closet of Illness" in the *Journal of Medical Humanities*, "A Perspective on the Role of Stories as a Mechanism of Meta-Healing" in *Psychoanalysis and Narrative Medicine*, "From Expatriate to Establishment: Medicine and the Literary Corpus of Dr. Abraham Verghese," and "Patient Pathography #8," a version of her essay in this collection, which was a finalist for the 2004 *Journal of General Internal Medicine* national creative writing prize. Kimberly is frequently invited to speak about issues in medical humanities to diverse audiences, and she has won numerous awards for university teaching, including the President's Award for Excellence in Teaching, the Provost's Award for Undergraduate Research/Creativity Mentoring, and Distinguished University Educator for the state of Montana.

Patricia O'Hara is Professor of English at Franklin & Marshall College, where she teaches creative writing and Victorian literature. She is the former editor of *Nineteenth Century Studies*. Her academic writings have appeared in *Victorian Studies*, *Victorian Literature and Culture*, *Nineteenth Century Contexts* and *Victorian Encounters*. Her creative writing (poetry, essays, fiction) has appeared in *The Bellevue Literary Review*, *The Sycamore Review*, *The Southwest Review*, *Harpur Palate*, *The Cortland Review*, *Brevity*, *ducts.org*, *Alehouse Poetry Review*, *Newsweek*, *Annals of Psychiatric Nursing*, and *Yale Journal for the Humanities in Medicine*. She is working on a collection of essays.

Ellin Ronee Pollachek has published two novels (*Seasons* and *Midnight Sins*) as well as dozens of articles, short stories and essays. Her doctoral dissertation in Culture and Communications from New York University examined the responses of scholars and critics to transgressive works of literature and photography. She teaches "Writing as a Healing Art" through Poets & Writers and has taught all levels of writing, world literature, and English as a Second Language at NYU, Hostos Community College, Pace University, College of Mt. St. Vincent, CUNY and Westchester Community College. Her best teaching experience was leading a week-long seminar at Yale University on the Beat poets. Her environmental portraits and travel photography have appeared in *Robb Report*, *Travel-Holiday*, *India Today*, *FollowMe*, *Soma*, *Modern Bride* and *Catskill Mountain Guide*. Her landscapes and environmental portraits have been shown in galleries in the Hudson River Valley region, Manhattan and Nepal. Ellin is interested in collaborating with a researcher to write about the relationship between being a caretaker and getting cancer. For further contact: email: EllinsPlace@aol.com; web: www.ellinpollachek.com; web: http://members2.authorsguild.net/epollachek/.

Rebecca A. Pope, Ph.D., MMQ is co-author with Susan J. Leonardi of *The Diva's Mouth: Body, Voice, Prima Donna Politics* and the forthcoming *It's Been Marvelous: The Life and Times of Holocaust Rescuers Ida and Louise Cook.* She is also the author of many essays and reviews. After teaching literature and medicine at a university in Washington D.C. for many years, she retrained in Medical Qigong,the most ancient branch of Chinese Medicine. She is now a certified Medical Qigong therapist and holds the rank of Master of Medical Qigong. She lives, teaches Qigong, and maintains a private practice in Davis, California.

Althea E. Rhodes is an Assistant Professor of Rhetoric at the University of Arkansas—Fort Smith. She completed her M.A. and Ph.D. in Rhetoric and Composition at Southern Illinois University at Carbondale with minors in Modern American Literature and Gender Issues in the Teaching of English. Her dissertation, *Finding the Ties That Bind—Writers in Transition: Moving Between Academic and Nonacademic Discourse Communities,* grew out of her need to help writers become more comfortable with their writing process and with different writing contexts. Dr. Rhodes has presented her research at local and regional conferences, including the National Council of Teachers of English, the Conference on College Composition and Communication, the College English Association, and the Midwest Modern Language Association. Currently, Dr. Rhodes is the Director of the UA-Fort Smith Writing Task Force.

Roxana Robinson is a fiction writer, biographer and essayist. She is the author of three novels: *Summer Light, This Is My Daughter,* and *Sweetwater;* three collections of short stories: *A Glimpse of Scarlet, Asking for Love,* and *A Perfect Stranger;* and the biography *Georgia O'Keeffe: A Life.* Four of these have been chosen as *New York Times* Notable Books; the most recent, *A Perfect Stranger,* was a *New York Times* Editors' Choice. She is an environmentalist, gardener and nature writer, and her work in this field has appeared in *The Boston Globe, House and Garden, Horticulture,* and in blogs for the NRDC. A scholar of American painting, her essays have appeared in *Artforum, Art News,* and in catalogues published by the Metropolitan Museum of Art and other institutions. Her fiction has appeared in *The New Yorker, The Atlantic, Harper's, Daedalus, One-Story, Best American Short Stories,* and elsewhere. Her nonfiction has appeared in *The New York Times, The Boston Globe, The Chicago Tribune, Vogue, The Wall Street Journal, The Washington Post,* and elsewhere. Her stories and essays have been anthologized and broadcast on NPR, and her books have been published in England, France, Germany, Holland and Spain. Roxana Robinson has received fellowships from the NEA, the MacDowell Colony and the Guggenheim Foundation and was named a Literary Lion by the New York Public Library. She has served on the board of the NHC and of PEN, and now serves on the Council of the Authors' Guild. Ms. Robinson has taught at the University of Houston and Wesleyan University; she now teaches at the New School for Social Research. She lives in New York City and in Maine.

Laurie Rosenblatt, M.D. is Assistant Professor of Psychiatry at Harvard Medical School and practices at Dana Farber Cancer Institute/Brigham and Women's Hospital. Dr. Rosenblatt's research focuses on stories of illness told by doctors and patients, and the uses of those narratives for medical education. She has published articles and book chapters on end of life care, grief, the psychological effects of political torture, and medical decision-making under managed care. She wrote a monthly column on contractual and medical staff issues for the Group Practice Journal when she was Associate Chief of Staff at the Cleveland Clinic Florida. Dr. Rosenblatt has published poems in *JAMA*, *Academic Medicine*, *The Bellevue Literary Review*, *Ibbetson Street*, and *Borderlands: Texas Poetry Review*, among others.

Michael Rowe is an Associate Clinical Professor in the Yale School of Medicine, Department of Psychiatry and Institution for Social and Policy Studies. He is also Co-Director of the Yale Program for Recovery and Community Health, and Director of the Program on Community Interventions for the Division of Law and Psychiatry, Yale Department of Psychiatry and Connecticut Mental Health Center. A medical sociologist with training in ethnographic and qualitative methods, he conducts research on homelessness and mental illness, community integration for persons with psychiatric disabilities, and medical humanities/narrative medicine. In addition to being the author of many articles and book chapters in these areas, he is the author of two books. *Crossing the Border: Encounters Between Homeless People and Outreach Workers*, is the only full-length study of mental health outreach work to homeless persons. *The Book of Jesse: A Story of Youth, Illness, and Medicine*, is a literary memoir about his son, who died in 1995 from complications of a liver transplant. Currently, he is conducting a qualitative study of doctors', patients', and family members' responses to medical errors. This study uses in-depth interviews to explore the feelings, thoughts, actions and inaction that stem from participating in, observing, or being the recipient of a perceived medical error that leads to patient harm.

Ellen Samuels is the author of a poetry chapbook, *December Morning*, and the co-editor of *Out of the Ordinary: Essays on Growing Up with Gay, Lesbian, and Transgender Parents*. Her poetry and creative nonfiction have been published in numerous journals and anthologies, including *The American Voice*, *Journal of the American Medical Association*, *Nimrod*, *Sojourner*, and *Women's Studies Quarterly*, and her writing awards include an Academy of American Poets Prize, two Lambda Literary Awards, and a Pushcart nomination. She earned a B.A. from Oberlin College, an M.F.A. from Cornell University, and a Ph.D. in English Literature from the University of California at Berkeley. In 2006–2007, as an Ed Roberts Postdoctoral Fellow in Disability Studies at U.C. Berkeley, she will teach creative writing workshops for people with disabilities and chronic illnesses.

Jane E. Schultz is Professor of English, American Studies, and Women's Studies at Indiana University-Purdue University-Indianapolis, the urban medical campus of Indiana University. She comes to the medical humanities by way of an interest in narrative forms and the hospital as a site of social interaction. *Women at the Front*, her study of gender and relief work in Civil War military hospitals, was a finalist for the 2005 Lincoln Prize. She has completed

This Birth Place of Souls, an annotated edition of one of the last extant nursing diaries from the Civil War, and is at work on *Performing Modesty: War, Commemoration, and the Sexual Politics of Publicity* in the History Department at Sydney University, where she is visiting scholar for the 2006–07 school year. Schultz is a veteran of two episodes of cancer, having survived pseudomyxoma peritonei only to be diagnosed with an unrelated breast cancer in 2004. After more surgery, more chemotherapy, radiation, and baldness, she has returned from a dark place and currently seeks the light.

Evelyn Scott has worked as a writing consultant, a classroom teacher, and a college composition instructor. Her personal essays appear in *Agora, Peepshow, Swing!, The Best of Both Worlds, Diverse Words, Whores and Other Feminists*, and *First Person Sexual*. "All Stripped Off" (*Whores and Other Feminists*) has been taught in college courses on the West Coast and in Texas. The fiction Scott contributed to the Herotica series garnered praise from magazines as divergent as *Publishers Weekly* and *Elle*. *The Oy of Sex* and *Leather, Lace, and Lust* as well as magazines such as *Dare, Mind Caviar*, and *Peacockblue* also feature Scott's sexy short stories. She has spoken at the University of Texas at Austin and at Eastern Illinois University on women's health, a topic on which she has also been interviewed by *InSite Magazine*. In addition to reading her stories at book signings, she has spoken on the craft of composing erotica for the Modern Language Association. Scott now writes for Custom Erotica Source and tutors troubled children.

Christopher R. Smit, Ph.D. is Assistant Professor for the Communication Arts and Sciences Department at Calvin College in Grand Rapids, Michigan. His edited collection, *Screening Disability: Essays on Cinema and Disability*, was published in 2001 by the University Press of America. Smit's essays on disability, media, popular music, and culture can be found in *Disability Studies Quarterly, Studies in Popular Culture, Journal of Popular Culture*, and several edited collections.

Maggie Griffin Taylor earned a Ph.D. from Texas Tech University in the field of Rhetoric and Composition. Her dissertation, entitled "The Rhetoric of Healing," explored the challenges of integrating alternative and biomedicine. She currently teaches at New Mexico Tech University.

Wendy Marie Thompson is a Ph.D. candidate in American Studies at the University of Maryland at College Park. She is currently working on a dissertation project that looks at racial hybridity, popular cultures, historic sites, and transnational ritual performance as they relate to Chinese diaspora communities in the Americas. Also of interest to her are narratives of trauma within immigrant families and families of color.

Ting Man Tsao holds a Ph.D. from the State University of New York at Stony Brook and is Assistant Professor of English at LaGuardia Community College of the City University of New York. His dissertation, "Representing China to the British Public in the Age of Free Trade, c. 1833–1844," examines the intersections between Britain's popular representations of China and its imperial policy during the Opium War period. His research interests include colonial discourse analysis and the scholarship of teaching and learning. His articles appear in *The History Teacher, In Transit: The LaGuardia Journal on Teaching and Learning*, and *Victorians Institute Journal*. Besides "More Than a Case," he has published a short story, "Ways to Carry a Baby," in *Writing Macao: Creative Text and Teaching*. Before joining academia, he worked in the not-for-profit world in several capacities—as a social worker at a child welfare agency, and as an ESL teacher and grant writer for organizations serving immigrant communities.

Michael Verde grew up in east Texas, where he played football, raised show pigs, and read so much that it alarmed his high school counselor. In 1985, he won first prize in *Guideposts* magazine's National Youth Writing Contest with a story about his grandfather, who at that time had not been diagnosed with AD. He graduated with honors from the Plan II Honors Program at University of Texas. He has an M.A. in literary studies from University of Iowa, and an M.A. in theology from the University of Durham, England, graduating first in his international class. He has taught English at the high school and university level for ten years. In 1997, he was named Lamar University's Teacher of the Year. His short story, "Weasel Loves," which explores the intractability of love and memory, was published in the nationally award-winning short story anthology, *Texas Short Stories*. His story was recognized in the *Houston Chronicle*, the *Dallas Morning Herald*, and the *San Antonio Times* as one of the best in the collection. Michael's abiding intellectual interests are in the areas of literature and religion, the verbal and cultural construction of selfhood, and the embodiments of memory. He currently directs the Foundation for Alzheimer's and Cultural Memory and lives in Chicago, Illinois.

Abraham Verghese, M.D., D.Sc., M.F.A., is the Director of The Center for Medical Humanities and Ethics at the University of Texas Health Science Center at San Antonio and is also Marvin Forland Distinguished Professor of Medicine. A graduate of Madras University, Verghese trained as a resident and chief resident in internal medicine at East Tennessee State University, and as a fellow in infectious diseases at Boston University. He has served on the faculty at East Tennessee State University, the University of Iowa, and Texas Tech University. From 1991 to 2002, he was Professor of Medicine at the Texas Tech University Health Sciences Center, El Paso, where he was Grover E. Murray Distinguished Professor. He is board certified in internal medicine, pulmonary diseases and infectious diseases. In 1990–91, Verghese attended the Iowa Writers Workshop at the University of Iowa, where he obtained a Master of Fine Arts degree. His first book, *My Own Country*, about AIDS in rural Tennessee, was a finalist for the National Book Critics Circle Award for 1994 and was made into a movie. His second book, *The Tennis Partner*, was a *New York Times* Notable Book and a national bestseller. Verghese's writing has appeared in *The New Yorker, Sports Illustrated, The Atlantic Monthly, Esquire, Granta, The New York Times Magazine, The Wall Street Journal*, and elsewhere. He has also published extensively in medical journals, including *Journal of the American Medical Association* and *New England Journal of Medicine*.

Andrea T. Wagner earned a Ph.D. from the University of Pennsylvania's Annenberg School for Communication. Interested in performance and cultural studies, narrative medicine, and qualitative methods, Wagner has published in the *Journal of Medical Humanities*, created multimedia ethnographic performances about the body and illness, and presented papers and performances at numerous conferences.

Index of Illnesses